ADDRESSING SICKLE CELL DISEASE

A STRATEGIC PLAN AND BLUEPRINT FOR ACTION

Committee on Addressing Sickle Cell Disease:
A Strategic Plan and Blueprint for Action

Marie McCormick, Henrietta Awo Osei-Anto, and
Rose Marie Martinez, *Editors*

Board on Population Health and Public Health Practice

Health and Medicine Division

A Consensus Study Report of

The National Academies of

SCIENCE   ENGINEERING   MEDICINE

THE

www.nap.edu

THE NATIONAL ACADEMIES PRESS   500 Fifth Street, NW   Washington, DC 20001

This activity was supported by Contract/Task Order No. HHSP233201400020B/HHSP23337086 between the National Academy of Sciences and the Office of the Assistant Secretary for Health, an operating agency of the U.S. Department of Health and Human Services. Any opinions, findings, conclusions, or recommendations expressed in this publication do not necessarily reflect the views of any organizations or agency that provided support for this project.

International Standard Book Number-13: 978-0-309-66960-3
International Standard Book Number-10: 0-309-66960-X
Digital Object Identifier: http://doi.org/10.17226/25632
Library of Congress Control Number: 2020943342

Additional copies of this publication are available from the National Academies Press, 500 Fifth Street, NW, Keck 360, Washington, DC 20001; (800) 624-6242 or (202) 334-3313; www.nap.edu.

Suggested citation: National Academies of Sciences, Engineering, and Medicine. 2020. *Addressing sickle cell disease: A strategic plan and blueprint for action*. Washington, DC: The National Academies Press. http://doi.org/10.17226/25632.

The National Academies of
SCIENCES · ENGINEERING · MEDICINE

The **National Academy of Sciences** was established in 1863 by an Act of Congress, signed by President Lincoln, as a private, nongovernmental institution to advise the nation on issues related to science and technology. Members are elected by their peers for outstanding contributions to research. Dr. Marcia McNutt is president.

The **National Academy of Engineering** was established in 1964 under the charter of the National Academy of Sciences to bring the practices of engineering to advising the nation. Members are elected by their peers for extraordinary contributions to engineering. Dr. John L. Anderson is president.

The **National Academy of Medicine** (formerly the Institute of Medicine) was established in 1970 under the charter of the National Academy of Sciences to advise the nation on medical and health issues. Members are elected by their peers for distinguished contributions to medicine and health. Dr. Victor J. Dzau is president.

The three Academies work together as the **National Academies of Sciences, Engineering, and Medicine** to provide independent, objective analysis and advice to the nation and conduct other activities to solve complex problems and inform public policy decisions. The National Academies also encourage education and research, recognize outstanding contributions to knowledge, and increase public understanding in matters of science, engineering, and medicine.

Learn more about the National Academies of Sciences, Engineering, and Medicine at **www.nationalacademies.org**.

The National Academies of
SCIENCES · ENGINEERING · MEDICINE

Consensus Study Reports published by the National Academies of Sciences, Engineering, and Medicine document the evidence-based consensus on the study's statement of task by an authoring committee of experts. Reports typically include findings, conclusions, and recommendations based on information gathered by the committee and the committee's deliberations. Each report has been subjected to a rigorous and independent peer-review process and it represents the position of the National Academies on the statement of task.

Proceedings published by the National Academies of Sciences, Engineering, and Medicine chronicle the presentations and discussions at a workshop, symposium, or other event convened by the National Academies. The statements and opinions contained in proceedings are those of the participants and are not endorsed by other participants, the planning committee, or the National Academies.

For information about other products and activities of the National Academies, please visit www.nationalacademies.org/about/whatwedo.

COMMITTEE ON ADDRESSING SICKLE CELL DISEASE: A STRATEGIC PLAN AND BLUEPRINT FOR ACTION

MARIE CLARE McCORMICK (*Chair*), Sumner and Esther Feldberg Professor (Emerita), Department of Social and Behavioral Sciences, Professor of Pediatrics, Harvard University

GILDA BARABINO, Dean and Daniel and Frances Berg Professor, The Grove School of Engineering, The City College of New York

MARY CATHERINE BEACH, Professor, General Internal Medicine and Berman Bioethics Institute, Johns Hopkins University

LORI E. CROSBY, Professor of Pediatrics, Cincinnati Children's Hospital

AMY DAWSON, Associate Director, Medical Director, Fort Wayne Medical Education Program

DARIUS LAKDAWALLA, Quintiles Chair in Pharmaceutical Development and Regulatory Innovation, Director of Research, University of Southern California

BERNARD (BERNIE) LOPEZ, Professor and Executive Vice Chair, Department of Emergency Medicine, Sidney Kimmel Medical College, Thomas Jefferson University

JONATHAN D. MORENO, David and Lyn Silfen University Professor, Professor of Medical Ethics and Health Policy, Professor of History and Sociology of Science, and Professor of Philosophy, University of Pennsylvania

ENRICO M. NOVELLI, Associate Professor of Medicine, University of Pittsburgh; Director, Adult Sickle Cell Program, and Chief, Section of Benign Hematology, University of Pittsburgh Medical Center

J. ANDREW ORR-SKIRVIN, Associate Clinical Professor, School of Pharmacy, and Interim Department Chair, Department of Pharmacy and Health System Sciences, Northeastern University

IFEYINWA (IFY) OSUNKWO, Hematologist–Oncologist Director, Sickle Cell Program, Atrium Health

SUSAN PAULUKONIS, Program Director, California Rare Disease Surveillance Program, Tracking California

CHARMAINE ROYAL, Associate Professor, Department of African and African American Studies, Duke University

KIM SMITH-WHITLEY, Clinical Director, Division of Hematology, Director, Comprehensive Sickle Cell Center, Children's Hospital of Philadelphia, University of Pennsylvania

Staff

HENRIETTA AWO OSEI-ANTO, Study Director
KAREN M. ANDERSON, Senior Program Officer
T. CHERI BANKS, Associate Program Officer
(*September 2018–December 2019*)
AHMED MOUER, Research Assistant (*July 2019–January 2020*)
PAMELA RAMEY-McCRAY, Senior Program Assistant
(*December 2018–March 2019*)
CYNDI TRANG, Research Associate (*from June 2019*)
HAYAT YUSUF, Senior Program Assistant (*March 2019–February 2020*)
ROSE MARIE MARTINEZ, Senior Director, Board on Population
Health and Public Health Practice

Consultant

ROBERT POOL, Deliberate Practice Consulting

Reviewers

This Consensus Study Report was reviewed in draft form by individuals chosen for their diverse perspectives and technical expertise. The purpose of this independent review is to provide candid and critical comments that will assist the National Academies of Sciences, Engineering, and Medicine in making each published report as sound as possible and to ensure that it meets the institutional standards for quality, objectivity, evidence, and responsiveness to the study charge. The review comments and draft manuscript remain confidential to protect the integrity of the deliberative process.

We thank the following individuals for their review of this report:

SHAWN BEDIAKO, University of Maryland, Baltimore County
CHANCELLOR E. DONALD, Tulane University School of Medicine and University Medical Center, New Orleans
JAMES ECKMAN, Emory University School of Medicine
TITILOPE FASIPE, Baylor College of Medicine and Texas Children's Cancer and Hematology Centers
JOHNSON HAYNES, JR., University of South Alabama
HOXI JONES, Senior Adult Consumer Advocate
JULIE KANTER, University of Alabama at Birmingham
PATRICIA KAVANAGH, Boston University
CATO T. LAURENCIN, University of Connecticut
TIMOTHY J. LEY, Washington University School of Medicine in St. Louis

GWENDOLYN POLES, University of Pittsburgh Medical Center Pinnacle and South Central PA Sickle Cell Council
JOSEPH TELFAIR, Jiann-Ping Hsu College of Public Health, Georgia Southern University

Although the reviewers listed above provided many constructive comments and suggestions, they were not asked to endorse the conclusions or recommendations of this report, nor did they see the final draft before its release. The review of this report was overseen by **OTIS W. BRAWLEY,** Johns Hopkins University, and **MAXINE HAYES,** University of Washington. They were responsible for making certain that an independent examination of this report was carried out in accordance with the standards of the National Academies and that all review comments were carefully considered. Responsibility for the final content rests entirely with the authoring committee and the National Academies.

Acknowledgments

The study committee and the Health and Medicine Division project staff take this opportunity to recognize and thank the many individuals who shared their time and expertise to support the committee's work and inform its deliberations.

This study was sponsored by the Office of Minority Health at the Office of the Assistant Secretary for Health at the U.S. Department of Health and Human Services. We thank Admiral Brett Giroir and Captain David Wong for their support and guidance.

The committee benefited greatly from discussions with the individuals who presented at and attended the committee's open sessions: Lakiea Bailey, Zyekevious (Zye) Barnes, Edward Benz, Jr., Beatrice Bowie, Brynn Bowman, Stephen Cha, Cheryl Damberg, Bernard Dauvergne, Tracie Bullock Dickson, Brian M. Elliott, ADM Brett P. Giroir, Jeffrey Glassberg, Gregory Green, Jonathan Hamilton, Elijah Henry, Tony Ho, Mary Hulihan, Charles Jonassaint, Ronald M. Kline, Ruth Krystopolski, Ted W. Love, Marc Manley, Donna McCurry, Emily Riehm Meier, Shirley Miller, Betsy Myers, Jennifer Nsenkyire, Tosin Ola, Derek Robertson, Kathryn Sabadosa, Carmen Sánchez, Adrienne Bell-Cors Shapiro, Amy Shapiro, Barbara Speller-Brown, James G. Taylor VI, Michael Thomas, Alexis Thompson, Sara van Geertruyden, Mark Walters, Richard P. Weishaupt, Shauna H. Whisenton, Wanda Whitten-Shurney, Celia Witten, Teonna Wolford, and CAPT David Wong. The committee would also like to thank all participants who attended the committee's open sessions and all others who made or submitted comments or materials for the committee's consideration. The committee is grateful to these presenters for volunteering to share their expertise, knowledge, data, and opinions not only with the committee but also with the members of the public who participated in the committee's open sessions. The committee also appreciates the efforts of numerous individuals who assisted project staff in identifying the presenters. We would like to thank and acknowledge organizations who supported and provided us with invaluable information to consider for this report, including the staff at the American Society of Hematology, the Association of Public Health Laboratories, the Centers for Disease Control and Prevention, and the Health Resources and Services Administration.

Furthermore, we acknowledge the many staff within the Health and Medicine Division who provided support in various ways to this project, including Stephanie Hanson, Aimee Mead, Sophie Yang, Rebecca Chevat, Dionna Ali, and Anne Styka; Nicole Joy and Greta Gorman from the communications office; Lauren Shern and Taryn Young, who provided support during the review process; Misrak Dabi, financial associate for the project; the late Daniel Bearss, senior research librarian, who conducted and compiled all of the literature searches; Jorge Mendoza-Torres, senior research librarian, who assisted with additional searches; Robert Pool, for his editorial assistance provided in preparing the final report; and Andrea Matthews of the Children's Sickle Cell Foundation, Inc., Pittsburgh, Pennsylvania, for sharing her expertise and personal experience to inform the report. Finally, we want to thank our consultants, Anna Hood, Jenny Park, Shantanu Srivatsa, and Jeffrey Yu, who assisted committee members with identifying information for this report.

Preface

This consensus study report was commissioned by the Office of Minority Health at the Office of the Assistant Secretary for Health at the U.S. Department of Health and Human Services to provide a comprehensive approach to the management and potential interventions for sickle cell disease (SCD), a genetic condition affecting approximately 100,000 people in the United States and millions worldwide.[1] While the molecular basis for the symptoms and complications of SCD and screening techniques to identify newborns with the disease have been known for decades, the development of interventions to improve the quality of life for these individuals, as well as the organization of health care systems to deliver appropriate care, has lagged. There has been substantial success in increasing the survival of children with SCD, but this success had not been translated to similar care as they now become adults. As will be argued in the report, a factor contributing to the slow progress is the fact that SCD is largely a disease of African Americans and as such exists in a context of racial discrimination, mistrust of the health care system, and the effects of poverty. In addition, there is substantial evidence that those with SCD may receive poorer quality of care. Finally, it should be noted that for a condition for which the presenting symptom may be acute and chronic pain, receipt of appropriate treatment is also influenced by the opioid crisis.

The report sets forth a substantial agenda beginning with the important need for information across the life span to characterize the trajectory

---

[1] This text has changed since the prepublication release of this report to more accurately reflect the estimates of prevalence of sickle cell disease identified in the literature.

of SCD and the antecedents of later complications. In parallel is the need to organize health care delivery and other services at the local, state, and global levels with a knowledgeable workforce to address the multiple needs of those with SCD, including engaging with the educational system and community-based groups. Although there is evidence of several important therapies in the pipeline, greater investment in research is needed into both more of these therapies and the dissemination of effective care into the affected population, especially in view of historical mistrust. This is not an impossible agenda; examples from other inborn conditions indicate that it can be done. The resilience of individuals living with SCD and the dedication of their families and communities that support them should also be harnessed as part of the solution.

I wish to express my gratitude for the excellent and demanding work done by the committee and staff members. However, special thanks are due to the individuals and organizations who shared often searing accounts of living with SCD, underscoring the urgency of the recommendations in the report.

Marie Clare McCormick, *Chair*
Committee on Addressing Sickle Cell Disease:
A Strategic Plan and Blueprint for Action

Contents

Boxes, Figures, and Tables

TABLES

Acronyms and Abbreviations

AAFP	American Academy of Family Physicians
AAHIVM	American Academy of HIV Medicine
AAP	American Academy of Pediatrics
AAPT	Analgesic, Anesthetic, and Addiction Clinical Trial Translations Innovations Opportunities and Networks (ACTTION) American Pain Society Pain Taxonomy
ACA	Patient Protection and Affordable Care Act
ACEP	American College of Emergency Physicians
ACGME	Accreditation Council for Graduate Medical Education
ACO	accountable care organization
ACOG	American College of Obstetricians and Gynecologists
ACP	American College of Physicians
ACS	acute chest syndrome
AHRQ	Agency for Healthcare Research and Quality
APHL	Association of Public Health Laboratories
ASCQ-Me	Adult Sickle Cell Quality of Life Measurement Information System
ASH	American Society of Hematology
ASPHO	American Society of Pediatric Hematology/Oncology
BDI	Beck Depression Inventory
CAHPS	Consumer Assessment of Healthcare Providers and Systems
CAM	complementary and alternative medicine
CBO	community-based organization

CBT	cognitive behavioral therapy
CC	consultative- or co-management-centered
CCM	Chronic Care Model
CCNC	Community Care of North Carolina
CDC	Centers for Disease Control and Prevention
CDU	clinical decision unit
CF	cystic fibrosis
CFC	cystic fibrosis carrier
CFF	Cystic Fibrosis Foundation
CHW	community health worker
CIBD	Center for Inherited Blood Disorders
CIRM	California Institute for Regenerative Medicine
CKD	chronic kidney disease
CMC	children with medical complexity
CMMI	Center for Medicare & Medicaid Innovation
CMS	Centers for Medicare & Medicaid Services
CPC+	comprehensive primary care plus
CRTI	Clinical Research Training Institute
CS	central sensitization
CSHCN	children with special health care needs
CVS	chorionic villus sampling
DALY	disability-adjusted life-year
DVT	deep vein thrombosis
EB	episode-based
ECHO	Extension for Community Healthcare Outcomes
ED	emergency department
EDSC[3]	Emergency Department of SCD Care Coalition
EHI	exertional heat illness
EHR	electronic health record
EPSDT	Early Periodic Screening, Diagnosis and Treatment
FDA	U.S. Food and Drug Administration
GBT	Global Blood Therapeutics
GERD	gastroesophageal reflux disease
GRADE	Grading of Recommendations Assessment, Development and Evaluation
GVHD	graft-versus-host-disease
HCV	hepatitis C virus
HFA	Hemophilia Federation of America

HHS	U.S. Department of Health and Human Services
HIPAA	Health Insurance Portability and Accountability Act
HLA	human leukocyte antigen
HOPE	Hematology–Oncology Psycho-Educational Needs Assessment
HPLC	high-performance liquid chromatography
HPSA	health professional shortage area
HRQOL	health-related quality of life
HRSA	Health Resources and Services Administration
HSA	Health Services Administration
HSCT	hematopoietic stem cell transplantation
HTC	hemophilia treatment center
HU	hydroxyurea
HUMLO	Hemoglobinopathy Uniform Medical Language Ontology
ICD	*International Classification of Diseases*
ICER	Institute for Clinical and Economic Review
IDEA	Individuals with Disabilities Education Act
IEF	isoelectric focusing
iHOMES	Improving Health Outcomes and Medical Education for Sickle Cell Disease
IOM	Institute of Medicine
IQ	intelligence quotient
IUGR	intrauterine growth restriction
IVF	in vitro fertilization
JHH	Johns Hopkins Hospital
JUH	Jefferson University Hospitals
KPMAS	Kaiser Permanente Mid-Atlantic States
LRP	loan repayment program
LV	lentiviral vector
MASAC	Medical and Scientific Advisory Council
MCHB	Maternal and Child Health Bureau
MRI	magnetic resonance imaging
MSH	Multicenter Study of Hydroxyurea
NBS	newborn screening
NCAA	National Collegiate Athletic Association
NHF	National Hemophilia Foundation
NHLBI	National Heart, Lung, and Blood Institute

NHSC	National Health Service Corps
NICE	National Institute for Health and Care Excellence
NICHQ	National Institute for Children's Health Quality
NIH	National Institutes of Health
NO	nitric oxide
NORD	National Organization for Rare Diseases
NQF	National Quality Forum
NSAID	non-steroidal anti-inflammatory drug
OASH	Office of the Assistant Secretary for Health
OIH	opioid-induced hyperalgesia
OUD	opioid use disorder
OWS	opioid withdrawal syndrome
PASCPN	Pennsylvania Sickle Cell Provider's Network
PBRS	performance-based risk-sharing
PCC	primary care-centered
PCMH	patient-centered medical home
PCORI	Patient-Centered Outcomes Research Institute
PCP	primary care provider
PCV	pneumococcal conjugate vaccine
PGD	pre-implantation genetic diagnosis
PiSCES	Pain in Sickle Cell Epidemiology Study
P-MAP	Pediatric Measure Application Partnership
PPSV (or PPV)	pneumococcal polysaccharide vaccine
PRES	posterior reversible encephalopathy syndrome
PRIDE	Program to Increase Diversity Among Individuals Engaged in Health-Related Research
PRO	patient-reported outcome
PTSD	posttraumatic stress disorder
QALY	quality-adjusted life-year
QI	quality improvement
QOL	quality of life
RBC	red blood cell
RC	Research Collaborative
REM	rapid eye movement
ROS	reactive oxygen species
RuSH	Registry and Surveillance System for Hemoglobinopathies
SCA	sickle cell anemia
SCCC	Sickle Cell Community Consortium

SCD	sickle cell disease
SCDAA	Sickle Cell Disease Association of America
SCDAAMI	Sickle Cell Disease Association of America, Michigan Chapter, Inc.
SCDAI	Sickle Cell Disease Association of Illinois
SCDC	Sickle Cell Data Collection
SCDFC	Sickle Cell Disease Foundation of California
SCDTDRCP	Sickle Cell Disease Treatment Demonstration Regional Collaborative Program
SCFGA	Sickle Cell Foundation of Georgia
SCI	silent cerebral infarct
SCT	sickle cell trait
SDM	shared decision making
SSA	Social Security Administration
SSDI	Social Security Disability Insurance
SSI	Supplemental Security Income
STEP	Solutions to Empower Patients
SUD	substance use disorder
TCD	transcranial Doppler
TRV	tricuspid regurgitant velocity
USPSTF	U.S. Preventive Services Task Force
VOC	vaso-occlusive crisis
VOE	vaso-occlusive episode
VTE	venous thromboembolism
WBDR	World Bleeding Disorders Registry
WFH	World Federation of Hemophilia

Summary[1]

There are approximately 100,000 people living with sickle cell disease (SCD) in the United States and millions more globally. Sickle cell trait (SCT) is even more prevalent and occurs in 1–3 million Americans and 8–10 percent of African Americans in the United States. Current estimates indicate that about 300,000 people are born with SCD each year worldwide and that more than 100 million people across the globe live with SCT. The sickle gene is found in every ethnic group, not just among those of African descent.

Since its discovery in 1910 by James Herrick, SCD has received relatively little attention and few resources from the scientific, clinical, and public health communities compared with other genetic disorders, such as cystic fibrosis (CF). Until December 2018 there was only one drug approved by the U.S. Food and Drug Administration (FDA) for the condition. A contributing factor to this lack of awareness and resources is that the affected population, which is primarily composed of racial and ethnic minorities, contends with persistent discrimination in the health care system and racism in society at large. As described by Keith Wailoo, a medical historian who has extensively studied the history of SCD, "Sickle cell disease is a microcosm of how issues of race, ethnicity, and identity come into conflict with issues of health care." Thus, individuals with SCD have suffered from a lag in the development of treatments and cures as well as an often strained relationship with health care providers and limited resources for advocacy efforts.

---

[1] Citations and references for all facts and figures mentioned in the Summary are included in the subsequent chapters of this report.

1

To accelerate progress for those living with SCD, the Office of Minority Health at the Office of the Assistant Secretary for Health (OASH) at the U.S. Department of Health and Human Services (HHS) asked the Health and Medicine Division of the National Academies of Sciences, Engineering, and Medicine (the National Academies) to develop a strategic plan and blueprint to address SCD in the United States. (The full charge to the committee [Statement of Task] is provided in Box S-1.) This report is the answer to that request.

BOX S-1
Committee's Statement of Task

An ad hoc committee will be convened to develop a strategic plan and blueprint for addressing sickle cell disease (SCD) in the United States. In conducting its work, the committee will examine:

- the epidemiology, health outcomes, genetic implications, and societal factors associated with SCD and sickle cell trait (SCT), including serious complications of SCD such as stroke, kidney and heart problems, acute chest syndrome, and debilitating pain crises;
- current guidelines and best practices for the care of patients with SCD;
- to the extent possible, the economic burden associated with SCD; and
- current federal, state, and local programs related to SCD and SCT, including screening, monitoring and surveillance, treatment and care programs, research, and others.

The committee will provide guidance on priorities for programs, policies, and research and make recommendations as appropriate regarding:

- limitations and opportunities for developing national SCD patient registries and/or surveillance systems;
- barriers in the health care sector associated with SCD and SCT, including access to care and quality of care, workforce development, pain management, and transitions from pediatric to adult care;
- needed innovations in research, particularly for curative treatments, such as gene replacement/gene editing, and increasing awareness and enrollment of SCD patients in clinical trials; and
- the expanded and optimal role of patient advocacy and community engagement groups.

Committee guidance should be formulated around strategic objectives (strategic plan) and action steps (blueprint). Throughout all the deliberations, the committee will give consideration to ethical issues related to SCD and SCT.

SCD and SCT status are currently identified at birth through universal newborn screening (NBS) in all 50 states, the District of Columbia, and U.S. territories. NBS has been highly successful at ensuring early access to much needed care, such as prophylactic penicillin for young children to avoid sepsis, which has saved countless children's lives. Despite the effectiveness of NBS, there are wide variations in states' short- and long-term follow-up practices regarding screening results (see Chapter 3). Most states also track individuals only if they remain within the same state, thus missing those who move out of the state. Additionally, while NBS identifies newborns who have SCT, there are currently no standardized practices for short- and long-term follow-up for carriers. This has important implications because of emerging evidence that SCT status might be a risk factor for certain clinical complications and because it is important for reproductive decision making. NBS also misses a large proportion of the SCD and SCT population who was born outside of the United States or before universal NBS was implemented in the country.

The genetic mutation responsible for SCD causes an individual's red blood cells to distort into a C or sickle shape, reducing their ability to transport oxygen throughout the body. These sickled red blood cells break down rapidly, become very sticky, and develop a propensity to clump together, which causes them to become stuck and cause damage within blood vessels. The result is reduced blood flow to distal organs, which leads to physical symptoms of incapacitating pain, tissue and organ damage, and early death.

Pain is the hallmark of SCD, and individuals with SCD experience both acute and chronic pain. SCD pain is complex because it can be influenced by the disease pathophysiology as well as by psychological and social factors. The disease can also affect every organ in the body, as discussed in Chapter 4. While death rarely occurs among children with SCD in the United States, with 98 percent surviving to 18 years of age, SCD has a persistently high mortality rate in adults, and end-organ damage is the major driver of this mortality. Fatigue and emotional distress, such as anxiety and depression, become more prevalent with age and, along with chronic pain, pose a high burden and cause significant disability, which is under-recognized. In addition, childhood mortality for SCD remains very high in resource-poor countries.

Care delivery for SCD is inadequate. This stems in part from the fact that for most of the 20th century SCD was considered primarily a childhood disease because most affected individuals did not survive into adulthood. High childhood mortality rates for SCD led to an increased emphasis on improving the infrastructure for pediatric care in the United States and conducting research to prevent early death from infections.

The emphasis on early interventions for SCD led to seminal studies that provided the evidence base for clinical guidelines for the prevention and management of pediatric complications, such as the implementation of guidelines for prophylaxis against pneumococcal sepsis and stroke. Unfortunately, over the years there has not been a parallel development of guidelines and infrastructure for care delivery to adults living with SCD. Persistent gaps in the understanding of the natural history of SCD, predictors and biomarkers of morbidity and mortality, and the pattern of emergence of organ damage and other sources of disability persist, thus limiting optimal care delivery, particularly for adults (see Chapter 4).

Individuals who are transitioning from pediatric to adult SCD care are at a particularly high risk for morbidity and mortality because the robust care delivery systems available to pediatric patients are not replaced by matching or adequate resources for the adult patients (see Chapters 5 and 6). The lack of dedicated facilities and personnel caring for adult patients is compounded by the rising complexity of the disease, the emergence of comorbidities, and the vulnerability of individuals through the challenging period of adolescence and young adulthood. Young adults with SCD report being unprepared to engage optimally with and navigate the adult health care system independently after years of support in the pediatric care system. Areas of particular unmet need center on the domains of independence, self-care, vocation, and insurance coverage. When these factors are coupled with the aforementioned stigma, racism, and discrimination within the health care setting and society more broadly, individuals living with SCD often find themselves facing a solitary battle. This battle includes having to advocate for themselves in the health care and public sectors, at work, in schools, and sometimes even in their families.

Finally, even when interventions are well established, the delivery of appropriate and comprehensive care is uneven (see Chapter 6). Some of this may reflect payment mechanisms that do not support coordinated care. The majority of those with SCD are publicly insured, and covered services may vary across states. Furthermore, health care providers may not be well versed in accessing appropriate and available enabling services,[2] or such enabling services may not exist. There is a lack of awareness among providers, especially those who do not regularly encounter patients with SCD, of the available clinical practice guidelines for evidence-based SCD care, which leads to inconsistent or substandard care. Members of a health care team may also be unaware of the implicit biases that influence their interactions with and medical decision making for those individuals living with SCD (see Chapters 2 and 6).

---

[2] Enabling services are defined as patient services that are intended to improve access to health care and create better health outcomes. Some examples include health education, case management, and transportation.

Improving the organization of care delivery can help ensure that individuals have access to appropriate services and can also enhance the quality of the care that is delivered, in turn improving the overall quality of life (QOL) for individuals living with SCD while increasing their access to new therapies. Two therapeutic products have been recently approved by FDA (voxelotor and crizanlizumab), and researchers are actively pursuing improved curative options by broadening access to stem cell transplant and developing gene therapy protocols (see Chapter 7). In addition to increasing access to new interventions, service delivery should be restructured by creating multidisciplinary care teams that can support delivery of whole-person care necessary to improve physical and social functioning and QOL for individuals with SCD.

The restructuring of care delivery would also provide a platform for patient advocacy groups and community-based organizations (CBOs) that have played an integral role in driving policy and much needed programming for the SCD population. These groups provide education about SCD and SCT, genetic support, psychosocial support, camps, care coordination, case referral, and transition assistance, among other services. However, it should be noted that patient advocacy groups and CBOs are under-resourced and are thereby limited in their ability to serve their constituents. Furthermore, there are no guidelines or unified infrastructure for the operation of these organizations and advocacy groups. Despite their key role for the SCD population, they also have traditionally not been recognized as part of the SCD care delivery system (see Chapter 8).

One challenge that has stifled progress in SCD is the lack of funding. To successfully garner attention and resources for those affected by SCD and SCT, there is a need for public education and awareness about the disease and the burden it places on individuals and the health care system. The contribution of racism, discrimination, mistrust of the health care system, socioeconomic disadvantage, and inadequate services across many sectors experienced by ethnic minorities in the United States cannot be overemphasized. However, the problems of access to high-quality health and social services are not exclusive to SCD, and the strategies developed to address them in other conditions can serve as a guide. CF and hemophilia, for instance, which are both rare and inheritable diseases, have well-organized and well-funded health care delivery systems despite there being smaller numbers of affected individuals (approximately 30,000 and 20,000, respectively, in the United States). Amyotrophic lateral sclerosis attracted widespread public attention and efforts fueled by social media, which resulted in dramatically increased funding. Other rare diseases have also benefited from an infusion of federal and private funding. These diseases set valuable precedents for addressing the needs of the SCD population.

SCOPE OF WORK

Charge to the Committee

The Office of Minority Health at OASH at HHS commissioned the National Academies' Health and Medicine Division to develop a strategic plan and blueprint to address SCD in the United States. A committee was formed to direct the study titled Addressing Sickle Cell Disease: A Strategic Plan and Blueprint for Action. The charge to the committee (Statement of Task) is shown in Box S-1.

The Committee's Approach

To accomplish its task, the committee focused the report to address the most salient issues surrounding SCD and SCT in the United States. Thus, most of the literature reviewed for the report originates from the United States. However, because the majority of the SCD population resides outside of the United States, seminal evidence and developments from other countries were included in the report where necessary. The bulk of the report focuses on the needs of the SCD population because this is the area of greatest need.

Conceptual Framework

Life-span approach In its assessment, the committee considered the needs and specific challenges at different stages in life. While most SCD complications are common to both children and adults, specific ones may be more prevalent at different ages. For example, dactylitis (painful swelling of the hands and feet), stroke, and enlarged spleen are all common in children, whereas retinopathy, pulmonary hypertension, heart failure, chronic leg ulcers, and cognitive burdens are more prevalent in the adult population.

The non-health-related needs of younger and older individuals with SCD may also vary. For instance, children who experience overt or silent strokes as a result of SCD develop cognitive impairment that may warrant additional educational support in order to increase the chances for academic success. With age, these cognitive challenges coupled with the additional burden of chronic organ damage may necessitate vocational rehabilitation support, specific workplace accommodations, or support to facilitate changes in vocation. Finally, the life-span approach is appropriate because existing resources for children and adults with SCD vary. High-quality care is currently better established for children, although there is room for improvement; quality indicators for adults with SCD are significantly underdeveloped and clinical guidelines for high-quality care lack a strong evidence base. As individuals with SCD survive into adulthood, information is needed about the appropriate service needs, and this need may require longitudinal

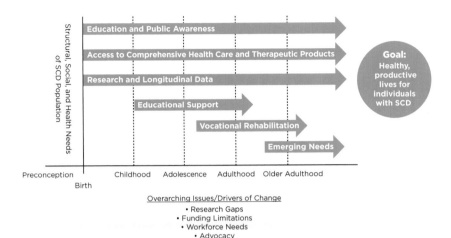

FIGURE S-1 A life-span approach to understanding and addressing the needs of the SCD population.
NOTE: SCD = sickle cell disease.

data systems that will inform evolving care and service needs over time. The committee conceptualized the life-span approach in Figure S-1 in order to represent the need for targeted interventions at different life stages.

It is also critical to include a focus on QOL factors and on understanding how QOL may change over a lifetime; this is a common approach in the study of other chronic conditions, such as cancer and cardiovascular diseases.

Person-centric SCD care SCD is a genetic lifelong condition; as the survival rate continues to improve for children, it must be managed as a chronic disease, which requires an ongoing person-centric, collaborative approach to care management. Building on previous National Academies work on epilepsy, another debilitating medical condition diagnosed in childhood, the SCD committee based its recommendations at least in part on the epilepsy model of care (see Figure S-2), which is built on Wagner's Chronic Care Model. Wagner's model emphasizes the foundational partnership between the care team and an activated and empowered patient as being crucial for care delivery. The model also underscores the importance of family members and community service providers in the care delivery system. This is especially relevant for the SCD population, which relies heavily on services provided by advocacy groups and CBOs.

The main focus for any model of care should be the individuals with SCD and their families, rather than the health care system. Bearing in mind

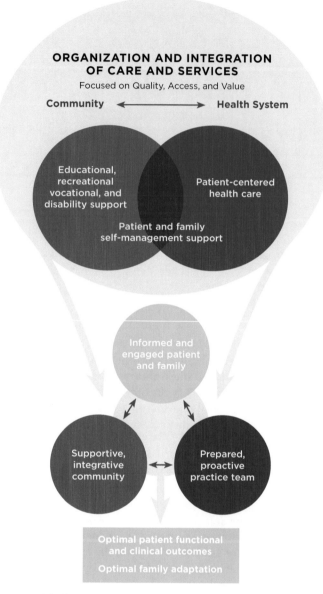

FIGURE S-2 Model of person-centric care for SCD.
NOTE: SCD = sickle cell disease.
SOURCES: IOM, 2012; originally adapted from Wagner, 1998. Republished with permission of American College of Physicians - Journals from Chronic Disease Management: What Will It Take to Improve Care for Chronic Illness?, E. H. Wagner, volume 1, 1998; permission conveyed through Copyright Clearance Center, Inc.

the individual's preferences, needs, and values, systemic efforts are required to facilitate access to comprehensive care and empower individuals to self-manage and remove barriers to treatment. Health care and social services are designed to benefit patients and improve their health outcomes, QOL, and ability to be productive. The engaged, supported, and empowered patients are then able to work collaboratively with the care delivery team and community resources to effectively manage their care.

There is also a need to establish acceptable minimum standards for the delivery of the complex care that individuals living with SCD require across the life span. Several centers of excellence in SCD have made efforts to establish learning collaboratives that define these care delivery standards, leveraging quality improvement measures to ensure that every patient has access to standardized care at all times, with ongoing data monitoring to track the processes' effectiveness. For example, the SCD Emergency Department Learning Collaborative recently supported quality improvement interventions across three sites to improve time to first analgesia for acute SCD pain, and the Hemoglobinopathy Learning Collaborative has focused on strategies that result in more coordinated and appropriate care in order to achieve fewer complications, acute care visits, and hospitalizations; enhanced QOL; and more compassionate and respectful treatment from the health care system. Expanding the reach of such collaboratives will help spread nationally agreed-upon standards of care to other sites, with ongoing efforts to improve the consistency and ultimately the quality of care for individuals living with SCD. (See Chapter 6 for more information.)

RECOMMENDATIONS

Against the contextual backdrop described in the preceding sections, the committee developed a strategic plan and blueprint for SCD action and identified strategies and specific actions (or recommendations) for improving care and outcomes. The vision for the strategic plan is to ensure "long, healthy, productive lives for those living with SCD and those with SCT." The committee found that the core message of the Institute of Medicine report *Crossing the Quality Chasm: A New Health System for the 21st Century* still holds true today for the SCD population, which has not benefited from medical science advances as much as the general population or even at the same rate as those living with other rare and heritable diseases, such as CF and hemophilia. There is insufficient up-to-date information about the SCD population to appropriately inform programming and policies that address the population's specific needs. Finally, evidence-based interventions (preventative, acute, and post-acute services) that apply to the general population are not always available to individuals living with SCD.

The committee determined that, at minimum, the strategic plan and blueprint should ensure that the SCD population receives the same high-quality care that every American is entitled to. The committee based the foundational principles for action on the six aims for the health care system identified in the *Crossing the Quality Chasm* report, namely that health care be safe, effective, patient-centered, timely, efficient, and equitable. According to the authors of the report, "a health care system that achieves major gains in these six areas would be far better at meeting patient needs." The committee felt that, due to the history of marginalization and racism experienced by the majority of the affected population, it was important to add a seventh principle: that health care be ethical.

The strategic plan (see Figure S-3) is made up of a strategic vision, eight overarching strategies or "pillars" that support the vision, and foundational

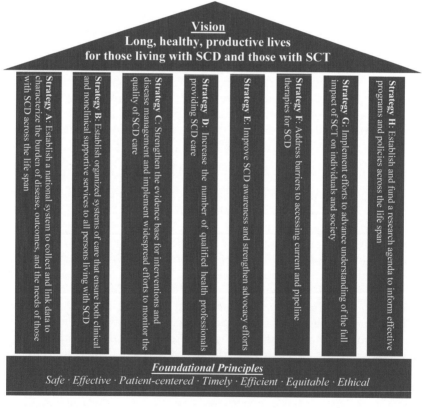

Vision
Long, healthy, productive lives
for those living with SCD and those with SCT

Strategy A: Establish a national system to collect and link data to characterize the burden of disease, outcomes, and the needs of those with SCD across the life span

Strategy B: Establish organized systems of care that ensure both clinical and nonclinical supportive services to all persons living with SCD

Strategy C: Strengthen the evidence base for interventions and disease management and implement widespread efforts to monitor the quality of SCD care

Strategy D: Increase the number of qualified health professionals providing SCD care

Strategy E: Improve SCD awareness and strengthen advocacy efforts

Strategy F: Address barriers to accessing current and pipeline therapies for SCD

Strategy G: Implement efforts to advance understanding of the full impact of SCT on individuals and society

Strategy H: Establish and fund a research agenda to inform effective programs and policies across the life span

__Foundational Principles__
Safe · Effective · Patient-centered · Timely · Efficient · Equitable · Ethical

FIGURE S-3 Strategic plan for improving SCD care and outcomes in the United States. NOTE: SCD = sickle cell disease; SCT = sickle cell trait.

principles, which undergird the strategic plan. The strategies take into account the multifaceted needs of the SCD and SCT population and the equally multidimensional interventions required to meet these needs. The strategies are equally important and need to be approached with the same amount of urgency.

The committee has also proposed a blueprint for implementing the strategic plan. The blueprint offers recommended actions for each of the strategies in the strategic plan. These action steps are the recommendations identified in the report's various chapters after a thoughtful review of the available evidence. The action steps or recommendations are enumerated with the chapter that contains the supporting evidence and listed in order of implementation timeframe. The committee offers timeframes for accomplishing each of the recommendations. The timeframes take into account the complexity of the activity, the level of resources needed to accomplish the task, and the existence of current programs that can serve as vehicles for advancing action. Activities are also prioritized by actions that need to occur sequentially.

In order to make meaningful and sustained progress on the strategic plan, OASH at HHS should appoint an oversight body with members from across HHS agencies to oversee the roll-out of the strategic plan and blueprint. The appointment of the oversight body should be immediate, and the current HHS Sickle Cell Disease Workgroup, which has representation from 11 HHS agencies, would be one option for such an interagency group.

Finally, to ensure continued progress, the oversight body should conduct regular assessments of the implementation of the strategic plan, with the first evaluation occurring no more than 5 years after the release of this report.

Chapter 9 includes a complete description of the components of the strategic plan and blueprint.

Strategy A: Establish a national system to collect and link data to characterize the burden of disease, outcomes, and the needs of those with SCD across the life span. This can be accomplished by building on current and previous data collection efforts by the Centers for Disease Control and Prevention, developing a clinical registry for SCD, and linking existing datasets on the SCD population as described below.

Recommendation 3-1: The Centers for Disease Control and Prevention should work with all states to develop state public health surveillance systems to support a national longitudinal registry of all persons with sickle cell disease.
Timeframe: 1–2 years

Recommendation 3-2: The Health Resources and Services Administration, the National Institutes of Health, and the Agency for Healthcare Research and Quality should develop a clinical data registry for sickle cell disease. The registry would allow for identifying best practices for care delivery and outcomes.
Timeframe: 1–2 years

Recommendation 3-3: The Office of the Assistant Secretary for Health should establish a working group to identify existing and disparate sources of data that can be immediately linked and mined. These data can be used to provide needed information on sickle cell disease health care services usage and costs in the short term.
Timeframe: 1–2 years

Strategy B: Establish organized systems of care that ensure both clinical and nonclinical supportive services to all persons living with SCD. Such systems would ensure access to high-quality, evidence-based, comprehensive primary and specialty (acute and chronic) care delivered by a multidisciplinary team; supplemental enabling services; and behavioral health and social services. The following action steps are recommended to achieve this strategy.

Recommendation 2-1: The Social Security Administration should review disability insurance qualifications to ensure that the qualification criteria reflect the burden of the disease borne by individuals with sickle cell disease.
Timeframe: 1–2 years

Recommendation 2-2: States should expand and enhance vocational rehabilitation programs for individuals with sickle cell disease who need additional training in order to actively participate in the workforce.
Timeframe: 2–3 years

Recommendation 5-1: The Office of the Assistant Secretary for Health, through the Office of Minority Health, should convene a panel of relevant stakeholders to delineate the elements of a comprehensive system of sickle cell disease (SCD) care, including community supports to improve health outcomes, quality of life, and health inequalities. Relevant stakeholders may include the National Minority Quality Forum, National Medical Association, American Society of Pediatric Hematology/Oncology, American Academy of Pediatrics, American Board of Pediatrics, American College of Physicians, American Society of Hematology, Sickle Cell Disease Association of America Inc., Sickle

Cell Adult Provider Network, and other key clinical disciplines and stakeholders engaged in SCD care; health systems; and individuals living with SCD and their families.
Timeframe: 2–3 years

Recommendation 5-2: The Centers for Medicare & Medicaid Services should work with state Medicaid programs to develop and pilot reimbursement models for the delivery of coordinated sickle cell disease health care and support services.
Timeframe: 3–4 years

Recommendation 5-3: The U.S. Department of Education should collaborate with state departments of health and education and local school boards to develop educational materials to provide guidance for teachers, school nurses, school administrators, and primary care providers to support the medical and academic needs of students with sickle cell disease.
Timeframe: 1–2 years

Strategy C: Strengthen the evidence base for interventions and disease management and implement widespread efforts to monitor the quality of SCD care. Existing evidence to support the care and management of SCD needs to be updated to reflect the current evolution of the SCD population, where individuals are living into adulthood and contending with complications that arise later in life. Excess mortality can be attributed to not receiving appropriate care. There also needs to be widespread efforts to track and improve the quality of care that accredited comprehensive SCD centers (as described in Strategy B) provide. This strategy can be accomplished through the following recommended action steps.

Recommendation 4-1: Private and public funders and health professional associations should fund and conduct research to close the gaps in the existing evidence base for sickle cell disease care to inform the development of clinical practice guidelines and indicators of high-quality care.
Timeframe: 3–5 years

Recommendation 5-4: The National Heart, Lung, and Blood Institute; Health Resources and Services Administration; Centers for Disease Control and Prevention; and U.S. Food and Drug Administration should collaborate with the American Society for Hematology, Pediatric Emergency Care Applied Research Network, Patient-Centered Outcomes

Research Institute, and private funders of quality improvement initiatives to foster the development of quality improvement collaboratives.
Timeframe: 3–5 years

Recommendation 6-1: Federal agencies including the Agency for Healthcare Research and Quality; National Heart, Lung, and Blood Institute; Health Resources and Services Administration; Centers for Disease Control and Prevention; and U.S. Food and Drug Administration should work together with and fund researchers and professional associations to develop and track a series of indicators to assess the quality of sickle cell disease care including the patient experience, the prevention of disease complications, and health outcomes.
Timeframe: 1–2 years (to identify and develop list of quality indicators); 3–5 years (to implement monitoring program to track performance of those indicators)

Recommendation 6-2: The Centers for Medicare & Medicaid Services and private payers should require the reporting of expert consensus-driven sickle cell disease (SCD) quality measures and other metrics of high-quality health care for persons with SCD.
Timeframe: 3–5 years

Recommendation 6-3: The U.S. Department of Health and Human Services should fund efforts to identify and mitigate potentially modifiable disparities in mortality and health outcomes. Specific subgroups to consider include young adults in transition from pediatric to adult care, pregnant women, and older adults.
Timeframe: 1–2 years

Strategy D: Increase the number of qualified health professionals providing SCD care by enhancing existing health professional training and accreditation programs and incentivizing providers to provide compassionate and high-quality care. This strategy can be achieved through the following recommended action steps.

Recommendation 6-4: The National Institutes of Health should disseminate information on loan repayment opportunities to incentivize health care professionals interested in conducting research on sickle cell disease (SCD). The Health Resources and Services Administration should add populations with SCD as a designated population health professional shortage area under the National Health Service Corps program and create a loan repayment program for health care professionals working with SCD populations.

Timeframe: 1–2 years (disseminate information about existing programs); 3–5 years (develop criteria for loan repayment and similar programs for health professionals working specifically with the SCD population)

Recommendation 6-5: Health professional associations (American Society of Hematology, American College of Obstetricians and Gynecologists, American College of Emergency Physicians, American Academy of Family Physicians,[3] American Academy of Pediatrics, National Medical Association, American College of Physicians) and organizations for other relevant health professionals such as advanced practice providers, nurses, and community health workers should convene an Academy of Sickle Cell Disease Medicine (SCD) to support SCD providers through education, credentialing, networking, and advocacy.
Timeframe: 2–3 years

Recommendation 6-6: Health professional associations and graduate and professional schools should develop early and effective mentoring programs to link early career health professionals with seasoned providers to generate interest in sickle cell disease care.
Timeframe: 3–5 years

Strategy E: Improve SCD awareness and strengthen advocacy efforts through targeted education and strategic partnerships among HHS, health care providers, advocacy groups and community-based organizations, professional associations, and other key stakeholders (e.g., media and state health departments). Strategic partnerships with advocacy groups and CBOs will enhance their capacity to provide supportive services and acknowledge their value as partners in promoting patient-centered policies and programs. The following recommended action steps will be necessary to achieve this strategy.

Recommendation 2-3: The U.S. Department of Health and Human Services should engage with media to improve awareness about the disease and address misconceptions about the disease and those affected.
Timeframe: 1–2 years

Recommendation 8-1: The U.S. Department of Health and Human Services, in collaboration with health professional associations, health care providers, and other key stakeholders, should partner with

---

[3] This text was revised since the prepublication release of this report to correct American Association of Family Practitioners to American Academy of Family Physicians.

community-based organizations and patient advocates to translate and disseminate emerging clinical research information to people living with sickle cell disease and their families in order to improve health literacy and empower them to engage in the care and treatment decision-making process.
Timeframe: 2–3 years

Recommendation 8-2: The U.S. Department of Health and Human Services, in collaboration with state health departments and health care providers, should partner with community-based organizations and community health workers to engage the sickle cell disease (SCD) population in designing educational and advocacy programs and policies and in disseminating information on health and community services to individuals living with SCD and their caregivers.
Timeframe: 1–2 years

Strategy F: Address barriers to accessing current and pipeline therapies for SCD, with the goal of ensuring widespread patient access to beneficial therapies. The following recommended action steps will be necessary to achieve this strategy.

Recommendation 7-1: The Centers for Medicare & Medicaid Services in collaboration with private payers should identify approaches to financing the up-front costs of curative therapies.
Timeframe: 2–3 years

Recommendation 7-2: The U.S. Department of Health and Human Services should encourage and reimburse the practice of shared decision making and the development of decision aids for novel, high-risk, potentially highly effective therapies for individuals living with sickle cell disease.
Timeframe: 1–2 years (to identify and synthesize criteria for the use of new medications); 3–5 years (to develop guidance for shared decision making and tools for implementation)

Recommendation 7-3: The National Institutes of Health, U.S. Food and Drug Administration, pharmaceutical industry, and research community should establish an organized, systematic approach to encourage participation in clinical trials by including affected individuals in the design of trials, working with community-based organizations to disseminate information and recruit participants, and conducting other targeted activities.
The Patient-Centered Outcomes Research Institute, American Society of Hematology, FDA, and National Institutes of Health all have

existing activities to foster patient-centric clinical trials design. Lessons and best practices from these disparate efforts need to be standardized, scaled, and adopted for inclusion in every clinical trial involving individuals living with SCD.
Timeframe: 2–3 years

Strategy G: Implement efforts to advance understanding of the full impact of SCT on individuals and society. The committee recommends the following action steps but cautions that all activities pertaining to collecting and using data to raise awareness and improve interventions should be performed so as not to stigmatize those living with SCT in any way.

Recommendation 3-4: The Health Resources and Services Administration should work with states to standardize the communication of and use of newborn screening positive results in genetic counseling and should create a mechanism for communicating this information across the life span and ensuring access to needed support and services.
Timeframe: 2–3 years

Recommendation 4-2: The National Institutes of Health should fund research to elucidate the pathophysiology of sickle cell trait.
Timeframe: 2–3 years

Recommendation 4-3: The Office of the Assistant Secretary for Health should partner with community-based organizations, the media, and other relevant stakeholders to disseminate information to promote awareness and education about the potential risks associated with sickle cell trait.
Timeframe: 1–2 years

Strategy H: Establish and fund a research agenda to inform effective programs and policies across the life span. Federal and private funders should collaborate to provide funding to clinician scientists and scholars with expertise in SCD, race, and stigma to advance research on pressing topics. The oversight body established by OASH at HHS should collaborate with health professional associations, researchers, individuals living with SCD, and funders to develop a robust research agenda with priority topics that need to be studied.
Timeframe: 1–2 years (to develop research agenda); 3–5 years (to disseminate funding opportunities for researchers)[4]

---

[4] This text was revised since the prepublication of the report to include the timeline for implementation of this strategy. The prepublication version of the report listed the timeline as "Ongoing."

1

Introduction

*Every single day that you get up out of bed, you're fighting a
battle, and when you take that first breath ... it's a breath of
pain. You assess mentally. Okay, where are all the places that
are hurting right now ... and you actually have to take several
deep breaths to push the circulation through your body.*

—Tosin O. (Open Session Panelist)

Sickle cell disease (SCD) refers to a group of inherited red blood cell
(RBC) disorders resulting from a mutation in hemoglobin, which impedes
regular blood flow and leads to painful vaso-occlusive episodes and other
severe complications (CDC, 2017b). Present at birth, SCD causes lifelong acute and chronic complications throughout the whole body. This
debilitating, multi-system condition affects approximately 100,000 people
in the United States and millions globally[1] (ASH, 2016; Mulumba and
Wilson, 2015). Childhood mortality due to SCD has declined in the United
States due to medical advances and preventive services, but despite this
progress life expectancy and quality of life for people living with SCD are
lower than for those without the disease (Lubeck et al., 2019; Piel et al.,
2017), necessitating action to improve health and outcomes and reduce
this disparity.

---

[1] This text has changed since the prepublication release of this report to more accurately
reflect the estimates of prevalence of sickle cell disease identified in the literature.

SCOPE OF WORK

Charge to the Committee

The Office of Minority Health at the Office of the Assistant Secretary for Health at the U.S. Department of Health and Human Services (HHS) requested that the National Academies of Sciences, Engineering, and Medicine (the National Academies) convene a committee to develop a strategic plan and blueprint to address SCD in the United States. The Committee on Addressing Sickle Cell Disease: A Strategic Plan and Blueprint for Action was established in response to this request. As part of its work, the committee was asked to develop a framework that provides guidance on the best approaches to addressing pertinent issues in SCD such as health care disparities, stigma, race and biases, access to care, workforce development, transitions in care, innovations needed, curative treatments, and the role of patient advocacy and community engagement. Box 1-1 shows the committee's Statement of Task. In addressing the Statement of Task, the committee defined its scope as addressing challenges of SCD and sickle cell trait (SCT)[2] in the United States and creating an action plan for prolonging healthy lives through the delivery of high-quality and equitable care to individuals with SCD. The committee found it necessary to acknowledge the global burden of the disease in low- and middle-income countries in order to display the full context of its impact; this was especially important for areas where research and findings from other countries were essential to fill in knowledge gaps in the United States. The committee also addressed ethical concerns pertaining to areas such as screening, treatment, and research.

STUDY PROCESS AND INFORMATION GATHERING

This section presents the process that the committee used to identify and evaluate the scientific literature related to SCD and the Statement of Task, committee areas of expertise, how the literature search was conducted, and the evaluation criteria used to screen and categorize literature for the chapters.

Committee Expertise and Meetings

The National Academies appointed a team of 14 multidisciplinary experts to the Committee on Addressing Sickle Cell Disease: A Strategic Plan and Blueprint for Action; their expertise spanned epidemiology,

---

[2] SCT is not a disease but refers to when an individual inherits one sickle gene from one parent and a normal gene from another parent. SCT carriers live normal lives and do not experience symptoms associated with SCD.

BOX 1-1
Committee's Statement of Task

An ad hoc committee will be convened to develop a strategic plan and blueprint for addressing sickle cell disease (SCD) in the United States. In conducting its work, the committee will examine:

- the epidemiology, health outcomes, genetic implications, and societal factors associated with SCD and sickle cell trait (SCT), including serious complications of SCD such as stroke, kidney and heart problems, acute chest syndrome, and debilitating pain crises;
- current guidelines and best practices for the care of patients with SCD;
- to the extent possible, the economic burden associated with SCD; and
- current federal, state, and local programs related to SCD and SCT, including screening, monitoring and surveillance, treatment and care programs, research, and others.

The committee will provide guidance on priorities for programs, policies, and research and make recommendations, as appropriate, regarding:

- limitations and opportunities for developing national SCD patient registries and/or surveillance systems;
- barriers in the health care sector associated with SCD and SCT, including access to care and quality of care, workforce development, pain management, and transitions from pediatric to adult care;
- needed innovations in research, particularly for curative treatments such as gene replacement/gene editing and increasing awareness and enrollment of SCD patients in clinical trials; and
- the expanded and optimal role of patient advocacy and community engagement groups.

Committee guidance should be formulated around strategic objectives (strategic plan) and action steps (blueprint). Throughout all the deliberations, the committee will give consideration to ethical issues related to SCD and SCT.

---

hemoglobinopathies, pediatrics, hematology, oncology, emergency medicine, psychology, care management and delivery, pain management, health disparities, health economics, health policy, ethics, treatment of diseases associated with SCD, research, and workforce development.

The committee convened five times; it held public information-gathering sessions at each of those meetings and invited panelists to present on specific topics of interest to the committee. Full descriptions of the open session panels are included in Appendix A. The first meeting included the presentation of the charge to the committee by the Assistant Secretary for Health and Office of Minority Health. Between the in-person meetings, committee members held deliberative sessions to review the literature, discuss the evidence base, and write the report.

Literature Search

The committee conducted a comprehensive literature search through the National Academies Research Center. The search encompassed a wide array of terms related to SCD and its complications, as detailed in Appendix B. The search was restricted to 1990–2019 except for the search terms: bias, stigma, discrimination, and racism, which had no date bounds to capture the experiences of minority populations in the health care system. The committee performed additional targeted searches, as needed, to supplement the landscape literature review and expanded their search to related patient populations when information on certain topics could not be found for SCD. Because there have been relatively few large, rigorous studies conducted on SCD and SCT, the committee decided not to employ specific criteria for including/excluding literature that was evaluated as part of this report, thus allowing for smaller, observational, and qualitative studies to be included in the committee's analysis. The committee also examined abstracts of conference presentations to allow for inclusion of emerging research on SCD and SCT.

Conceptual Approaches for Information Gathering

Life-Span Approach

SCD causes various challenges at different stages in life, so the committee conceptualized the tasks for this report by assessing the needs of people living with SCD over the life span. For example, dactylitis occurs mainly in children, whereas heart failure and chronic leg ulcers typically affect adults. Age compounds the complications and impact of SCD on the affected individual's body (Oyedeji et al., 2019; Quinn et al., 2010; Sandhu and Cohen, 2015; Swanson et al., 2011). Children may also experience strokes, which can negatively affect cognitive function, impede their performance in school, and explain long-term cognitive function limitations in adulthood, which can manifest as poor pain coping or non-adherence to prescribed treatments (Crosby et al., 2015; Gold et al., 2008; Greenham et al., 2016; Swanson et al., 2011). These long-term cognitive limitations could be a contributing factor to the high rate of unemployment in the SCD population (Swanson et al., 2011). Taking a life-span approach provides the

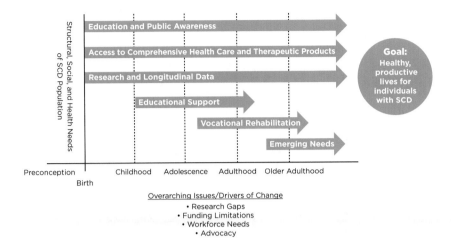

FIGURE 1-1 A life-span approach to understanding and addressing the needs of the SCD population.
NOTE: SCD = sickle cell disease.

opportunity to identify specific areas for continued research and policy to improve care for individuals as they transition from pediatric to adult care and into old age. Figure 1-1 provides a graphical representation of some of the categories of interventions that the committee identified as crucial at different stages of life.

Person-Centric SCD Care Approach

Considering that more people with SCD are living into adulthood, it is important to understand how to manage this chronic disease across the life span, with collaborative input from physicians, those living with SCD and their families, and relevant community stakeholders. The committee decided that effective management of SCD needs to happen in the context of a team-based comprehensive care model that places the patient and his or her needs at the center. Consequently, the committee referred to a previous National Academies report titled *Epilepsy Across the Spectrum* (IOM, 2012) that provides a detailed description of a model used to provide care for epilepsy, which in turn was based on the so-called Chronic Care Model (see Figure 1-2). Developed by Edward Wagner and his colleagues, this model emphasizes the need for transformation in the health care delivery system to proactively keep individuals with chronic diseases healthy. Both

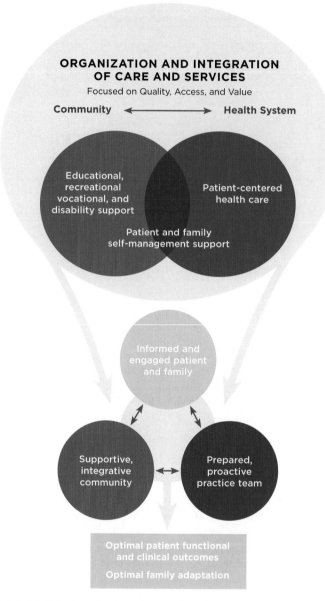

FIGURE 1-2 Model of person-centric care for SCD.
NOTE: SCD = sickle cell disease.
SOURCES: IOM, 2012; originally adapted from Wagner, 1998. Republished with permission of American College of Physicians - Journals from Chronic Disease Management: What Will It Take to Improve Care for Chronic Illness?, E. H. Wagner, volume 1, 1998; permission conveyed through Copyright Clearance Center, Inc.

the health system and the community have key roles to play in equipping individuals with chronic conditions such as SCD to self-manage their conditions in pursuit of optimal outcomes (IOM, 2012; Wagner, 1998; Wagner et al., 2001, 2005). Similar care models for a variety of chronic diseases have been implemented, such as for cystic fibrosis (CF), which is discussed in Chapter 5, while others are being piloted by the Centers for Medicare & Medicaid Services and can be adapted for the SCD population.

OVERVIEW OF SCD AND SCT

SCD is a group of genetic blood disorders. A point mutation in the gene that codes for beta globin, one of the two types of amino acid chains that compose the adult hemoglobin, leads to an abnormal hemoglobin named hemoglobin S (HbS). HbS polymerizes under low oxygen states, forming elongated structures within the RBCs that deform their shape from a bi-concave, donut-shaped disc to a sickle or crescent shape, from which the name of the disease derives (Booth et al., 2010; CDC, 2017b; Malowany and Butany, 2012; Mentzer and Wang, 1980; NHLBI, n.d.; Telen et al., 2019). James Herrick first discovered and named SCD in Chicago in 1910; he described the sickle RBCs he was examining as "peculiar, elongated and sickle-shaped red blood corpuscles" (ASH, 2008; Herrick, 1910, p. 517). In 1949 Linus Pauling postulated that SCD was caused by the presence of an abnormal hemoglobin molecule (ASH, 2008), representing the first identification of a molecular disease (Eaton, 2003).

The inheritance of a single copy of the mutation leads to SCT (heterozygous carrier), a mostly benign condition, while the inheritance of two copies of the mutation (HbSS) or one copy of the HbS mutation in combination with a copy of certain other hemoglobin mutations leads to SCD (see Figure 1-3). Thus, SCD is an autosomal recessive disease, because only the individual that inherits two mutated beta globin chains is affected. Table 1-1 describes SCT and the common SCD genotypes and provides the appropriate nomenclature.

SCD collectively denotes a set of syndromes that, if untreated, can be highly morbid and deadly (Dampier, 2019; Habara and Steinberg, 2016; NIH, 2019; Quinn, 2016; Williams and Weatherall, 2012).

The homozygous inheritance of HbS, also known as sickle cell anemia (SCA), is the most prevalent and severe form of the disease and also the most researched (Dampier, 2019; Habara and Steinberg, 2016). SCD also occurs as compound heterozygotes for HbS and other hemoglobin variants, including HbC, HbE, HbD, and HbO/Arab or beta thalassemia mutations (Habara and Steinberg, 2016; Serjeant, 2013; Williams and Weatherall, 2012). Hemoglobin Sβ^0 –thalassemia (HbSβ^0) is clinically similar to HbSS and sometimes jointly referred to as SCA (NHLBI, 2014). HbSC has

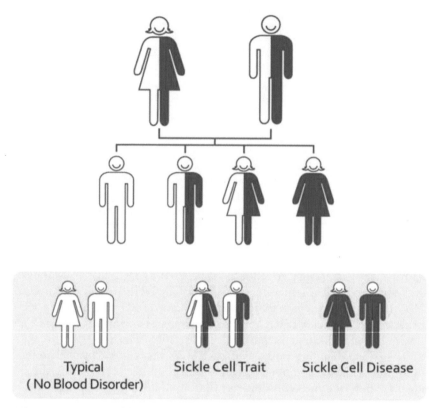

FIGURE 1-3 How sickle cell trait and sickle cell disease are inherited.
SOURCE: CDC, 2017b.

moderate clinical severity, and HbSβ⁺ is generally a milder genotype, although all individuals with SCD, regardless of the genotype, are at risk of severe complications (NIH, 2019; Quinn, 2016).

    If both parents have SCT, each child will have a 50 percent chance of inheriting SCT and a 25 percent chance of inheriting SCD, while there is a 25 percent chance that the child will inherit neither SCT nor SCD and have non-mutated hemoglobin.

    The origins of the sickle gene have been traced to sub-Saharan Africa (with earlier theories hypothesizing an independent, additional origin of the gene elsewhere). HbS confers partial protection from *Plasmodium falciparum* malaria, a major infectious killer in the tropics; hence, the mutation provides a survival advantage to individuals with SCT and has been conserved throughout evolution (Luzzatto, 2012; Williams and Weatherall, 2012). The trans-Atlantic slave trade and, later, global migration patterns

TABLE 1-1 Common SCD Genotypes, Nomenclature, and Mutational Products

Genotype	Common Diagnostic Term	Types of Beta Globin Gene Mutation Product
Homozygous SS	Hemoglobin SS disease; sickle cell anemia	Two hemoglobin S genes (HbSS)
Compound Heterozygous SC	Hemoglobin SC disease	One hemoglobin S gene and one hemoglobin C gene (HbSC)
Compound Heterozygous SD	Hemoglobin SD disease	One hemoglobin S gene and one hemoglobin D gene (HbSD)
Compound Heterozygous SE	Hemoglobin SE disease	One hemoglobin S gene and one hemoglobin E gene (HbSE)
Compound Heterozygous SO	Hemoglobin SO disease	One hemoglobin S gene and one hemoglobin O gene (HbSO)
Compound Heterozygous S Beta Thalassemia Zero	S/B^0 thalassemia Hemoglobin S/B^0 thalassemia	One hemoglobin S gene and one hemoglobin beta thalassemia zero gene (HbSβ^0-thalassemia)
Compound Heterozygous S Beta Thalassemia Plus	S/B plus thalassemia Hemoglobin S/B$^+$ thalassemia	One hemoglobin S gene and one hemoglobin beta thalassemia plus gene (HbSβ$^+$-thalassemia)
Sickle Cell Trait (*Not a form of sickle cell disease*)	Sickle Trait Hemoglobin AS	One hemoglobin A gene and one hemoglobin S gene (HbAS)

contributed to the spread of the disease across the world (Dampier, 2019; Piel et al., 2010; Schroeder et al., 1990; Solovieff et al., 2011; Williams and Weatherall, 2012).

The HbS gene can now be found among every ethnic group, with the highest prevalence seen in individuals from sub-Saharan Africa and India and their descendants across the world; other areas of relatively high prevalence are the Middle East and Mediterranean basin (CDC, 2017a; Williams and Weatherall, 2012).

Epidemiology of SCD and SCT in the United States

An estimated 100,000 Americans are affected by SCD, and approximately 1 million to 3 million individuals in the United States are carriers of SCT, including approximately 8 to 10 percent of African Americans (ASH, n.d.; Hassell, 2010). Each year, 1,800 to 2,000 infants are born with SCD, including every 1 out of 365 African American births and 1 out of 16,300 Hispanic American births (CDC, 2018). An analysis of 2010 data from state newborn screening (NBS) programs found that the incidence of SCT in participating states was 15.5 cases per 1,000 newborns overall, including

73.1 cases per 1,000 African American newborns; 6.9 cases per 1,000 Hispanic newborns; 3.0 cases per 1,000 Caucasian American newborns; and 2.2 cases per 1,000 Asian, Native Hawaiian, or other Pacific Islander newborns (Ojodu et al., 2014). The total number of babies born with SCT in 2010 was estimated to be greater than 60,000 (CDC, 2018). Although SCD is relatively rare in the United States, there are millions of affected individuals across the globe.

The population living with SCD is concentrated along Southern and Eastern states in the United States (see Figure 1-4). This distribution has implications for access to care and state programming and policies. The map in Figure 1-4, which is based on a publication from almost 10 years ago, uses data estimated from NBS and therefore does not account for individuals with SCD born outside of those states or before universal NBS was implemented.

The mortality rate from SCD has historically been high, with most people not living past childhood due to a lack of access to proper care and a lack of treatment. However, in recent decades the mortality rate for children with SCD has been steadily decreasing, which can be attributed to preventative services, such as pneumococcal vaccines and the use of prophylactic penicillin to prevent sepsis. The Centers for Disease Control and Prevention

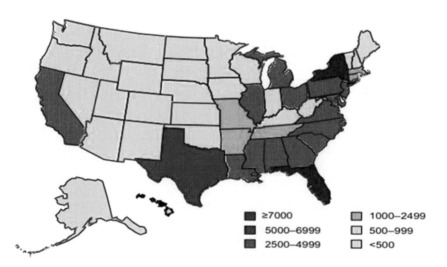

FIGURE 1-4 Geographic distribution of SCD by state using data derived from the National Newborn Screening Information System.
SOURCE: Reprinted from the *American Journal of Preventive Medicine*, 38 (4 Suppl), K. L. Hassell, Population Estimates of Sickle Cell Disease in the U.S., S512–S521, Copyright (2010), with permission from Elsevier.

reported that SCD-related deaths for African American children aged 4 and younger decreased by 42 percent between 1999 and 2002 (CDC, 2017a). Despite medical advances, however, individuals living with SCD continue to experience barriers to access care and knowledgeable providers, and their average life expectancy remains 20–30 years lower than that of the average American (Lubeck et al., 2019; Piel et al., 2017). A recent simulation modeling study showed that projected quality-adjusted life expectancy for individuals with SCD was 33 years, compared with 67 years for the non-SCD cohort (Lubeck et al., 2019).

Diagnosis of SCD

SCD can be easily diagnosed by blood testing. The classical blood test is hemoglobin electrophoresis, which identifies and measures different types of hemoglobin, including HbS, in the blood (Mentzer and Wang, 1980). However, there are numerous other tests that are more suitable in specific situations or in determined subpopulations. For instance, most NBS programs employ high-performance liquid chromatography or isoelectric focusing to identify children with SCD (Naik and Haywood, 2015). Typically, a positive result by NBS is followed by a confirmatory test by the same or different method.

Prenatal diagnosis through chorionic villus sampling of fetal DNA and amniocentesis are also available (Mentzer and Wang, 1980; Yenilmez and Tuli, 2016). These tests may pose some risks and raise ethical and social concerns, as discussed in Chapter 3. Point-of-care diagnostic strategies for SCD and SCT are being developed and may be particularly advantageous in settings with limited resources (McGann and Hoppe, 2017; Steele et al., 2019).

Clinical Complications and Comorbidities

RBCs harboring high levels of HbS have a shorter life span (approximately 20 days versus approximately 120 days for normal RBCs), which results in hemolysis, the premature destruction of RBCs. Hemolysis in turn results in anemia when the production of RBCs cannot compensate for their premature destruction (NHLBI, n.d.). In recent decades, thanks to in vitro studies and mouse models of SCD, multiple mechanisms of disease have been elucidated. Because of hemolysis and other changes to the integrity of RBCs, SCD results in a chronic inflammatory state that affects multiple other cell types. RBCs, white clood cells, platelets, and endothelial cells become hyperadhesive, causing them to stick to each other and to the walls of the blood vessels, thereby impeding blood flow to the organs and causing ischemia (lack of oxygen) and infarction (death of tissues). Chronic and acute ischemia and the rapid restoration of blood flow lead to a cascade of downstream effects that predispose individuals with SCD to numerous complications (Sundd et al., 2019; Telen et al., 2019).

The severe, acute pain episodes that result from the sickling of RBCs and vaso-occlusion are known as the most common complication of SCD; however, SCD is also a complex multi-system disease, characterized by other acute and chronic clinical complications, which are discussed in Chapter 4.

Causes of Death for SCD Patients

Individuals in the United States with SCD have a life expectancy that is 30 years less than their same-ethnicity peers (Platt et al., 1994). While childhood mortality rates have declined to the point that 98 percent of children now survive to at least age 18, one study found that adult (> 19 years) mortality rates increased at a rate of 1 percent per year during the study period (1979–2005) (Lanzkron et al., 2013). Early death occurs in all SCD genotypes, including the compound heterozygous sickle cell syndromes, particularly during the delicate transition period from pediatric to adult care (Blinder et al., 2013).

Advances in the science, treatment, and management of SCD have led to improvements in survival, with most children living to at least 18 years of age (Hulihan et al., 2017). Despite this progress, morbidity and mortality remain high, especially among adults. A proportion of SCD deaths can be attributed to acute chest syndrome, stroke, pulmonary hypertension, and infection (Fitzhugh et al., 2005). However, a large proportion of deaths are sudden and undefined. A study of 306 autopsies conducted on patients with SCD found that almost 41 percent had experienced sudden and unexpected deaths (Manci et al., 2003). This incidence is slightly higher than that recorded in another study of 141 adults treated by a single physician at one institution. That study, which also used autopsy reports to determine the cause of death, classified approximately 24 percent of those deaths as sudden. The leading causes of death were determined to be pulmonary hypertension, renal failure, sepsis, thromboembolism, and cirrhosis (Darbari et al., 2015). In a recent study of 486 individuals identified from the California SCD Data Collection Program who died at a median age of 45 years, most were in the hospital (63 percent) and emergency department (15 percent), signaling that they may have been receiving care for an acute event that became life threatening (Johnston et al., 2020).

Health-Related Burden

Data from the Global Burden of Disease project suggest that sickle cell disorders in the United States alone are annually responsible for 744 deaths,

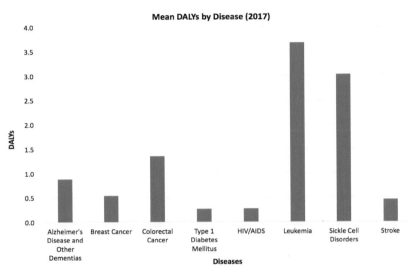

FIGURE 1-5 Mean disease burden in the United States among individuals with certain diseases.
NOTE: DALY = disability-adjusted life-year.
SOURCE: Global Health Data Exchange, 2019.

29,284 years of life lost, and 3,984 disability-adjusted life-years (DALYs) lost (Coles and Mensah, 2017). In terms of DALYs, the burden of SCD on individual patients exceeds that of numerous other severe illnesses, including Alzheimer's disease, breast cancer, colorectal cancer, type 1 diabetes mellitus, HIV/AIDS, leukemia,[3] and stroke (Global Health Data Exchange, 2019) (see Figure 1-5). DALYs measure the potential years of life lost due to premature death and the years of healthy life lost due to disease or disability (WHO, 2006a). Another way of thinking of DALYs is as the additional expected years of life and healthy years of life that a patient would have enjoyed if he or she had never been diagnosed with the disease in question.

Available data suggest that SCD imposes a significant mortality and morbidity burden, but the quality and completeness of these data could be improved. Paulukonis et al. (2016) report SCD deaths using SCD surveillance data and find that about half of them are not captured by government mortality databases. It is unclear whether SCD patients who are invisible to government statistics die at higher or lower rates than their peers. This uncertainty suggests the value of expanding existing SCD surveillance and

---

[3] This category includes acute lymphoid leukemia, acute myeloid leukemia, chronic lymphoid leukemia, and chronic myeloid leukemia.

patient registries to capture more complete data on health-related burden and other key metrics of patient well-being.

United States Versus Global Burden

In 2006 the World Health Organization declared SCD a global health issue and challenged countries to identify solutions to aid individuals living with the disease (WHO, 2006b). As mentioned before, available estimates indicate that 100,000 Americans currently have SCD. Globally, about 300,000 people are born with SCD each year (ASH, 2016; Thien and Thien, 2016). There are approximately 100,000,000 people worldwide who carry the SCT gene (ASH, n.d.). In some African countries, approximately 10–40 percent of the population carry the gene (ASH, 2016).

In developing countries, the burden of SCD is high; 90 percent of children do not live into adulthood (Sickle Cell Disease Coalition, n.d.). A systematic review conducted by Wastnedge et al. (2018) identified 67 studies (from literature published from 1980 through 2017) on incidence and mortality data in children under age 5. Africa experiences the highest SCD birth prevalence and mortality rate. The birth prevalence in Africa was 1,125 per 100,000 live births, compared with 43 per 100,000 live births in Europe (Wastnedge et al., 2018). Mortality data for SCD in children are limited; only 15 of the identified studies in the systematic review contained mortality data. Wastnedge et al. (2018) reported a pooled estimate of mortality per 100 years of child observation of 7.30 for Africa, 0.11 for Europe, and 1.06 for the United States (Wastnedge et al., 2018). The burden of SCD has been decreasing in the United States, especially in children; from 1999 through 2002 the mortality rate decreased by 68 percent for 0- to 3-year-olds, 39 percent for 4- to 9-year-olds, and 24 percent for 10- to 14-year-olds (CDC, 2017a). The child survival rate has increased to 94 percent in the United States. Even with this progress, the U.S. survival rate still lags behind the rate in Britain, which has a 99 percent survival rate for SCD, with an estimated median age of survival of 67 years (DeBaun et al., 2019; Gardner et al., 2016).

The economic costs associated with SCD also present a significant burden. In the United States, from 1989 through 1993 the 75,000 hospitalizations per year among people with SCD were estimated to cost $475 million annually (Ashley-Koch et al., 2000). SCD-related costs in the United States have now risen to $2 billion per year (CDC Foundation, 2019). In developing countries, information on the economic burden is limited. Proper care management for SCD in the United States and internationally needs to be addressed in an effort to decrease mortality rates and medical expenditures.

THE SICKLE CELL PATIENT AND THE HEALTH CARE SYSTEM

SCD has long been considered a childhood disease because survival to adulthood was uncommon due to the high rates of fatal infections in early childhood. Efforts to understand and address the disease have thus been focused on the pediatric population, which has resulted in an improved survival into young adulthood; for example, between 1999 and 2002 mortality rates decreased by 42 percent among African American children under the age of 4, thanks in part to the introduction of a vaccine against invasive pneumococcal disease (CDC, 2017a). However, mortality and morbidity rates increase dramatically as individuals transition into young adulthood and adulthood, likely because there is no standardized system to appropriately transition children into adult care. Other likely factors contributing to this increase are individuals' lack of necessary knowledge and skills to make effective decisions about their care as they get older and their anxiety over receiving care from an unfamiliar provider (described in Chapter 6). Finally, health care personnel issues and resources play a role, as SCD-expert-led, multidisciplinary health care teams focusing on comprehensive care appear to be more prevalent and accessible in pediatrics than in adult care (Treadwell et al., 2011).

The health care needs of individuals living with SCD have been neglected by the U.S. and global health care systems, causing them and their families to suffer (Bahr and Song, 2015). Many of the complications that afflict individuals with SCD, particularly pain, are invisible. Pain is only diagnosed by self-reports, and in SCD there are few to no external indicators of the pain experience. Nevertheless, the pain can be excruciatingly severe and requires treatment with strong analgesics. Individuals with SCD often face discrimination by health care providers who do not see visible signs to corroborate the reports of pain and, with the frequent recurrence of crisis, tend to characterize the repeat acute care visits by individuals with SCD, a majority of whom are African American, as "drug-seeking" behavior (Jenerette and Brewer, 2010).

The SCD community has developed a significant lack of trust in the health care system due to the nearly universal stigma and lack of belief in its reports of pain, a lack of trust that has been further reinforced by historical events, such as the Tuskegee experiment, in which researchers deliberately withheld treatment from African Americans with syphilis in order to track the progression of the disease (CDC, 2015). This pervasive disengagement of an entire disease population from health care and research is partly responsible for the absence of new treatments to help improve care (Braveman and Gottlieb, 2014).

The neglect of SCD by the health care system extends to research into the natural history of the condition and the utility of different interventions as well as to a lack of investigation into new treatments. There have been significant disparities in research funding for SCD compared with similar rare genetic disorders of childhood, as discussed for CF later in this chapter.

The decrease in survival rates for SCD following transition into adult care is fueled by the lack of evidence-based clinical practice guidelines across the life span, particularly for aging adults who continue to experience accelerated mortality. This has led to the current situation in which there is a pressing need to address treatment options for SCD, to improve the delivery of care and ensure optimal access to high-quality care with treatments to prevent subsequent morbidity and mortality, and to develop curative therapies. There is also an imperative to establish an informed workforce to apply these interventions.

POLICY MAKING AND FUNDING FOR SCD

Legislative Activity

Since the discovery of SCD, relatively few federal legislations with direct or indirect impact on SCD care, research, and funding have been enacted (see Figure 1-6).

The first landmark legislation for SCD was the National Sickle Cell Anemia Control Act of 1972 (Public Law 92-294), which authorized funding for screening and counseling programs, research programs for health care professionals, and medical training on SCD treatment and prevention. It also authorized the creation of comprehensive sickle cell research and treatment centers (Manley, 1984) and education clinics under the National Institutes of Health (NIH).

The Rare Diseases Act of 2002 (Public Law 107-280) was created to amend the Public Health Service Act; it authorized the creation of an Office of Rare Diseases under NIH. The purpose of this act was to provide a national research agenda, to offer educational opportunities for researchers, and to increase the development of diagnostics and treatments for those with rare diseases such as SCD (Public Law 107-280).

In 2004 the American Jobs Creation Act of 2004 (Public Law 108-357) was signed into law, amending Title XIX (Medicaid) of the Social Security Act. Section 712 of the act authorized primary and secondary medical services and treatment for individuals with SCD as medical assistance under the Medicaid program. It also directed the administrator of the Health Resources and Services Administration (HRSA) to conduct a demonstration program to develop and establish systemic mechanisms, including a national coordinating center, to improve the prevention and treatment of SCD. This act established the Sickle Cell Disease Treatment Demonstration Program, with the purpose of funding regional coordinating centers that

35

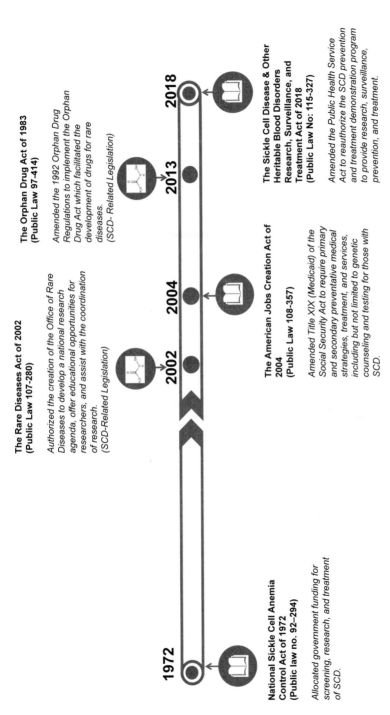

1972

National Sickle Cell Anemia Control Act of 1972 (Public law no. 92–294)

Allocated government funding for screening, research, and treatment of SCD.

2002 **2004**

The Rare Diseases Act of 2002 (Public Law 107-280)

Authorized the creation of the Office of Rare Diseases to develop a national research agenda, offer educational opportunities for researchers, and assist with the coordination of research.
(SCD-Related Legislation)

The American Jobs Creation Act of 2004 (Public Law 108-357)

Amended Title XIX (Medicaid) of the Social Security Act to require primary and secondary preventative medical strategies, treatment, and services, including but not limited to genetic counseling and testing for those with SCD.

2013 **2018**

The Orphan Drug Act of 1983 (Public Law 97-414)

Amended the 1992 Orphan Drug Regulations to implement the Orphan Drug Act which facilitated the development of drugs for rare diseases.
(SCD- Related Legislation)

The Sickle Cell Disease & Other Heritable Blood Disorders Research, Surveillance, and Treatment Act of 2018 (Public Law No: 115-327)

Amended the Public Health Service Act to reauthorize the SCD prevention and treatment demonstration program to provide research, surveillance, prevention, and treatment.

FIGURE 1-6 Timeline of key SCD-related milestones.
NOTE: SCD = sickle cell disease.

would work to form networks that would support processes to improve and treat SCD (Public Law 108-357).

In 2013 the Orphan Drug Act of 1983 (Public Law 97-414) was amended to address and encourage the development of drugs for people with rare diseases. This amendment provided clarity concerning the regulatory language used and suggested improvements for the drug designation process; drugs such as hydroxyurea that were previously only available to adults were made available to children. The amendment also paved the way for the development of Endari, the second drug approved for SCD by the U.S. Food and Drug Administration (FDA). In late 2019 FDA approved two additional drugs for SCD: Adakveo (crizanlizumab) and Oxbryta (voxelotor) (Global Blood Therapeutics, 2019; Novartis, 2019). Figure 1-7 provides a timeline of all FDA approvals of drugs for treating SCD.

The most recent legislative action for SCD took place on December 18, 2018, with the signing into law of the Sickle Cell Disease and Other Heritable Blood Disorders Research, Surveillance, Prevention, and Treatment Act of 2018 (Public Law 115-327). That act amended part A of Title XI of the Public Health Service Act to reauthorize HHS to support data collection on SCD and promote public health activities on heritable blood disorders. The legislation seeks to improve SCD treatment, research, monitoring, and prevention. As of the development of this report, the section of the legislation related to data collection on certain blood disorders had not yet been funded by Congress.

Funding

Funding for SCD has historically been low and has decreased over the years. For example, appropriations for the National Sickle Cell Anemia Control Act of 1972 (Public Law 92-294) authorized $85 million, and the American Jobs Creation Act of 2004 (Public Law 108-357) authorized $50 million over 5 years, for medical services and treatment for individuals with SCD.

It is also well documented that SCD receives less federal and private funding than other conditions. Some attribute this difference to the history of discrimination against the racial and ethnic minority population most affected by SCD (Haywood et al., 2014). Figure 1-8 compares NIH funding between 2008 and 2016 for SCD with its funding for CF, which mostly affects white Americans and affects fewer people (approximately 30,000). Average annual NIH funding per affected individual for CF was almost four times more than the average annual funding per affected individual for SCD during the period under review (Farooq and Strouse, 2018). The funding difference was even more stark for funds from private foundations ($342 million for CF compared with $6.4 million for SCD between 2008 and 2012) (Farooq and Strouse, 2018) (see Figure 1-9).

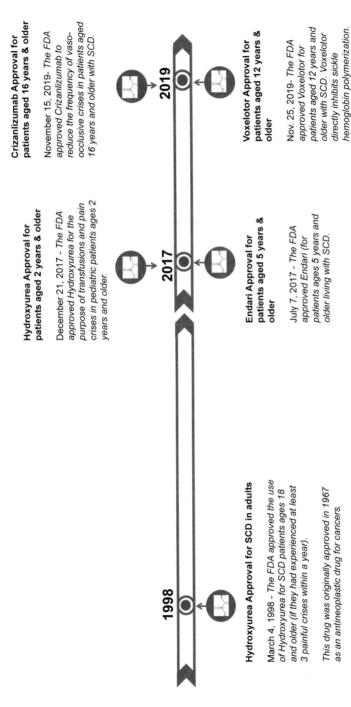

Hydroxyurea Approval for SCD in adults

March 4, 1998 - *The FDA approved the use of Hydroxyurea for SCD patients ages 18 and older (if they had experienced at least 3 painful crises within a year).*

This drug was originally approved in 1967 as an antineoplastic drug for cancers.

Hydroxyurea Approval for patients aged 2 years & older

December 21, 2017 - *The FDA approved Hydroxyurea for the purpose of transfusions and pain crises in pediatric patients ages 2 years and older.*

Endari Approval for patients aged 5 years & older

July 7, 2017 - *The FDA approved Endari (for patients ages 5 years and older living with SCD.*

Crizanlizumab Approval for patients aged 16 years & older

November 15, 2019- *The FDA approved Crizanlizumab to reduce the frequency of vaso-occlusive crises in patients aged 16 years and older with SCD.*

Voxelotor Approval for patients aged 12 years & older

Nov. 25, 2019- *The FDA approved Voxelotor for patients aged 12 years and older with SCD. Voxelotor directly inhibits sickle hemoglobin polymerization.*

1998   2017   2019

FIGURE 1-7 Timeline of SCD drug approvals.
NOTE: FDA = U.S. Food and Drug Administration; SCD = sickle cell disease.
SOURCE: Data from ClinicalTrials.gov.

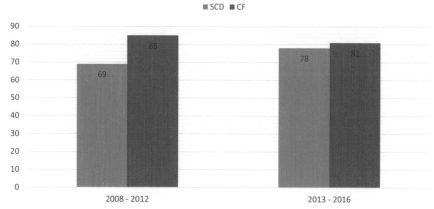

FIGURE 1-8 National Institutes of Health funding for SCD versus cystic fibrosis.
NOTE: CF = cystic fibrosis; SCD = sickle cell disease.
SOURCE: Adapted from Farooq and Strouse, 2018.

KEY SCD ACTORS

There are several actors actively engaged in SCD research, treatment, and advocacy. This section provides a brief description of such actors, including the federal and state governments, health care providers, payers, health professional associations, and industry as well as other stakeholders from the scientific community, advocacy groups, and patients and families (see Table 1-2).

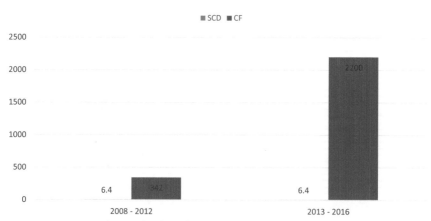

FIGURE 1-9 Foundation funding for SCD versus cystic fibrosis.
NOTE: CF = cystic fibrosis; SCD = sickle cell disease.
SOURCE: Adapted from Farooq and Strouse, 2018.

TABLE 1-2 Description of SCD Key Actors

Stakeholder	Description
Federal Government	Federal agencies' work in sickle cell disease (SCD) includes • The Centers for Disease Control and Prevention's programs focus on collecting and tracking SCD statistics (see Chapter 3); • The Health Resources and Services Administration currently funds programs for children with inheritable disorders, such as SCD, including the Sickle Cell Disease Treatment Demonstration Program and the Newborn Screening Follow-up Program (see Chapter 3); • The National Institutes of Health, through the National Heart, Lung, and Blood Institute, conducts clinical trials and research and also funds extramural research on SCD and launched the Cure Sickle Cell Initiative in 2018 with the goal of accelerating the development of genetic therapies for SCD; • The U.S. Food and Drug Administration (FDA) is working with multiple stakeholders to accelerate the development of SCD treatments through a fast-track designation. FDA also gives certain drugs orphan status which designates them to be used for individuals with rare diseases (see Chapter 7); and • The Social Security Administration lists SCD as a condition eligible for Social Security Disability Insurance or Supplemental Security Income and determines eligibility requirements for qualification (see Chapter 2).
Health Care Providers	Health care systems, including multi-hospital systems and stand-alone community clinics, have programs that provide services to individuals with SCD. Large academic health systems, which are located primarily in urban areas, may run specialized sickle cell centers or clinics. A wide variety of health care providers, including doctors, nurses, and allied health professionals are also key to care delivery (see Chapters 5 and 6).
Payers	Public and private payers, together with individuals with SCD and their families, bear the substantial costs associated with SCD care (see Chapter 2).
Health Professional Associations	Professional associations and organizations, specifically for medical specialties that often treat SCD patients such as the American Society of Hematology and the American College of Emergency Physicians, have efforts to promote awareness of SCD and to provide ongoing education of members and other activities to improve care for individuals with SCD (see Chapter 6).
Industry	Several pharmaceutical and biopharmaceutical companies are actively developing therapeutic products for SCD (see Figure 1-7 for approved SCD therapies and Chapter 7 and Appendix I for therapeutic products in development). Some of these companies also partner with stakeholders for advocacy and fund services for individuals with SCD and their families.

TABLE 1-2 Continued

Stakeholder	Description
Research Community	Beyond federal agencies, other entities fund or conduct SCD research. A couple of examples are the Patient-Centered Outcomes Research Institute, which has funded a robust portfolio of SCD projects (PCORI, n.d.) and the California Institute for Regenerative Medicine, which was created by the state of California to fund research on stem cell–based therapies for multiple diseases, including SCD (CIRM, n.d.). Researchers at several large academic medical centers are also actively conducting research and enrolling patients in clinical trials.
State Agencies	Multiple state agencies, including departments of health, education, and social work, among others, run programs that benefit individuals with SCD. The availability and types of such programs vary by state. Some states also have detailed state-level SCD action plans even though the status of the implementation of these programs is unclear, per publicly available information.
Patient Advocacy Groups and Community-Based Organizations	Patient advocacy groups and community-based organizations may function at the federal, state, local, or even community level and may take on various structures, such as virtual organizations or being based at a health care institution. The roles of these organizations also vary and are discussed in Chapter 8.
Patients and Families	Individuals living with SCD and their families are integral to improving SCD care because of their lived experience with the disease. They have a role to play in SCD research, health care, and advocacy.

ORGANIZATION OF THE REPORT

This report contains 9 chapters and 14 appendixes. Chapter 2 presents background information on the societal, individual, and environmental factors that affect SCD patients; the impact of SCD on mental health; the economic burden on people living with SCD and their families; and the distribution of both private and public insurance for patients. Chapter 3 provides a detailed description of screening, registries, and surveillance. This chapter examines the importance of communication for screening results, the use of that data, the ethical implications of screening, and the limitations and strengths of using surveillance, screening, or registries. Chapter 4 summarizes management approaches for SCD care as it pertains to disease-modifying agents, therapies, the treatment of complications, mental health, non-pharmacologic therapies, psychosocial support, and disease self-management education. This chapter describes evidence-based strategies, the effectiveness of current therapeutics approaches, and the opportunities for maximizing the use of current resources; it also summarizes the available evidence on SCT. Chapter 5 reviews the organization and delivery of SCD care. This chapter delves into how and where people with SCD should receive care and what types of care they should receive; the issues with the transition from pediatric to adult care; what comprehensive SCD care encompasses; and the geographic, financial, and socioeconomic barriers to care. Chapter 6 addresses the current state of quality of SCD care and the workforce needs to deliver high-quality care. This chapter provides details on the transition of care, the indicators for high-quality care, how to engage health care professionals, the attitudes of health care providers, and the opportunities for training programs for health professionals. Chapter 7 centers on innovative and curative therapies. This chapter highlights the perspectives of those with SCD, current therapies, the process for clinical trials, reimbursement policies and lifetime costs, and the reform of health care delivery. Chapter 8 focuses on the landscape of patient organizations advocating for and providing services to the SCD population, community engagement, and the importance of education and awareness for people with SCD and the public. Chapter 9 presents the strategic plan and blueprint for action created by the committee to address SCD. The recommended actions detailed in the blueprint are linked to the conclusions and recommendations in the chapters.

The committee's conclusions and recommendations are presented at the end of each chapter. The references used follow each chapter. Appendix A contains the agendas of the open meetings and a list of presentation topics. Appendix B describes the literature review strategy with the terms used by the National Academies Research Center. Appendix C provides the committee and staff biographies. Appendix D details the results of a brief survey that the Association of Public Health Laboratories conducted on behalf of the committee. Appendixes E, F, and G give brief descriptions of the California SCD Data Collection Program, the 24-hour sickle cell program at Grady Memorial Hospital, and the Emory Adult Cystic Fibrosis Program Protocol, respectively. Appendix H provides information on SCD programs funded by HRSA. Appendix I lists select treatments that are currently under development. Appendix J provides information on other models for training hematologists. Appendix K provides a list of some of the community-based organizations and patient advocacy groups in the United States. Appendix L is a summary of the committee's strategic plan and blueprint for action. Appendix M is a guide of the chapters in this report that discuss SCT. Finally, Appendix N is a glossary of key terms used in the field of SCD and research and referenced in this report.

REFERENCES

ASH (American Society of Hematology). 2008. *Milestones in sickle cell disease.* https://www. hematology.org/About/History/50-Years/1533.aspx (accessed June 5, 2019).

ASH. 2016. *State of sickle cell disease.* http://www.scdcoalition.org/pdfs/ASH%20State%20 of%20Sickle%20Cell%20Disease%202016%20Report.pdf (accessed June 5, 2019).

ASH. n.d. *Sickle cell trait.* https://www.hematology.org/Patients/Anemia/Sickle-Cell-Trait.aspx (accessed June 5, 2019).

Ashley-Koch, A., Q. Yang, and R. Olney. 2000. Sickle hemoglobin (Hb S) allele and sickle cell disease: A huge review. *American Journal of Epidemiology* 151(9):839–845.

Bahr, N. C., and J. Song. 2015. The effect of structural violence on patients with sickle cell disease. *Journal of Health Care for the Poor and Underserved* 26(3):648–661.

Blinder, M. A., F. Vekeman, M. Sasane, A. Trahey, C. Paley, and M. S. Duh. 2013. Age-related treatment patterns in sickle cell disease patients and the associated sickle cell complications and healthcare costs. *Pediatric Blood & Cancer* 60(5):828–835.

Booth, C., B. Inusa, and S. K. Obaro. 2010. Infection in sickle cell disease: A review. *International Journal of Infectious Disease* 14(1):e2–e12.

Braveman, P., and L. Gottlieb. 2014. The social determinants of health: It's time to consider the causes of the causes. *Public Health Reports* 129(Suppl 2):19–31.

CDC (Centers for Disease Control and Prevention). 2015. *U.S. Public Health Service syphilis study at Tuskegee: The Tuskegee timeline.* https://www.cdc.gov/tuskegee/timeline.htm (accessed August 1, 2019).

CDC. 2017a. *Data & statistics on sickle cell disease.* https://www.cdc.gov/ncbddd/sicklecell/ data.html (accessed June 5, 2019).

CDC. 2017b. *What is sickle cell disease?* https://www.cdc.gov/ncbddd/sicklecell/facts.html (accessed June 5, 2019).

CDC. 2018. *Incidence of sickle cell trait in the U.S.* https://www.cdc.gov/ncbddd/sicklecell/ features/keyfinding-trait.html (accessed June 5, 2019).

CDC Foundation. 2019. *Improving the lives of people with sickle cell disease.* https://www. cdcfoundation.org/sites/default/files/files/2019CDCFSickleCell.pdf (accessed June 5, 2019).

CIRM (California Institute for Regenerative Medicine). n.d. *Stem cell gene therapy for sickle cell anemia.* https://www.cirm.ca.gov/our-progress/video/stem-cell-gene-therapy-sickle-cell-anemia-donald-kohn (accessed June 5, 2019).

Coles, E., and G. A. Mensah. 2017. The burden of heart, lung, and blood diseases in the United States, 1990 to 2016: Perspectives from the National Heart, Lung, and Blood Institute. *Global Heart* 12(4):349–358.

Crosby, L. E., N. E. Joffe, M. K. Irwin, H. Strong, J. Peugh, L. Shook, K. A. Kalinyak, and M. J. Mitchell. 2015. School performance and disease interference in adolescents with sickle cell disease. *Physical Disabilities: Education and Related Services* 34(1):14–30.

Dampier, C. 2019. New and emerging treatments for vaso-occlusive pain in sickle cell disease. *Expert Review of Hematology* 12(10):857–872.

Darbari, D. S., J. Kwagyan, S. Rana, V. R. Gordeuk, and O. Castro. 2015. 47 causes of death in adult sickle cell disease patients at Howard University. *Journal of Investigative Medicine* 53(2):S395.

DeBaun, M., D. Ghafuri, M. Rodeghier, P. Maitra, S. Chaturvedi, A. Kassim, and K. Ataga. 2019. Decreased median survival of adults with sickle cell disease after adjusting for left truncation bias: A pooled analysis. *Blood* 133(6):615–617.

Eaton, W. A. 2003. Linus Pauling and sickle cell disease. *Biophysical Chemistry* 100(1–3):109–116.

Farooq, F., and J. Strouse. 2018. Disparities in foundation and federal support and development of new therapeutics for sickle cell disease and cystic fibrosis. *Blood* 132(Suppl 1):4687.

Fitzhugh, C., N. Lauder, J. Jonassaint, F. R. Gilliam, M. J. Telen, and L. M. De Castro. 2005. Morbidity and associated sudden death in sickle cell disease. *Blood* 106(11):2348.

Gardner, K., A. Douiri, E. Drasar, M. Allman, A. Mwirigi, M. Awogbade, and S. Thein. 2016. Survival in adults with sickle cell disease in a high-income setting. *Blood* 128(10):1436–1438.

Global Blood Therapeutics. 2019. *FDA approves Oxbryta™ (voxelotor), the first medicine specifically targeting the root cause of sickle cell disease.* https://ir.gbt.com/news-releases/news-release-details/fda-approves-oxbrytatm-voxelotor-first-medicine-specifically (accessed February 19, 2020).

Global Health Data Exchange. 2019. *Secondary global health data exchange—GBD results tool 2019.* http://ghdx.healthdata.org/gbd-results-tool (accessed June 10, 2019).

Gold, J. I., C. B. Johnson, M. J. Treadwell, N. Hans, and E. Vichinsky. 2008. Detection and assessment of stroke in patients with sickle cell disease: Neuropsychological functioning and magnetic resonance imaging. *Pediatric Hematology and Oncology* 25(5):409–421.

Greenham, M., A. Gordon, V. Anderson, and M. T. Mackay. 2016. Outcome in childhood stroke. *Stroke* 47(4):1159–1164.

Habara, A., and M. H. Steinberg. 2016. Minireview: Genetic basis of heterogeneity and severity in sickle cell disease. *Experimental Biology and Medicine (Maywood)* 241(7):689–696.

Hassell, K. 2010. Population estimates of sickle cell disease in the U.S. *American Journal of Preventive Medicine* 38(4):S512–S521.

Haywood, C., Jr., M. Diener-West, J. Strouse, C. P. Carroll, S. Bediako, S. Lanzkron, J. Haythornthwaite, G. Onojobi, and M. C. Beach. 2014. Perceived discrimination in health care is associated with a greater burden of pain in sickle cell disease. *Journal of Pain and Symptom Management* 48(5):934–943.

Herrick, J. 1910. Peculiar elongated and sickle-shaped red blood corpuscles in a case of severe anemia. *JAMA* (formerly Archives of Internal Medicine) 6(5):517–521.

Hulihan, M., K. L. Hassell, J. L. Raphael, K. Smith-Whitley, and P. Thorpe. 2017. CDC grand rounds: Improving the lives of persons with sickle cell disease. *Morbidity and Mortality Weekly Report* 66(46):1269–1271.

IOM (Institute of Medicine). 2012. *Epilepsy across the spectrum: Promoting health and understanding.* Washington, DC: The National Academies Press.

Jenerette, C. M., and C. Brewer. 2010. Health-related stigma in young adults with sickle cell disease. *Journal of the National Medical Association* 102(11):1050–1055.

Johnston, E. E., O. O. Adesina, E. Alvarez, H. Amato, S. Paulukonis, A. Nichols, L. J. Chamberlain, and S. Bhatia. 2020. Acute care utilization at end of life in sickle cell disease: Highlighting the need for a palliative approach. *Journal of Palliative Medicine* 23(1):24–32.

Lanzkron, S., C. P. Carroll, and C. Haywood, Jr. 2013. Mortality rates and age at death from sickle cell disease: U.S., 1979–2005. *Public Health Reports* 128(2):110–116.

Lubeck, D., I. Agodoa, N. Bhakta, M. Danese, K. Pappu, R. Howard, M. Gleeson, M. Halperin, and S. Lanzkron. 2019. Estimated life expectancy and income of patients with sickle cell disease compared with those without sickle cell disease. *JAMA Network Open* 2(11):e1915374.

Luzzatto, L. 2012. Sickle cell anaemia and malaria. *Mediterranean Journal of Hematology and Infectious Diseases* 4(1):e2012065.

Malowany, J., and J. Butany. 2012. Pathology of sickle cell disease. *Seminars in Diagnostic Pathology* 29(1):49–55.

Manci, E. A., D. E. Culberson, Y. M. Yang, T. M. Gardner, R. Powell, J. Haynes, Jr., A. K. Shah, V. N. Mankad, and Investigators of the Cooperative Study of Sickle Cell Disease. 2003. Causes of death in sickle cell disease: An autopsy study. *British Journal of Haematology* 123(2):359–365.

Manley, A. F. 1984. Legislation and funding for sickle cell services, 1972–1982. *The American Journal of Pediatric Hematology/Oncology* 6(1):67–71.

McGann, P. T., and C. Hoppe. 2017. The pressing need for point-of-care diagnostics for sickle cell disease: A review of current and future technologies. *Blood Cells Molecules and Diseases* 67:104–113.

Mentzer, W., and W. Wang. 1980. Sickle-cell disease: Pathophysiology and diagnosis. *Pediatric Annals* 9(8):10–22.

Mulumba, L. L., and L. Wilson. 2015. Sickle cell disease among children in Africa: An integrative literature review and global recommendations. *International Journal of Africa Nursing Sciences* 3:56–64.

Naik, R. P., and C. Haywood, Jr. 2015. Sickle cell trait diagnosis: Clinical and social implications. *Hematology* 2015:160–167.

NHLBI (National Heart, Lung, and Blood Institute). 2014. *Evidence-based management of sickle cell disease: Expert panel report, 2014.* Bethesda, MD: National Heart, Lung, and Blood Institute.

NHLBI. n.d. *Hemolytic anemia.* https://www.nhlbi.nih.gov/health-topics/hemolytic-anemia (accessed January 9, 2020).

NIH (National Institutes of Health). 2019. *Your guide to understanding genetic conditions: Sickle cell disease.* https://ghr.nlm.nih.gov/condition/sickle-cell-disease#inheritance (accessed June 5, 2019).

Novartis. 2019. *New novartis medicine Adakveo® (crizanlizumab) approved by FDA to reduce frequency of pain crises in individuals living with sickle cell disease.* https://www.novartis.com/news/media-releases/new-novartis-medicine-adakveo-crizanlizumab-approved-fda-reduce-frequency-pain-crises-individuals-living-sickle-cell-disease (accessed August 1, 2019).

Ojodu, J., M. M. Hulihan, S. N. Pope, and A. M. Grant. 2014. Incidence of sickle cell trait—United States, 2010. *Morbidity and Mortality Weekly Report* 63(49):1155–1158.

Oyedeji, C., J. J. Strouse, R. D. Crawford, M. E. Garrett, A. E. Ashley-Koch, and M. J. Telen. 2019. A multi-institutional comparison of younger and older adults with sickle cell disease. *American Journal of Hematology* 94(4):e115–e117.

Paulukonis, S. T., J. R. Eckman, A. B. Snyder, W. Hagar, L. B. Feuchtbaum, M. Zhou, A. M. Grant, and M. M. Hulihan. 2016. Defining sickle cell disease mortality using a population-based surveillance system, 2004 through 2008. *Public Health Reports* 131(2):367–375.

PCORI (Patient-Centered Outcomes Research Institute). n.d. *Explore our portfolio of funded projects.* https://www.pcori.org/research-results?keywords=sickle+cell#search-results (accessed August 1, 2019).

Piel, F. B., A. P. Patil, R. E. Howes, O. A. Nyangiri, P. W. Gething, T. N. Williams, D. J. Weatherall, and S. I. Hay. 2010. Global distribution of the sickle cell gene and geographical confirmation of the malaria hypothesis. *Nature Communications* 1(1):104.

Piel, F. B., M. H. Steinberg, and D. C. Rees. 2017. Sickle cell disease. *New England Journal of Medicine* 377(3):305.

Platt, O. S., D. J. Brambilla, W. F. Rosse, P. F. Milner, O. Castro, M. H. Steinberg, and P. P. Klug. 1994. Mortality in sickle cell disease. Life expectancy and risk factors for early death. *New England Journal of Medicine* 330(23):1639–1644.

Quinn, C. T. 2016. Minireview: Clinical severity in sickle cell disease: The challenges of definition and prognostication. *Experimental Biology and Medicine (Maywood)* 241(7):679–688.

Quinn, C. T., Z. R. Rogers, T. L. McCavit, and G. R. Buchanan. 2010. Improved survival of children and adolescents with sickle cell disease. *Blood* 115(17):3447–3452.

Sandhu, M. K., and A. Cohen. 2015. Aging in sickle cell disease: Co-morbidities and new issues in management. *Hemoglobin* 39(4):221–224.

Schroeder, W., E. Munger, and D. Powars. 1990. Sickle cell anaemia, genetic variations, and the slave trade to the United States. *The Journal of African History* 31(2):163–180.

Serjeant, G. R. 2013. The natural history of sickle cell disease. *Cold Spring Harbor Perspectives in Medicine* 3(10):a011783.

Sickle Cell Disease Coalition. n.d. *Spread the word.* http://www.scdcoalition.org/get-involved/spread-the-word.html (accessed June 5, 2019).

Solovieff, N., S. W. Hartley, C. T. Baldwin, E. S. Klings, M. T. Gladwin, J. G. Taylor, G. J. Kato, L. A. Farrer, M. H. Steinberg, and P. Sebastiani. 2011. Ancestry of African Americans with sickle cell disease. *Blood Cells, Molecules, and Diseases* 47(1):41–45.

Steele, C., A. Sinski, J. Asibey, M. D. Hardy-Dessources, G. Elana, C. Brennan, I. Odame, C. Hoppe, M. Geisberg, E. Serrao, and C. T. Quinn. 2019. Point-of-care screening for sickle cell disease in low-resource settings: A multi-center evaluation of HemoTypeSC, a novel rapid test. *American Journal of Hematology* 94(1):39–45. https://doi.org/10.1002/ajh.25305.

Sundd, P., M. Gladwin, and E. Novelli. 2019. Pathophysiology of sickle cell disease. *Annual Review of Pathology: Mechanisms of Disease* 14:263–292.

Swanson, M. E., S. D. Grosse, and R. Kulkarni. 2011. Disability among individuals with sickle cell disease: Literature review from a public health perspective. *American Journal of Preventive Medicine* 41(6):S390–S397.

Telen, M. J., P. Malik, and G. M. Vercellotti. 2019. Therapeutic strategies for sickle cell disease: Towards a multi-agent approach. *Nature Reviews Drug Discovery* 18(2):139–158.

Thein, M. S., and S. L. Thein. 2016. World Sickle Cell Day 2016: A time for appraisal. *Indian Journal of Medical Research* 143(6):678–681.

Treadwell, M., J. Telfair, R. W. Gibson, S. Johnson, and I. Osunkwo. 2011. Transition from pediatric to adult care in sickle cell disease: Establishing evidence-based practice and directions for research. *American Journal of Hematology* 86(1):116–120.

Wagner, E. H. 1998. Chronic disease management: What will it take to improve care for chronic illness? *Effective Clinical Practice* 1(1):2–4.

Wagner, E. H., B. T. Austin, C. Davis, M. Hindmarsh, J. Schaefer, and A. Bonomi. 2001. Improving chronic illness care: Translating evidence into action. *Health Affairs* 20(6):64–78.

Wagner, E. H., S. M. Bennett, B. T. Austin, S. M. Greene, J. K. Schaefer, and M. Vonkorff. 2005. Finding common ground: Patient-centeredness and evidence-based chronic illness care. *Journal of Alternative and Complementary Medicine* 11(Suppl 1):S7–S15.

Wastnedge, E., D. Waters, S. Patel, K. Morrison, M. Goh, D. Adeloye, and I. Rudan. 2018. The global burden of sickle cell disease in children under five years of age: A systematic review and meta-analysis. *Journal of Global Health* 8(2):021103.

WHO (World Health Organization). 2006a. *Years of life lost (percentage of total).* https://www.who.int/whosis/whostat2006YearsOfLifeLost.pdf (accessed June 5, 2019).

WHO. 2006b. *Fifty-Ninth World Health Assembly: Resolutions and decisions, annexes: WHA59/2006/REC/1.* Geneva, Switzerland: World Health Organization.

Williams, T. N., and D. J. Weatherall. 2012. World distribution, population genetics, and health burden of the hemoglobinopathies. *Cold Spring Harbor Perspectives in Medicine* 2(9):a011692.

Yenilmez, E. D., and A. Tuli. 2016. New perspectives in prenatal diagnosis of sickle cell anemia. In B. Inusa, ed. *Sickle cell disease: Pain and common chronic complications.* London: IntechOpen.

2

Societal and Structural
Contributors to Disease Impact

*I grew up in West Africa, where having sickle cell disease is not
something that is shared. You don't go around telling people that you
have sickle cell disease, even though it is not my fault that I have the
disease. But it is a stigma attached to having that disease. You don't
go around telling people.*

—Jenn N. (Open Session Panelist)

Chapter Summary

- In addition to disease-related factors, there are numerous sociocultural, environmental, individual, and economic factors that influence outcomes across the life span for those living with sickle cell disease (SCD).
- Historically, the population affected by SCD has contended with racism and implicit bias within and outside the health care system; socially, they are stigmatized because of cultural beliefs and the lack of general understanding of the disease.
- Individuals living with SCD rely on certain coping mechanisms, including religion and spirituality, which have been shown to have some positive effects. These personal strategies, combined with meaningful policy and programmatic interventions, could help counter the sociocultural and economic burden of the disease.
- While health needs take precedence, individuals living with SCD have non-health needs that should be addressed to improve overall outcomes for the population.

INTRODUCTION

Chapter 1 highlighted the fact that the needs of those affected by sickle cell disease (SCD) have been overlooked by the health care system. However, these needs extend beyond the health care system itself. It is impossible to view SCD as simply a medical condition without an understanding of the sociopolitical and cultural context. In the United States, SCD disproportionately affects African Americans, which has implications for health care access, delivery, and outcomes.

The experience of SCD is shaped by sociocultural factors, environmental factors, and socioeconomic factors, which can exacerbate the disease's impact for people from racial and ethnic minority groups living with the disease. Because of systemic racism, unconscious bias, and the stigma associated with the diagnosis, the disease brings with it a much broader burden. Socioeconomically, African American children living with SCD are more likely to be in a household below the federal poverty level (Boulet et al., 2010). The additive effects of adverse health outcomes and the associated costs magnify the economic burden.

Complications associated with the disease may also affect the mental health of individuals living with SCD by increasing the risk of depression and overwhelming their coping reserves. For adolescents and children these effects may extend to educational achievement, and for adults they may extend to employment, thus affecting opportunities across the life span.

Environmental factors also affect the experience of people living with SCD. For example, children exposed to environmental hazards are more at risk for low cognitive functioning (Liu and Lewis, 2014). These exposures also contribute to comorbid conditions, such as asthma.

Despite the disproportionate burdens of living with SCD, many individuals are highly resilient. They develop strong coping skills and often have a strong spiritual or faith-based foundation. Individuals from cohesive families also have demonstrated resilience.

This chapter will discuss a variety of non-medical risk factors, describe how they affect individuals living with SCD, and explain the importance of and strategies for mitigating these risks as part of a comprehensive approach to addressing whole-person needs.

SOCIETAL FACTORS

A variety of societal factors tend to add to the burden of SCD. Those factors include the stigma associated with SCD, implicit bias, and racism. Given that most SCD and sickle cell trait (SCT) studies in the United States have focused on African Americans, the available evidence on the impact of these societal factors on other populations in the United States (the "emerging populations") is very limited. The discussion in this section therefore focuses primarily on the African American population. As the body of literature on SCD in global populations increases, so should research with the emerging populations in the United States.

Stigma and Bias

Stigma is one of the burdens borne by individuals with SCD. Health-related stigma refers to "a social process or related personal experience characterized by exclusion, rejection, blame, or devaluation that results from experience or reasonable anticipation of an adverse social judgment about a person or group identified with a particular health problem" (Weiss and Ramakrishna, 2006, p. 536). Stigma may also have health-related impacts if it results in individuals having limited access to beneficial services because they are socially judged or excluded because of their identity, such as race and ethnicity, socioeconomic status, and sexual orientation (Weiss et al., 2006). Stigma can create serious barriers to care, intensify existing physiological symptoms, and impose a severe psychological burden. Research has found that stigmatized individuals with SCD have decreased quality of life (QOL) and face numerous mental health challenges (Bediako et al., 2016; Wakefield et al., 2017).

The stigma associated with SCD can be traced to various sources, including racism, disease status, socioeconomic status, and pain episodes that require treatment with opioids (Bediako and Moffitt, 2011; Bulgin et al., 2018; Jenerette and Brewer, 2010; Wakefield et al., 2018), and it can be expressed by family, friends, and medical professionals (Bulgin et al., 2018; Wesley et al., 2016). In the United States, health care providers may ascribe negative characteristics to individuals living with SCD, such as labeling them as drug seekers (patients who use manipulative and demanding tactics to obtain prescription medication [Copeland, 2020]), which reflects and exacerbates the stigma and compromises health care use and quality of care (Bediako and Moffitt, 2011; Bediako et al., 2016; Bulgin et al., 2018; Jenerette and Brewer, 2010; Wakefield et al., 2018). Many patients report experiencing social isolation and a fear of disclosing their disease status because of the stigma associated with the disease (Leger et al., 2018).

Internalized stigma can heighten individuals' concerns about their employability and, if their disease status is known, affect their ability to interact regularly with others. Stigma can also affect an individual's use of health care and provider–patient interaction. SCD patients report fearing being viewed by providers as drug seekers and as seeking "unnecessary" pain treatment (Anderson and Asnani, 2013; Glassberg et al., 2013).

SCD-related stigma is a global problem. A study in Nigeria found that individuals with SCD who reported depressive or suicidal symptoms often reported also having experienced stigma or discriminatory remarks (Ola et al., 2016). The psychosocial impact of stigma also includes the fear of being devalued or viewed as less worthy by others, including close friends and relatives. In Saudi Arabia, SCD patients reported having experienced stigma from health care providers, with some stating that they were called addicts for seeking treatment for their acute vaso-occlusive pain (Asiri et al., 2017). Such experiences prompted some patients to seek consultations on-line from international clinicians.

Stigma can also affect intimate relationships because of the fear of being viewed differently; the various physiological complications of SCD, such as pain episodes and delayed pubertal development, can magnify the effects of stigma on a relationship (Cobo et al., 2013). In India, a study of 52 adolescents (25 with sickle cell anemia, a specific form of SCD; 12 with SCT; and 15 with neither) found that stigma had tremendous impact on the QOL of the children with SCD (Patel and Pathan, 2005). The children included in the study reported experiencing stigma and perceiving themselves to be a burden on their family. Furthermore, children with SCD—and, to a lesser extent, SCT—were found to have a lower QOL across all domains: physical, cognitive, and psychosocial. Stigma was postulated as being a central factor causing the perceived lack of support and disinterest from teachers for students with SCD.

SCD stigma also affects non-black individuals with the disease. According to a study in New York, health outreach workers at a community-based organization reported a perceived stigma associated with having an "African" disease among Dominicans and that family members requested that knowledge of their SCT status be kept within the family (Siddiqui et al., 2012). Perceptions of SCD as a "black disease" can cause Latinx people and other ethnicities to avoid accessing health care appropriately (Gallo et al., 2010; Siddiqui et al., 2012).

Implicit Bias

Unconscious bias, also known as "implicit bias," refers to attitudes or stereotypes that are outside one's awareness but that affect understanding, interactions, and decisions (Staats et al., 2016). Individuals' ability to quickly and automatically categorize people is a fundamental quality of the human mind: "Categories give order to life, and people group other people into categories based on social and other characteristics daily. This is the foundation of stereotypes, prejudice, and, ultimately, discrimination" (Teaching Tolerance, n.d.).

Researchers have found that all people harbor unconscious associations—both positive and negative—about other people based on characteristics such as race, ethnicity, gender, age, social class, and appearance (Kirwan Institute, 2017). These associations may influence people's feelings and attitudes and result in involuntary discriminatory practices, especially under demanding circumstances (Kirwan Institute, 2017). Studies show that people can be consciously committed to promoting equal rights and opportunities for all while still harboring hidden negative prejudices or stereotypes (The Joint Commission, 2016).

Despite progress made against overt bias in medicine, unconscious biases still pose barriers to achieving a diverse and equitable health care system (White, 2011). Considerable research has confirmed that unconscious bias in health care delivery has detrimental effects on patient health outcomes (IOM, 2003).

The medical literature shows that a patient's race can influence clinical decision making, including decisions to offer joint replacement, cardiovascular interventions, and chronic and acute pain management (Katz, 2016; Mody et al., 2012; Wyatt, 2013; Zhang et al., 2016). Nelson and Hackman (2013) used a survey adapted from the Centers for Disease Control and Prevention's 2008 Behavioral Risk Factor Surveillance System and the Sickle Cell Transfer Questionnaire with specific questions regarding race, racism, and health care delivery in order to investigate the experience of perceived bias among patients, their families, and health care staff at the Sickle Cell Center at Children's Hospital and Clinics of Minnesota. Half of the patients and their families responding to the survey (a majority of whom identified as black) reported that they saw race as affecting health care, whereas less than one-third of staff (the majority of whom identified as white) felt the same. Based on these findings, the authors suggested that providers' unconscious attitudes contribute to continued health care disparities (Nelson and Hackman, 2013). A variety of efforts are under way to help reduce provider bias in health care, including the use of social–cognitive psychology and outreach to minority communities (Burgess et al., 2007; Joseph, 2018), but there is a need for studies that evaluate implicit bias against the SCD population.

Racism

Those affected by SCD often also face racism, which is related to but distinct from stigma and implicit bias. Racism is an overarching bias that is responsible for many barriers to SCD care and a social factor that must be addressed as part of a strategic plan for SCD. Because SCD is found mostly among black individuals globally, it is inevitably linked to racism and health inequity.

At the system level, racism manifests in the form of unequal levels of funding and national attention for SCD. One perceived impact of racism is lower funding support for SCD—and the resulting lessened research output—compared with diseases that affect predominantly white individuals, such as cystic fibrosis (CF) (Strouse et al., 2013). Bahr and Song (2015) argue that SCD should be considered a "neglected disease" based on WHO definitions, as structural violence imposed by racial and economic factors has led to stagnation in treatment advancements. Despite patient interest in participating in clinical trials, more attention is given to CF and other diseases with a lower prevalence (Bahr and Song, 2015). A module embedded in the 2011 Cooperative Congressional Electoral Study to assess perceptions about SCD among participants and how these perceptions were associated with support for government spending on SCD found that white participants supported significantly less funding for SCD than non-white participants did (Bediako and King-Meadows, 2016). This situation affects SCD treatment downstream in the form of stagnant research and development and limited resources for treatment.

At the individual level, some providers express racial biases that result in offering a significantly lower quality of care to African Americans and, by default, individuals living with SCD. There are both similarities and differences among countries with the unique burden imposed by racism. For example, in the United States it is nearly impossible to separate the effects of stigma from racism, as much of the literature does not distinguish between the two. Racism poses an additional burden on the individual and compounds the barriers to treatment and care. In countries with predominantly black populations, racism may still affect treatment, along with related factors, such as colorism or discrimination related to skin color or shade (Bulgin et al., 2018).

Racism and the Treatment of SCD Pain

Acute and chronic pain treatment is affected by racism at an individual level because of provider biases (discussed further in Chapters 5 and 7). The literature shows that many in the medical community hold false beliefs regarding biological differences in perceptions of pain between black and white patients. This perception dates back to the era of slavery (Savitt, 2002). Racist medical knowledge produced during the early 19th century about the black body in pain was used to reinforce existing racialized power structures and justify the U.S. slave system. Clinicians claimed that blacks were built to endure harsh labor conditions due to their limited emotional response capacity. This belief was part of a divisive racial biology that included claims that blacks possess a relative immunity to certain diseases and that they are less sensitive to physical suffering than whites (Hoberman, 2012).

These racist ideas about biological differences between black and white people still persist to a certain degree and affect modern medical practice. In a study of 121 participants with no medical training, the white participants (92) rated the pain that black people would feel across 18 scenarios (e.g., slamming a hand in a car door, hitting the head, or getting a paper cut) lower than what a white person would experience (Hoffman et al., 2016). Even white medical students and residents are not immune to these misconceptions and may harbor false beliefs about biological differences between white and black bodies, some of which may relate to racial bias in pain perception (Hoffman et al., 2016).

As a result of these racist beliefs about pain, African Americans are more likely to receive a lower quality of pain management than white patients and may be perceived as having drug-seeking behavior. African American patients are significantly less likely to receive pain relief than white patients, even with the same reported levels of pain (Burgess et al., 2006; Tait and Chibnall, 2014), and they may be prescribed fewer pain medications than whites (Green and Hart-Johnson, 2010; Hoffman et al., 2016). People living with SCD may have their pain exacerbated by the emotional distress of not being believed, excessive wait times to get pain relief, insufficient medication, and stigma related to health care use (Haywood et al., 2013).

The racism experienced by individuals with SCD coupled with the longstanding racism in health care and the historical medical exploitation experienced by the African American population has contributed to a mistrust of providers among individuals and families affected by SCD (Stevens et al., 2016; Zempsky, 2010).

The few studies available allude to an association between the experiences of racism and bias and the overall well-being of individuals with SCD. In a 2007 qualitative study, researchers questioned 10 women affected by SCD about their disease-related experiences of stress, perceived racism, and unfair treatment in the health care system and the workplace (Cole, 2007). These underlying risk factors are known to affect African American women to a greater degree, particularly when coping strategies or tools are limited (Cole, 2007). In a very small, non-random sample, eight women reported experiencing stress in the health care system, especially relating to their experience of pain. The women reported that experiences in the emergency department (ED) were a particular trigger for these feelings. As the author stated, "In order to help patients with SCD deal with depression and anxiety, we need to know the source of stress: Is it the disease, the living conditions of the patient, or both?" (Cole, 2007, p. 36).

Lack of Public Awareness

Although public awareness of SCD has increased in recent years, studies indicate that globally there are still significant gaps in knowledge and that individuals living with the disease continue to face stigma. A cross-sectional study conducted in Uganda found that a majority of study participants had heard of SCD but did not know the causes or whether they had the disease or trait. Close to 70 percent of study respondents stated that they would never marry a person with SCD, indicating high levels of stigma (Tusuubira et al., 2018). Another study of 20- to 32-year-old graduates from Nigerian tertiary educational institutions found a deficit in knowledge about SCD transmission and their carrier status (Adewuyi, 2000).

In the United States, public awareness and misinformation follow similar trends. Individuals with SCD typically lack information about how it is inherited and their carrier status, although they are more likely to be informed if a family member also has the disease (Harrison et al., 2017; Siddiqui et al., 2012). Women are likely to be more knowledgeable than men. This may be because women are provided with genetic counseling during prenatal care (Adewuyi, 2000; Al Arrayed and Al Hajeri, 2010; Harrison et al., 2017; Siddiqui et al., 2012). There are efforts to improve national and international awareness of SCD such as the adoption of June 19 as World Sickle Cell Day by the United Nations General Assembly and the designation of September as National Sickle Cell Month by the U.S. Congress. Despite these milestones, there is a need for activities and public education to promote widespread awareness of SCD and SCT.

INDIVIDUAL FACTORS

The effects of SCD vary based on its severity and a number of individual factors that affect how—and how effectively—an individual deals with SCD. These factors include health literacy, demographic variables, cognitive deficits, mental health challenges (e.g., depression), and coping mechanisms.

Health Literacy Issues

Health literacy is the "degree to which an individual has the capacity to obtain, communicate, process, and understand basic health information and services to make appropriate health decisions" (IOM, 2004, p. 32). Factors such as language barriers, communication challenges, and cultural differences can influence health literacy within and across groups. Health literacy skills include recognizing critical symptoms, managing medications, and making decisions about treatments, as well as other important needs. One study found that most of the caretakers of individuals with SCT who received in-person education as part of the study interventions improved their SCT knowledge over a 6-month period. The caregivers who did not achieve high SCT knowledge after education were those who had lower health literacy at baseline (Creary et al., 2017). In a study of adolescents living with SCD, Perry et al. (2017) found that their health literacy scores were lower than expected for their respective average grades. Examples of poor health literacy range from misunderstanding providers' instructions to not understanding the biological bases of SCD or the importance of medication adherence. Although the findings do not suggest that SCD is the cause of poor health literacy, they could be indicative of a need to increase SCD health literacy in the affected population so as to increase adherence to treatment, the likelihood of keeping appointments, and the ability to improve QOL and health outcomes (Adediran et al., 2016; Khemani et al., 2018).

The educational tools that are developed to improve health literacy should include information on not only SCD, managing medications, and making decisions about treatments but also curative therapies, such as hematopoietic stem cell transplantation (HSCT), gene transfer, and genome editing. They should be culturally appropriate and written with the appropriate attention to literacy levels for laypersons. In considering HSCT as a potential option, for example, patients must undertake a complex decision-making process that requires knowledge about disease-related complications, the availability of donors, relationships with caregivers, and numerous other factors (Khemani et al., 2018). Globally, knowledge about HSCT for SCD is low, indicating a need for educational tools aimed at increasing literacy on this topic among caregivers and patients as well as the general population (Adediran et al., 2016; Bugarin-Estrada et al., 2019). Interestingly, adequately informed patients tend to overestimate the effectiveness of HSCT, whereas patients and caregivers who lack information have less acceptance and belief in its efficacy (Adediran et al., 2016; Bugarin-Estrada et al., 2019).

Impact of Cognitive Deficits from Stroke and Anemia in the Population

Individuals with SCD have been shown to be at a higher risk for cognitive impairments according to a meta-analysis on the topic (Prussien et al., 2019). These impairments include reductions in attention, memory, language, and general cognitive function and may result from not only the highly prevalent stroke and silent cerebral infarcts (SCIs) but also from the impact of chronic illness and chronic anemia that reduce overall oxygen delivery to vital organs, including the brain. Even in individuals without a history of stroke or silent infarcts, cognitive deficits are visible early in childhood, possibly because of the disruption of cerebral blood flow. In studies examining various levels of cognitive function, individuals with SCD who had no history of stroke still performed worse on tests of cognitive function than controls (Kawadler et al., 2016; Prussien et al., 2019; Sanger et al., 2016). Tailoring interventions to address cognitive function early in childhood may increase cognitive capacity following overt strokes and could be included in the vocational rehabilitation services provided for adults with SCD, who may continue to experience SCIs.

Neurocognitive deficits may have a positive feedback effect (causing symptoms to worsen faster). One study found that cognitive impairment was related to adult SCD patients' inability to adhere to hydroxyurea (HU) therapy (Merkhofer et al., 2016), which could further worsen physiological and psychosocial symptoms. Some researchers have theorized that poor adherence to treatment in older adults may stem from neurocognitive deficits from early childhood that went unrecognized, such as impairments in episodic memory (Kawadler et al., 2016; Merkhofer et al., 2016). These early cognitive deficits and impairments to processing may also be associated with an increased risk for unemployment later in life (Sanger et al., 2016). Thus, a model for chronic care designed to preserve and optimize cognitive function should be implemented starting in early childhood, with continued support across the life span.

One such model involves the use of community health workers (CHWs) to successfully manage chronic disease treatment and aid in self-management and positive decision-making behaviors targeted to support medically identified cognitive deficits (Hsu et al., 2016). CHWs have been integrated into several SCD programs in the United States, and they aid in finding adolescents and young adults who have been lost to follow-up. Additional CHW-specific services include reminding patients to adhere to medical appointments and HU treatment and helping families overcome social barriers to care. Although long-term follow-up will be necessary to fully examine the efficacy of CHWs, this model can be used to ensure continuous chronic care support for individuals with SCD and to reduce the negative behavioral and social impact of neurocognitive impairments.

Mental Health Impacts

The family carries with it that guilt of the gene, and that heaviness, and that feeling from generation to generation of surrender to this thing that is constantly disrupting life: the feeling of helplessness.

—Adrienne S. (Open Session Panelist)

Research studies show that adults and children living with SCD experience mental health impacts from the condition, as discussed in Chapter 4. These studies have focused primarily on assessing such variables as anxiety, depression, coping, neurological complications, and QOL. The rest of the discussion in this section focuses on the mental health impacts of SCD on caregivers.

Adults who are providing care for children, adolescents, or life partners living with SCD also face impacts on their mental health. Parents and caregivers may have an overall negative perception of their child's QOL. Palermo et al. (2002) compared health-related quality-of-life (HRQOL) scores for children living with SCD to a sample of demographically similar healthy children without SCD using the Child Health Questionnaire–Parent Report Form. Caregivers of children living with SCD reported that their children had more limited psychological and social well-being than caregivers of healthy children reported for their charges. Caregivers of children living with SCD also reported to be more affected emotionally by their child's health. Panepinto et al. (2005) compared HRQOL scores for children living with SCD as reported by the children with the scores reported by their parents. Parents were more negative in their perceptions of health, self-esteem, and behavior of their children living with SCD than were the children themselves.

Caregivers of children with SCD were also reported to worry more than caregivers of children without the disease and to be more likely to have poorer mental health outcomes. Noll et al. (1998) compared the responses of 48 caregivers of children living with SCD to questions about their child-rearing practices with the responses of 48 caregivers of comparison peers. Only two items, both pertaining to parental concern or worry, were significantly different between the two groups of caregivers: "I worry about the health of my child" and "I don't want my child to be looked upon as different from others" (Noll et al., 1998). In a 2006 interview study of maternal caregivers of children living with SCD, mothers caring for children with SCD had higher depressive mood scores than mothers caring for healthy children (Moskowitz et al., 2007). The authors stated that "additional attention is warranted to developing adequate resources for caregivers of children with SCD to mitigate the stress of unexpected crises" (p. 64).

In a recent investigation of caregivers of adolescents living with SCD, based on focus group data, caregivers reported the perception of stigma about SCD across a variety of settings, such as academic, athletic, and medical settings (Wesley et al., 2016). Caregivers also reported internalized stigma and other negative feelings about the disease. Caregivers suggested more education for all individuals who work with children living with SCD and increased public awareness to improve the situation for individuals with SCD and their families (Wesley et al., 2016).

The mental health challenges experienced by caregivers for children living with SCD are understudied. Additionally, interventions designed to ensure that caregivers have an adequate understanding of SCD are needed. Support groups, information about financial assistance, and strong relationships with health care providers could all assist in meeting the needs of caretakers.

Coping Mechanisms

Because of the variability of the SCD phenotype, individuals have adopted different strategies for coping with the related physical and psychosocial complications. Many studies have attempted to identify and classify these strategies, which range from cognitive and behavioral strategies to religion and spirituality (Anderson and Asnani, 2013; Clayton-Jones and Haglund, 2016; Cotton et al., 2009; Gomes et al., 2019; Harrison et al., 2005; Hildenbrand et al., 2015). One study, for example, examined the utility of Roth and Cohen's "approach" versus "avoidance" coping framework, which has been used to categorize coping strategies for individuals with chronic diseases, to SCD (Hildenbrand et al., 2015). The approach model refers to strategies that directly deal with or mitigate a stressor, whereas the avoidance model includes strategies that attempt to distance the individual from a stressor. The study found that children with SCD and their parents use both "approach" and "avoidance" strategies to manage disease-related stressors, including pain episodes.

Cognitive behavioral therapy (CBT) is one effective method that has been used to help the SCD population reduce health care usage for pain and minimize the disruptions in their daily activities caused by pain (Schatz et al., 2015). CBT interventions typically involve psychoeducation, distraction strategies, and coping mechanisms. Recent studies show that introducing a CBT intervention through smartphone technology could increase coping skills and reduce SCD-related complications in children (Palermo et al., 2018; Schatz et al., 2015). Because the majority of pain episodes in children are typically managed at home (Yang et al., 1997), an easily accessible technology, such as mHealth, may be beneficial for promoting positive coping strategies. Cognitive and behavioral coping strategies have also been used by individuals living with SCD in Jamaica to reestablish control over their response to SCD, others' responses to SCD, and the physical manifestations of SCD (Anderson and Asnani, 2013).

In addition, individuals with SCD may develop various coping strategies and adaptive behaviors on their own to respond to their stressors. A study of adolescents found that building self-esteem, drawing on family support, and strengthening relationships with parents were key adaptations to SCD (Ziadni et al., 2011). Furthermore, as adolescents learned to self-manage their symptoms, their perceived self-competence and self-reliance increased. Understanding how individuals with SCD naturally develop their own coping strategies could aid in tailoring interventions to work in conjunction with natural adaptive behaviors.

Spirituality and Religiosity

Spirituality has been found to be a powerful coping mechanism for individuals with SCD, and struggles with spirituality and faith have been associated with poor mental health and psychological outcomes (Adegbola, 2011; Adzika et al., 2016; Bediako et al., 2011; Clayton-Jones and Haglund, 2016; Clayton-Jones et al., 2016; Harrison et al., 2005). Spirituality may allow individuals to decrease negative attitudes and mental states, such as fatalism and hopelessness, which are known to be key factors in pain perception, to be associated with poor self-efficacy, and to further compound issues in chronic care management (Adegbola, 2011; Jenerette and Murdaugh, 2008; Jenerette et al., 2005). Because of the power of religion as a support and coping mechanism and its cultural importance in navigating community and identity, individuals with SCD may find it useful to explore its benefits.

Managing SCD requires a holistic approach aimed both at decreasing hospitalizations and symptoms and increasing the overall QOL (Adegbola, 2011). Patients' self-reported religious coping is associated with fewer hospital admissions and decreased pain perception (Bediako et al., 2011; Harrison et al., 2005). It has been theorized that religion works by increasing access to social support, psychological resources, positive health behaviors, and a sense of coherence (Harrison et al., 2005). A study of adults living with SCD in Ghana revealed that strategies for coping with SCD included attending a place of worship and praying and that SCD pain was the main reason for using these strategies (Adzika et al., 2016). A 2015 review of the literature on the roles of spirituality and religiosity in adolescents and adults living with SCD confirmed that they are sources of coping associated with enhanced pain management and improved health care use and QOL (Clayton-Jones and Haglund, 2016). Nonetheless, few studies have examined the effects of spirituality and religiosity on SCD outcomes. More work is needed to understand their influences on SCD experiences and outcomes in diverse populations. Efforts may need to be directed at engaging and educating religious leaders in order to understand their potential role in increasing the coping ability of individuals with SCD and other serious illnesses through spirituality.

Other Protective Factors

Researchers have found that a number of other factors can protect against various harms associated with SCD. For instance, Ladd et al. (2014) found that high family cohesion, as measured by the Family Environment Scale via interviews with parents, was positively correlated with a lower likelihood for grade retention and might protect children with SCD against poor academic achievement. Thus, a positive family environment can serve as a protective factor for these children.

As described earlier in this chapter, Ziadni et al. (2011) looked at self-report data from 44 adolescents to consider the links among stress-processing variables (appraisals of hope and pain coping), QOL, adaptive behaviors, and coping strategies. Low QOL scores were significantly associated with less adaptive behaviors, while appraisals of hope were significantly associated with more adaptive behaviors. The authors concluded that "stress processing variables (coping and appraisals), essential to successful adaptation to the demands of sickle cell complications and disease course" (Ziadni et al., 2011, p. 341), are important elements of resilience for such adolescents.

ENVIRONMENTAL FACTORS

In addition to societal and individual factors, environmental factors also contribute to the variability in how SCD manifests clinically; however, the exact roles that such factors play in influencing symptoms and complications are not well understood. Environmental factors range from the physical, such as climate and temperature, to the socio-environmental, such as place of residence and discrimination. These factors are often interrelated. For instance, residential area is correlated with factors such as air quality, socioeconomic status, school and work environments, and access to healthy foods.

Studies have found exposure to cold or wind to be correlated with higher incidences of pain crises and emergency admissions (Tewari et al., 2014, 2015). Residential area also influences SCD symptoms. A study in Jamaica found that urban patients who lived closer to factories had more severe respiratory events and pain crises than rural patients (Asnani et al., 2017). Severe outcomes were associated with higher poverty and living further away from health care services. Place of residence not only influences access to care but also is related to such factors as socioeconomic status and exposure to pollutants that can initiate or exacerbate common comorbid conditions, such as asthma. Furthermore, socioeconomic stress, financial struggle, and poor parent and family functioning are associated with cognitive deficits in children (Bills et al., 2019; Yarboi et al., 2017). Additional studies are needed to explore modifiable socio-environmental factors and their association with cognitive function and long-term outcomes.

Leg ulcers are one of the most debilitating SCD complications; these are recurrent wounds that appear near the ankles and are challenging to manage for both patients and providers. A cyclical mechanism to explain ulcer formation, proposed by Minniti and Kato (2016), involves malnutrition and underlying vascular damage leading to inflammation and bacterial colonization. Environmental stress, discrimination, and depression can all contribute to heightened pain sensitization and increased inflammation, leading to further ulcer growth and inhibiting healing processes (Minniti and Kato, 2016).

Efforts to improve QOL and outcomes for individuals living with SCD must include attention to environmental contributors, which in general are more amenable to change than molecular and other biological contributors.

Harnessing public will and working with community-based organizations, urban/city planners, and government agencies (e.g., the U.S. Department of Housing and Urban Development) could be effective in addressing key environmental risk factors.

THE BURDEN OF SCD

Many individuals with SCD are twice burdened: first, by a debilitating health condition and, second, by socioeconomic disadvantage. African American children with SCD are about one-third more likely (47.8 percent versus 34.7 percent, $p < 0.05$) than other similarly aged African American children to reside in a household that lies below the federal poverty level (Boulet et al., 2010). While the study authors offer no explanation for this disparity, the findings suggest that socioeconomic status could have important implications for access to care and use of treatment for children with SCD. Thus, even if the disease imposed no additional economic burdens, children with SCD would, on average, be disadvantaged by their poorer socioeconomic status. The disease itself results in a range of adverse health outcomes that affect daily functioning and potential early mortality. This results in a constellation of disparate problems that contribute to the burden of the illness, which implies that an equally wide range of policy instruments must be deployed in response. Health insurance, disability insurance, employment accommodation, school-based interventions, and medical innovation all must play a role in addressing the SCD burden.

Health Care Cost Burden

One major part of the economic burden of SCD is the additional health care costs imposed on individuals and families, which are so high that they represent a major financial burden on most families. Some families are not able to pay for it all, which results in leaving some aspects of the disease untreated.

The Magnitude of the Health Care Cost Burden

Individuals living with SCD often have considerable unmet health needs, even compared with patients with other serious illnesses. They and their insurers also face substantial financial costs for the health care that they can access. Using data from individuals enrolled in the Florida Medicaid program during 2001–2005, researchers estimated that the lifetime cost per SCD patient with Medicaid coverage exceeds $460,000 for SCD-related and non-SCD-related health care use (Kauf et al., 2009). Given the inflation in medical prices since 2009, it seems probable that updating this decade-old estimate would result in a current cost of more than $700,000.[1] The Florida Medicaid data suggest that the total annual health care costs ranged from $10,704 for the youngest patients (under age 10) to nearly $31,000 for those aged 50–64 (Kauf et al., 2009). Even this is likely an underestimate, considering that Medicaid spending per patient is typically less than that for commercial payers, and Medicaid covers patients for only a portion of their lives (i.e., the low-income, elderly, and individuals with disabilities are covered) (Clemans-Cope et al., 2016; Rudowitz et al., 2019). For both of these reasons, Medicaid data will typically fail to reflect the full lifetime cost burden borne by a cohort of SCD patients.

According to an analysis using SCD epidemiological and claims data, third-party commercial insurers paid approximately $3 billion for SCD-related charges in 2015; more than half was attributable to inpatient costs (more than $15,000 per patient), and more than one-third to outpatient costs (more than $10,000 per patient) (Huo et al., 2018).

Another study estimates that lifetime cost per SCD patient, assuming a 50-year life expectancy, could be as high as $8,747,908 (not accounting for inflation) (Ballas, 2009). This amount was estimated from the true cost (charges) of care for SCD, as opposed to the amount reimbursed by insurers. The author also notes that this estimate does not include the costs of expensive procedures such as iron chelation therapy and blood exchange transfusion for a stroke patient, which occur repeatedly over the lifetime of an individual with SCD.

Truven Health MarketScan® data on Medicaid and commercial health insurance plans suggest that children with SCD annually accrue more than $11,000 on Medicaid plans and nearly $15,000 on commercial health plans (Mvundura et al., 2009). These costs are estimated to be approximately 6 and 11 times the costs incurred by children without SCD on Medicaid and commercial health plans, respectively (Amendah et al., 2010).

Health care costs are borne by patients and their health insurers. Among patients with commercial insurance, SCD is estimated to be associated with approximately $1,293 in additional annual out-of-pocket expenditures (Huo et al., 2018). The financial burden is expected to be even higher for uninsured patients and to worsen with age as chronic end-organ damage accumulates. Young adults with SCD are a particularly vulnerable group; they face a high risk of being uninsured when transitioning from child to adult insurance arrangements. Constructing and implementing registries with long-term follow-up could provide more robust evidence of how SCD patients transition across health insurance status over the life course and true lifetime costs of care.

---

[1] Estimate based on SCD committee's analysis.

Mitigating Poor Health Outcomes and the Health Care Cost Burden

Even the best managed SCD patient populations will suffer worse health outcomes than their typical non-SCD counterparts. Thus, eliminating the health-related burden of SCD will require medical innovation, a topic addressed later in this report. However, the evidence suggests that gains can likely also be made by using today's medical technologies more widely and appropriately.

SCD is a rare disease in the United States, affecting only about 100,000 individuals (Hassell, 2010). The small size of this population—compared with the more common chronic conditions in health care—makes it difficult to conduct empirical analyses that indisputably measure the effects of real-world policy interventions within this group. For example, it is impractical to demand natural experimental or randomized data on a range of plausible real-world interventions because there are too few patients to support such a body of evidence. Instead, policy makers will need to base their decisions on a body of suggestive studies rather than a handful of definitive ones.

A key question is whether expanding access to health insurance and the breadth of services covered can improve health outcomes. There is limited research in the SCD population with which to answer this question; the broader health economics literature reports mixed evidence regarding the ability of health insurance to improve health outcomes. While there are indisputable benefits in the form of greater financial security, there is relatively little evidence that health insurance coverage actually causes gains in health (Baicker and Finkelstein, 2011; Finkelstein et al., 2012; Levy and Meltzer, 2008). However, patients with chronic, severe diseases are an important exception. Research suggests that health insurance access can decrease the likelihood of death for patients with serious illnesses, such as HIV (Goldman et al., 2001). Thus, it is worth considering the idea that health insurance will improve health outcomes for those severely ill with SCD. Medicaid expansion, which has increased access to insurance for millions since the implementation of the Patient Protection and Affordable Care Act (ACA), is associated with greater access to care, more preventive care, and improved chronic disease management (Gruber and Sommers, 2019). Researchers caution, however, that these are process measures that may not actually affect health state (Allen and Sommers, 2019; Gruber and Sommers, 2019). In reviewing evidence from multiple studies, researchers found that a few studies found evidence that Medicaid expansion has been associated with improved health in low-income U.S. residents as measured by self-reported health, acute and chronic disease outcomes, and mortality reductions (Allen and Sommers, 2019).

The available evidence specific to SCD patients demonstrates that health insurance status clearly affects access to care. Research using the Nationwide Emergency Department Sample—a sample of ED visits—found that insurance affected whether SCD patients were admitted to the hospital when presenting at the ED (Krishnamurti et al., 2010). Insured patients were about 50 percent more likely (42.3 percent versus 30.5 percent) to be admitted. Among the insured, the commercially insured were the most likely to be admitted, followed by those insured by Medicaid and those insured by Medicare (45.4 percent, 42.0 percent, and 39.9 percent, respectively) (Krishnamurti et al., 2010).

While this evidence does not definitively prove a causal link between health insurance and health outcomes, there are at least two possible explanations, both of which suggest a role for health insurance as a policy lever. First, uninsured patients may be denied access to clinically appropriate inpatient care. This would be true if they either avoided presenting to the ED with acute exacerbations or, when they did arrive, they were similar in health status to the insured patients. If so, this would suggest that health insurance can expand access to appropriate care. On the other hand, uninsured patients may be using ED visits for less acute episodes, which would normally be handled by a routine source of care. If so, then the logical conclusion would be that insurance promotes access to routine care for SCD patients. This latter interpretation is indirectly supported by a study of California ED data (Wolfson et al., 2012), which found that patients living farther from a comprehensive SCD care provider ended up with more ED visits but a lower likelihood of inpatient admission in the wake of the ED visit.

There is also evidence for an underlying causal mechanism linking insurance status with health outcomes in the SCD population. First, insurance affects access to HSCT. Commercially insured patients were nearly three times as likely to receive HSCT as Medicaid and uninsured patients (Anand et al., 2017). A review of state Medicaid websites reveals that these programs are more likely to restrict HSCT coverage in various ways, including limiting coverage of donor search and standard transplant indications and imposing ceilings on the number of inpatient days allowed (Preussler et al., 2014). Bone marrow transplantation exhibits qualitatively similar patterns. Among transplant centers, 45 percent and 30 percent faced considerable issues with Medicaid and Medicare reimbursement rates, respectively. Issues with commercial payers were present but were less prevalent and severe (Silver, 2015).

This evidence suggests that access is best for commercial payers, next best for Medicare patients, and worst for Medicaid patients. While the literature contains no specific comparisons between patients with Medicaid and uninsured patients, this is likely due to low rates of uninsurance and the resulting small sample sizes—as discussed below, uninsurance rates are 1–7 percent, depending on the age group. Insurance status appears to covary with mortality rates in much the same way that it covaries with access. In an inpatient sample, uninsured patients and Medicaid patients were more likely to develop complications and die than were Medicare patients (Perimbeti et al., 2018). For example, uninsured patients were 3.5–7 times more likely to die from their complications than Medicare patients. This study controlled for demographic factors available in inpatient data, including race, age, sex, income, and comorbidities. Confounding from unobservable disease severity remains an issue, however.

Adverse outcomes for Medicaid patients are of particular concern, because Medicaid likely covers the majority of SCD patients. The committee was unable to find national estimates of health insurance coverage for SCD patients in the literature. However, surveillance data from California shared by the CDC Foundation with the committee provide some relevant insight. Among the sample of SCD patients who visited EDs in 2016, 56 percent had Medicaid, 21 percent had Medicare, 16 percent had commercial insurance, 4 percent were uninsured, and the remaining 3 percent had other types of coverage.[2] These data will be used to inform the below discussion of insurance status, with the caveat that the discussion is limited to the California ED population. This is another potential application of sickle cell registry data.

While the estimated 4 percent rate of uninsurance in the California ED population is below the national average, which was 10 percent for all non-elderly Americans in 2016 (Tolbert et al., 2019), the fact that 1 out of every 25 SCD patients lacks health insurance is still a concern. In addition, the average figure blurs differences across age groups. Wider access to Medicaid among children and to Medicare among older people often leaves other adults behind. The rates of uninsurance are 2 percent, 1 percent, and 1 percent for people under 10, 10–19, and over 60, respectively. On the other hand, 7 percent of 40- to 49-year-olds are uninsured, as are 4 percent of 20- to 29-year-olds, despite the ACA provisions that make it easier for young adults to remain on their parents' health insurance.

The rate of uninsurance for the SCD population is expected to vary nationwide. Using the California estimates, public insurance continues to be the highest source of insurance for this population, and most of the southern U.S. states, which have the highest estimated number of individuals with SCD, have not expanded Medicaid eligibility per provisions in the ACA (see Figure 2-1). It is worth noting that Medicaid insurance coverage is determined by the Social Security Disability Insurance (SSDI) and Supplemental Security Income (SSI) criteria, which are structured to required "disability" as a prerequisite for coverage, as discussed later in this chapter. This causes various problems as it precludes an individual from participating in the employment sector and being covered by Medicaid at the same time, thus contributing to the economic burden borne by the individual.

---

[2] Analysis derived from surveillance data for California for 2010–2016, shared with the committee by the CDC Foundation's Sickle Cell Data Collection program.

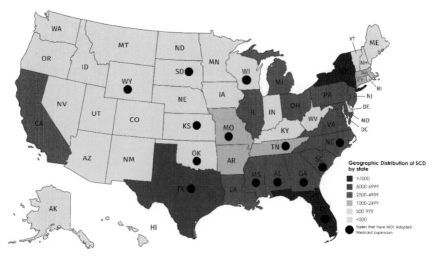

FIGURE 2-1 Estimated number of individuals with SCD across the United States and Medicaid non-expansion states.
NOTE: SCD = sickle cell disease.
SOURCE: Reprinted and modified from Hassell, 2010, with permission from Elsevier. Medicaid expansion data from KFF, 2019.

Taken as a whole, the evidence suggests that health insurance affects access to particular therapies, correlates with access to health care facilities, and correlates with mortality and outcomes in the same direction. It is not possible to rule out that poor health outcomes among, say, Medicaid and uninsured patients result from the patients' greater disadvantage status rather than from their insurance status. However, because health insurance affects access to effective therapies, it seems plausible that health gains could be made by expanding coverage.

Alongside its effects on health outcomes, health insurance also provides financial protection against catastrophic medical spending. Randomized evidence from the Oregon Medicaid experiment suggests that generous Medicaid coverage substantially reduced the likelihood of beneficiaries going into debt or skipping other bill payments in order to afford their medical care (Baicker and Finkelstein, 2011). While the Oregon experiment was not specific to SCD, it is plausible to believe that the benefits might be even larger for families facing SCD than for a representative sample of Oregonian families at or near Medicaid eligibility. Expanding the generosity of health insurance coverage (e.g., by reducing copayments, cost-sharing, and deductibles) would almost certainly improve financial security and ameliorate the social and psychological burden for families affected by SCD.

Economic Burden Beyond Health Care Costs

Because SCD is a debilitating disease that impairs functional status, affected individuals experience adverse effects on employment and education, which magnify the underlying health burden. The following discusses the magnitude of this burden and potential ways to mitigate it.

Disruptions in Employment

The committee could not find national estimates for unemployment rates in the SCD population. According to Sanger et al. (2016), various studies report that approximately 28–52 percent of individuals with SCD are unemployed. This proportion is substantially higher than the U.S. unemployment rate of 3.6 percent as of January 2020 (BLS, 2020). Several studies have researched the impact of SCD on employment. Sanger et al. (2016) considered the hypothesis that unemployment is related to cognitive deficits. The authors reviewed the charts of 50 individuals living with SCD for employment status and intelligence (as measured by the Wechsler Adult Intelligence Scale). The authors found an unemployment rate of nearly half (44 percent) and an association between lower educational attainment and higher odds of unemployment. It is unclear whether this link is due to cognitive impairment as a result of SCD, although the authors suggest that this may contribute to the risk of unemployment and argue for specific education and vocational services to be made available.

Idowu et al. (2013) compared 20 patients living with SCD to non-SCD siblings. Each patient completed a series of questionnaires about employment history and also answered questions concerning a sibling's employment history. The authors found that 75 percent of the siblings were employed (15 out of 20) but that only 20 percent of the individuals living with SCD were employed (4 out of 20). Fourteen of the individuals living with SCD received disability benefits, and 14 out of the 16 individuals with SCD who were not employed expressed a desire to have a job. The authors concluded that SCD has a major negative impact on successful employment, and they argue for developing workplace assistance interventions.

The treatment of SCD can also affect employment status. Ballas et al. (2010) compared employment status and changes therein for individuals receiving and responding to HU, individuals who did not respond to the treatment, and a placebo group, all participating in a multi-center study of HU for treating SCD. Although there were no statistically significant differences in employment among the groups, there was a general trend indicating more consistent employment in the HU group. The authors postulate that the lack of a significant difference between the treatment and placebo groups could also be attributed to the fact that most of the enrolled study participants had moderate to severe disease with significant complications.

The authors conclude that "it would be attractive to hypothesize that future treatment of young patients with HU could prevent or mitigate the incidence of complications of sickle cell anemia and, hence, improve the employment status of treated patients" (Ballas et al., 2010, p. 999).

The ability to successfully gain and maintain employment is an important factor in adult mental health. The Office of Disability Employment Policy in the U.S. Department of Labor offers guidelines for workplace accommodations for individuals living with SCD (JAN, 2019). These accommodations may include a flexible schedule that allows the individual to receive necessary medical treatment, an adjustable workstation, and an aide, if needed.

Facilitating employment can be a positive factor in managing health care use. Williams et al. (2018) followed 95 individuals living with SCD prospectively and found that employment was significantly associated with decreased health care interactions. Additional interventions to assist individuals in seeking employment are needed. Educational interventions for potential employers could also make a difference. This is an area for more public investments in research.

An additional factor to consider is that the mortality burden of SCD reduces lifetime income. A recent study estimates that premature mortality alone decreases lifetime earnings by about 40 percent; lifetime income is calculated to be $1.2 million for individuals living with SCD but $1.9 million to $2 million for matched controls (Agodoa et al., 2018).

Family caregivers also experience deficits in employment and income. They are burdened by the time they spend on diagnostic procedures, medication administration, care for in-dwelling tubes, and skin care (Moskowitz et al., 2007). Comprehensive estimates of time costs are not available for the SCD population specifically, but a study on children with special health care needs found that family caregivers for such children spend an average of 260 hours per year[3] on caregiving (Romley et al., 2017). This time commitment is estimated to be worth $3,200 per child per year (in 2015 dollars). Improving health insurance access and generosity might address out-of-pocket spending burdens, but there are few financial instruments available for insuring patients against this considerable time cost of caregiving.

Educational Attainment

Perhaps due to the combined effects of socioeconomic status and the disease itself, children with SCD have poorer educational outcomes than those without it. Depending on the severity and location of ischemic

---

[3] Approximately 5.6 million U.S. children with special health care needs received 1.5 billion hours annually of family-provided health care.

injury from strokes in SCD, overall intellectual capacity may be adversely affected as well as subdomains of attention and executive function, language, memory, and visuomotor skills (Berkelhammer et al., 2007; Boulet et al., 2010). Ladd et al. (2014) studied the neurocognitive effects due to strokes from SCD on poor academic performance using a nationally representative sample of 370 children and adolescents with SCD. The researchers assessed academic achievement via the Woodcock-Johnson tests of cognitive abilities and grade retention history. Parental reports indicated that 19 percent of the youth had been held back for at least one grade. Low math achievement and low reading achievement were both related to a higher likelihood of grade retention. Children with SCD may also experience higher rates of school problems because they disproportionately come from low-income, minority families; both factors that have been shown to confer independent risk for poor outcomes (NRC and IOM, 2000). This increased risk for academic difficulties may make children with SCD eligible for special educational assistance. Nearly one-third of children with SCD must repeat a grade or require special education services; this is more than double the corresponding rates for their non-SCD peers (Schatz, 2004). Herron et al. (2003) reported that in a sample of 26 high schoolers living with SCD in the St. Louis area, only 4 were on target to graduate on time. The authors surmised that these students were receiving inadequate educational support. A brief description of a second study of 39 students (Herron et al., 2003) reported that 28 percent had been held back for at least one grade. However, research on the efficacy of grade retention indicates that it is not an effective educational strategy (Peixoto et al., 2016). Additional resources may be needed to improve educational outcomes (Epping et al., 2013). A recently settled lawsuit was filed against Boston Public Schools to force the schools to provide more services for students with SCD, especially tutoring to keep up with classes (Irons, 2018).

Children with SCD are often ill and miss school. A number of studies have examined relationships between attendance and school performance among children living with SCD. Schwartz et al. (2009) assessed medical and school records and had 40 12- to 18-year-olds complete a series of self-reported measures of psychosocial functioning. They found that more than one-third (35 percent) had missed at least 1 month of school. Overall, these youth missed an average of 12 percent of the school year. Absenteeism was significantly associated with the health variables and psychosocial measures. The authors conclude that school absenteeism remains a significant problem and that there needs to be collaboration among schools, medical providers, and parents to better manage the academic achievement of students living with SCD. The finding was reinforced by a study by Peterson et al. (2005), which gave a brief needs assessment to 72 parents.

One-third of the parents indicated that their child experienced "frequent school absences" of more than 20 days per year.

Tools exist to assess the educational support needs of children with SCD; however, they appear to be underused, meaning that strategies to effectively address these needs are not appropriately deployed. In the afore-mentioned study by Peterson et al. (2005) the authors surveyed 72 parents of children (ages 5 to 17 years) living with SCD using the Hematology–Oncology Psycho-Educational Needs Assessment (HOPE) tool, which they developed. According to the HOPE survey results, more than half of all parents expressed concerns about their children's education and reported teacher concerns about the children's academic performance. Other data in-dicated that more than one-third of the children repeated at least one grade (36 percent) and that almost half failed to pass a statewide proficiency exam (47 percent). More than one-third had missed at least 20 days of school (35 percent); the authors also reported on behavioral issues noted by teachers (32 percent) and disciplinary consequences associated with these behavioral issues (38 percent). Less than two-thirds of these children had undergone testing for learning disabilities (64 percent), and even fewer had an individualized education plan in place (28 percent). This suggests that elementary and secondary schools need to better address the academic and functional needs of children living with SCD.

These childhood effects of SCD appear to result in long-term educa-tional costs. Based on retrospective reports, one study found that 85 percent of adults with SCD reported missing school once per week (Idowu et al., 2014). This is 6.5 times the corresponding rate of their counterparts with-out SCD ($p < 0.001$). Perhaps not surprisingly, SCD adults' college gradu-ation rates are less than half that of their siblings without SCD (15 percent versus 35 percent, $p < 0.001$).

Individuals living with SCD and their families also suffer employment costs as a result of the disease. Those who do secure gainful employment often suffer from poor educational attainment, which would depress their earnings.

Mitigating the Economic Burden

Early childhood development To ease the educational and economic impact of SCD, it is necessary to offer early-intervention programs, with ongoing targeted support across the life span to mitigate the long-term consequences of complications that occurred early in childhood. There are various pro-grams and policies designed to support early childhood development for children with special needs, but their comprehensiveness and participation are highly variable. For example, all children living with SCD (because they have special health care needs) are eligible for services under the Individuals with Disabilities Education Act, Part C, which covers young children with a recognized disability or at risk for developmental delay (discussed further in Chapter 5). However, there are sizable state-to-state differences in participation rates, and McManus et al. (2009, 2011, 2019) found that most children who access these services come from low-income households and that there is often a delay from diagnosis to receipt of services. There is a need to expand eligibility and shorten the time between application for and receipt of benefits to help mitigate some of these adverse outcomes.

Richardson et al. (2019) presented data indicating that children eligible for early-intervention services are not using these services as intensely as might be expected. Using an administrative database from a large early-intervention program, the authors reported that children appear to be receiving less substantive services than had previously been the case, and they hypothesized that this may be due to an overall decline in federal per child appropriations for early-intervention services.

Access to early-intervention services appears to be spotty at best and influenced by child and family characteristics, such as the primary language spoken in the home, race, and ethnicity. There are few large-scale studies of early-intervention services at a national level, primarily due to a lack of common data collection elements.

Young adulthood and beyond To optimize functional outcomes for adults living with SCD, it will be important to develop an understanding of how to improve the structure of existing programs and to remove obstacles so as to make the programs more accessible to these adults and their families. Health insurance does not cover the adverse employment and economic consequences of SCD. Instead, that lies within the traditional scope of disability insurance programs, such as SSDI and SSI. The goal of such programs is to provide partial income replacement to people suffering from disabilities that impair their ability to work.

The design of disability programs must account for the well-known trade-off between insurance and incentives for work. Very generous programs provide better insurance, but they also create incentives for moderately or mildly ill workers to opt out of the labor force and receive disability benefits instead, particularly for groups of workers facing bleaker wage prospects (Autor and Duggan, 2003). In contrast, strict programs provide worse insurance but fewer incentives for borderline workers to leave the labor force. Thus, such programs are, in principle, designed to screen out less severe illnesses that do not compromise the ability to work.

Unfortunately, the eligibility rules for SCD create a number of unintended consequences in their effort to screen out less severe cases. Section 7.05 of the U.S. Social Security Administration's "Blue Book" lists the four ways to qualify for SSI (SSA, n.d.):

1. Six pain crises in a 12-month period that required "narcotic medication" and were spaced at least 30 days apart;
2. Three or more hospitalizations of 48 hours or more for hemolytic anemia in a 12-month period;
3. Three episodes of hemoglobin below 7.0 grams per deciliter in a 12-month period, spaced at least 30 days apart; and
4. Beta thalassemia major that requires "life-long [red blood cell] transfusions at least once every 6 weeks to maintain life."

Notably, the first three criteria reward patients and their providers for poorly managing complications. Diligently managing anemia and pain crises could disqualify the patient for public assistance, including the insurance benefit that helped get the disease under control in the first place. The fourth does not suffer from the same drawback because it identifies a biomarker that cannot be altered by the patient or provider and that results in difficulty maintaining employment.

More generally, recent research in the economics literature on disability insurance programs—not specific to SCD—recommends expanding access to these programs and reducing the number of eligibility reassessments needed (Low and Pistaferri, 2018). The crux of the argument is that the existing disability insurance program involves a very high rate of rejecting worthy applicants and a correspondingly low rate of accepting unworthy applicants. In such an environment, moving toward more generosity can improve well-being because it admits more worthy applicants than unworthy ones.

CONCLUSIONS AND RECOMMENDATIONS

Conclusion 2-1: Stigma and racism have been shown to negatively affect access to care, treatment, psychological health, and disease outcomes of individuals with SCD in the United States and globally. However, their impacts are often conflated in the literature, and their mechanisms of action are poorly understood. Further studies are needed to understand the separate and combined influences of stigma and racism on individuals with SCD and to develop and implement strategies to address them.

Conclusion 2-2: Public awareness of SCD is still suboptimal, which further perpetuates stigma and bias against individuals with the disease and trait. There is a need for the development of multimedia (e.g., print, text, video, games, apps) educational materials for the general public and for individuals with SCD.

Conclusion 2-3: The SCD disability insurance criteria are restrictive, especially for young adults as they transition from childhood into adulthood. Loss of SSI has implications for transitioning youth, as it affects their eligibility for Medicaid insurance. The disability insurance eligibility criteria are dependent on the individual remaining disabled and unable to hold a job and underscores the need for better biomarkers of SCD severity that are objective and not easily modifiable by providers, patients, or payers. Such biomarkers would be more appropriate mechanisms for judging disability program eligibility.

Conclusion 2-4: Neurocognitive deficits are both a result and a cause of chronic symptoms in SCD. Neurocognitive deficits early in childhood may affect patients' abilities to manage their disease in the long term and result in missed appointments, poor treatment adherence, and suboptimal outcomes both clinically and throughout the life span.

Conclusion 2-5: SCD imposes psychological, social, and financial burdens on the individual, caregivers, and family.

Recommendation 2-1: The Social Security Administration should review disability insurance qualifications to ensure that the qualification criteria reflect the burden of the disease borne by individuals with sickle cell disease.

Recommendation 2-2: States should expand and enhance vocational rehabilitation programs for individuals with sickle cell disease who need additional training in order to actively participate in the workforce.

Recommendation 2-3: The U.S. Department of Health and Human Services should engage with media to improve awareness about the disease and address misconceptions about the disease and those affected.

REFERENCES

Adediran, A., M. B. Kagu, T. Wakama, A. A. Babadoko, D. O. Damulak, S. Ocheni, and M. I. Asuquo. 2016. Awareness, knowledge, and acceptance of haematopoietic stem cell transplantation for sickle cell anaemia in Nigeria. *Bone Marrow Research* 2016:7062630.

Adegbola, M. A. 2011. Using lived experiences of adults to understand chronic pain: Sickle cell disease, an exemplar. *i-manager's Journal on Nursing* 1(3):1–12.

Adewuyi, J. O. 2000. Knowledge of and attitudes to sickle cell disease and sickle carrier screening among new graduates of Nigerian tertiary educational institutions. *Nigerian Postgraduate Medical Journal* 7(3):120–123.

Adzika, V. A., D. Ayim-Aboagye, and T. Gordh. 2016. Pain management strategies for effective coping with sickle cell disease: The perspective of patients in Ghana. *Scandinavian Journal of Pain* 12(1):117.

Agodoa, I., D. Lubeck, N. Bhakta, M. Danese, K. Pappu, R. Howard, M. Gleeson, M. Halperin, and S. Lanzkron. 2018. Societal costs of sickle cell disease in the United States. *Blood* 132(Suppl 1):4706.

Al Arrayed, S., and A. Al Hajeri. 2010. Public awareness of sickle cell disease in Bahrain. *Annals of Saudi Medicine* 30(4):284–288.

Allen, H., and B. D. Sommers. 2019. Medicaid expansion and health: Assessing the evidence after 5 years. *JAMA* 322(13):1253–1254.

Amendah, D. D., M. Mvundura, P. L. Kavanagh, P. G. Sprinz, and S. D. Grosse. 2010. Sickle cell disease-related pediatric medical expenditures in the U.S. *American Journal of Preventative Medicine* 38(4 Suppl):S550–S556.

Anand, S., R. Theodore, A. Mertens, P. A. Lane, and L. Krishnamurti. 2017. Health disparity in hematopoietic cell transplantation for sickle cell disease: Analyzing the association of insurance and socioeconomic status among children undergoing hematopoietic cell transplantation. *Blood* 130(Suppl 1):4636.

Anderson, M., and M. Asnani. 2013. "You just have to live with it": Coping with sickle cell disease in Jamaica. *Qualitative Health Research* 23(5):655–664.

Asiri, E., M. Khalifa, S. A. Shabir, M. N. Hossain, U. Iqbal, and M. Househ. 2017. Sharing sensitive health information through social media in the Arab world. *International Journal for Quality in Health Care* 29(1):68–74.

Asnani, M. R., J. Knight Madden, M. Reid, L. G. Greene, and P. Lyew-Ayee. 2017. Socio-environmental exposures and health outcomes among persons with sickle cell disease. *PLOS ONE* 12(4):e0175260.

Autor, D. H., and M. G. Duggan. 2003. The rise in the disability rolls and the decline in unemployment. *Quarterly Journal of Economics* 118(1):157–206.

Bahr, N. C., and J. Song. 2015. The effect of structural violence on patients with sickle cell disease. *Journal of Health Care for the Poor and Underserved* 26(3):648–661.

Baicker, K., and A. Finkelstein. 2011. The effects of Medicaid coverage—Learning from the Oregon experiment. *New England Journal of Medicine* 365(8):683–685.

Ballas, S. K. 2009. The cost of health care for patients with sickle cell disease. *American Journal of Hematology* 84:320–322.

Ballas, S. K., R. L. Bauserman, W. F. McCarthy, and M. A. Waclawiw. 2010. The impact of hydroxyurea on career and employment of patients with sickle cell anemia. *Journal of the National Medical Association* 102(11):993–999.

Bediako, S., and T. King-Meadows. 2016. Public support for sickle-cell disease funding: Does race matter? *Race and Social Problems* 8.

Bediako, S. M., and K. R. Moffitt. 2011. Race and social attitudes about sickle cell disease. *Ethnicity and Health* 16(4–5):423–429.

Bediako, S. M., L. Lattimer, C. Haywood, Jr., N. Ratanawongsa, S. Lanzkron, and M. C. Beach. 2011. Religious coping and hospital admissions among adults with sickle cell disease. *Journal of Behavioral Medicine* 34(2):120–127.

Bediako, S. M., S. Lanzkron, M. Diener-West, G. Onojobi, M. C. Beach, and C. Haywood, Jr. 2016. The measure of sickle cell stigma: Initial findings from the Improving Patient Outcomes through Respect and Trust study. *Journal of Health Psychology* 21(5):808–820.

Berkelhammer, L. D., A. L. Williamson, S. D. Sanford, C. L. Dirksen, W. G. Sharp, A. S. Margulies, and R. A. Prengler. 2007. Neurocognitive sequelae of pediatric sickle cell disease: A review of the literature. *Child Neuropsychology* 13(2):120–131.

Bills, S. E., J. Schatz, S. J. Hardy, and L. Reinman. 2019. Social-environmental factors and cognitive and behavioral functioning in pediatric sickle cell disease. *Child Neuropsychology* 26(1):83–99.

BLS (Bureau of Labor Statistics). 2020. *Databases, tables & calculators by subject.* https://data.bls.gov/timeseries/LNS14000000 (accessed March 9, 2020).

Boulet, S. L., E. A. Yanni, M. S. Creary, and R. S. Olney. 2010. Health status and healthcare use in a national sample of children with sickle cell disease. *American Journal of Preventative Medicine* 38(4 Suppl):S528–S535.

Bugarin-Estrada, E., A. G. De León, J. M. Yáñez-Reyes, P. R. Colunga-Pedraza, and D. Gómez-Almaguer. 2019. Assessing patients' knowledge and attitudes towards HSCT in an outpatient-based transplant center in Mexico. *Biology of Blood and Marrow Transplantation* 25(3):S301.

Bulgin, D., P. Tanabe, and C. Jenerette. 2018. Stigma of sickle cell disease: A systematic review. *Issues in Mental Health Nursing* 39(8):675–686.

Burgess, D. J., M. van Ryn, M. Crowley-Matoka, and J. Malat. 2006. Understanding the provider contribution to race/ethnicity disparities in pain treatment: Insights from dual process models of stereotyping. *Pain Medicine* 7(2):119–134.

Burgess, D., M. van Ryn, J. Dovidio, and S. Saha. 2007. Reducing racial bias among health care providers: Lessons from social-cognitive psychology. *Journal of General Internal Medicine* 22(6):882–887.

Clayton-Jones, D., and K. Haglund. 2016. The role of spirituality and religiosity in persons living with sickle cell disease: A review of the literature. *Journal of Holistic Nursing* 34(4):351–360.

Clayton-Jones, D., K. Haglund, R. Belknap, J. Schaefer, and A. Thompson. 2016. Spirituality and religiosity in adolescents living with sickle cell disease. *Western Journal of Nursing Research* 38(6):686–703.

Clemans-Cope, L., J. Holahan, and R. Garfield. 2016. *Medicaid spending growth compared to other payers: A look at the evidence.* Washington, DC: Kaiser Family Foundation.

Cobo, V. A., C. A. Chapadeiro, J. B. Ribeiro, H. Moraes-Souza, and P. R. Martins. 2013. Sexuality and sickle cell anemia. *Revista Brasileira de Hematologia e Hemoterapia* 35(2):89–93.

Cole, P. L. 2007. Black women and sickle cell disease: Implications for mental health disparities research. *Californian Journal of Health Promotion* 5:24–39.

Copeland, D. 2020. Drug-seeking: A literature review (and an exemplar of stigmatization in nursing). *Nursing Inquiry* 27(1):e12329.

Cotton, S., D. Grossoehme, S. L. Rosenthal, M. E. McGrady, Y. H. Roberts, J. Hines, M. S. Yi, and J. Tsevat. 2009. Religious/spiritual coping in adolescents with sickle cell disease: A pilot study. *Journal of Pediatric Hematology/Oncology* 31(5):313–318.

Creary, S., I. Adan, J. Stanek, S. H. O'Brien, D. J. Chisolm, T. Jeffries, K. Zajo, and E. Varga. 2017. Sickle cell trait knowledge and health literacy in caregivers who receive in-person sickle cell trait education. *Molecular Genetics & Genomic Medicine* 5(6):692–699.

Epping, A. S., M. P. Myrvik, R. F. Newby, J. A. Panepinto, A. M. Brandow, and J. P. Scott. 2013. Academic attainment findings in children with sickle cell disease. *Journal of School Health* 83(8):548–553.

Finkelstein, A., S. Taubman, B. Wright, M. Bernstein, J. Gruber, J. P. Newhouse, H. Allen, and K. Baicker. 2012. The Oregon health insurance experiment: Evidence from the first year. *Quarterly Journal of Economics* 127(3):1057–1106.

Gallo, A. M., D. Wilkie, M. Suarez, R. Labotka, R. Molokie, A. Thompson, P. Hershberger, and B. Johnson. 2010. Reproductive decisions in people with sickle cell disease or sickle cell trait. *Western Journal of Nursing Research* 32(8):1073–1090.

Glassberg, J. A., P. Tanabe, A. Chow, K. Harper, C. Haywood, Jr., M. R. DeBaun, and L. D. Richardson. 2013. Emergency provider analgesic practices and attitudes toward patients with sickle cell disease. *Annals of Emergency Medicine* 62(4):293–302.

Goldman, D. P., J. Bhattacharya, D. F. McCaffrey, N. Duan, A. A. Leibowitz, G. F. Joyce, and S. C. Morton. 2001. Effect of insurance on mortality in an HIV-positive population in care. *Journal of the American Statistical Association* 96(455):883–894.

Gomes, M. V., A. Xavier, E. S. S. Carvalho, R. C. Cordeiro, S. L. Ferreira, and A. D. Morbeck. 2019. "Waiting for a miracle": Spirituality/religiosity in coping with sickle cell disease. *Revista Brasileria de Enfermagem* 72(6):1554–1561.

Green, C. R., and T. Hart-Johnson. 2010. The adequacy of chronic pain management prior to presenting at a tertiary care pain center: The role of patient socio-demographic characteristics. *Journal of Pain* 11(8):746–754.

Gruber, J., and B. D. Sommers. 2019. The Affordable Care Act's effects on patients, providers, and the economy: What we've learned so far. *Journal of Policy Analysis and Management* 38(4):1028–1052.

Harrison, M. O., C. L. Edwards, H. G. Koenig, H. B. Bosworth, L. Decastro, and M. Wood. 2005. Religiosity/spirituality and pain in patients with sickle cell disease. *Journal of Nervous and Mental Disease* 193(4):250–257.

Harrison, S. E., C. M. Walcott, and T. D. Warner. 2017. Knowledge and awareness of sickle cell trait among young African American adults. *Western Journal of Nursing Research* 39(9):1222–1239.

Hassell, K. L. 2010. Population estimates of sickle cell disease in the U.S. *American Journal of Preventive Medicine* 38(4 Suppl):S512–S521.

Haywood, C., Jr., P. Tanabe, R. Naik, M. C. Beach, and S. Lanzkron. 2013. The impact of race and disease on sickle cell patient wait times in the emergency department. *American Journal of Emergency Medicine* 31(4):651–656.

Herron, S., S. J. Bacak, A. King, and M. R. DeBaun. 2003. Inadequate recognition of education resources required for high-risk students with sickle cell disease. *Archives of Pediatrics and Adolescent Medicine* 157(1):104.

Hildenbrand, A. K., L. P. Barakat, M. A. Alderfer, and M. L. Marsac. 2015. Coping and coping assistance among children with sickle cell disease and their parents. *Journal of Pediatric Hematology/Oncology* 37(1):25–34.

Hoberman, J. 2012. *Black and blue: The origins and consequences of medical racism.* Berkeley, CA: University of California Press.

Hoffman, K. M., S. Trawalter, J. R. Axt, and M. N. Oliver. 2016. Racial bias in pain assessment and treatment recommendations, and false beliefs about biological differences between blacks and whites. *Proceedings of the National Academy of Sciences* 113(16):4296–4301.

Hsu, L. L., N. S. Green, E. Donnell Ivy, C. E. Neunert, A. Smaldone, S. Johnson, S. Castillo, A. Castillo, T. Thompson, K. Hampton, J. J. Strouse, R. Stewart, T. Hughes, S. Banks, K. Smith-Whitley, A. King, M. Brown, K. Ohene-Frempong, W. R. Smith, and M. Martin. 2016. Community health workers as support for sickle cell care. *American Journal of Preventive Medicine* 51(1):S87–S98.

Huo, J., H. Xiao, M. Garg, C. Shah, D. J. Wilkie, and A. I. Mainous. 2018. PSY10–The economic burden of sickle cell disease in the United States. *Value in Health* 21(Suppl 2):S108.

Idowu, M., O. Fawibe, P. Rowan, H. S. Juneja, and D. Brown. 2013. Occupational history for adults with sickle cell disease compared with healthy siblings. *Blood* 122(21):4937.

Idowu, M., S. Badejoko, P. Rowan, and H. S. Juneja. 2014. Academic achievement for adults with sickle cell disease compared with healthy siblings. *Blood* 124(21):4936.

IOM (Institute of Medicine). 2003. *Unequal treatment: Confronting racial and ethnic disparities in health care.* Washington, DC: The National Academies Press.

IOM. 2004. *Health literacy: A prescription to end confusion.* Washington, DC: The National Academies Press.

Irons, M. 2018. Boston public schools agree to recognize sickle cell disease as disability. *The Boston Globe*, February 7. https://www.bostonglobe.com/metro/2018/02/07/boston-public-schools-agree-recognize-sickle-cell-diseases/v6EHbwEbKSA46mbLTOMGLN/story.html (accessed January 5, 2020).

JAN (Job Accommodation Network). 2019. *Job Accommodation and compliance series: Employees with sickle cell anemia.* Morgantown, WV: Job Accommodation Network.

Jenerette, C. M., and C. Brewer. 2010. Health-related stigma in young adults with sickle cell disease. *Journal of the National Medical Association* 102(11):1050–1055.

Jenerette, C. M., and C. Murdaugh. 2008. Testing the theory of self-care management for sickle cell disease. *Research in Nursing and Health* 31(4):355–369.

Jenerette, C. M., M. Funk, and C. Murdaugh. 2005. Sickle cell disease: A stigmatizing condition that may lead to depression. *Issues in Mental Health Nursing* 26(10):1081–1101.

Joseph, P. 2018. Eliminating disparities and implicit bias in health care delivery by utilizing a hub-and-spoke model. *Research Ideas and Outcomes* 4:e26370.

Katz, J. N. 2016. Persistence of racial and ethnic differences in utilization and adverse outcomes of total joint replacement. *Journal of Bone and Joint Surgery* 98(15):1241–1242.

Kauf, T. L., T. D. Coates, L. Huazhi, N. Mody-Patel, and A. G. Hartzema. 2009. The cost of health care for children and adults with sickle cell disease. *American Journal of Hematology* 84(6):323–327.

Kawadler, J. M., J. D. Clayden, C. A. Clark, and F. J. Kirkham. 2016. Intelligence quotient in paediatric sickle cell disease: A systematic review and meta-analysis. *Developmental Medicine and Child Neurology* 58(7):672–679.

KFF (Kaiser Family Foundation). 2019. *Status of state Medicaid expansion decisions: Interactive map.* https://www.kff.org/medicaid/issue-brief/status-of-state-medicaid-expansion-decisions-interactive-map (accessed January 15, 2019).

Khemani, K., D. Ross, C. Sinha, A. Haight, N. Bakshi, and L. Krishnamurti. 2018. Experiences and decision making in hematopoietic stem cell transplant in sickle cell disease: Patients' and caregivers' perspectives. *Biology of Blood and Marrow Transplantation* 24(5):1041–1048.

Kirwan Institute. 2017. *Proceedings of the Diversity and Inclusion Innovation Forum: Unconscious bias in academic medicine.* Columbus, OH: Kirwan Institute for the Study of Race and Ethnicity, The Ohio State University.

Krishnamurti, L., R. Goel, and P. Viswanathan. 2010. Factors predicting hospital admission following a visit to the emergency room for sickle cell crisis. *Pediatric Blood & Cancer* 54(6):837.

Ladd, R. J., C. R. Valrie, and C. M. Walcott. 2014. Risk and resilience factors for grade retention in youth with sickle cell disease. *Pediatric Blood & Cancer* 61(7):1252–1256.

Leger, R. R., L. D. Wagner, and V. Odesina. 2018. Stigma in adults with sickle cell disease and family members: Scale development and pilot study in the USA and Nigeria. *International Journal of Africa Nursing Sciences* 9:23–29.

Levy, H., and D. Meltzer. 2008. The impact of health insurance on health. *Annual Review of Public Health* 29:399–409.

Liu, J., and G. Lewis. 2014. Environmental toxicity and poor cognitive outcomes in children and adults. *Journal of Environmental Health* 76(6):130–138.

Low, H., and L. Pistaferri. 2018. Disability insurance and the dynamics of the incentive insurance trade-off. *American Economic Review* 105(10):2986–3029.

McManus, B., M. C. McCormick, D. Acevedo-Garcia, M. Ganz, and P. Hauser-Cram. 2009. The effect of state early intervention eligibility policy on participation among a cohort of young CSHCN. *Pediatrics* 124(Suppl 4):S368–S374.

McManus, B. M., A. C. Carle, D. Acevedo-Garcia, M. Ganz, P. Hauser-Cram, and M. C. McCormick. 2011. Social determinants of state variation in special education participation among preschoolers with developmental delays and disabilities. *Health & Place* 17(2):681–690.

McManus, B. M., Z. Richardson, M. Schenkman, N. Murphy, and E. H. Morrato. 2019. Timing and intensity of early intervention service use and outcomes among a safety-net population of children. *JAMA Network Open* 2(1):e187529.

Merkhofer, C., S. Sylvester, M. Zmuda, J. Jonassaint, L. M. De Castro, G. J. Kato, M. A. Butters, and E. M. Novelli. 2016. The impact of cognitive function on adherence to hydroxyurea therapy in patients with sickle cell disease. *Blood* 128(22):2493.

Minniti, C. P., and G. J. Kato. 2016. Critical reviews: How we treat sickle cell patients with leg ulcers. *American Journal of Hematology* 91(1):22–30.

Mody, P., A. Gupta, B. Bikdeli, J. F. Lampropulos, and K. Dharmarajan. 2012. Most important articles on cardiovascular disease among racial and ethnic minorities. *Circulation: Cardiovascular Quality and Outcomes* 5(4):e33–e41.

Moskowitz, J. T., E. Butensky, P. Harmatz, E. Vichinsky, M. B. Heyman, M. Acree, J. Wrubel, L. Wilson, and S. Folkman. 2007. Caregiving time in sickle cell disease: Psychological effects in maternal caregivers. *Pediatric Blood & Cancer* 48(1):64–71.

Mvundura, M., D. Amendah, P. L. Kavanagh, P. G. Sprinz, and S. D. Grosse. 2009. Health care utilization and expenditures for privately and publicly insured children with sickle cell disease in the United States. *Pediatric Blood & Cancer* 53(4):642–646.

Nelson, S. C., and H. W. Hackman. 2013. Race matters: Perceptions of race and racism in a sickle cell center. *Pediatric Blood & Cancer* 60(3):451–454.

Noll, R. B., J. M. McKellop, K. Vannatta, and K. Kalinyak. 1998. Child-rearing practices of primary care children with sickle cell disease: The I of professionals and caregivers. *Journal of Pediatric Psychology* 23(2):131–140.

NRC and IOM (National Research Council and Institute of Medicine). 2000. *From neurons to neighborhoods: The science of early childhood development.* Washington DC: National Academy Press.

Ola, B. A., S. J. Yates, and S. M. Dyson. 2016. Living with sickle cell disease and depression in Lagos, Nigeria: A mixed methods study. *Social Science and Medicine* 161:27–36.

Palermo, T. M., L. Schwartz, D. Drotar, and K. McGowan. 2002. Parental report of health-related quality of life in children with sickle cell disease. *Journal of Behavioral Medicine* 25(3):269–283.

Palermo, T. M., W. T. Zempsky, C. D. Dampier, C. Lalloo, A. S. Hundert, L. K. Murphy, N. Bakshi, and J. N. Stinson. 2018. iCanCope with sickle cell pain: Design of a randomized controlled trial of a smartphone and web-based pain self-management program for youth with sickle cell disease. *Contemporary Clinical Trials* 74:88–96.

Panepinto, J. A., K. M. O'Mahar, M. R. DeBaun, F. R. Loberiza, and J. P. Scott. 2005. Health-related quality of life in children with sickle cell disease: Child and parent perception. *British Journal of Haematology* 130(3):437–444.

Patel, A. B., and H. G. Pathan. 2005. Quality of life in children with sickle cell hemoglobin-opathy. *Indian Journal of Pediatrics* 72(7):567–571.

Peixoto, F., V. Monteiro, L. Mata, C. Sanches, J. Pipa, and L. S. Almeida. 2016. "To be or not to be retained ... that's the question!" Retention, self-esteem, self-concept, achievement goals, and grades. *Frontiers in Psychology* 7:1550.

Perimbeti, S. P., K. Y. Hou, S. Ramanathan, A. Woodard, D. Kyung, Q. Wang, P. A. Crilley, K. Ward, and M. Styler. 2018. The effect of health care disparities on complications and mortality in sickle cell disease. *Blood* 132(Suppl 1):5886.

Perry, E. L., P. A. Carter, H. A. Becker, A. A. Garcia, M. Mackert, and K. E. Johnson. 2017. Health literacy in adolescents with sickle cell disease. *Journal of Pediatric Nursing* 36:191–196.

Peterson, C. C., T. M. Palermo, E. Swift, A. Beebe, and D. Drotar. 2005. Assessment of psycho-educational needs in a clinical sample of children with sickle cell disease. *Children's Health Care* 34(2):133–148.

Preussler, J. M., S. H. Farnia, E. M. Denzen, and N. S. Majhail. 2014. Variation in Medicaid coverage for hematopoietic cell transplantation. *Journal of Oncology Practice* 10(4):e196–e200.

Prussien, K. V., L. C. Jordan, M. R. DeBaun, and B. E. Compas. 2019. Cognitive function in sickle cell disease across domains, cerebral infarct status, and the lifespan: A meta-analysis. *Journal of Pediatric Psychology* 44(8):948–958.

Richardson, Z. S., M. A. Khetani, E. Scully, J. Dooling-Litfin, N. J. Murphy, and B. M. McManus. 2019. Social and functional characteristics of receipt and service use intensity of core early intervention services. *Academic Pediatrics* 19(7):722–732.

Romley, J. A., A. K. Shah, P. J. Chung, M. N. Elliott, K. D. Vestal, and M. A. Schuster. 2017. Family-provided health care for children with special health care needs. *Pediatrics* 139(1):e20161287.

Rudowitz, R., R. Garfield, and E. Hinton. 2019. *10 things to know about Medicaid: Setting the facts straight.* Washington, DC: Kaiser Family Foundation.

Sanger, M., L. Jordan, S. Pruthi, M. Day, B. Covert, B. Merriweather, M. Rodeghier, M. DeBaun, and A. Kassim. 2016. Cognitive deficits are associated with unemployment in adults with sickle cell anemia. *Journal of Clinical and Experimental Neuropsychology* 38(6):661–671.

Savitt, T. L. 2002. *Medicine and slavery: The diseases and health care of blacks in antebellum Virginia.* Champaign, IL: University of Illinois Press.

Schatz, J. 2004. Brief report: Academic attainment in children with sickle cell disease. *Journal of Pediatric Psychology* 29(8):627–633.

Schatz, J., A. M. Schlenz, C. B. McClellan, E. S. Puffer, S. Hardy, M. Pfeiffer, and C. W. Roberts. 2015. Changes in coping, pain, and activity after cognitive–behavioral training: A randomized clinical trial for pediatric sickle cell disease using smartphones. *Clinical Journal of Pain* 31(6):536–547.

Schwartz, L. A., J. Radcliffe, and L. P. Barakat. 2009. Associates of school absenteeism in adolescents with sickle cell disease. *Pediatric Blood & Cancer* 52(1):92–96.

Siddiqui, S., K. Schunk, M. Batista, F. Adames, P. Ayala, B. Stix, J. Rodriguez, M. McCord, and N. S. Green. 2012. Awareness of sickle cell among people of reproductive age: Dominicans and African Americans in northern Manhattan. *Journal of Urban Health* 89(1):53–58.

Silver, A. 2015. NMDP transplant center network survey of payer policy issues. *Biology of Blood and Marrow Transplantation* 21(2):S362–S363.

SSA (Social Security Administration). n.d. Disability evaluation under Social Security. 7.00 Hematological disorders—Adult. In *Blue book. Disability evaluation under Social Security: Listing of impairments—Adult listings (Part A).* https://www.ssa.gov/disability/professionals/bluebook/7.00-HematologicalDisorders-Adult.htm (accessed January 17, 2019).

Staats, C., K. Capatosto, R. A. Wright and V. W. Jackson. 2016. *State of the science: Implicit bias review 2016.* Columbus, OH: Kirwan Institute for the Study of Race and Ethnicity, The Ohio State University.

Stevens, E. M., C. A. Patterson, Y. B. Li, K. Smith-Whitley, and L. P. Barakat. 2016. Mistrust of pediatric sickle cell disease clinical trials research. *American Journal of Preventive Medicine* 51(1 Suppl 1):S78–S86.

Strouse, J. J., K. Lobner, S. Lanzkron, and C. Haywood, Jr. 2013. NIH and national foundation expenditures for sickle cell disease and cystic fibrosis are associated with PubMed publications and FDA approvals. *Blood* 122(21):1739.

Tait, R. C., and J. T. Chibnall. 2014. Racial/ethnic disparities in the assessment and treatment of pain: Psychosocial perspectives. *American Psychologist* 69(2):131–141.

Teaching Tolerance. n.d. *Test yourself for hidden bias.* https://www.tolerance.org/professional-development/test-yourself-for-hidden-bias (accessed March 9, 2020).

Tewari, S., F. Piel, V. Brousse, B. P. D. Inusa, P. Telfer, S. Menzel, M. De Montalembert, K. Gardner, G. Fuller, S. L. Thein, and D. Rees. 2014. A multicentre study of environmental factors on the severity of sickle cell disease. *Blood* 124(21):4841.

Tewari, S., V. Brousse, F. B. Piel, S. Menzel, and D. C. Rees. 2015. Environmental determinants of severity in sickle cell disease. *Haematologica* 100(9):1108–1116.

The Joint Commission. 2016. Implicit bias in health care. *Quick Safety* 23:1–4.

Tolbert, J., K. Orgera, N. Singer, and A. Damico. 2019. *Key facts about the uninsured population.* http://files.kff.org/attachment/Issue-Brief-Key-Facts-about-the-Uninsured-Population (accessed September 29, 2020).

Tusuubira, S. K., R. Nakayinga, B. Mwambi, J. Odda, S. Kiconco, and A. Komuhangi. 2018. Knowledge, perception and practices towards sickle cell disease: A community survey among adults in Lubaga division, Kampala, Uganda. *BMC Public Health* 18(1):561.

Wakefield, E. O., J. M. Popp, L. P. Dale, J. P. Santanelli, A. Pantaleao, and W. T. Zempsky. 2017. Perceived racial bias and health-related stigma among youth with sickle cell disease. *Journal of Developmental and Behavioral Pediatrics* 38(2):129–134.

Wakefield, E. O., W. T. Zempsky, R. M. Puhl, and M. D. Litt. 2018. Conceptualizing pain-related stigma in adolescent chronic pain: A literature review and preliminary focus group findings. *Pain Reports* 3(Suppl 1):e679.

Weiss, M. G., and J. Ramakrishna. 2006. Stigma interventions and research for international health. *Lancet* 367(9509):536–538.

Weiss, M. G., J. Ramakrishna, and D. Somma. 2006. Health-related stigma: Rethinking concepts and interventions. *Psychology, Health & Medicine* 11(3):277–287.

Wesley, K. M., M. Zhao, Y. Carroll, and J. S. Porter. 2016. Caregiver perspectives of stigma associated with sickle cell disease in adolescents. *Journal of Pediatric Nursing* 31(1):55–63.

White, A. A. 2011. Diagnosis and treatment: The subconscious at work. In *Seeing patients: Unconscious bias in health care.* Cambridge, MA: Harvard University Press. Pp. 199–210.

Williams, H., R. N. S. Silva, D. Cline, C. Freiermuth, and P. Tanabe. 2018. Social and behavioral factors in sickle cell disease: Employment predicts decreased health care utilization. *Journal of Health Care for the Poor and Underserved* 29(2):814–829.

Wolfson, J. A., S. M. Schrager, R. Khanna, T. D. Coates, and M. D. Kipke. 2012. Sickle cell disease in California: Sociodemographic predictors of emergency department utilization. *Pediatric Blood & Cancer* 58(1):66–73.

Wyatt, R. 2013. Pain and ethnicity. *Virtual Mentor* 15(5):449–454.

Yang Y., A. K. Shah, M. Watson, and V. N. Mankad. 1997. Comparison of costs to the health sector of comprehensive and episodic health care for sickle cell disease patients. *Public Health Reports* 110(1):80–86.

Yarboi, J., B. E. Compas, G. H. Brody, D. White, J. Rees Patterson, K. Ziara, and A. King. 2017. Association of social-environmental factors with cognitive function in children with sickle cell disease. *Child Neuropsychology* 23(3):343–360.

Zempsky, W. T. 2010. Evaluation and treatment of sickle cell pain in the emergency department: Paths to a better future. *Clinical Pediatric Emergency Medicine* 11(4):265–273.

Zhang, W., S. Lyman, C. Boutin-Foster, M. L. Parks, T.-J. Pan, A. Lan, and Y. Ma. 2016. Racial and ethnic disparities in utilization rate, hospital volume, and perioperative outcomes after total knee arthroplasty. *Journal of Bone and Joint Surgery* 98(15):1243–1252.

Ziadni, M. S., C. A. Patterson, E. R. Pulgaron, M. R. Robinson, and L. P. Barakat. 2011. Health-related quality of life and adaptive behaviors of adolescents with sickle cell disease: Stress processing moderators. *Journal of Clinical Psychology in Medical Settings* 18(4):335–344.

3

Screening, Registries, and Surveillance

The reason for collecting, analyzing, and disseminating information on a disease is to control that disease. (Foege et al., 1976)

—Mary H. (Open Session Panelist)

Chapter Summary

- While newborn screening is mandated in all 50 states, the District of Columbia, Puerto Rico, Guam, and the U.S. Virgin Islands, it is ineffective in capturing individuals living with sickle cell disease (SCD) who were born prior to universal screening or outside of the United States and its territories.
- Follow-up for positive sickle cell trait and SCD screens varies greatly by state; there is a need for standardization in follow-up (including who receives and communicates positive results) to ensure that all individuals with SCD across the United States are getting needed care as early as possible.
- Registries and public health surveillance systems hold great promise to provide valuable information about the SCD population—who they are and what their care and research needs are. Current efforts to collect these data need to be standardized and scaled at the national level.
- Attempts to gather data about the SCD population must be governed by strict patient privacy and confidentiality rules to ensure that the data are not used to discriminate against minority patients, who have a long history of mistreatment in the medical system.

Throughout this report, there are descriptions of gaps in information and understanding about sickle cell disease (SCD) and sickle cell trait (SCT), the populations living with the disease and carrier status, the treatments used, the impact of SCD on the health care system, access to health care and other services, health outcomes, and the overall impact of SCD and SCT. To address what the committee perceives to be significant problems for those living with SCD, it will be necessary to collect reliable information to define the problems clearly, promote measurable changes to address them, and monitor the progress of these interventions and changes in the health system.

Data are often collected to gain insights into defined populations receiving clinical interventions or participating in local programs to understand outcomes across an entire health care system. Such analyses are of high value in generalizing to subpopulations with SCD who are similar to those studied, and these research efforts should be supported and promoted. This chapter focuses on efforts to ethically and efficiently collect reliable, high-utility data from whole populations or representative samples thereof and to use those data in improving health and health outcomes. Such data may have been originally gathered for other purposes (as with newborn screening [NBS] data or passive surveillance systems drawn from existing data sources), or efforts may be made to collect the most useful information from a wide variety of persons affected by SCD, as with a registry.

This chapter discusses these approaches and combined approaches and presents models of data gathering and use from other, similar diseases to provide context. All of the data gathering and investigations described here have the same goals: to better understand and thus be able to more effectively address the health, health outcomes, quality of life (QOL), and challenges to receiving quality care that face those with SCD and to better understand and advise those individuals on health and reproductive decision making.

The most successful example of the collection and use of population-wide data on SCD is NBS for SCD and SCT in the United States, which is now universal across all 50 states and the District of Columbia. NBS allows parents with SCD-positive newborns to gain quick access to knowledgeable hematologic care providers and should ensure that children receive standard-of-care treatment, such as prophylactic penicillin to prevent sepsis, appropriate immunizations, SCD screening to assess the risk of stroke, and hydroxyurea to reduce complications. NBS for SCT should help ensure that those with carrier status receive appropriate information as they reach reproductive age, and it may help health care providers monitor for health conditions associated with SCT. The promise of NBS is not consistently fulfilled, however. There is more to be done in sharing and translating positive results to caregivers and health care providers, and gaps remain in follow-up care.

Registries and surveillance systems have been in development for SCD for some time, and they show great promise for capturing much needed information about those living with the disease, their care, and their outcomes. But there are challenges, merits, and deficits in collecting data for these important purposes. Furthermore, all efforts to gather health information face formidable ethical challenges and considerations; this chapter briefly discusses those considerations and concludes with suggestions for improving the collection, capture, and use of data from the different types of systems discussed.

This chapter is concerned with three approaches to gathering and analyzing information on those living with SCD and SCT. All three are ways of understanding the problem of SCD or SCT, but they address the disease and trait through different lenses and methodologies. The chapter uses the following definitions:

- *Screening* is the act of identifying the presence or absence of a disease or carrier state in a person. With respect to SCD in the United States, such screening typically takes place either at birth (NBS) or in the prenatal period. Screening may also be done for SCT at birth or any time throughout the life course. Symptomatic people who were not screened at birth may receive diagnostic testing for SCD.
- A *disease registry* is a system of data collection and communications with individuals affected by a particular disease. Such systems may be sponsored by government, disease advocacy organizations, pharmaceutical or device companies, or other entities. Patients typically consent to participate and share identifying and health information with the sponsor. Sponsors may provide benefits, such as education and information, access to health records, or information about clinical trials.
- *Public health surveillance* has been defined as "the ongoing, systematic collection, analysis, and interpretation of health-related data needed for the planning, implementation, and evaluation of public health practice" (CDC, 1986, p. ii). In particular, surveillance is aimed at evaluating and improving health at the population level and supporting and improving research and the care provided at the individual and clinical levels. Public health surveillance of SCD in the United States is typically conducted by state governments.

SCREENING FOR SCD AND SCT

Screening has long been recognized as an important tool for early disease detection, and as technological advances have improved the ability to screen for an increasing number of diseases, screening rationales and criteria have also evolved. Even with these advances, however, it remains important to exercise caution and judgment beforehand and to make sure that there are adequate resources for follow-up and treatment (NRC, 1975; Wilson and Jungner, 1968). During the early developmental stages of genetic and other types of screening, the proposed criteria typically included the importance of the condition, acceptability of the treatment, availability of care facilities, cost effectiveness, and an agreement on the progression of the condition (Andermann et al., 2008; Wilson and Jungner, 1968).

Over the past 40 years, researchers and providers have adapted these original criteria to reflect new knowledge of genetic diseases in order to increase the effectiveness of screening programs (Andermann et al., 2008; Grosse et al., 2010; Simopoulos and Committee for the Study of Inborn Errors of Metabolism, 2009). Newer criteria tend to emphasize equity, informed choice and autonomy, and evidence-based criteria (Andermann et al., 2008; Ross, 2012). More specifically, newer adaptations of the 1960s era Wilson and Jungner criteria take into account the effects on family members and parents, the importance of screening for rare diseases despite unfavorable cost–benefit analyses, the need for confidentiality concerning trait/disease status, and genetic counseling (Grosse et al., 2010). Although current programs vary in their methodologies and outputs, many describe their aim as providing results that can inform future reproductive choices, provide long-term care, and offer implications for family members (Andermann et al., 2008). The shift away from broad, blanket programs covering everyone to ensuring personalized, informed choice from all participants has sparked ethical debate and will continue to shape future genetic screening criteria (Grosse et al., 2010; NRC, 1975).

Types of Screening for SCD and SCT

The most common methods of screening include hemoglobin electrophoresis, isoelectric focusing (IEF), high-performance liquid chromatography (HPLC), and sickle solubility tests (Naik and Haywood, 2015). These tests all involve dried blood spots or whole liquid blood from a heel prick and check for red blood cell (RBC) count or hemoglobin variants. Electrophoresis is a classic method for identifying hemoglobinopathies; it uses an electric field to separate hemoglobins based on their charge. Further separation is possible by changing the pH and support medium. This method is the cheapest, but it is time and labor intensive (McGann and Hoppe, 2017). IEF and HPLC both separate hemoglobin based on net charge on a gel medium at particular pH levels. IEF requires more labor and time, whereas HPLC has rapid output and can be automated to run thousands of samples in minutes. However, HPLC is also cost intensive and requires high levels of technical expertise (McGann and Hoppe, 2017; Naik and Haywood, 2015). Because of issues with false positives and false negatives, confirmatory testing following the initial screening is generally required (APHL and CDC, 2015). Sickle solubility tests may be unreliable and are known to yield false negatives in patients with severe anemia, in those with sickle hemoglobin (HbS) below a specific percentage, or in patients with high levels of fetal hemoglobin (HbF) (e.g., newborns less than 6 months old) (CDC, n.d.; Tubman and Field, 2015). Due to the cost and resources required for IEF, electrophoresis, and HPLC, they are usually not feasible options in low-resource settings. Point-of-care testing methods are being developed and may be particularly advantageous in both the United States and in settings with limited resources (McGann and Hoppe, 2017; Steele et al., 2019).

Screening for SCT and SCD involve similar sample collections; however, certain techniques are required to differentiate between SCT and SCD by discriminating among hemoglobin variants (Naik and Haywood, 2015). Solubility testing only detects the presence or absence of sickled hemoglobin and thus cannot discriminate between SCT and SCD (Tubman and Field, 2015). IEF, electrophoresis, and HPLC quantify hemoglobin and so can discriminate, making them the primary methods for NBS programs and confirmatory testing. Because these methods are more costly, they are usually not the first choice in low-resource settings. A study in Uganda found that the sickling test followed by confirmation with electrophoresis was a sensitive and cost-effective method for screening children (Okwi et al., 2009). Because of gaps in follow-up and the optimal communication of results both in the United States and globally, there is a pressing need for a point-of-care testing method to deliver results within minutes to hours, rather than days to weeks (McGann and Hoppe, 2017). Several point-of-care tests with high sensitivity and specificity in SCT and SCD detection have been developed in recent years and used in various low-resource countries (Alvarez et al., 2019; Nnodu et al., 2019; Segbena et al., 2018). Some continue to have the barrier of being unable to detect hemoglobins aside from HbS or normal hemoglobin, HbA (Mukherjee et al., 2019).

Prenatal Screening

Prenatal diagnoses and other means of determining whether a fetus has SCD are medical procedures designed to inform parents so that they may prepare for raising the child or decide whether to terminate a pregnancy. In the United States, prenatal screening for SCD is not universal, and its occurrence depends on individual desires, insurance coverage, and the family's history of disease (Gallo et al., 2010). The procedures used as part of prenatal screening include amniocentesis and chorionic villus sampling (CVS), both of which are invasive and conducted early in the pregnancy— between the 10th and 12th week of the pregnancy for CVS and the 14th and 20th week for amniocentesis (Yenilmez and Tuli, 2016). These tests pose minor risks of miscarriage or complications; researchers have piloted new methods of non-invasive prenatal diagnosis, such as cell-free fetal DNA tests where fetal DNA that is found in the mother's blood is tested for genetic conditions for use in prenatal SCD diagnosis. Infants born with SCD after such screening are identified and recorded as a part of routine NBS in the United States.

The results of prenatal screening and information about whether the pregnancy came to term may or may not be transferred to the state's NBS program; practices differ by state. For example, California has a sickle cell surveillance program which compiles data from numerous sources, including NBS programs, Medicaid, emergency department (ED) admissions, clinic care, and vital records (Feuchtbaum et al., 2013). While prenatal diagnosis can be an important part of early pregnancy care, it is not yet useful as a data source for tracking SCD at a population level due to the small sample size and lack of integration with other medical records (Housten et al., 2016; Savage et al., 2015).

Newborn Screening

Because of the high morbidity and mortality associated with SCD, universal NBS offers substantial payoffs in addressing comorbidities and reducing mortality (Vichinsky et al., 1988). NBS followed by confirmatory screening is recommended by 2 months of age so that, if necessary, it is possible to initiate treatment and follow-up care promptly. Early prophylactic treatment with penicillin is essential to combat what would otherwise be a high rate of mortality from infections (Lin, 2009). More generally, it is crucial to establish care early in life to manage complications and build a continuum of care.

Among U.S. territories NBS began in the U.S. Virgin Islands in 1987 and in Puerto Rico in 1977 (Morales et al., 2009). By 2006 universal NBS screening was implemented in all 50 states and the District of Columbia (Benson and Therrell, 2010). Today, NBS has been highly successful in most states, providing critical information to parents, pediatricians, and pediatric hematology care providers that enables young children to avoid most of the severe complications, which are major contributors to infant and childhood mortality (AAP Newborn Screening Task Force, 2000). In particular, the high rate of uptake of prophylactic penicillin for young children has saved countless children; thus, universal NBS has proven to be a cost-effective, life-saving intervention in the United States (El-Haj and Hoppe, 2018). This screening can also provide valuable information on the incidence of SCD in that jurisdiction. On the other hand, screening is usually not intended to be longitudinal, nor does it capture information on treatments, complications, or other health outcomes for those diagnosed. NBS is also expensive, but the cost is typically shared by state agencies and insurers, and it is seen to have a reasonable cost–benefit ratio in lives saved and health care resources conserved by keeping children healthy.

In most states, NBS also identifies newborns who are SCT carriers. Although it was initially thought that SCT status had virtually no clinical implications beyond reproductive decision making, recent studies have shown that some individuals with SCT are at risk for a variety of clinical complications (Alvarez, 2017; Alvarez et al., 2015; Elliott and Bruner, 2019; Naik and Haywood, 2015; Shetty and Matrana, 2014) (further addressed in Chapter 4). These complications include exertional rhabdomyolysis (muscle breakdown), cardiac dysfunction, sudden death, chronic renal disease, cancer, splenic infarction, and venous thromboembolism (Key et al., 2015; Naik and Haywood, 2015; Naik et al., 2018). Therefore, knowledge of carrier status is important to increase individuals' awareness of these rare but serious potential complications and to help guide reproductive decisions in adulthood. Unfortunately, the transfer of knowledge from a state NBS program, parents, or providers to the teens and young adults who ultimately need it to make informed life choices is not systematic. Promoting knowledge of SCT carrier status in young adults should be a high priority, but no states are currently known to track the health status or reproductive outcomes of those with SCT.

SCD-related legislation and programs and federal funding vary by state. Studies show that 18 states had no legislation and that states received funding from a variety of federal agencies such as the National Institutes of Health (NIH), Health Resources and Services Administration (HRSA), and Centers for Disease Control and Prevention (CDC) (Benson and Therrell, 2010; Minkovitz et al., 2016).

According to information available from the Association of Public Health Laboratories' (APHL's) website, roughly half of U.S. states conduct some long-term follow-up care coordination when NBS identifies SCD (NewSTEPs, 2020). Practices vary widely, however, and persons with SCD are typically tracked up to 5 years—but only if they stay within the state of birth (APHL and CDC, 2015; NewSTEPs, 2020). Furthermore, there are no standard requirements for data storage for any specified length of time. For example, the Maryland Department of Health is required by law to keep newborn samples for 25 years so that tests can be replicated, if needed (Maryland Department of Health, n.d.). By comparison, dried blood spots in Texas may be kept by law for 2 years unless a parent provides consent for longer storage (Texas Department of State Health Services, 2019). California's surveillance program was able to track individuals with SCD by location and report the prevalence of complications, health care use, and distribution of haplotypes from records between 2004 and 2008 (Feuchtbaum et al., 2013). Challenges in synthesizing all of these data include variability in data source, duplicate records, and limited access to data sources conducive to research. Similar long-term program development in different states may face these same challenges of fragmentation and variability.

These inadequacies can be tied to the structural racism surrounding SCD, which results in fewer funding sources and incentives to develop interventions (Bediako and King-Meadows, 2016). Furthermore, there is high variability in state screening programs, although it is unclear whether this is influenced by differences in prevalence across states or specific structural factors (Minkovitz et al., 2016).

One study of postpartum women found a poor understanding of NBS, indicating a need to educate parents about NBS and its importance (Lang et al., 2009). In states with few state-led initiatives or policies, individuals, families, and the general public may not have a clear understanding of the necessity for screening and appropriate follow-up.

Subpopulation Screening for SCT

In light of the emerging knowledge of complications that may be associated with SCT, as discussed in Chapter 4, there are various subpopulations for whom screening for SCT makes particular sense.

A key subpopulation is pregnant women, given the current technologies that allow for genetic testing before birth. The discussion earlier in this chapter established the importance and opportunities to ensure that pregnant women are educated about SCD and SCT and know their status. Studies have found that pregnant women generally fall into three categories: those who wish to carry the child to term regardless of status, those who choose medical termination of a pregnancy with positive results, and those who do not wish to be screened at all (Gallo et al., 2010; Smith and Aguirre, 2012). The women who refuse screening may be basing this choice on the fear of being rejected by their partner, their religious beliefs, or the stigma surrounding discussing SCT status openly (Asgharian et al., 2003).[1]

Exertional sickling and exertional heat illnesses (EHIs) are also of great concern, particularly for members of the U.S. military. In the 1970s, the first military cases of exercise-induced death without a pre-existing condition were identified and classified as sudden death induced by sickling (Jones et al., 1970). Early studies of military recruits found that those with SCT had an increased risk of exercise-induced sudden death in basic training (Charache, 1988; Kark et al., 1987).

In recent years, as knowledge of the risks associated with SCT has grown, debates about how best to handle training for recruits with SCT

---

[1] Both studies collected data on women in the United Kingdom rather than the United States.

have resumed (Mitchell, 2018). Case reports of the deaths of two soldiers with undetected SCT who collapsed as they attempted to finish a 2-mile run demonstrated that rhabdomyolysis caused by intense exercise could be fatal (Ferster and Eichner, 2012). A study of active-duty soldiers with SCT found an increased risk for exertional rhabdomyolysis, similar in magnitude to the effect of tobacco use (Nelson et al., 2016).

Currently, the U.S. military has no standardized protocol for dealing with service members with SCT; Air Force and Navy recruits wear armbands to indicate that they have SCT throughout training, for example, whereas Marine Corps recruits are not identified (Webber and Witkop, 2014). The U.S. Army currently uses SCT screening only for specific combat deployments and specialties, such as high-altitude work (Nelson et al., 2016). Furthermore, there are no protocols for handling physical activity or mitigating risk for identified individuals. Instead, the Army uses broad precautions to reduce the risk of dehydration and EHIs in all military personnel.

Even though the risks to military members with SCT are well understood, mandated screening is a highly contentious topic because of concerns about discrimination and stigmatization and because of doubts concerning the benefits of screening (Kark et al., 2010; Nelson et al., 2016; Singer et al., 2018b; Webber and Witkop, 2014). The theorized benefits of universal SCT testing include a reduction in exercise-induced sickling deaths, increased knowledge of SCT complications, and decreases in risky behaviors that can lead to exercise-induced illness. Proponents of mandatory military screening argue that knowledge of SCT status could lead recruits to change their behavior; an aware trainee would be more likely to end a workout early rather than persisting through the pain (Jones et al., 1970; Webber and Witkop, 2014). It is however important to note that at least one study of 48,000 soldiers, 3,500 of whom had SCT, found that while carrier status is associated with a higher risk of exertional rhabdomyolysis, it is not associated with a higher risk of death (Nelson et al., 2016).

National Collegiate Athletic Association (NCAA) student-athletes are another subpopulation targeted for SCT screening. In people with SCD, extreme exertion and heat and high altitudes can lead to sickling, which may present as normal exhaustion or heat-related illness (Anderson et al., 2011; Baker et al., 2018) but can result in mortality if it is not detected and treated appropriately. As discussed above, intense exercise can also lead to exertional rhabdomyolysis (Nelson et al., 2016). Between 2000 and 2011 there were 16 non-traumatic football deaths among NCAA athletes, of which 10 were attributed to exertional sickling (Anderson et al., 2011). Furthermore, in an examination of NCAA student-athletes, SCT was found to be associated with a 37-fold higher risk for exertional death (Harmon et al., 2012). Concerns over exertion-related deaths in

student-athletes led to an NCAA screening policy designed to identify SCT
and prevent catastrophic consequences from acute sickling events associated with physical exertion.

A 2018 survey of NCAA staff and athletes found that staff members
were more supportive of SCT screening than were student-athletes (Baker
et al., 2018). The athletes' concerns included relevance to their racial status,
fear of being treated differently by coaches, and poor understanding of the
necessity of screening. At least one student felt that athletes should know
their trait status before college, rendering college screening unnecessary.
In addition, many white athletes felt that they did not need to be screened
because they believed SCT did not affect white individuals. The study also
revealed various challenges to implementation, including the financial costs
to institutions, variability in implementation and follow-up, and long wait
times for the results (Baker et al., 2018). The coaches were most concerned
that waiting for the test results would contribute to time lost for playing,
conditioning, and practice. Several organizations have also raised concerns
about athlete screening.

In 2012 the American Society of Hematology (ASH) issued a policy
statement that opposed mandatory screening by the NCAA, citing concerns
over stigmatizing individuals and recommending universal interventions to
prevent exertion-related deaths instead, regardless of carrier status. Another
frequently raised concern is genetic discrimination, especially because the
NCAA is not covered under federal genetic anti-discrimination laws (Jordan
et al., 2011). Invasions of genetic privacy are also possible, given that mandatory testing of athletes reveals their genetic status and information on the
carrier status of their parents and relatives (Jordan et al., 2011). A recent
study found that mandated screening could identify only up to one-third
of individuals with SCT who were at risk for EHIs (Singer et al., 2018a).
Critics of universal screening point to potential inefficiency, discrimination,
and the lack of evidence-based research to support such a policy (Singer
et al., 2018a; Webber and Witkop, 2014).

Missed Opportunities for Screening

There are specific groups that can be—and often are—missed within
the spectrum of SCD care, especially screening. For instance, immigrants
to the United States are not often screened in their respective countries,
and the United States lacks a cohesive policy on screening immigrants for
sickle cell status, so data are limited on the follow-up of immigrant adults
and children (Faro et al., 2016). In some countries, such as Germany, rising
immigration rates corresponding with increasing prevalence of SCD have
prompted calls for increased screening of immigrants and general education for providers (Kunz et al., 2017). The ethical and legal implications of

such policies are currently being debated, as the German Genetic Testing Act allows individuals the right to know—and to not know—their individual genetic status for a particular disease. Furthermore, health care in Germany is not currently set up to handle SCD care, and thus a functioning infrastructure must be developed before adopting any SCD-specific screening policy (Frommel et al., 2014). In the Netherlands a study found that approximately 27 percent of new pediatric patients were immigrants, a majority of whom were diagnosed in the Netherlands for the first time (Peters et al., 2010). The lack of data on SCD and SCT in immigrant populations is a known information gap. Global immigration patterns should inform policies in the United States and other countries in order to effectively screen and treat immigrants in need of care and follow-up.

In addition, individuals born in the United States before the adoption of NBS protocols are at risk of falling through the cracks if they are not screened as adults. Research shows that most adults are not aware of their personal SCT status and that many do not wish to be screened, indicating that there is a need to reach out to older populations to assess their risk (Harrison et al., 2017). In the case of individuals unaware of their status, it may be effective to have them screened by ED providers when they present for any condition (Wright et al., 1994).

Adult screening for SCT can be problematic. For example, researchers found that in St. Louis "no coordinated agency exists to provide systematic trait testing or genetic counseling for individuals at risk for SCT" (Housten et al., 2016, p. 2). The same researchers also found that 10.5 percent of adults recruited at eight different community sites who were asked to participate in a screening test for SCT declined (Housten et al., 2016). Additionally, follow-up with genetic counseling did not routinely occur; in the sample only 56 percent of those tested chose to meet with a genetic counselor. Study participants under the age of 30 were least likely to follow up with genetic counseling (Housten et al., 2016).

COMMUNICATING SCREENING RESULTS

Despite the importance of effectively screening and following up on SCD and SCT screening results, there is a notable lack of guidelines and policies advising providers on how to effectively communicate disease or carrier status to affected people or their parents. Initially, NBS was not designed to communicate carrier status, and identifying SCT was solely a by-product of SCD testing (Pecker and Naik, 2018). Consequently, there was little direction given to clinicians about communicating SCT status discovered during NBS. Today, the communication of neonatal screening results on SCD (and on SCT where conducted) varies by state, with many states providing the results to providers but not to parents.

Once a dried blood spot from NBS is sent to the laboratory, the tests are generally performed within 72 hours, followed, if necessary, by confirmatory testing. The results are then sent to the primary care provider (PCP), who is left to decide the appropriate way to communicate with the family and specialists (El-Haj and Hoppe, 2018). One study of NBS programs found that only 40 percent and 37 percent of families were directly informed of their child's SCD or SCT status, respectively (Kavanagh et al., 2008). However, most NBS programs shared results with primary care clinicians (100 percent and 88 percent for SCD and SCT, respectively) and with the hospitals of birth (73 percent and 63 percent for SCD and SCT, respectively) so that they could give the results to the families (Kavanagh et al., 2008). Family notification rates varied widely from state to state, indicating greater issues with communicating screening results in some birth locations.

Effective communication of SCD and SCT testing results is extremely important because parents who discover that their child tested positive will often experience mental distress, ranging from anxiety to depression (Farrell and Christopher, 2013). Studies indicate that providers may use a great deal of scientific jargon, which hampers parental understanding and limits effective decision making (Farrell and Christopher, 2013). It has been suggested that communicating SCT status to parents could be more effective if PCPs treated SCT as more than an incidental finding and if an effort was made to connect providers with families through calls (Christopher et al., 2012). Following up on screening results has been found to require minimal effort if NBS programs have adequate funding to connect families with local providers.

In addition, a community-based screening program was found to be effective in increasing knowledge of SCT/SCD status and increasing the likelihood of follow-up genetic counseling, indicating that such interventions may be beneficial if tailored to specific communities (Housten et al., 2016). State programs looking to build patient registries and increase their capacity for patient–data linkage have explored linking medical records (Abhyankar et al., 2010; Hinton et al., 2014; Posnack, 2015). Health care professionals are now focusing on standardizing an approach to care due to the current gaps in patient follow-up, the lack of information on the impact of screening and treatment, and the absence of a cohesive policy on communicating genetic screening results (Abhyankar et al., 2010; Hinton et al., 2014, 2016; Hoots, 2010). This standardization will help to reduce miscommunications among laboratories, providers, and patients and improve care. One proposed method would be to link individuals' screening results to their birth certificates (Hinton et al., 2016; Posnack, 2015; Zuckerman, 2009). This could potentially decrease the loss to follow-up that occurs across state lines. It would also provide records of population-level information and allow for potential access to data on usage and socioeconomic information. Although current screening communication is inadequate in terms of its outreach and quality, standardizing protocols for screening and collecting data could improve the efficiency of care and communication.

State-Level Approaches to Screening and Communicating Results

State-funded screening programs usually source money from third-party programs, such as Medicaid, Title V, or federal allocations (Blood-Siegfried et al., 2006). This results in great variability in screening and communication procedures (Blood-Siegfried et al., 2006; Hoff and Hoyt, 2006; Kavanagh et al., 2008). As Table 3-1 shows, this variation means that numerous stakeholders are not informed about SCT and SCD results, including hematologists, PCPs, and families (Kavanagh et al., 2008). Of those providers who do communicate results, a small percentage report that they lack the competency to adequately do so.

The National Academies SCD committee contacted APHL to obtain updated results on states' follow-up procedures for SCD- and SCT-positive screens. In response, APHL fielded a brief survey (see Appendix D) to members of their hemoglobinopathies workgroup and obtained responses from six state NBS programs (Colorado, Connecticut, Florida, New Jersey, Tennessee, and Washington). All of the programs that took part in the survey had standardized protocols (written/formal versus informal) for SCD screening, turnaround time for communicating results, and follow-up (see Appendix D). Although communication protocols varied, all programs had a turnaround time ranging from 1 day to a few weeks. Furthermore, 98–100 percent of babies who screened positive for SCD received follow-up within 1 year. All six NBS programs had a standardized protocol for informing parents of their children's SCT status, and five programs had a required turnaround time (1–6 weeks).

The five NBS programs with follow-up protocols for SCT were not able to provide the percent of newborns who screen positive and receive follow-up in 1 year. These programs distribute letters to parents or PCPs or both, and the NBS program does not receive additional information after that. One program provides SCT results to requests from any properly authorized university or organization. These preliminary findings show possible improvements in screening procedures since 2008. Larger and more comprehensive studies are needed to confirm this and to fill the knowledge gaps about state NBS screening procedures. Further research will also help identify areas that still need to be addressed to optimize the quality and impact of NBS.

TABLE 3-1 Stakeholders Informed by Newborn Screening Programs

State	Sickle Cell Disease	Sickle Cell Trait
Alabama	PCP, heme., hospital, sickle cell org.	PCP, public health nurse, sickle cell org.
Alaska	PCP[a], heme.,[a] hospital[b]	PCP,[a] hospital[b]
Arizona	PCP, heme., family, sickle cell org.	PCP, family, sickle cell org.
Arkansas	PCP, heme., hospital	PCP, family, hospital
California	PCP, heme., family, hospital	PCP, family, hospital
Colorado	PCP, heme., family	PCP
Connecticut	PCP, heme., family	PCP, family, hospital, sickle cell org
Delaware	PCP, heme., family, hospital, Child Development Watch (with permission)	PCP, family, hospital
District of Columbia	PCP, heme., family, hospital, sickle cell org.	PCP, heme., family, hospital, sickle cell org.
Florida	PCP, heme., family, hospital	Family
Georgia (Grady)	PCP, public health nurse	
Georgia (MCG)	PCP, public health nurse	
Hawaii	PCP,[a] heme.,[a] public health RN,[a] family,[a] hospital,[b] Hawaii Community Genetics	PCP,[a] hospital[b]
Idaho	PCP,[a] heme.,[a] hospital[b]	PCP,[a] hospital[b]
Illinois	PCP, sickle cell org.	PCP, sickle cell org.
Indiana	PCP, heme., family, hospital, sickle cell org.	PCP, sickle cell org.
Iowa	PCP, heme., hospital	PCP, heme., hospital
Kansas	PCP, family	PCP
Kentucky	PCP, heme., hospital	PCP, hospital
Louisiana	PCP, heme., family, hospital, sickle cell org.	Family
Maine	PCP, heme., hospital	PCP, heme., hospital
Maryland	PCP, heme., family, hospital[b]	PCP,[b] hospital[b]
Massachusetts	PCP, heme., hospital	PCP, family, hospital
Michigan	PCP, heme., family, hospital, sickle cell org	PCP, family, hospital, sickle cell org.
Minnesota	PCP, heme., hospital	PCP, hospital
Mississippi	PCP, heme., public health RN, family, hospital[b]	PCP, public health RN, family, hospital[b]
Missouri	PCP, heme., family, hospital	PCP, heme., family, hospital

TABLE 3-1 Continued

State	Sickle Cell Disease	Sickle Cell Trait
Montana	PCP[b]	PCP[b]
Nebraska	PCP, heme., hospital	PCP, family, hospital
Nevada	PCP,[a] heme.,[a] hospital[a]	PCP[a]
New Hampshire	PCP	PCP
New Jersey	PCP, heme., family, hospital[b]	family, hospital[b]
New Mexico	PCP, heme., public health RN, family, hospital, sickle cell org.	PCP, public health RN, hospital, sickle cell org.
New York	PCP, heme., public health RN, hospital	PCP, hospital
North Carolina	PCP, sickle cell org., sickle cell educator	PCP,[b] sickle cell org.,[b] sickle cell educator
North Dakota	PCP,[a] heme.[a]	PCP,[a] heme.[a]
Ohio	PCP, heme., hospital	PCP, hospital, sickle cell org
Oklahoma	PCP, heme., hospital, sickle cell org.	PCP, family, sickle cell org
Oregon	PCP, heme., hospital	PCP, hospital
Pennsylvania	PCP, heme., hospital	PCP[a], heme.[a]
Rhode Island	PCP, heme.	PCP
South Carolina	PCP, hospital	PCP, hospital, sickle cell org.[b]
South Dakota	PCP[a], heme.,[a] hospital[b]	PCP,[a] heme.,[a] hospital[b]
Tennessee	PCP, heme, family, hospital	PCP, family, hospital
Texas	PCP, public health RN, family, hospital	PCP,[b] hospital[b]
Utah	PCP, hospital	PCP, hospital
Vermont	PCP, heme., family	PCP, hospital
Virginia	PCP, heme., hospital,[b] sickle cell org.	PCP, family
Washington	PCP, heme., hospital, sickle cell org.	PCP, hospital, sickle cell org.
West Virginia	PCP, heme.	PCP, family
Wisconsin	PCP, heme., public health RN, hospital	PCP, hospital
Wyoming	PCP, heme., family	PCP

NOTE: heme. = hematologist; MCG = Medical College of Georgia; org. = organization; PCP = primary care provider; RN = registered nurse.

[a] Contracts with outside laboratory/program.

[b] Information provided by state laboratory only.

SOURCE: Kavanagh et al., 2008.

A lack of funds can also be a significant barrier to screening; the patient can incur a cost ranging from relatively low (e.g., $10) to a high of $130, depending on the state (Blood-Siegfried et al., 2006). Budget cuts to health programs mean that state-level priorities for SCD- and SCT-related activities are low compared with other public health investments, and improving the quality of neonatal care for SCD may require greater advocacy (Minkovitz et al., 2016).

THE USE OF SCREENING DATA

NBS data can be used in a variety of ways to improve the lives of individuals with SCD and SCT. Doing so will require that the information is made available to all of those who should receive it, including family members and relevant clinicians, and that the people who do receive it understand what it means and are equipped to make effective decisions based on it.

Genetic Counseling

If parents are to understand the implications of SCD and SCT for their children and themselves, it is important that they receive screening for hemoglobinopathy and genetic counseling (Chudleigh et al., 2016). As noted in the previous section, while providers, hospitals, or even families may be informed of a child's status, there is little indication for how these individuals are referred to genetic counselors or for communicating information about their status from birth through adolescence and adulthood, especially for SCT (Taylor et al., 2014). A study conducted in Michigan to examine the prevalence of genetic counseling provided by PCPs found that the physicians surveyed reported that they were more likely to provide some genetic counseling to parents of children who are cystic fibrosis carriers (CFCs) than to parents of children with SCT (92 percent versus 80 percent; $p < 0.01$) (Moseley et al., 2013). Parents of children with CFC were also more likely to be counseled by genetic counselors or specialty centers than parents of children with SCT (85 percent versus 60 percent; $p < 0.01$) (Moseley et al., 2013). A lack of available counselors, parents declining counseling, and the physician not recommending counseling were all cited as reasons that contributed to the disparities.

Reproductive Decision Making

Because SCD is life threatening, it has important implications for reproductive decisions. With the advent of prenatal genetic testing for SCD, parents with SCT can now learn relatively early in a pregnancy whether their child will have SCD, which offers them options, including medical termination. Parents must carefully weigh this decision based on their assessment of their potential child's likely QOL and their personal values. Both prenatal and postnatal counseling must be provided appropriately, taking into account the child's SCD and SCT status and specific follow-up and treatment needs. Whether or not parents choose to terminate an SCD-positive fetus, they should receive appropriate counseling to deal with the impacts of their decision (Pecker and Naik, 2018).

There are various barriers to parents making informed decisions. One issue is the vast amount of misinformation and misunderstanding that surrounds the topic, some of which may be perpetuated by health care providers. A Hispanic participant in a qualitative interpretive meta-synthesis study reported that her health care provider had told her that SCD was an African American disease (Smith and Aguirre, 2012). Additionally, some men denied their SCT status and tried to convince women that they were not positive, perhaps because of the history of discrimination associated with the disease and a fear of stigma if their status was revealed (Smith and Aguirre, 2012). One study that examined health beliefs regarding counseling and testing found that African American women strongly believed in the severity of SCD and the benefits of counseling but did not believe that they were at risk of having a child with SCD (Gustafson et al., 2007). Genetic counseling offers a missed opportunity for educating individuals with SCT and their families and providers about the benefits of counseling and standardizing referrals to counselors.

Some parents avoid prenatal genetic testing because of the cost or because of a fear that the test might be painful (Gustafson et al., 2007). When designing interventions to increase genetic screening rates, fee waivers and effective reproductive counseling strategies may help eliminate concerns about financial burden or pain (Mayo-Gamble et al., 2018).

Additionally, it is important for all prospective parents to understand and be aware of the potential to use pre-implantation genetic diagnosis (PGD) in conjunction with in vitro fertilization (IVF). Hemoglobinopathies can be diagnosed very early with PGD via a cell biopsy from the embryo or zygote (Vrettou et al., 2018), making it possible to decide whether to implant an embryo based on the results of the test. The first published case of a successful unaffected pregnancy using PGD in conjunction with IVF was in the late 1990s (Xu et al., 1999). Since then, this procedure has remained an option for informed pregnancies and also makes it possible for families that already have affected children to have another child who is a potential match as a donor for human stem cell transplantation (Vrettou et al., 2018).

Families are, however, confronted with a major financial hurdle with this option because public and private insurance coverage for PGD is variable and may be tied to coverage for infertility treatment, leaving some couples to cover the test out of pocket. Currently, only 16 states in the

---

United States have laws that require insurers to cover or offer coverage for infertility treatment (NCSL, 2019). A qualitative study with 18 genetic high-risk couples found that the study participants were concerned about the costs associated with PGD but ultimately prioritized the opportunity to not pass on a genetic disorder to their offspring (Drazba et al., 2014). Most families who have a child with SCD report an interest in learning about PGD and say that they would consider using it in a future pregnancy (Darbari et al., 2018).

Parents who oppose IVF with PGD often cite ethical or religious concerns (Schultz et al., 2014). Unfortunately, a small study of 19 parents with a child with SCD in the United States found that less than half (44 percent) of the parents surveyed knew about PGD as an option (Darbari et al., 2018). Thus, providing access to preconception counseling and education on both PGD and IVF may be an important future direction for parents with SCT.

Long-Term Follow-Up for SCT- and SCD-Positive Individuals

The long-term follow-up of individuals with SCT represents a significant gap in the overall spectrum of care and also a public health problem, as these individuals have a lifelong risk of passing on the sickle cell variant to their children or having children affected by SCD. These individuals may be predisposed to the emerging risk of certain conditions (discussed in Chapter 4) (Grant et al., 2011). Children with SCD are sometimes followed as long as they remain within the state, but they are no longer tracked if they cross state lines. State-level tracking of individuals with SCT is extremely disjointed, and there is little communication between states (Kavanagh et al., 2008; Minkovitz et al., 2016).

The accessibility of SCT status results later in life varies across states as well, but the committee was unable to find documentation about specific state practices. The committee was also unable to find any known long-term follow-up of health conditions or outcomes for those with positive SCT status in the United States, despite growing evidence of an increased risk for certain chronic health conditions (Alvarez, 2017; Alvarez et al., 2015; Elliott and Bruner, 2019; Naik and Haywood, 2015; Naik et al., 2018; Shetty and Matrana, 2014). While a first priority should be population-based surveillance for those living with SCD, given the severity of the disease, a focus on SCT as an emerging public health problem may be an important future policy initiative. Framing SCT as a public health concern may help increase funding, advocacy, and research for both SCD and SCT.

Even when NBS programs are highly effective, comprehensive follow-up and care for those diagnosed with SCD (SCD-positive individuals) are still required to ensure that these individuals receive quality care to reduce SCD-related morbidity. Assessing the quality of this care is important in order to develop and implement policies universally. A 2016 study identified key indicators that could be used to assess the quality of care for individuals with SCD and SCT (Faro et al., 2016). High-quality care provided early genetic counseling, timely reporting of results, screening for immigrants, and penicillin prophylaxis. A 1998 study in California, Illinois, and New York found that follow-up from NBS was lacking in the areas of treatment and compliance (CDC, 2000). Antibiotics are still underused, and there are adherence issues being reported (Cober and Phelps, 2010; Reeves et al., 2018; Teach et al., 1998).

In a national CDC study, 76 percent of doctors reported providing penicillin prophylaxis, but only 44 percent of patients followed through (CDC, 2000). Several other studies found similar trends in treatment and adherence among providers and patients, respectively (Cober and Phelps, 2010; Reeves et al., 2018; Teach et al., 1998). A study synthesizing the effects of NBS programs found that surveillance information was needed to obtain longitudinal data and carry out follow-up programs (Yusuf et al., 2011). One NBS program in New York had a 12 percent loss to follow-up among children, indicating that these gaps in follow-up care must be addressed to ensure the effectiveness of these programs (Yusuf et al., 2011).

Other Approaches to Educating the Public About SCD

One way to communicate the importance for SCD and SCT screening is to include it within public health education focused on other areas. One program in Zambia, for instance, integrated screening into a dental hygiene program that provided free toothbrushes and toothpaste and informed rural residents of tooth decay (Chunda-Liyoka et al., 2018). Combining several health interventions within a single program or roll-out allows for increased reach and access that a single program might not have. Other possible education methods would be to work through registered nurses, who are already heavily involved in the care and case management of individuals with SCD (Arhin, 2019), or with community-based organizations (CBOs) and patient advocacy groups.

PATIENT REGISTRIES

Patient disease registries, which vary widely in their structure, scope, and purpose, are distinguished by their common approach: they collect information from a subset of people with a particular disease to develop a generalizable picture of who has the disease, what effects they are experiencing, and how they are being cared for (AHRQ, 2014). That information typically includes the registrants' characteristics, clinical data and test results, and health status over time. Like clinical trial databases, registries typically aim to collect highly reliable and precise data. Depending on the sponsorship and intended goal, patient registries are likely to provide valuable information to researchers, drug and device developers, clinicians, and sometimes the patients themselves (AHRQ, 2014).

Registries typically require a high level of resources to recruit, consent, and collect detailed data. Registries may be sponsored and funded by grants or government contracts, pharmaceutical companies or device developers, professional associations, or CBOs. There can be significant overlap between patient registries and clinical trial data collection in the types of data collected and their use (Forrest et al., 2011). Registries may or may not be long-term or longitudinal, and the sponsors may or may not widely share the results of data analysis.

Registry participants may be rewarded in various ways, including receiving a stipend for their time, being connected with clinical trials, or receiving education or support in forums or from trained community health workers. Registries for rare diseases that include clinical data can be helpful for researchers tracking clinical outcomes related to specific treatments or preventative measures.

By their nature, registries collect identifiable and sensitive information about patients and are typically designed so that patients (or their legal guardians) must explicitly consent to take part by sharing their information directly or providing access to their medical records. Although some registries capture information from the majority of patients (e.g., state cancer registries), there are always nonparticipants—due to challenges related to consent, access to the registry portal or the data collection interview, or simple unwillingness— and this can create bias in results derived from registry data if those results are assumed to apply to all of those living with the disease.

Examples of SCD Patient Registries

Multisite clinical registries have been used to track the specific outcomes or sequelae of the complications of SCD. These may be considered extensions of the clinical trial model.

A granting agency may conceive and fund federally supported registries, with research institutions performing the work of obtaining patient consent, collecting data, analyzing the data, and disseminating the results. These efforts may be funded to develop methodologies through pilot programs or to implement registry systems on a larger scale. NIH's National Heart, Lung, and Blood Institute (NHLBI) implemented the Comprehensive Sickle Cell Centers Collaborative Data collection effort from 2005 to 2008, which gathered data from 3,640 persons with SCD nationwide via clinical interviews and medical record extraction (Dampier et al., 2011; NHLBI, 2007). NHLBI currently supports the Sickle Cell Disease Implementation

Consortium, begun in 2016, which includes a patient registry with participants recruited from the participating centers. The goal of this SCD registry is to collect data on 2,400 adolescent and adult patients (SCDIC, n.d.).

Multiple Private-Sector Efforts to Collect and Use Data on Individuals with SCD

CBOs frequently collect records of the health of their clients, whether formally or informally. For example, the Sickle Cell Disease Association of America (SCDAA), the largest national CBO focused on SCD, launched its patient registry, Get Connected, in 2018 with multiple aims: providing patients with the storage of and easy access to their medical information, offering information and resources to patients and their families, and helping with clinical research planning and recruitment. As of June 2018, the registry, which had been promoted by SCDAA since 2015, had collected data on nearly 6,128 persons, 4,984 of whom had SCD and another 633 with SCT. The remaining enrollees are non-patients (Pena, 2018).

Professional organizations may also support or host data collection systems for those affected by the focal conditions. In 2018, for example, ASH launched the ASH Research Collaborative (RC) Data Hub, which functions as a data repository with information on hematologic diseases and which was set up to facilitate clinicians' and researchers' access to patient data. This effort may be of particular use to researchers studying rare hematologic diseases, which may not otherwise have a centralized data collection system. The RC Data Hub can collect prospective and retrospective data from both U.S. and international sources, including inpatient and outpatient clinical systems, industry and government datasets, patients, and other existing registries (ASH RC, 2019). The data include genomic or molecular correlates, clinical and laboratory data, patient-reported outcomes, information on population health, and social determinants. The RC Data Hub automates data collection when necessary and allows for information on new diseases to be captured. In addition, automation allows researchers and medical personnel to promptly retrieve data that can be used to answer certain research questions through advanced querying.

In 2019, ASH launched the Sickle Cell Disease Clinical Trials Network, which provides a framework for finding and categorizing patient cohorts for clinical trials, placing trial sponsors with sites, and recruiting eligible patients. It collects information from the RC Data Hub to assist with identifying areas of research and treatment that could benefit from additional data. The mission of the network is to "improve outcomes for individuals with SCD by expediting therapy development and facilitating innovation in clinical trial research" (ASH RC, 2018).

Expanded Registries

In countries that are disproportionately affected by a specific genetic disease, registries may be sponsored by the national government; one such example is Greece's hemoglobinopathy registry, established in 2009. Because this registry includes everyone diagnosed with SCD and follows these individuals over time with the goal of conducting longitudinal surveillance, it may be considered a public health surveillance effort; in this context, it offers a possible model for developing state- or even national-level universal registries in the United States (Voskaridou et al., 2019). There are similar registries within the United States for other severe diseases, which have been successful in gathering data on nearly all affected patients and tracking them over their lifetimes. An example is the cystic fibrosis (CF) registry, which includes nearly every person with the disease living in the United States. Registrants are monitored by staff at clinical sites, which ensures that the patient data are entered into the system accurately and in a timely manner. The registry receives support from private funding, including the Cystic Fibrosis Foundation, and other sources (CFF, 2018).

Hemophilia treatment centers (HTCs), sites of high-quality care for those living with hemophilia in the United States, also participate in a lifelong data collection system, Community Counts. This effort is a collaboration among HTCs participating in the U.S. Hemophilia Treatment Center Network, CDC, HRSA, and the American Thrombosis and Hemostasis Network. The system tracks the clinical visits of those living with hemophilia through the HTC Population Profile and tracks these individuals over their life course (including mortality) through the Registry for Bleeding Disorders Surveillance (Manco-Johnson et al., 2018).

Standardizing Data Collection and Patient Registries

Researchers developing registries, data collection systems for clinical research, and other systems for outcomes data may be frustrated with the lack of standardization and comparability across such efforts. If patient outcomes are defined differently in different settings, it is difficult to compare the results of interventions or methods changes. NHLBI convened a steering committee of those involved in SCD research to develop standards for data collection as a part of the PhenX Toolkit (consensus measures for **Phen**otypes and e**X**posures) (Eckman et al., 2017; Hamilton et al., 2011). All researchers and scientists participating in SCD-related data collection efforts are encouraged to design their measures around these common data elements and standards to improve data usefulness and consistency.

PUBLIC HEALTH SURVEILLANCE

As noted above, public health surveillance is the ongoing and systematic collection, analysis, and interpretation of health-related data, with a particular emphasis on the timely dissemination of the data and results in order to make them as useful as possible (Foege et al., 1976; Thacker and Berkelman, 1988). Wide-ranging surveillance efforts provide data on a large number of patients, typically with low bias in the cohort examined (i.e., nearly everyone is captured, with little difference in characteristics between those followed and those not). Depending on the methodologies used, surveillance systems can provide excellent "bird's eye view" data on population-level disease prevalence, health outcomes, mortality, access to care, and cost of care. Such data can augment other data collection efforts, such as NBS or registries (Choi, 2012).

Suggested surveillance systems as described here can be distinguished from many registries by the former's aim to be universal in scope, capturing all of those with the disease of interest along with longitudinal data on the population, and by the relatively low resources needed to establish surveillance systems (compared to far-reaching registries). However, the data used to define the population living with SCD were not originally intended for surveillance and do not approach the reliability of clinical trials data or registries. Furthermore, surveillance systems' purpose and scope vary from those of registries. Specifics such as laboratory values, biomarkers, and QOL measures (e.g., employment or educational achievement) are generally not known, and there are different gaps in data in every system across states or regions. Administrative data may also be more prone to errors than NBS or registry data, although such errors are unlikely to be biased (and thus are unlikely to affect conclusions). Complete information on the cost of care and treatments that may not be billed (e.g., clinical trials or charity care) or bundled as part of managed care may be missing.

Surveillance is typically defined geographically, with efforts at a state or national level. Rare disease surveillance is increasingly seen as a necessary tool to understand the complications, comorbidities, uptake of treatments, and health outcomes for diseases that may otherwise be difficult to track, given their small population sizes and widely dispersed care. In 2007 the American Society of Pediatric Hematology/Oncology convened the Sickle Cell Disease Summit, a meeting of stakeholders in hemoglobinopathies, to settle on a unified approach to health care and research disparities for SCD. One key finding was that there is a critical need for population-based surveillance to track outcomes (Hassell et al., 2009).

The creation of the Registry and Surveillance System for Hemoglobinopathies (RuSH), a cooperative agreement among CDC, NHLBI, and seven states with significant populations of people living with SCD and thalassemia, was one outcome of this summit and its recommendations. This 2010–2012 effort was intended to develop and test methodologies for public health surveillance in these disorders at the state level. It was originally intended to be developed and validated over 4 years, but funding was ultimately provided for only 2 years. Although some states had already begun to gather data on their Medicaid populations or to follow NBS-diagnosed cases of SCD, RuSH was the first large-scale attempt to conduct public health surveillance for SCD in the United States. Information on incidence and prevalence in RuSH states produced by these efforts was novel and intended to be helpful to researchers and policy makers in those states (Hulihan et al., 2015; Paulukonis et al., 2014).

California, Georgia, and CDC have continued this work with the Sickle Cell Data Collection (SCDC) program, which has been funded privately by the CDC Foundation since 2015. The two states collect NBS-identified cases, hospital discharge data, ED data, vital records death data, Medicaid claims for all claimants with SCD diagnostic codes, and reports from SCD care clinics on patient genotype. These data are used to support policy decisions at the state and federal level, inform researchers and providers via published manuscripts, and educate those living with the disease, their families and communities, and health care providers on the disease and the latest research on it (Paulukonis et al., 2015).

Several states have also implemented or expanded public health surveillance of SCD. In 2019, CDC, through the CDC Foundation's SCDC, awarded grants to train seven additional states—Alabama, Indiana, Michigan, Minnesota, North Carolina, Tennessee, and Virginia—on how to implement comprehensive data collection programs for SCD. No data will be collected under the grant, but the states will receive training on the conduct of longitudinal data collection and surveillance for SCD (CDC, 2019). Tennessee's St. Jude Children's Research Hospital gathers data from multiple sources and uses them to support research and policy (St. Jude Children's Research Hospital, 2019).

Each state or other geographic region that attempts surveillance efforts in SCD or any rare disease will by necessity use varying methodologies. Access to data differs by location and the program's relationship to data stewards, and the data sources, patient identifiers, and underlying programs vary widely. Still, most states that have attempted such an endeavor have found that it yields fruitful and novel information; improves communication across agencies, providers, insurers, and patients living with the disease; and supports policy change that can improve access to high-quality care and health outcomes for those with SCD. Collectively these surveillance programs have used data to publish manuscripts on epidemiology and health outcomes among those with SCD, to support grants, to connect health care providers with resources and support, and to support policy change (CDC, 2018).

Public health surveillance may use fewer resources than more intensive methods of gathering information on the SCD population, particularly when considered as cost per patient or per year of data included. It is best suited to provide information to support policy change and new research programs that can gather reliable individual-level data. The Sickle Cell Disease and Other Heritable Blood Disorders Research, Surveillance, Prevention, and Treatment Act of 2018 explicitly authorizes grants to conduct public health surveillance for SCD and other heritable blood disorders. Appropriations have not yet been made, however. Support of this law and its appropriate funding will be critical for public health surveillance in SCD in coming years.[2]

As noted above, organizations dealing with diseases similar to SCD have successfully integrated public health surveillance and registry approaches and data. When the majority of the affected population finds benefit in sharing health information and receives consistent, high-quality care, as with the CF and hemophilia communities (discussed in Chapter 8), the value of the registry data for tracking health care and health outcomes over time is dramatically increased. As SCD registry and surveillance systems in the United States become more established and successful, merging data and methods across these systems and incorporating information from NBS will be an ideal model for which to strive. A merged system would provide valuable information about individuals over the life course to participants, health care providers, researchers, and policy makers.

ETHICAL IMPLICATIONS AND PRIVACY CONSIDERATIONS

When individuals with SCD interact with clinicians or researchers, there are a variety of ethical and privacy issues that must be taken into account. The issues are particularly relevant for African Americans because of the history of medical and research establishments in the United States treating them unethically.

Perceptions of Who Is Affected

The widespread presence of SCT in people of African origin is due largely to an accident of evolutionary biology, as it confers a survival advantage in areas with a high prevalence of malaria. As many as 40 percent of individuals in parts of sub-Saharan Africa may be affected, but SCT may also be found in people in southern Europe, Saudi Arabia, and India—a result of centuries of genetic diffusion (Serjeant, 2013). The slave trade brought

---

[2] Sickle Cell Disease and Other Heritable Blood Disorders Research, Surveillance, Prevention and Treatment Act of 2018, Public Law 115-327, 115th Congress (December 18, 2018).

vast numbers of people to the Americas and the Caribbean, parts of the world where the genetically conferred resistance was largely irrelevant but where the disease took root, with its greatest prevalence today among those with African ancestry.

However, the resulting widespread belief in the United States that SCD is an African American disease is not only incorrect but can create additional challenges (e.g., some people assume they can judge the likelihood of someone having SCT solely by looks). Skin color has been shown to be a poor marker of African descent (Crawford et al., 2017), and it is not uncommon for SCT to be found in people who do not present as African American, including Caucasians and Latinos. For these people, the notion that SCD is an African American disease may present special obstacles to care. See Box 3-1 for the perspective of a Hispanic individual living with SCD.

A History of Discrimination

Throughout the 19th century and more than halfway through the 20th century, diseases that particularly affected African Americans received significantly less attention than diseases that were of more concern to white Americans. For example, a historian of medicine wrote that at the outset of the 20th century, the sickle cell population was "clinically invisible" (Wailoo, 2017). After 1910, the disorder was understood to be caused by physically distorted RBCs. However, correct diagnosis was infrequent, and the common symptoms, such as infections and pain, were often attributed to other conditions, especially when diseases with similar symptoms were endemic, such as malaria in Memphis (Wailoo, 2001). World War II investigators in the growing field of molecular biology recognized that a corrective therapy for the hemoglobin molecule could theoretically be devised, but in practice providers relied mainly on antibiotics (Wailoo, 2017). Although the providers' actions did decrease mortality, they did nothing to identify methods to treat the hemoglobin molecule directly.

Beginning in the 1960s, the civil rights movement, media coverage, and grassroots civic engagement, such as that of the Black Panthers, helped stimulate public awareness of SCD (Bassett, 2016). The new political and medical science environments led to the passage of the Sickle Cell Anemia Control Act of 1972. No longer clinically invisible, patients with SCD did benefit from longer life spans made possible by continually improving antibiotics. Nevertheless, the overall progress continues to be slow.

Furthermore, suggestions that those with the gene should be aggressively identified in order to prevent it from being passed on were reminiscent of earlier eugenic efforts (Bowman, 1996). Despite the benefits of PGD and genetic counseling discussed in earlier sections, these options need to

BOX 3-1
A Patient's Voice: A Changing Perspective

Servio Astacio was born in the Dominican Republic and diagnosed with sickle cell disease (SCD) when his parents noticed the yellow tone of his skin and sporadic episodes of rigidness shortly after his birth. Astacio said the diagnosis had affected his personal life in many ways, including occupationally, educationally, and mentally. As the grandson of military members, Astacio had always aspired to join the military and eventually work for the National Aeronautics and Space Administration or the Central Intelligence Agency. He stated, "I had my life planned out," but when "I went to the Army, Navy, and Marine recruitment centers, they told me no. They told me they don't accept people with my condition." He explained that this rejection had made him "depressed for some time. It really changed my views. It made me lose hope."

Astacio noted that he would sometimes experience these periods of depression, but "no one has helped me with my depression. I had to deal with it on my own. Getting professional treatment for depression never occurred to me." At that time, he did not even know he was depressed; "it was just sadness," and his clinicians did not ask him about depression. Furthermore, Astacio said that he has experienced discrimination and ageism in the medical setting. He explained "that when I am dressed [formally] like I just came out of work, then I don't get treated with a hard time." However, if "I am dressed in shorts, t-shirt, and tennis shoes, then people will want to determine if I have a legitimate need to pain medication and if I am really in pain." Astacio added that he "is not surprised with difficulties other people may be having [in the medical setting] due to their ethnicity." Astacio also sometimes faces ageism in the medical setting due to his young facial features. He shared that "once, when two nurses were trying to explain a medical term to me, one nurse told the other nurse 'you have to explain it to him because he is a baby. He doesn't know.'"

To treat his signs and symptoms, including depression, Astacio found that keeping a positive mindset can make a difference. He also recommends "staying hydrated, taking medications appropriately, knowing your limits, and tackling health issues immediately" to maintain proper health. He advises others with SCD: "Always be confident about you being able to take care of your health. Always keep up with your medication, a healthy diet, and not overworking your body."

Although SCD has greatly limited some of his personal goals, Astacio said that being diagnosed "has given me more ambition to educate myself in school and to work harder to afford medical treatment." He noted that the disease had eventually "inspired me to do better, because I have a family, objectives, and goals. I'm hopeful of the future." He added, "eventually, I found another purpose in life, another passion,"

continued

be approached with sensitivity in light of the history of racial discrimination in the United States. Elsewhere in the world, there have been such eugenics-type efforts. In Bahrain genotyping and counseling has reduced the births of affected infants (Almutawa and Alqamish, 2009), and mandatory premarital screening for couples has led to voluntary cancellations of marriage proposals in Saudi Arabia (Alotaibi, 2017). Such programs would raise complications in the United States, however, because of its history of racial discrimination.

In recent years, individuals living with SCD in the United States have been entangled in the controversy around pain management and opiates, with the added complication that pain reported by those perceived as African Americans has been taken less seriously than when reported by other patients (Hoffman et al., 2016). In addition, African Americans are particularly vulnerable to the stigma of suspected addictive behavior. Patients with SCD continue to encounter controversies and difficulties that are often more societal than scientific.

Patient Privacy Concerns

Patient privacy and confidentiality are core values of medical ethics. They are even cited in the Hippocratic Oath (Hajar, 2017). But unlike in the ancient world, where one clinician interacted with one patient, modern health care systems have extensive medical records combined with patient care provided by a health care team. This presents many opportunities for others to access personal health information. The Institute of Medicine defines privacy as follows:

Privacy addresses the question of who has access to personal informa-tion and under what conditions. Privacy is concerned with the collection, storage, and use of personal information, and examines whether data can be collected in the first place, as well as the justifications, if any, under which data collected for one purpose can be used for another (secondary) purpose. An important issue in privacy analysis is whether the indi-vidual has authorized particular uses of his or her personal information. (IOM, 2009)

Rarely are there objections to caregivers viewing necessary medical information to provide the best patient care, but illegitimate access must be prevented. Protecting against this may be especially important for pa-tients who are members of historically discriminated groups or liable to be stigmatized because of their disease, both of which apply to many people affected by SCD.

The Health Insurance Portability and Accountability Act of 1996 (HIPAA) safeguards the privacy of medical information in addition to ensuring that health coverage cannot be denied when someone loses or changes a job and providing protections against the denial of coverage because of certain diseases and pre-existing conditions (OCR, 2013). How-ever, in practice HIPAA may also create confusion about information shar-ing among those with a "need to know" basis, particularly with regard to mental health information (IOM, 2009). In brief, a mental health profes-sional may share information with a patient's personal representative and also family, friends, or caregivers insofar as that information is relevant to the patient's caregiving (and without patient objection). If the patient lacks or has impaired decision-making capabilities, a therapist may share relevant information with others who can make medical decisions based on the patient's best interests.

Federal law specifically requires the confidentiality of SCD-related medical records that are held by the U.S. Department of Veterans Affairs.[3] Patients should be confident that learning their SCD status from genetic testing will not subject them to discriminatory practices. This became a public issue in the early 1970s, when some states required that African Americans be tested to identify both carriers and SCD-positive individuals. In response, Congress enacted the National Sickle Cell Anemia Control Act in 1972, which withheld federal funds from states that mandated testing. Thus, the experience with SCD served as a precursor to the 2008 Genetic Information Nondiscrimination Act, which protects individuals

---

[3] Veterans Health Administration. 2016. VHA Directive 1605.01. Privacy and Release of Information. Washington, DC: Veterans Health Administration, U.S. Department of Veterans Affairs. See https://www.va.gov/vhapublications/ViewPublication.asp?pub_ID=5456 (accessed March 3, 2020).

from any sort of genetic discrimination in health insurance and employment (Feldman, 2012).

Data Protection Considerations

Neither participants in research studies nor patients in clinical care typically have ownership rights to any data collected from them; in particular, they do not have a financial interest in any commercial products that may be developed based on those data. Rather, the data in data banks and registries typically are owned by health care providers and insurance plans, funding agencies for registry projects, research institutions, and government agencies. However, following several legal cases, such as the Henrietta Lacks case (Shah, 2010), there is now widespread agreement that patients and research participants should at least be clearly informed, in advance, that they will not have rights to any data collected. It is also understood that the privacy and confidentiality of patients providing data should be carefully protected (e.g., by "de-identification"), which makes it difficult, if not impossible, for the information to be traced back to the patients.

In 1979, the National Commission for the Protection of Human Subjects of Biomedical and Behavioral Research issued the *Belmont Report*, which offered three principles to guide research involving human participants: respect for persons, beneficence, and justice (National Commission for the Protection of Human Subjects of Biomedical and Behavioral Research, 1979). These principles remain the core values of the U.S. biomedical research enterprise. In the context of data protection, respect requires that participants' privacy and dignity be preserved and that patients should be able to give their informed consent for the way their data are collected and used. Beneficence requires that harm to participants and relevant groups be minimized and benefits maximized, including the harm and benefits of information in a data registry. Justice requires that no particular group be involved in the research enterprise more than any other and that the benefits of the research be shared equitably. Considering that the National Commission was partly a response to the controversy from the U.S. Public Health Service Syphilis Study (CDC, 2015), these principles have special resonance for African Americans, who suffer a disproportionate burden of SCD.

The movement for personalized medicine in the era of big data suggests that in the future it will be increasingly more difficult to distinguish regular clinical care from research. Data registries and machine-learning systems that use sophisticated and continuously revised algorithms will increasingly be part of the regular clinical experience. If the identification of people with SCD can be improved and their clinical experiences entered into these systems, those patients stand to benefit. Still, the ethical protections that apply to data protection should continue to be respected.

Public Health Surveillance and Research

Public health surveillance is crucial to tracking the distribution of a disease to improve access to health care resources in areas with health disparities. For SCD, improved surveillance is particularly important because of current data limitations, including the exact percentage of affected African Americans. Recognizing that SCD research and treatment lags behind research for other chronic illnesses, the Sickle Cell Disease and Other Heritable Blood Disorders Research, Surveillance, Prevention, and Treatment Act of 2018[4] reauthorized an SCD prevention and treatment program and provides grants for research, surveillance, prevention, and treatment of heritable blood disorders. As of the development of this report, the section of the legislation related to data collection on certain blood disorders had not yet been funded by Congress. Although the focus of public health surveillance is improving the well-being of populations, the ethics of public health also requires respecting the health and dignity of individuals.

While public health surveillance essentially consists of data collection and analysis that generates hypotheses (Thacker and Berkelman, 1988), public health research builds on that information to test which hypotheses provide the most effective interventions for population-level prevention and treatment. Individuals' interests must be balanced against the value of a public health intervention to the community, taking into account the benefits and costs. Surveillance and research depend on each other to be effective in promoting population health (Lussier et al., 2012). Public trust is crucial for both approaches, so every reasonable effort should be made to communicate goals and explain the relevant practices to the affected population.

Especially in cases of chronic social vulnerability, as with the communities most likely to be affected by SCD, members of representative civic and religious organizations should be closely involved in every phase of the surveillance and intervention. Among African Americans, trust in the medical establishment has justifiably been a topic of intense concern, particularly considering the history of exploitive experiments and surveillance studies. Yet there is evidence that African Americans are interested in participating in clinical trials, though that interest may not be accommodated in enrollment processes. As for any subpopulation, appropriate arrangements should be made in the prior review (e.g., institutional review board representation) and consent phases (e.g., clarity about the prospects of commercializing any important research result) (Hamel et al., 2016).

NBS raises specific ethical and social issues. The World Health Organization recommends screening if diagnosis and treatment will benefit the

---

[4] Sickle Cell Disease and Other Heritable Blood Disorders Research, Surveillance, Prevention and Treatment Act of 2018, Public Law 115-327, 115th Congress (December 18, 2018).

newborn. The classical example that meets this test is phenylketonuria screening. For selective screening to be useful, the affected communities must be part of the program (Avard et al., 2006).

Blood donations are sometimes screened for SCD as part of public health surveillance and to protect the blood supply. Incidental findings, such as the discovery of SCT, raise the question of whether donors should be informed of their status, about which they may not be aware. One option is to inform potential donors that their blood may be screened for SCT and give them the choice of whether to be notified, along with being informed about the medical and reproductive health implications of a positive result. Responsible regulatory agencies and community organizations need to collaborate to address concerns about stigma and discrimination while also protecting public health (Lee and Marks, 2014).

Electronic Informed Consent Issues

Electronic informed consent has been defined as "the use of electronic systems and processes that may employ multiple electronic media, including text, graphics, audio, video, podcasts, passive and interactive Web sites, biological recognition devices, and card readers, to convey information related to the study and to obtain and document informed consent" (FDA, 2016, p. 2). No matter how informed consent is obtained, the same ethical requirements apply. Specifically, the individual must have the capacity to give consent, the information provided must be complete and understandable enough that the patient can make an informed decision, and the participant's or patient's consent must be verified. Furthermore, with consent processes that involve only remote interactions by electronic means, care must be taken that the participant or patient has the same opportunities to have any questions and concerns addressed in person.

CONCLUSIONS AND RECOMMENDATIONS

Conclusion 3-1: There are gaps in information for SCD that do not exist for similar diseases. Robust and well-supported longitudinal data collection systems that include the majority of those living with the disease will provide the information and evidence needed for decision making and facilitate the evaluation of changes in SCD care.

Conclusion 3-2: Communication of SCD results to parents/guardians, the pediatrician of record, a referred pediatric hematologist, and other relevant care providers as well as follow-up once diagnosed are inconsistent across state NBS programs.

Therefore, newborns with SCD and their families do not receive standardized quality care and familial support across different state programs in a timely manner.

Conclusion 3-3: Follow-up and communication of positive SCT status to parents, the pediatrician of record, other relevant care providers, and young adults seeking trait status from NBS systems are not consistent across state NBS programs. Thus, some people with SCT are unaware of their status despite a confirmed determination by NBS. This may affect future reproductive decisions and/or health.

Recommendation 3-1: The Centers for Disease Control and Prevention should work with all states to develop state public health surveillance systems to support a national longitudinal registry of all persons with sickle cell disease.

Recommendation 3-2: The Health Resources and Services Administration, the National Institutes of Health, and the Agency for Healthcare Research and Quality should develop a clinical data registry for sickle cell disease. The registry would allow for identifying best practices for care delivery and outcomes.

Recommendation 3-3: The Office of the Assistant Secretary for Health should establish a working group to identify existing and disparate sources of data that can be immediately linked and mined. These data can be used to provide needed information on sickle cell disease health care services usage and costs in the short term.

Recommendation 3-4: The Health Resources and Services Administration should work with states to standardize the communication of and use of newborn screening positive results in genetic counseling and should create a mechanism for communicating this information across the life span and ensuring access to needed support and services.

REFERENCES

AAP (American Academy of Pediatrics) Newborn Screening Task Force. 2000. Serving the family from birth to the medical home. *Pediatrics* 106(Suppl 2):389.

Abhyankar, S., M. A. Lloyd-Puryear, R. Goodwin, S. Copeland, J. Eichwald, B. L. Therrell, and C. J. McDonald. 2010. Standardizing newborn screening results for health information exchange. *AMIA Annual Symposium Proceedings* 2010:1–5.

AHRQ (Agency for Healthcare Research and Quality). 2014. AHRQ methods for effective health care. In R. E. Gliklich, N. A. Dreyer, and M. B. Leavy (eds.), *Registries for evaluating patient outcomes: A user's guide.* Rockville, MD: Agency for Healthcare Research and Quality.

Almutawa, F. J., and J. R. Alqamish. 2009. Outcome of premarital counseling of hemoglobinopathy carrier couples attending premarital services in Bahrain. *Journal of the Bahrain Medical Society* 21(1):217–220.

Alotaibi, M. M. 2017. Sickle cell disease in Saudi Arabia: A challenge or not. *Journal of Epidemiology and Global Health* 7(2):99–101.

Alvarez, O. A. 2017. Renal medullary carcinoma: The kidney cancer that affects individuals with sickle cell trait and disease. *Journal of Oncology Practice* 13(7):424–425.

Alvarez, O., M. M. Rodriguez, L. Jordan, and S. Sarnaik. 2015. Renal medullary carcinoma and sickle cell trait: A systematic review. *Pediatric Blood & Cancer* 62(10):1694–1699.

Alvarez, O. A., T. Hustace, M. Voltaire, A. Mantero, U. Liberus, and R. Saint Fleur. 2019. Newborn screening for sickle cell disease using point-of-care testing in low-income setting. *Pediatrics* 144(4):e20184105.

Andermann, A., I. Blancquaert, S. Beauchamp, and V. Dery. 2008. Revisiting Wilson and Jungner in the genomic age: A review of screening criteria over the past 40 years. *Bulletin of the World Health Organization* 86(4):317–319.

Anderson, S. A., J. Doperak, and G. P. Chimes. 2011. Recommendations for routine sickle cell trait screening for NCAA Division I athletes. *PM&R* 3(2):168–174.

APHL (Association of Public Health Laboratories) and CDC (Centers for Disease Control and Prevention). 2015. *Hemoglobinopathies: Current practices for screening, confirmation and follow-up.* https://www.aphl.org/aboutAPHL/publications/Documents/NBS_HemoglobinopathyTesting_122015.pdf (accessed January 9, 2020).

Arhin, A. O. 2019. Knowledge deficit of sickle cell trait status: Can nurses help? *Critical Care Nursing Quarterly* 42(2):198–201.

Asgharian, A., K. A. Anie, and M. Berger. 2003. Women with sickle cell trait: Reproductive decision-making. *Journal of Reproductive and Infant Psychology* 21(1):23–34.

ASH RC (American Society of Hematology Research Collaboration). 2018. *Sickle Cell Disease Clinical Trials Network.* https://www.ashresearchcollaborative.org/sites/default/files/2018-12/ASH_Research_Collaborative_CTN_Handout.pdf (accessed March 10, 2020).

ASH RC. 2019. *Data Hub.* https://www.ashresearchcollaborative.org/s/data-hub (accessed March 10, 2020).

Avard, D., L. Kharaboyan, and B. Knoppers. 2006. Newborn screening for sickle cell disease: Socio-ethical implications. In S. A. M. McLean (ed.), *First do no harm: Law, ethics and healthcare.* Aldershot, England: Ashgate. Pp. 493–507.

Baker, C., J. Powell, D. Le, M. S. Creary, L. A. Daley, M. A. McDonald, and C. D. Royal. 2018. Implementation of the NCAA sickle cell trait screening policy: A survey of athletic staff and student-athletes. *Journal of the National Medical Association* 110(6):564–573.

Bassett, M. T. 2016. Beyond berets: The Black Panthers as health activists. *American Journal of Public Health* 106(10):1741–1743.

Bediako, S., and T. King-Meadows. 2016. Public support for sickle-cell disease funding: Does race matter? *Race and Social Problems* 8(2).

Benson, J. M., and B. L. Therrell, Jr. 2010. History and current status of newborn screening for hemoglobinopathies. *Seminars in Perinatology* 34(2):134–144.

Blood-Siegfried, J., H. S. Lieder, and K. Deary. 2006. To screen or not to screen: Complexities of newborn screening in the 21st century. *Journal for Nurse Practitioners* 2(5):300–307.

Bowman, J. E. 1996. The road to eugenics. *The University of Chicago Law School Roundtable* 3(2):7.

CDC (Centers for Disease Control and Prevention). 1986. *Comprehensive plan for epidemiologic surveillance*. Atlanta, GA: U.S. Department of Health and Human Services.

CDC. 2000. Update: Newborn screening for sickle cell disease—California, Illinois, and New York, 1998. *Morbidity and Mortality Weekly Report* 49(32):729–731.

CDC. 2015. *U.S. Public Health Service syphilis study at Tuskegee: The Tuskegee timeline*. https://www.cdc.gov/tuskegee/timeline.htm (accessed January 9, 2020).

CDC. 2018. *Sickle cell data collection program report: Data to action introduction*. https://www.cdc.gov/ncbddd/hemoglobinopathies/data-reports/2018-summer/index.html (accessed January 9, 2020).

CDC. 2019. *CDC awards funds to learn more about people with sickle cell disease*. https://www.cdc.gov/media/releases/2019/p0925-cdc-awards-funds-sickle-cell.html (accessed March 11, 2020).

CDC. n.d. *Get screened to know your sickle cell status*. https://www.cdc.gov/ncbddd/sicklecell/documents/Factsheet_ScickleCell_Status.pdf (accessed March 10, 2020).

CFF (Cystic Fibrosis Foundation). 2018. *2017 annual report*. Bethesda, MD: Cystic Fibrosis Foundation.

Charache, S. 1988. Sudden death in sickle trait. *American Journal of Medicine* 84(3, Part 1):459–461.

Choi, B. C. 2012. The past, present, and future of public health surveillance. *Scientifica (Cairo)* 2012:875253.

Christopher, S. A., J. L. Collins, and M. H. Farrell. 2012. Effort required to contact primary care providers after newborn screening identifies sickle cell trait. *Journal of the National Medical Association* 104(11–12):528–534.

Chudleigh, J., S. Buckingham, J. Dignan, S. O'Driscoll, K. Johnson, D. Rees, H. Wyatt, and A. Metcalfe. 2016. Parents' experiences of receiving the initial positive newborn screening (NBS) result for cystic fibrosis and sickle cell disease. *Journal of Genetic Counseling* 25(6):1215–1226.

Chunda-Liyoka, C., A. A. Kumar, P. Sambo, F. Lubinda, L. Nchimba, T. Humpton, P. Okuku, C. Miyanda, J. Im, K. Maguire, G. M. Whitesides, and T. P. Stossel. 2018. Application of a public health strategy to large-scale point-of-care screening for sickle cell disease in rural sub-Saharan Africa. *Blood Advances* 2(Suppl 1):1–3.

Cober, M. P., and S. J. Phelps. 2010. Penicillin prophylaxis in children with sickle cell disease. *Journal of Pediatric Pharmacology and Therapeutics* 15(3):152–159.

Crawford, N. G., et al. 2017. Loci associated with skin pigmentation identified in African populations. *Science* 358(6365):eaan8433.

Dampier, C., P. LeBeau, S. Rhee, S. Lieff, K. Kesler, S. Ballas, Z. Rogers, W. Wang, and Comprehensive Sickle Cell Centers Clinical Trial Consortium Site Investigators. 2011. Health-related quality of life in adults with sickle cell disease (SCD): A report from the Comprehensive Sickle Cell Centers Clinical Trial Consortium. *American Journal of Hematology* 86(2):203–205.

Darbari, I., J. E. O'Brien, S. J. Hardy, B. Speller-Brown, L. Thaniel, B. Martin, D. S. Darbari, and R. S. Nickel. 2018. Views of parents of children with sickle cell disease on pre-implantation genetic diagnosis. *Pediatric Blood & Cancer* 65(8):e27102.

Drazba, K. T., M. A. Kelley, and P. E. Hershberger. 2014. A qualitative inquiry of the financial concerns of couples opting to use preimplantation genetic diagnosis to prevent the transmission of known genetic disorders. *Journal of Genetic Counseling* 23(2):202–211.

Eckman, J. R., K. L. Hassell, W. Huggins, E. M. Werner, E. S. Klings, R. J. Adams, J. A. Panepinto, and C. M. Hamilton. 2017. Standard measures for sickle cell disease research: The PhenX Toolkit sickle cell disease collections. *Blood Advances* 1(27):2703–2711.

El-Haj, N., and C. C. Hoppe. 2018. Newborn screening for SCD in the USA and Canada. *International Journal of Neonatal Screening* 4(4):36.

Elliott, A., and E. Bruner. 2019. Renal medullary carcinoma. *Archives of Pathology and Laboratory Medicine* 143(12):1556–1561.

Faro, E. Z., C. J. Wang, and S. O. Oyeku. 2016. Quality indicator development for positive screen follow-up for sickle cell disease and trait. *American Journal of Preventive Medicine* 51(1 Suppl 1):S48–S54.

Farrell, M. H., and S. A. Christopher. 2013. Frequency of high-quality communication behaviors used by primary care providers of heterozygous infants after newborn screening. *Patient Education and Counseling* 90(2):226–232.

FDA (U.S. Food and Drug Administration). 2016. *Use of electronic informed consent questions and answers: Guidance for institutional review boards, investigators, and sponsors.* https://www.fda.gov/media/116850/download (accessed January 9, 2020).

Feldman, E. A. 2012. The Genetic Information Nondiscrimination Act (GINA): Public policy and medical practice in the age of personalized medicine. *Journal of General Internal Medicine* 27(6):743–746.

Ferster, K., and E. R. Eichner. 2012. Exertional sickling deaths in army recruits with sickle cell trait. *Military Medicine* 177(1):56–59.

Feuchtbaum, L., S. Paulukonis, and N. Rosenthal. 2013. Sickle cell disease surveillance in California: Methods, findings, and challenges. In *Newborn Screening and Genetic Testing Symposium.* Atlanta, GA: Association of Public Health Laboratories.

Foege, W. H., R. C. Hogan, and L. H. Newton. 1976. Surveillance projects for selected diseases. *International Journal of Epidemiology* 5(1):29–37.

Forrest, C. B., R. J. Bartek, Y. Rubinstein, and S. C. Groft. 2011. The case for a global rare-diseases registry. *The Lancet* 377(9771):1057–1059.

Frommel, C., A. Brose, J. Klein, O. Blankenstein, and S. Lobitz. 2014. Newborn screening for sickle cell disease: Technical and legal aspects of a German pilot study with 38,220 participants. *BioMed Research International* 2014:695828.

Gallo, A. M., D. Wilkie, M. Suarez, R. Labotka, R. Molokie, A. Thocmpson, P. Hershberger, and B. Johnson. 2010. Reproductive decisions in people with sickle cell disease or sickle cell trait. *Western Journal of Nursing Research* 32(8):1073–1090.

Grant, A. M., C. S. Parker, L. B. Jordan, M. M. Hulihan, M. S. Creary, M. A. Lloyd-Puryear, J. C. Goldsmith, and H. K. Atrash. 2011. Public health implications of sickle cell trait: A report of the CDC meeting. *American Journal of Preventive Medicine* 41(6 Suppl 4):S435–S439.

Grosse, S. D., W. H. Rogowski, L. F. Ross, M. C. Cornel, W. J. Dondorp, and M. J. Khoury. 2010. Population screening for genetic disorders in the 21st century: Evidence, economics, and ethics. *Public Health Genomics* 13(2):106–115.

Gustafson, S. L., E. A. Gettig, M. Watt-Morse, and L. Krishnamurti. 2007. Health beliefs among African American women regarding genetic testing and counseling for sickle cell disease. *Genetics in Medicine* 9(5):303–310.

Hajar, R. 2017. The physician's oath: Historical perspectives. *Heart Views* 18(4):154–159.

Hamel, L. M., L. A. Penner, T. L. Albrecht, E. Heath, C. K. Gwede, and S. Eggly. 2016. Barriers to clinical trial enrollment in racial and ethnic minority patients with cancer. *Cancer Control* 23(4):327–337.

Hamilton, C. M., L. C. Strader, J. G. Pratt, D. Maiese, T. Hendershot, R. K. Kwok, J. A. Hammond, W. Huggins, D. Jackman, H. Pan, D. S. Nettles, T. H. Beaty, L. A. Farrer, P. Kraft, M. L. Marazita, J. M. Ordovas, C. N. Pato, M. R. Spitz, D. Wagener, M. Williams, H. A. Junkins, W. R. Harlan, E. M. Ramos, and J. Haines. 2011. The PhenX toolkit: Get the most from your measures. *American Journal of Epidemiology* 174(3):253–260.

Harmon, K. G., J. A. Drezner, D. Klossner, and I. M. Asif. 2012. Sickle cell trait associated with a RR of death of 37 times in National Collegiate Athletic Association football athletes: A database with 2 million athlete-years as the denominator. *British Journal of Sports Medicine* 46(5):325–330.

Harrison, S. E., C. M. Walcott, and T. D. Warner. 2017. Knowledge and awareness of sickle cell trait among young African American adults. *Western Journal of Nursing Research* 39(9):1222–1239.

Hassell, K., B. Pace, W. Wang, R. Kulkarni, N. Luban, C. S. Johnson, J. Eckman, P. Lane, and W. G. Woods. 2009. Sickle Cell Disease Summit: From clinical and research disparity to action. *American Journal of Hematology and Oncology* 84(1):39–45.

Hinton, C. F., C. T. Mai, S. K Nabukera, L. D. Botto, L. Feuchtbaum, P. A. Romitti, Y. Wang, K. N. Piper, and R. S. Olney. 2014. Developing a public health-tracking system for follow-up of newborn screening metabolic conditions: A four-state pilot project structure and initial findings. *Genetic Medicine* 16(6):484–490.

Hinton, C. F., C. J. Homer, A. A. Thompson, A. Williams, K. L. Hassell, L. Feuchtbaum, S. A. Berry, A. Comeau, B. L.Therrell, A. Brower, K. B. Harris, C. Brown, J. Monaco, R. J. Ostrander, A.E. Zuckerman, C. Kaye, D. Dougherty, C. Greene, N. S. Green, and the Follow-up and Treatment Sub-Committee of the Advisory Committee on Heritable Disorders in Newborns and Children (ACHDNC). 2016. A framework for assessing outcomes from newborn screening: On the road to measuring its promise. *Molecular Genetics and Metabolism* 118(4):221–229.

Hoff, T., and A. Hoyt. 2006. Practices and perceptions of long-term follow-up among state newborn screening programs. *Pediatrics* 117(6):1922–1929.

Hoffman, K. M., S. Trawalter, J. R. Axt, and M. N. Oliver. 2016. Racial bias in pain assessment and treatment recommendations, and false beliefs about biological differences between blacks and whites. *Proceedings of the National Academy of Sciences* 113(16):4296–4301.

Hoots, W. K. 2010. The registry and surveillance in hemoglobinopathies: Improving the lives of individuals with hemoglobinopathies. *American Journal of Preventive Medicine* 38(4 Suppl):S510–S511.

Housten, A. J., R. A. Abel, T. Lindsey, and A. A. King. 2016. Feasibility of a community-based sickle cell trait testing and counseling program. *Journal of Health Disparities Research and Practice* 9(3):1.

Hulihan, M. M., L. Feuchtbaum, L. Jordan, R. S. Kirby, A. Snyder, W. Young, Y. Greene, J. Telfair, Y. Wang, W. Cramer, E. M. Werner, K. Kenney, M. Creary, and A. M. Grant. 2015. State-based surveillance for selected hemoglobinopathies. *Genetics in Medicine* 17(2):125–130.

IOM (Institute of Medicine). 2009. *Beyond the HIPAA privacy rule: Enhancing privacy, improving health through research*. Washington, DC: The National Academies Press.

Jones, S. R., R. A. Binder, and E. M. Donowho, Jr. 1970. Sudden death in sickle-cell trait. *New England Journal of Medicine* 282(6):323–325.

Jordan, L. B., K. Smith-Whitley, M. J. Treadwell, J. Telfair, A. M. Grant, and K. Ohene-Frempong. 2011. Screening U.S. college athletes for their sickle cell disease carrier status. *American Journal of Preventive Medicine* 41(6 Suppl 4):S406–S412.

Kark, J. A., D. M. Posey, H. R. Schumacher, and C. J. Ruehle. 1987. Sickle-cell trait as a risk factor for sudden death in physical training. *New England Journal of Medicine* 317(13):781–787.

Kark, J. A., R. J. Labotka, J. W. Gardner, and F. T. Ward. 2010. Prevention of exercise-related death unexplained by preexisting disease (EDU) associated with sickle cell trait (SCT) without hemoglobin (Hb) screening or Hb specific management. *Blood* 116(21):945.

Kavanagh, P. L., C. J. Wang, B. L. Therrell, P. G. Sprinz, and H. Bauchner. 2008. Communication of positive newborn screening results for sickle cell disease and sickle cell trait: Variation across states. *American Journal of Medical Genetics. Part C: Seminars in Medical Genetics* 148C(1):15–22.

Key, N. S., P. Connes, and V. K. Derebail. 2015. Negative health implications of sickle cell trait in high income countries: From the football field to the laboratory. *British Journal of Haematology* 170(1):5–14.

Kunz, J. B., H. Cario, R. Grosse, A. Jarisch, S. Lobitz, and A. E. Kulozik. 2017. The epidemiology of sickle cell disease in Germany following recent large-scale immigration. *Pediatric Blood & Cancer* 64(7).

Lang, C. W., A. P. Stark, K. Acharya, and L. F. Ross. 2009. Maternal knowledge and attitudes about newborn screening for sickle cell disease and cystic fibrosis. *American Journal of Medical Genetics, Part A* 149A(11):2424–2429.

Lee, L. M., and P. Marks. 2014. When a blood donor has sickle cell trait: Incidental findings and public health. *Hastings Center Report* 44(4):17–21.

Lin, K. W. 2009. Screening for sickle cell disease in newborns. *American Family Physician* 79(6):507–508.

Lussier, M.-T., C. Richard, T.-L. Bennett, T. Williamson, and A. Nagpurkar. 2012. Surveillance or research: What's in a name? *Canadian Family Physician/Medecin de Famille Canadien* 58(1):117.

Manco-Johnson, M. J., V. R. Byams, M. Recht, B. Dudley, B. Dupervil, D. J. Aschman, M. Oakley, S. Kapica, M. Voutsis, S. Humes, R. Kulkarni, A. M. Grant, and U.S. Haemophilia Treatment Center Network. 2018. Community counts: Evolution of a national surveillance system for bleeding disorders. *American Journal of Hematology* 93(6):E137–E140.

Maryland Department of Health. n.d. *Newborn screening—Frequently asked questions.* https://health.maryland.gov/laboratories/Pages/nbs-faq.aspx (accessed March 10, 2020).

Mayo-Gamble, T. L., S. E. Middlestadt, H. C. Lin, J. Cunningham-Erves, P. Barnes, and P. B. Jackson. 2018. Identifying factors underlying the decision for sickle cell carrier screening among African Americans within middle reproductive age. *Journal of Genetic Counseling* 27(5):1302–1311.

McGann, P. T., and C. Hoppe. 2017. The pressing need for point-of-care diagnostics for sickle cell disease: A review of current and future technologies. *Blood Cells, Molecules, and Diseases* 67:104–113.

Minkovitz, C. S., H. Grason, M. Ruderman, and J. F. Casella. 2016. Newborn screening programs and sickle cell disease: A public health services and systems approach. *American Journal of Preventive Medicine* 51(1 Suppl 1):S39–S47.

Mitchell, B. L. 2018. Sickle cell trait and sudden death. *Sports Medicine—Open* 4(1):19.

Morales, A., A. Wierenga, C. Cuthbert, S. Sacharow, P. Jayakar, D. Velazquez, J. Loring, and D. Barbouth. 2009. Expanded newborn screening in Puerto Rico and the U.S. Virgin Islands: Education and barriers assessment. *Genetics in Medicine* 11(3):169–175.

Moseley, K. L., S. Z. Nasr, J. L. Schuette, and A. D. Campbell. 2013. Who counsels parents of newborns who are carriers of sickle cell anemia or cystic fibrosis? *Journal of Genetic Counseling* 22(2):218–225.

Mukherjee, M. B., R. B. Colah, P. R. Mehta, N. Shinde, D. Jain, S. Desai, K. Dave, Y. Italia, B. Raicha, and E. Serrao. 2019. Multicenter evaluation of HemoTypeSC as a point-of-care sickle cell disease rapid diagnostic test for newborns and adults across India. *American Journal of Clinical Pathology* 153(1):82–87.

Naik, R. P., and C. Haywood, Jr. 2015. Sickle cell trait diagnosis: Clinical and social implications. *Hematology* 2015:160–167.

Naik, R. P., K. Smith-Whitley, K. L. Hassell, N. I. Umeh, M. de Montalembert, P. Sahota, C. Haywood, Jr., J. Jenkins, M. A. Lloyd-Puryear, C. H. Joiner, V. L. Bonham, and G. J. Kato. 2018. Clinical outcomes associated with sickle cell trait: A systematic review. *Annals of Internal Medicine* 169(9):619–627.

National Commission for the Protection of Human Subjects of Biomedical and Behavioral Research. 1979. *The Belmont report: Ethical principles and guidelines for the protection of human subjects of research.* https://www.hhs.gov/ohrp/regulations-and-policy/belmont-report/read-the-belmont-report/index.html (accessed January 9, 2020).

NCSL (National Conference of State Legislatures). 2019. *State laws related to insurance coverage for infertility treatment.* https://www.ncsl.org/research/health/insurance-coverage-for-infertility-laws.aspx (accesssed January 9, 2020).

Nelson, D. A., P. A. Deuster, R. Carter, 3rd, O. T. Hill, V. L. Wolcott, and L. M. Kurina. 2016. Sickle cell trait, rhabdomyolysis, and mortality among U.S. Army soldiers. *New England Journal of Medicine* 375(5):435–442.

NewSTEPs. 2020. *Data visualizations: State profiles.* Silver Spring, MD: Association of Public Health Laboratories. https://www.newsteps.org/data-visualizations (accessed January 9, 2020).

NHLBI (National Heart, Lung, and Blood Institute). 2007. *Establishing a database of people with sickle cell disease (Comprehensive Sickle Cell Centers Collaborative Data Project, C-Data).* https://ClinicalTrials.gov/show/NCT00529061 (accessed January 9, 2020).

Nnodu, O., H. Isa, M. Nwegbu, C. Ohiaeri, S. Adegoke, R. Chianumba, N. Ugwu, B. Brown, J. Olaniyi, E. Okocha, J. Lawson, A. A. Hassan, I. Diaku-Akinwumi, A. Madu, O. Ezenwosu, Y. Tanko, U. Kangiwa, A. Girei, Y. Israel-Aina, A. Ladu, P. Egbuzu, U. Abjah, A. Okolo, N. Akbulut-Jeradi, M. Fernandez, F. B. Piel, and A. Adekile. 2019. HemoTypeSC, a low-cost point-of-care testing device for sickle cell disease: Promises and challenges. *Blood Cells, Molecules, and Diseases* 78:22–28.

NRC (National Research Council). 1975. *Genetic screening: Programs, principles, and research.* Washington, DC: National Academy of Sciences.

OCR (Office for Civil Rights). 2013. *Summary of the HIPAA security rule.* https://www.hhs.gov/hipaa/for-professionals/security/laws-regulations/index.html (accessed March 11, 2020).

Okwi, A. L., W. Byarugaba, C. M. Ndugwa, A. Parkes, M. Ocaido, and J. K. Tumwine. 2009. Knowledge gaps, attitude and beliefs of the communities about sickle cell disease in eastern and western Uganda. *East African Medical Journal* 86(9):442–449.

Paulukonis, S. T., W. T. Harris, T. D. Coates, L. Neumayr, M. Treadwell, E. Vichinsky, and L. B. Feuchtbaum. 2014. Population based surveillance in sickle cell disease: Methods, findings and implications from the California Registry and Surveillance System in Hemoglobinopathies project (RuSH). *Pediatric Blood & Cancer* 61(12):2271–2276.

Paulukonis, S., F. Raider, and M. Hulihan. 2015. *Longitudinal data collection for sickle cell disease in California: History, goals and challenges.* https://trackingcalifornia.org/cms/file/sickle-cell-disease/scd-in-cali (accessed March 11, 2020).

Pecker, L. H., and R. P. Naik. 2018. The current state of sickle-cell trait: Implications for reproductive and genetic counseling. *Blood* 132(22):2331–2338.

Pena, A. 2018. Sickle cell disease association launches first patient-powered registry. *Sickle Cell Disease News*, June 21. https://sicklecellanemianews.com/2018/06/21/sickle-cell-disease-association-launches-first-patient-powered-registry (accessed April 1, 2020).

Peters, M., K. Fijnvandraat, X. W. van den Tweel, F. G. Garre, P. C. Giordano, J. P. van Wouwe, R. R. Pereira, and P. H. Verkerk. 2010. One-third of the new paediatric patients with sickle cell disease in the Netherlands are immigrants and do not benefit from neonatal screening. *Archives of Disease in Childhood* 95(10):822–825.

Posnack, S. 2015. *Connecting health and care for the nation: A shared nationwide interoperability roadmap.* https://ncvhs.hhs.gov/wp-content/uploads/2015/10/Day-2-NCVHS-Dept-Update-POSNACK.pdf (accessed March 10, 2020).

Reeves, S. L., A. C. Tribble, B. Madden, G. L. Freed, and K. J. Dombkowski. 2018. Antibiotic prophylaxis for children with sickle cell anemia. *Pediatrics* 141(3):e20172182.

Ross, L. F. 2012. Newborn screening for sickle cell disease: Whose reproductive benefit? *European Journal of Human Genetics* 20(5):484–485.

Savage, W. J., G. R. Buchanan, B. P. Yawn, A. N. Afenyi-Annan, S. K. Ballas, J. C. Goldsmith, K. L. Hassell, A. H. James, J. John-Sowah, L. Jordan, R. Lottenberg, M. H. Murad, E. Ortiz, P. J. Tanabe, R. E. Ware, and S. M. Lanzkron. 2015. Evidence gaps in the management of sickle cell disease: A summary of needed research. *American Journal of Hematology* 90(4):273–275.

SCDIC (Sickle Cell Disease Implementation Consortium). n.d. *Home page.* https://scdic.rti.org (accessed January 9, 2020).

Schultz, C. L., T. Tchume-Johnson, T. Jackson, H. Enninful-Eghan, M. Schapira, and K. Smith-Whitley. 2014. Reproductive decisions in families affected by sickle cell disease. *Blood* 124(21):2175.

Segbena, A. Y., A. Guindo, R. Buono, I. Kueviakoe, D. A. Diallo, G. Guernec, M. Yerima, P. Guindo, E. Lauressergues, A. Mondeilh, V. Picot, and V. Leroy. 2018. Diagnostic accuracy in field conditions of the sickle SCAN® rapid test for sickle cell disease among children and adults in two West African settings: The DREPATEST study. *BMC Hematology* 18:26.

Serjeant, G. R. 2013. The natural history of sickle cell disease. *Cold Spring Harbor Perspectives in Medicine* 3(10):a011783.

Shah, S. 2010. Henrietta Lacks' story. *The Lancet* 375(9721):1154.

Shetty, A., and M. R. Matrana. 2014. Renal medullary carcinoma: A case report and brief review of the literature. *Ochsner Journal* 14(2):270–275.

Simopoulos, A. P., and Committee for the Study of Inborn Errors of Metabolism. 2009. Genetic screening: Programs, principles, and research-thirty years later. Reviewing the recommendations of the Committee for the Study of Inborn Errors of Metabolism (SIEM). *Public Health Genomics* 12(2):105–111.

Singer, D. E., C. Byrne, L. Chen, S. Shao, J. Goldsmith, and D. W. Niebuhr. 2018a. Risk of exertional heat illnesses associated with sickle cell trait in U.S. Military. *Military Medicine* 183(7–8):e310–e317.

Singer, D. E., L. Chen, S. Shao, J. Goldsmith, C. Byrne, and D. W. Niebuhr. 2018b. The association between sickle cell trait in U.S. service members with deployment, length of service, and mortality, 1992–2012. *Military Medicine* 183(3–4):e213–e218.

Smith, M., and R. T. Aguirre. 2012. Reproductive attitudes and behaviors in people with sickle cell disease or sickle cell trait: A qualitative interpretive meta-synthesis. *Social Work in Health Care* 51(9):757–779.

St. Jude Children's Research Hospital. 2019. *Genomic and clinical data for the sickle cell research community.* https://sickle-cell.stjude.cloud (accessed January 9, 2020).

Steele, C., A. Sinski, J. Asibey, M. D. Hardy-Dessources, G. Elana, C. Brennan, I. Odame, C. Hoppe, M. Geisberg, E. Serrao, and C. T. Quinn. 2019. Point-of-care screening for sickle cell disease in low-resource settings: A multi-center evaluation of HemoTypeSC, a novel rapid test. *American Journal of Hematology* 94(1):39–45.

Taylor, C., P. Kavanagh, and B. Zuckerman. 2014. Sickle cell trait—Neglected opportunities in the era of genomic medicine. *JAMA* 311(15):1495–1496.

Teach, S. J., K. A. Lillis, and M. Grossi. 1998. Compliance with penicillin prophylaxis in patients with sickle cell disease. *Archives of Pediatrics and Adolescent Medicine* 152(3):274–278.

Texas Department of State Health Services. 2019. *Newborn screening—Use and storage of dried blood spots after NBS.* Last modified March 1, 2019. https://www.dshs.texas.gov/lab/nbsbloodspots.shtm (accessed March 10, 2020).

Thacker, S. B., and R. L. Berkelman. 1988. Public health surveillance in the United States. *Epidemiologic Reviews* 10:164–190.

Tubman, V. N., and J. J. Field. 2015. Sickle solubility test to screen for sickle cell trait: What's the harm? *Hematology* 2015(1):433–435.

Vichinsky, E., D. Hurst, A. Earles, K. Kleman, and B. Lubin. 1988. Newborn screening for sickle cell disease: Effect on mortality. *Pediatrics* 81(6):749–755.

Voskaridou, E., A. Kattamis, C. Fragodimitri, A. Kourakli, P. Chalkia, M. Diamantidis, E. Vlachaki, M. Drosou, S. Lafioniatis, K. Maragkos, F. Petropoulou, E. Eftihiadis, M. Economou, E. Klironomos, F. Koutsouka, K. Nestora, I. Tzoumari, O. Papageorgiou, A. Basileiadi, I. Lafiatis, E. Dimitriadou, A. Kalpaka, C. Kalkana, G. Xanthopoulidis, I. Adamopoulos, P. Kaiafas, A. Mpitzioni, A. Goula, I. Kontonis, C. Alepi, A. Anastasiadis, M. Papadopoulou, P. Maili, D. Dionisopoulou, A. Tsirka, A. Makis, S. Kostaridou, M. Politou, I. Papassotiriou, and Greek Haemoglobinopathies Study Group. 2019. National registry of hemoglobinopathies in Greece: Updated demographics, current trends in affected births, and causes of mortality. *Annals of Hematology* 98(1):55–66.

Vrettou, C., G. Kakourou, T. Mamas, and J. Traeger-Synodinos. 2018. Prenatal and preimplantation diagnosis of hemoglobinopathies. *International Journal of Laboratory Hematology* 40(Suppl 1):74–82.

Wailoo, K. 2001. *Dying in the city of the blues: Sickle cell anemia and the politics of race and health*. Chapel Hill, NC: University of North Carolina Press.

Wailoo, K. 2017. Sickle cell disease—A history of progress and peril. *New England Journal of Medicine* 376(9):805–807.

Webber, B. J., and C. T. Witkop. 2014. Screening for sickle-cell trait at accession to the United States military. *Military Medicine* 179(11):1184–1189.

Wilson, J. M., and Y. G. Jungner. 1968. Principles and practice of mass screening for disease. *Boletín de la Oficina Sanitaria Panamericana (Pan American Sanitary Bureau)* 65(4):281–393.

Wright, S. W., M. H. Zeldin, K. Wrenn, and O. Miller. 1994. Screening for sickle-cell trait in the emergency department. *Journal of General Internal Medicine* 9(8):421–424.

Xu, K., Z. M. Shi, L. L. Veeck, M. R. Hughes, and Z. Rosenwaks. 1999. First unaffected pregnancy using preimplantation genetic diagnosis for sickle cell anemia. *JAMA* 281(18):1701–1706.

Yenilmez, E. D., and A. Tuli. 2016. New perspectives in prenatal diagnosis of sickle cell anemia. In B. Inusa (ed.), *Sickle cell disease: Pain and common chronic complications*. London: IntechOpen.

Yusuf, H. R., M. A. Lloyd-Puryear, A. M. Grant, C. S. Parker, M. S. Creary, and H. K. Atrash. 2011. Sickle cell disease: The need for a public health agenda. *American Journal of Preventive Medicine* 41(6 Suppl 4):S376–S383.

Zuckerman, A. E. 2009. The role of health information technology in quality improvement in pediatrics. *Pediatric Clinics of North America* 56(4):965–973.

4

Complications of Sickle Cell Disease and Current Management Approaches

A lot of ... clinical knowledge is not captured in research yet....
[W]e are still defining value in a context that really only looks at what
the existing literature is.

—Sara v. G. (Open Session Panelist)

Chapter Summary

- Sickle cell disease (SCD) is a multi-organ blood and blood vessel disease, with pain (both acute and chronic) being its most prominent aspect.
- Individuals with SCD experience recurrent but unpredictable episodes of debilitating acute pain that, over time, evolve into daily chronic pain.
- Individuals with SCD also experience severe disease complications, with or without accompanying pain.
- Lifelong debilitating multi-system organ damage occurs in individuals with SCD and is responsible for the continued high morbidity and mortality associated with the disease. Currently there is a lack of predictors for identifying individuals at risk for the most severe complications.
- Tremendous strides have been made in the past few decades in the care of children with SCD, which have led to almost all children in high-income settings surviving to adulthood.

continued

123

- People with SCD are living longer, into late adulthood; however, disease management is still based on limited clinical information in adults.
- Further research is needed on evidence-based management approaches, particularly those that improve quality of life, increase longevity by preventing chronic organ damage, and mitigate acute and chronic complications in both adults and children.

INTRODUCTION

Sickle cell disease (SCD) is a multi-system disorder resulting from the complex interplay among hemolysis (the destruction of red blood cells [RBCs]), chronic inflammation, and systemic vascular damage. Its main presenting symptom is pain. Unpredictable, recurrent, and excruciating episodes of acute pain—often referred to as "pain crises"—and the various consequences of chronic pain are responsible for most of the psychosocial devastation of the disease and are also the primary reason for the use of health care (Borhade and Kondamudi, 2019). However, despite its importance, pain is perhaps the least understood complication of SCD and thus will be considered first in this chapter, separately from the disease's other complications.

In addition to acute and chronic pain, SCD also has profound effects on every organ and system of the body, as discussed later in the chapter. Managing SCD requires paying attention to its complex pathophysiology and its nuanced effects on general medical comorbidities, which are becoming increasingly common as individuals survive into adulthood. The SCD population has benefited from research that generated evidence-based guidelines to prevent infections and strokes (which were the primary reason for early mortality in the 1970s and 1980s).

However, although it has been more than 70 years since the precise genetic defect responsible for this disorder was identified (Ingram, 2004), life expectancy for individuals with SCD remains more than 20 years less than that of the general population, according to research conducted at two academic medical centers (DeBaun et al., 2019). The characterization of the full range of morbidity and the identification of efficacious interventions for managing the disease have both come much more slowly than for other inherited disorders of childhood (e.g., hemophilia and cystic fibrosis). Biomarker development to guide clinical care and identify outcome measures for clinical trials has also proceeded at a slow pace, partly due to the complexity of the disease.

There is a desperate need for new and ongoing research to identify and widely implement modern, effective, and comprehensive management approaches that will improve both longevity and the quality of life (QOL) in children and adults with SCD by preventing chronic complications and end-organ damage. Research is also required to identify and deploy strategies to mitigate the intense suffering and morbidity from SCD pain.

PAIN IN SCD

Pain is the prototypical symptom of SCD and the most common reason to seek acute or ambulatory care. It is associated with increased morbidity, mortality, and health care costs (Ballas et al., 2012a). Acute vaso-occlusive episodes (VOEs, also known as pain crises, pain episodes, or vaso-occlusive crises) are acute episodes of intense pain and are underpinned by a complex pathophysiology. VOEs are multifactorial and may stem from a variety of causes, and a high rate of VOEs is typically associated with early mortality from multi-organ damage. Individuals living with SCD also experience daily chronic pain. Pain may occur from chronic end-organ or nerve damage from SCD as a result of treatments (e.g., opioid-induced hyperalgesia [OIH]) or from non-SCD medical comorbidities, such as osteoarthritis, gout, or rheumatoid arthritis (Dampier et al., 2017).

Pain is, in a sense, an "invisible" complication of SCD. There are often no objective physical signs or biomarkers of either acute or chronic SCD pain. The lack of an objective tool to accurately predict and characterize pain in SCD and to guide clinicians to the appropriate therapeutic intervention remains a significant research gap, as discussed in Chapter 7 (Darbari and Brandow, 2017).

The complex pathophysiology of acute and chronic pain in SCD is poorly understood, which may be one of the reasons why its treatment remains suboptimal. There is insufficient understanding of the interplay among (1) the pathophysiology of pain in SCD, (2) the cumulative effects of recurrent pain episodes, (3) the individual variability in pain perception and coping, and (4) the influence of pain treatments (particularly the chronic exposure to opioids). As a growing number of individuals with SCD have now survived into adulthood, the cumulative burden of opioid-related side effects, including OIH, is emerging and will need to be further investigated.

Finally, but also importantly, socioeconomic factors relating to race and social milieu that are characteristic of the affected population complicate the experience and treatment of pain. Sociodemographic factors have been shown to influence pain perception, expression, and response to treatment (Clark et al., 1999). Individuals with SCD report higher levels of pain compared with cancer patients of either the same or a different race (Ezenwa et al., 2018). When individuals living with SCD perceive discrimination from physicians or nurses on account of their race or socioeconomic status, they exhibit poor coping strategies (Ezenwa et al., 2017) and more intense stress and pain (Ezenwa et al., 2015; Haywood et al., 2014).

The Epidemiology of Pain in SCD

Acute Pain in SCD

VOEs are characterized by severe and unpredictable acute pain. Diggs described the typical acute VOE as being of sudden onset; involving the lower back, joints, or extremities; either localized or migratory; and often continuous and throbbing (Ballas et al., 2012a; Diggs, 1956). The Analgesic, Anesthetic, and Addiction Clinical Trial Translations Innovations Opportunities and Networks–American Pain Society Pain Taxonomy (AAPT) initiative has recently established diagnostic criteria for acute SCD pain (Dampier et al., 2017). According to AAPT criteria, acute SCD pain is new-onset pain that lasts ≥ 2 hours but that has not been present for more than 10 days or two standard deviations above the mean length of an acute pain episode in adults with SCD (based on the Pain in Sickle Cell Epidemiology Study [PiSCES] cohort) (Field et al., 2019). This definition aims to distinguish acute pain from transient and chronic pain but may not adequately capture pain syndromes that represent a transition from acute to chronic pain.

Acute pain in SCD happens when the rapid breakdown of the sickled RBCs leads to increased inflammation by depleting the body of anti-inflammatory molecules that also help maintain blood vessel integrity. When the cells making up the lining of the blood vessels (i.e., the endothelium) are damaged, any inflammation makes it easier for sickled RBCs to obstruct the blood flow through the vessels. As a result there is an oxygen deficit to the downstream organs, which causes pain in tissues and nerves (Ballas et al., 2012a). The chronically heightened inflammatory state of SCD leads to activation of white blood cells, platelets, and endothelial cells as well as of the clotting pathways and, ultimately, multicellular adhesion or clumping, which results in vaso-occlusion (the obstruction of blood vessels) and ischemia–reperfusion injury, which is the damage created by reoxygenation after a period of oxygen deprivation (Kalogeris et al., 2012).

When an organ's blood flow is compromised (ischemia), the resultant injury to the body's pain-sensing (nociceptive) tissue results in acute pain (Ballas et al., 2012a). In the bone marrow, inflammation and death of cells (necrosis) occur, leading to pain that may be nociceptive, inflammatory, or neuropathic and is experienced acutely but can also persist, evolving into chronic pain (Charache and Page, 1967; Conran et al., 2009; Zhang et al., 2016).

Repetitive bouts of excruciating pain have a profoundly negative impact on all aspects of health-related quality of life (HRQOL) across the life span (Dampier et al., 2011). Pain rates (measured in episodes per year) in SCD vary by age, with the highest rates in the 20- to 29-year-old cohort (Platt et al., 1991). A study by Brousseau et al. (2010) found that 21,112 patients had a total of 109,344 acute care encounters, which yields an acute care use rate of 2.59. This means that, on average, the individuals included in the study had approximately three acute care encounters per year; the majority of these were for pain (Brousseau et al., 2010).

Acute care use for pain is responsible for a large proportion of health care spending for SCD. Using data from 4,294 Florida Medicaid enrollees with SCD, Kauf et al. (2009) determined that the approximately 100,000 affected individuals in the United States use approximately $1.1 billion in medical care; this number is believed to be a conservative estimate (Kauf et al., 2009).

Patient-reported VOE pain has been found to be an independent predictor of mortality in individuals with SCD (Darbari et al., 2013). Frequent admissions (three or more per year) for acute painful events have been demonstrated to correlate with increased mortality (Elmariah et al., 2014). An investigation into the causes of death for 209 individuals with SCD revealed that 33 percent who were free of organ damage died during VOEs (Platt et al., 1994). These findings highlight the link between the symptom of pain and its underlying pathophysiology and related complications and their attendant morbidity and mortality.

Current treatment approaches are aimed at rapidly relieving pain and investigating and mitigating its triggers (Ballas et al., 2012a; Uwaezuoke et al., 2018). The most common triggers include dehydration, infection, extreme emotional distress, physical overexertion, and exposure to ambient temperature extremes (Ballas and Smith, 1992; Ballas et al., 2012a; Yale et al., 2000). Most individuals report that they can sense when a crisis is imminent and often resort to mindfulness-based and supportive management strategies, such as liberal oral hydration, rest, relaxation, massage of the affected area, or walking to increase circulation in an effort to abort the symptoms (Simmons et al., 2019; Williams et al., 2017). This is in line with the findings of multiple studies and anecdotal evidence that the majority of acute pain in SCD is managed at home, with acute care use occurring in only a minority (3–5 percent) of cases (Smith et al., 2008).

Once an individual presents to an acute care setting, the initial phase of the VOE treatment is focused on relieving the acute distress and intense pain by quickly offering effective analgesia. A typical approach is to provide parenteral opioids (typically through an intravenous injection), with or without non-steroidal anti-inflammatory drugs (NSAIDs), and supportive hydration (Puri et al., 2018; Uwaezuoke et al., 2018; Yale et al., 2000). After the initial relief of intense pain is achieved, the clinician maintains pain relief by frequent repeat dosing of analgesia while also treating the underlying trigger, if identifiable, until the pain begins to resolve. Acute pain episodes may last from a few hours to a few days, to more than 1 week (Okwerekwu and Skirvin, 2018). As acute pain enters the resolving phase, it is important to gradually decrease the daily doses of opioids to avoid both rebound pain and withdrawal symptoms (Carroll, 2020). There are significant research gaps concerning the most effective way to apply the current understanding of the pathophysiology of SCD and knowledge of opioid pharmacogenomics to develop management strategies for acute pain in VOE (Puri et al., 2018).

The acute pain experience is characterized by the current episode of pain superimposed on the numerous prior acute pain episodes, plus the contribution of any chronic pain condition (Field et al., 2019). Thus, it is unrealistic to expect pain in SCD to be unidimensional in either presentation or response to treatment. The complexity and multifactorial nature of pain in SCD are difficult to dissect by patients, who may struggle to describe pain to health care providers, and by the providers, who may not completely understand it and thus inadequately treat it.

Chronic SCD Pain

In addition to acute pain, as individuals with SCD age they increasingly develop chronic pain. Chronic pain in SCD is defined as pain lasting more than 3 months, according to a National Institutes of Health (NIH) expert panel report (NHLBI, 2014). Among adolescents with SCD, this type of pain has been observed to change from intermittent acute pain that fully resolves between episodes to insidious daily pain with intermittent acute exacerbations, with the exacerbations perceived as becoming more intense over time (Smith and Scherer, 2010). The PiSCES study reported pain in 54.5 percent of 31,017 analyzed patient-days among adults with SCD; nearly 30 percent of the study participants reported experiencing pain on more than 95 percent of the days surveyed (Smith et al., 2008). The prospective Examining Sickle Cell Acute Pain in the Emergency vs. Day Hospital trial reported 68 percent of participants with chronic pain (Lanzkron et al., 2018), underscoring the high prevalence of this complication. Chronic pain in SCD often occurs in more than one location in the body (Franck et al., 2002), may have a neuropathic component (Wilkie et al., 2010), and often is accompanied by comorbid anxiety and depressive symptoms (Jonassaint et al., 2016).

The AAPT initiative attempted to better capture the multiple facets of chronic pain in SCD by developing an evidence-based classification system (Dampier et al., 2017). The new AAPT taxonomy defines chronic SCD pain as occurring on most days, lasting more than 6 months, and evidenced by at least one sign of pain sensitivity or chronic disease complication (e.g., a skin ulcer, splenic infarct, or bone infarction) associated with the location of the pain. The taxonomy defines three specific chronic pain subtypes: with contributory disease complications (e.g., gallstones, avascular necrosis, bone infracts), without contributory disease complications, and mixed (see Box 4-1). The new taxonomy can now be applied to address research gaps in the epidemiology, pathophysiology, and treatment of SCD chronic pain.

BOX 4-1
American Pain Society Pain Taxonomy Diagnostic Criteria
for Chronic Pain Associated with SCD (Chronic SCD Pain)

Dimension 1: Core Diagnostic Criteria
1. Diagnosis of SCD confirmed by laboratory testing
2. Reports of ongoing pain present on most days over the past 6 months either in a single location or in multiple locations
3. Must display at least 1 sign
   - Palpation of the region of reported pain elicits focal pain or tenderness
   - Movement of the region of reported pain elicits focal pain
   - Decreased range of motion or weakness in the region of reported pain
   - Evidence of skin ulcer in the region of reported pain
   - Evidence of hepatobiliary or splenic imaging abnormalities (eg, splenic infarc, chronic pancreatitis) consistent with the region of reported pain
   - Evidence of imaging abnormalities consistent with bone infarction or avascular necrosis in the region of reported pain
4. There is no other diagnosis that better explains the signs and symptoms

Chronic SCD pain diagnostic modifiers:
   We propose 3 diagnostic modifiers to indicate subtypes of chronic SCD pain.
1. Chronic SCD pain without contributory disease complications is used if there is no evidence of contributory SCD complications on the basis of either clinical signs (eg, presence of leg ulcers) or test results (eg, imaging abnormalities)
2. Chronic SCD pain with contributory disease complications should be used if there is evidence of contributory SCD complications on the basis of clinical signs or mixed results
3. Chronic SCD pain with mixed pain types should be used if there is evidence of contributory SCD complications (eg, avascular necrosis) on the basis of clinical signs or test results and there is pain also occurring in unrelated sites (eg, arms, back, chest, or abdominal pain)

SOURCE: Dampier et al., 2017, p. 492.

Neuropathic Pain

Neuropathic pain in SCD is not fully understood, but it likely arises from damage to the peripheral or central nervous systems (somatosensory system) during or following a VOE (Wilkie et al., 2010). As a result, it may be characterized by peripheral nociceptive sensitization or hypersensitivity that results in hyperalgesia and allodynia. Hyperalgesia is a heightened perception of severe pain generated by stimuli that are typically only mildly painful (Colloca et al., 2013; McMahon et al., 2013) and occurs in SCD with the onset of chronic pain. With allodynia, there is perception of severe pain from repeated stimuli that are usually painless; there is a need for additional research to understand its origin, prevention, and treatment in SCD (Ballas et al., 2012a).

Neuropathic pain occurs in 25–40 percent of individuals living with SCD (Brandow et al., 2014; Ezenwa et al., 2016); this is a significantly higher prevalence than in the general pain population although comparable to the prevalence in people with cancer (36–39 percent) (Brandow et al., 2014; Rayment et al., 2013). Patients describe neuropathic pain as numbness, tingling, and lancinating pain that is paroxysmal and often intense (Wilkie et al., 2010). Thermal pain sensitivity documented by quantitative sensory testing is indicative of neuropathic pain and has been reported in both children and adults (Brandow et al., 2013; Ezenwa et al., 2016; O'Leary et al., 2014). Despite the fact that neuropathic pain is a common archetype of chronic SCD pain, only 14 percent of adults with SCD and chronic pain in one study reported being prescribed adjuvant drugs that may target neuropathic pain pathways; the majority of the study participants received opioids only (Brandow et al., 2014; WHO, 2018; Wilkie et al., 2010).

Central Sensitization

Central sensitization (CS) refers to an increase in sensitivity to pain and in the responsiveness of neurons; it causes individuals with SCD to regularly experience clinical pain and other chronic pain syndromes (Ballas et al., 2012a; Campbell et al., 2016; Cataldo et al., 2015). Nociceptive signals from the periphery assault the central nervous system and alter the spinal cord and brain, causing chronic amplification of pain sensations (Woolf, 2011). One study reported CS in approximately 17–35 percent of chronic pain patients (Schliessbach et al., 2013); by contrast, CS is reportedly present in approximately 25–90 percent of individuals with SCD and chronic pain, according to two other studies (Campbell et al., 2016; Ezenwa et al., 2015). A higher degree of CS is associated with more clinical pain, more VOE pain, poor sleep, higher rates of pain catastrophizing, and negative mood (Campbell et al., 2016). It is believed that chronic exposure to opioids can result in CS (Cohen et al., 2008; Hay et al., 2009). Additional predisposing factors include genetics (Smith et al., 2012), psychosocial and behavioral comorbidities (Finan et al., 2013; Smith and Scherer, 2010), and neuropsychological factors (Cruz-Almeida et al., 2013).

Opioid-Induced Hyperalgesia

OIH refers to the paradoxical increased sensitivity to pain and heightened perception of pain that occurs after repeated/chronic exposure to opioids (Angst and Clark, 2006). With OIH even harmless stimuli can trigger an exaggerated pain response that worsens with increasing doses of opioids. This is an important differential diagnosis of exclusion; OIH is confirmed when pain perception and experience improve after ending opioid therapy (Lee et al., 2011; Ramasubbu and Gupta, 2011). While discontinuing opioids is a common approach in treating OIH, it should be undertaken with care because it may precipitate opioid withdrawal (Fishbain and Pulikal, 2019; Lee et al., 2011).

Opioid-Related Cyclical Withdrawal Syndrome

Unfortunately, the most common complication associated with opioids, opioid withdrawal syndrome (OWS), has been largely ignored in the management of SCD (Carroll et al., 2016). The committee was unable to find any published articles describing cyclic OWS and SCD, even though this clinical phenomenon is commonly experienced by individuals with SCD. OWS commonly occurs after VOE resolves and patients are transitioned to oral opiates without an appropriate taper or parenteral-to-oral dose adjustment. The resulting OWS may be interpreted as a new acute VOE, often leading to readmission and a vicious cycle of increased tolerance, higher opioid doses, and worse OWS.

Triggers and Psychological Impact of Pain

You can think of any life event, and I can tell you a story of how sickle cell disease impacted it.

—Tosin O. (Open Session Panelist)

Pain Catastrophizing

Pain catastrophizing is the tendency to worry and obsess about pain, leading to feelings of helplessness that interfere with function and adversely affect QOL (Van Damme et al., 2002). The PiSCES study reported a significantly higher degree of catastrophizing among adults with SCD than among those with other temporal chronic pain conditions (Citero et al., 2007) and also found an inverse relationship between mood and QOL ($p < 0.001$) (Citero et al., 2007). A study by Sil et al. (2016) showed that when a child and his or her parents express a large number of negative thoughts with a mindset of impending doom about the pain experience (pain catastrophizing), the child is more likely to also experience significant levels of functional disability (Sil et al., 2016). A failure to address thought patterns about pain can result in treatment failure.

Anxiety and Anticipatory Pain

The unpredictability and anticipation of SCD pain may trigger anxiety, as do repeated experiences of undertreatment of pain or inconsistent interactions with health care providers during acute pain exacerbations (Schlaeger et al., 2019). Some individuals may become anxious or stressed that they will have pain and miss an important activity, a life milestone (e.g., graduating from high school), or social activities with friends. Heightened anxiety is associated with increased pain sensitivity and can trigger VOEs. The relationship between anxiety and pain is discussed in more detail later in this chapter.

Treatment of Pain

Acute SCD Pain Management

The National Heart, Lung, and Blood Institute's evidence-based consensus guidelines (NHLBI, 2014) provide a general philosophy for managing acute SCD pain. The guidelines recommend prompt oral or intravenous analgesia for rapid relief. The recommended drugs to treat acute VOE pain at home include oral mild to moderate opioids, such as hydrocodone, oxycodone, morphine, or hydromorphone. Once oral therapy has failed, the recommendation is to proceed to intravenous or subcutaneous administration of morphine or hydromorphone or intranasal or intravenous administration of fentanyl. Pain relief should be paired with a thorough assessment of the cause or trigger of the pain event—including infections, dehydration, or acidosis—and then prompt treatment of the identified triggers and any other complications identified. Ideally, the prompt treatment of acute SCD pain should take place in a dedicated SCD day hospital, observation unit, or infusion center with trained personnel who follow standardized treatment plans with individualized dosing, when possible.

Chronic SCD Pain Management

Management of SCD chronic pain in the United States has traditionally been unidimensional and involved opioid titration and rotation; there are very few studies to identify best practices for treating chronic pain. Without evidence-based recommendations for treating chronic pain in SCD, the committee borrowed best practices from the general chronic pain literature and the recent Centers for Disease Control and Prevention (CDC) guidelines for opioid prescribing to manage chronic pain. The guidelines recommend non-pharmacological therapies due to the lack of proven efficacy and demonstrated harm associated with long-term opioid therapy (Dowell et al., 2016). Additionally, existing guidelines prescribe a structured approach to the use of opioids for chronic pain, including realistic goal setting between provider and patient after discussion of risk and benefits of opioids, with regular reappraisal; use of the lowest effective dose of preferably short-acting opioids, with caution when escalating doses over recommended morphine equivalent per day limits; minimal use of long-acting opioids when possible; not co-prescribing opioids with other sedating medications (benzodiazepines); the use of risk mitigation strategies (including reviewing the state prescription drug monitoring database for controlled substance prescription history); urine drug testing; and supporting evidence-based treatment for substance use disorder (SUD) when identified (Dowell et al., 2016).

While these guidelines seem intuitive, they are outside of the usual scope of practice of hematologists who care for individuals with SCD. The complications associated with long-term exposure to opioids have been overlooked, and individuals with SCD are poorly informed about the potential contribution of chronic opioids to their current and prior medical comorbidities (Benyamin et al., 2008). Delayed puberty, gastrointestinal complaints, and OIH are examples of complications that patients and health care providers may not always recognize as opioid-related.

The management of SCD chronic pain remains an area of frustration and dissatisfaction for providers and people living with SCD. Insurance plans typically limit access to non-pharmacologic therapies, which are, as a consequence, often overlooked in SCD. With the obvious need to de-emphasize the use of opioids in chronic pain management, there have not been commensurate evidence-based recommendations for alternative approaches.

Non-Opioid Medications

Acetaminophen Oral acetaminophen has been widely used in multimodal pain management strategies in SCD with variable efficacy (Shah et al., 2019). Intravenous acetaminophen is rarely used because of cost considerations, but it has been found to reduce acute pain in children with SCD (Baichoo et al., 2019).

Non-steroidal anti-inflammatory drugs While ketorolac and other NSAIDS have been routinely incorporated in the management of acute pain in SCD, studies about their effectiveness in controlling SCD pain have shown mixed results (Beiter et al., 2001; Hardwick et al., 1999; Perlin et al., 1994; Wright et al., 1992). Importantly, caution is paramount when using NSAIDs in SCD because kidney dysfunction may exist even in the presence of a normal serum creatinine and, therefore, remain undiagnosed. Acute kidney injury with ketorolac use has been reported in SCD (Baddam et al., 2017; Simckes et al., 1999).

Cannabis Cannabis use is prevalent in SCD, with one small study showing that 18 percent of the study participants (all of whom had SCD) had positive urine test for cannabis alone and 5 percent tested positive in combination with cocaine/phencyclidine (Roberts et al., 2018). The majority of cannabis users with SCD report that cannabis helps them relax and alleviates insomnia (Howard et al., 2005). A minority state that they use cannabis only for non-medical reasons and recreationally. The regulatory framework around marijuana is becoming more lax in the United States, and marijuana for medical use can be obtained legally under certain qualifying conditions in 33 states and the District of Columbia (Procon.org, 2019); SCD is a qualifying medical condition in several U.S. states.

In spite of the increased availability of medical marijuana, evidence for its efficacy and safety in SCD is limited. A study conducted on patients with SCD using recreational cannabis showed that cannabis use was associated with increased hospitalizations (Ballas, 2017), but causality could not be inferred because sicker patients may have been more prone to using cannabis to relieve their symptoms. Studies in sickle mice show that cannabinoids may reduce pain by reducing mast cell activation and inflammation (Vincent et al., 2016), but controlled studies in people with SCD are lacking. Thus, efforts should be made to rapidly close the research gaps on the therapeutic effects and risks associated with marijuana and other cannabinoids in treating pain in SCD (NASEM, 2017).

Topical lidocaine Topical lidocaine has been associated with improved pain control in small studies (Rasolofo et al., 2013), but it is not generally approved by insurance plans and is rarely used for home management.

Ketamine Intravenous ketamine is emerging as an alternative to morphine for acute pain management in SCD and may lead to lower opioid consumption (Lubega et al., 2018; Puri et al., 2019). However, neurological and psychiatric side effects are likely to limit its widespread use in the future.

Drugs targeting neuropathic pain Neuropathic pain is difficult to treat and is usually refractory to opioid and non-opioid analgesics (e.g., acetaminophen, NSAIDS). Tricyclic antidepressants, gabapentin, and pregabalin have been extensively used to treat neuropathic pain in other diseases but are underused in SCD (Sharma and Brandow, 2020). In a pediatric administrative dataset, neuropathic pain-targeting drugs were prescribed to only 2.9 percent of children, and their use was associated with older age, female gender, and longer length of stay (Brandow et al., 2015).

Partial Agonist Opioids

Buprenorphine Buprenorphine is a recently approved opioid with lower risk for misuse, withdrawal symptoms, and cravings for opioids as well as reduced risk of overdose. Recent data showed successful conversion to buprenorphine in patients with chronic pain and high opioid doses with a decrease in pain scores and acute care use, and increase in QOL measurements (Osunkwo et al., 2019).

SCD and the Opioid Epidemic

It is important to draw a clear distinction between the appropriate pain management used to address "acute-on-chronic" pain conditions like VOE in SCD and the overprescribing of pain medications that has led to the opioid epidemic in the United States. CDC has recently updated its opioid overuse prescribing guidelines to acknowledge that the pendulum has swung too far in the direction of restricting access, to the point that patients with a clear need for long-term opioids are being denied appropriate care (ASH, 2019; Meghani and Vapiwala, 2018). Because the opioid epidemic has become a major public health concern, the messaging to providers has tended to emphasize documenting the pain source, carrying out an appropriate workup, developing functional goals for pain, using a state registry to track controlled substance prescriptions, and monitoring prescriptions appropriately (Dowell et al., 2016). While all of these procedures are reasonable, the proliferation of high-profile provider indictments has resulted in a reluctance on the part of physicians to prescribe opioids for pain, further restricting access for vulnerable groups.

The committee believes that the unintended consequence of the new opioid-adverse climate could be a decreased access to opioids for SCD patients in need, such as those who are managing or recovering from acute VOE or have previously been maintained on daily opioids; pharmacies may not stock opioids in underserved communities perceived to have high rates of "opioid-using individuals" or risk of robbery, and some may require a 72-hour hold to allow time to investigate the appropriateness of the prescription. This climate has reflected on patients' perceptions of discrimination; people living with SCD have reported feeling increased stigma regarding their diagnosis and medication profile both within the hospital and at the pharmacy (Meghani and Vapiwala, 2018).

Non-Pharmacological Treatments of Pain in SCD

Non-Pharmacological Approaches

Various non-opioid-based treatments have been proposed for reducing acute pain and the duration of pain and for preventing pain in SCD; these treatments should be incorporated into a multidisciplinary pain control strategy whenever possible (Niscola et al., 2009). Because uncontrolled depression, anxiety, emotional trauma, and poor self-efficacy can worsen pain perception and control, behavioral and psychiatric comorbidities should be addressed as part of pain control strategies.

Oxygen In acute VOEs, oxygen has been used to shorten the duration of VOE and to prevent complications, but its indiscriminate use in non-hypoxic settings could be detrimental (Helmerhorst et al., 2015). Importantly, while oxygen is helpful in treating acute hypoxemia, small studies have shown no additional benefit in terms of reducing the duration or severity of a VOE (Niscola et al., 2009). Large studies on this topic are lacking.

Topical heat and massage There is low-quality evidence (i.e., primarily pilot studies with convenience samples) indicating that both heat and massage have moderate efficacy in pain control. Massage in adults and children living with SCD holds promise for reducing pain (Bodhise et al., 2004; Myers et al., 1999) and may lead to reduced use of pain medication and emergency department (ED) visits (Bodhise et al., 2004). The committee found one randomized controlled trial that evaluated massage in pediatric SCD (Lemanek et al., 2009); youth receiving the massage intervention had lower levels of pain, decreased anxiety and depression, and better overall functioning. More research is needed to understand the impact of massage in SCD.

Hydration Hydration has been a cornerstone of VOE prevention (Okomo and Meremikwu, 2007), but its benefits have been challenged in recent years because overhydration carries a risk of pulmonary edema, acute lung injury, and cardiac complications (Barabino et al., 2010; Gaartman et al., 2019). Intuitively, hypotonic solutions may ameliorate RBC dehydration in SCD and reduce sickle hemoglobin (HbS) polymerization and sickling, but recent publications have demonstrated that hypertonic fluid may have a negative impact on red cell deformability in in vitro microfluidic models and result in poorer pain control in pediatric patients presenting to the ED for acute VOE pain (Carden et al., 2017, 2019). Large, controlled clinical studies are needed to determine the optimal intravenous fluid solution and the rate and volume of administration.

Incentive spirometry Using an incentive spirometer (a device that tracks and promotes slow, deep breathing) has been shown to reduce the risk of pulmonary complications in VOE (Bellet et al., 1995; Yawn et al., 2014); all hospitalized patients with VOE should be encouraged to use an incentive spirometer throughout the hospital stay.

Complementary and Alternative Medicine

Complementary and alternative medicine (CAM) is a catch-all category for treatments that reside outside traditional medical science, such as hypnosis, yoga, acupuncture, massage, and prayer. Mind–body techniques such as mindfulness mediate endogenous pain at the supraspinal level. Studies have found that individuals with SCD frequently use CAM, including prayer, acupuncture, dietary supplements, relaxation, massage, and exercise (Niscola et al., 2009; Thompson and Eriator, 2014).

Acupuncture Acupuncture involves placing needles into defined points on the body to relieve symptoms. There are reports of reduced pain with acupuncture in SCD (Bhushan et al., 2015; Sinha et al., 2019), while another study found no difference in SCD pain after acupuncture or control treatment (needles placed randomly) (Co et al., 1979). A recent study conducted at the NIH Clinical Center found that people living with SCD and receiving acupuncture while hospitalized or in the outpatient setting demonstrated reductions in pain (Lu et al., 2014). Recent evidence showed that children with SCD receiving acupuncture to treat acute SCD pain in an ED experienced decreased pain scores post-treatment (Tsai et al., 2018).

Further studies are needed to confirm the clinical benefit of acupuncture, particularly on different types of SCD pain (e.g., neuropathic) (Lu et al., 2014). It is also important to note that this treatment may not be covered by insurance plans, making it difficult for individuals to access (Sinha et al., 2019).

Yoga Yoga, a practice that incorporates physical positions, mindfulness, relaxation, and breathing exercises, has been shown to reduce chronic and acute pain in adults, although there are limited data concerning its use for the treatment of SCD pain. The only randomized controlled trial of yoga as a treatment for acute SCD pain for children hospitalized with VOE supported its feasibility, acceptability, and potential for reducing pain (Moody et al., 2017). However, the committee was unable to find similar studies for adults.

Folk remedies As discussed in Chapter 2, African Americans' mistrust of the health care establishment and perceived discrimination by providers may lead to discounting care providers' recommendations and resorting to using home or "folk" remedies. Quandt et al. (2015) found that older, rural African Americans were more likely to use both food- and non-food remedies than were older, rural whites and that these remedies were sometimes used in place of prescription medications. The authors note that these home remedies "can potentially interfere with biomedical treatments" (Quandt et al., 2015, p. 121), thereby warranting further research.

Behavioral Treatment

Behavioral treatment can modulate the pathway between nociceptive pain and emotional responses to pain in the limbic system, hypothalamus, and amygdala, thus potentially reducing the perception of pain.

Cognitive behavioral therapy As discussed in Chapter 2, cognitive behavioral therapy (CBT) has been shown to be effective in the SCD population by addressing coping strategies and normalizing chronic pain. In CBT, individuals learn to differentiate emotional and behavioral reactions from a triggering event, such as pain (Anie and Green, 2015; Schatz et al., 2018). This method addresses thought distortions, working to de-catastrophize pain and address automatic negative thoughts associated with pain.

Mindfulness Mindfulness is a treatment that involves heightening one's level of awareness by intentionally attending to the present in an accepting and non-judgmental way (Kabat-Zinn, 2009). Mind–body techniques, such as mindfulness meditation, mediate endogenous pain at the supraspinal level. Mindfulness-based interventions led to reduction in chronic pain (Reiner et al., 2013). A 4-week guided imagery intervention improved self-efficacy in children with SCD (Dobson and Byrne, 2014). A study of children and adults found that self-hypnosis over 18 months reduced pain frequency and improved sleep but did not affect rates of school absenteeism (Dinges et al., 1997). An ongoing, randomized trial of a telephone-delivered mindfulness intervention for adults with SCD is examining the impact of mindfulness on pain catastrophizing (Williams et al., 2017).

OVERVIEW OF SCD COMPLICATIONS

SCD affects multiple organs over the life span. The earliest complications develop at the age of 6 months and coincide with the almost complete replacement of fetal hemoglobin with adult hemoglobin in RBCs (Kanter and Kruse-Jarres, 2013). Some of the most common complications in children are splenomegaly (an enlarged spleen), dactylitis (painful inflammation of fingers and toes), and jaundice. Some complications may appear in childhood and persist through adulthood, while others, especially those pertaining to organ failure, may manifest later in adulthood. SCD complications are best understood when grouped according to whether they are acute or chronic and based on the systems they affect. General medical comorbidities can have a negative effect on SCD outcomes, with the reverse being also true. Very little data have been published on the impact of general medical comorbidities in SCD, particularly among adults.

Table 4-1 summarizes the complications of SCD by the affected organ system, describing the signs and symptoms experienced acutely and chronically. The table also highlights the comorbidities that often occur as a cause or consequence of these complications and must be considered in the overall management of SCD. The table is followed by a brief description of available evidence on some of the most common complications. These complications are also discussed by Ballas et al. (2012b) and Ballas (2018).

System- or Organ-Specific Complications of SCD

Cardiovascular System

SCD is a chronic hemolytic anemia and can lead to various cardiopulmonary and circulatory disorders. Cardiac hypertrophy (enlargement of the heart) develops early in life in response to chronic anemia. Diastolic dysfunction, possibly from myocardial fibrosis, is relatively common (Gladwin, 2017). Risk factors for increased cardiovascular mortality among individuals with SCD include systemic hypertension, pulmonary hypertension, heart attack, and possibly subclinical electrical instability (Haywood, 2009).

Central Nervous System

SCD causes acute and chronic neurological complications. Research conducted using data from patients enrolled in the Cooperative Study of Sickle Cell Disease shows that the chances of having a cerebrovascular accident (defined as transient ischemic attack, completed infarctive stroke, and hemorrhagic stroke) for the first time by age 20 years is 11 percent and by age 45 years is 24 percent for those with HbSS (i.e., the form of SCD in which a child inherits a sickle cell hemoglobin gene from each parent) (Ohene-Frempong et al., 1998).

Rates of silent strokes (ischemic lesions detectable by magnetic resonance imaging [MRI] that do not cause symptoms of acute stroke) are even higher: 21 percent in children (Pegelow et al., 2002) and more than 50 percent in adults (Kassim et al., 2016). Hemorrhagic strokes are also more prevalent in individuals

TABLE 4-1 Summary of SCD Complications by Affected Organ or System (Alphabetical Order)

| Organ System | Manifestations (Signs/Symptom Burden) | | Comorbid Conditions |
	Acute	Chronic	
Cardiovascular	• Sudden death • Fatigue • Dyspnea • Syncope • Relative systolic hypertension • Myocardial infarction	• Sickle cardiomyopathy • Left ventricular hypertrophy • Diastolic dysfunction • Heart failure with preserved ejection fraction • Iron-induced cardiomyopathy and dysrhythmias • Endothelial dysfunction/autonomic dysfunction • Prolonged QT interval • Pulmonary hypertension	• Cardiac iron toxicity • Methadone related prolonged QT interval[a] • Hyperlipidemia • Obesity-related cardiovascular complications • Venous thromboembolism
Central Nervous System	• Headache • Infarctive stroke • Hemorrhagic stroke • Ruptured aneurysms • Moyamoya syndrome • Silent cerebral infarcts • Sino-venous thrombosis	• Chronic headaches • Neurocognitive disorders due to silent cerebral infarcts/overt cerebrovascular accidents or strokes and chronic anemia • Poor executive functioning • Memory deficits • Increased cerebral blood flow • Cerebral vasculopathy and Moyamoya syndrome • Cerebral aneurysms	• Posterior reversible encephalopathy syndrome • Pre-/post-eclampsia • Arnold Chiari malformation • Cerebral aneurysms
Dental	• Dental abscess • Dental crown fracture • Dental pulp fracture	• Dental caries • Gingivitis • Cracked teeth • Early dental loss • Misaligned dentition	• Cardiovascular risk • Dental cavities, gingival disease, malocclusion
Endocrine	• Pain around menses, pregnancy, and menopause	• Growth hormone deficiency • Hypogonadism • Disturbances in cortisol levels • Delayed puberty • Premature menopause	• Diabetes and thyroid disease from iron overload • Early menopause and bone health • Hypo/hyperthyroidism

Gallbladder/ Pancreas	• Cholelithiasis • Cholecystitis • Common bile duct obstruction • Acute pancreatitis	• Chronic gallbladder sludge • Dyspepsia • Chronic cholecystitis • Chronic pancreatitis	• Pancreatitis with comorbid alcohol misuse
General Gastrointestinal	• Mesenteric infarcts	• Chronic abdominal pain • Constipation • Irritable bowel syndrome • GERD • Increased abdominal girth due to shortened trunk and barrel chest (sickle-habitus)	• Constipation (opioid induced and VOE related) • Ileus • Cyclic vomiting syndrome • Drug-induced nausea and vomiting
Genitourinary	• Priapism • Enuresis • Hematuria • Menses-induced VOE	• Erectile (sexual) dysfunction • Postcoital pain • Enuresis/nocturia • Hematuria	• Menorrhagia leading to worsening anemia • Dysmenorrhea with increased acute care use
Hematopoietic System (excluding spleen)	• Acute anemia • Aplastic crisis • Sequestration crises • Functional asplenia • Indirect hyperbilirubinemia • Scleral icterus • Hemostatic activation[b]	• Chronic hemolysis[c] • Chronic anemia • Extramedullary hematopoiesis • Leukocytosis • Thrombocytosis • Splenomegaly • Hypersplenism • Conjunctival pallor • Scleral icterus • Hemostatic activation[b] • Thrombophilia	• Delayed hemolytic transfusion reactions • Parvovirus B19 infection • CKD, suppressing erythropoiesis • Hypoplastic anemia from CKD
Hepatic	• Hyperbilirubinemia • Hepatic sequestration • Hepatitis • Acute intrahepatic cholelithiasis/cholestasis • Transaminitis	• Hepatomegaly • Hepatic congestion/chronic congestive hepatopathy • Portal hypertension	• Hepatic hemosiderosis and fibrosis • Infectious hepatitis • Hepatorenal syndrome • Autoimmune/chemical (drug-induced) hepatitis • Gilberts Syndrome

continued

TABLE 4-1 Continued

| Organ System | Manifestations (Signs/Symptom Burden) | | Comorbid Conditions |
	Acute	Chronic	
Immune System	• Bacteremia/sepsis • Meningitis • Hepatitis • Osteomyelitis • Pyelonephritis • Influenza	• Osteomyelitis • Hepatitis • Dental abscesses • Gingivitis • Leg ulcer super infection	• Transfusion-associated infection—babesiosis, parvovirus, hepatitis, HIV • Salmonella osteomyelitis • Sexually transmitted infections
Musculoskeletal	• Bony infarction • Dactylitis • Acute VOE	• Avascular necrosis • Vertebral body endplate changes, including vertebral compression fractures • Maxillary hyperplasia and bony changes associated with extramedullary hematopoiesis • Gout • Osteopenia/osteoporosis from increased bone turnover • Vitamin D deficiency/rickets	• Hypovitaminosis D • Orbital bone infarction, mental nerve impingement (numb chin syndrome) • Osteonecrosis or avascular necrosis of the jaw, particularly when exposed to bisphosphonates • Increased risk of pathological fractures
Ophthalmic	• Retinal detachment • Retinal artery occlusion • Vitreous hemorrhage • Macular infarction	• Sickle retinopathy (proliferative and nonproliferative) • Maculopathy	• Early cataracts • Early glaucoma • Increased intraocular pressure with posttraumatic hyphema
Pulmonary	• Acute chest syndrome • Pneumonia • Pulmonary fat embolism syndrome • Airway hyperreactivity • Atelectasis from hypoventilation • Pulmonary embolism	• Chronic lung disease • Chronic hypoxemia/hypoxia • Nocturnal hypoxemia • Chronic pulmonary embolism	• In situ pulmonary thrombosis • Asthma • Adenotonsillar enlargement • Obstructive sleep apnea • Right middle lobe syndrome

Renal	• Acute kidney injury (recurrent) • Hematuria • Papillary necrosis	• Hypertension • Glomerular hyperfiltration • Proteinuria/microalbuminuria • Hyposthenuria • CKD • End-stage renal disease • Renal tubular acidosis • Renal osteodystrophy	• Acute increase in blood pressure with acute pain • Susceptibility to dehydration • NSAID and contrast nephropathy
Reproductive	• Spontaneous abortion/miscarriages • Intrauterine growth retardation • Early fetal demise • Pre- and post-eclampsia • Severe dilutional anemia • Other maternal-fetal complications	• Low sperm counts/poor sperm function • Post-pregnancy chronic pain	• Hypospermia from hydroxyurea use • Infertility from conditioning regimens from SCT
Skin	• Leg ulcers	• Leg ulcers • Varicosity	• Melanonychia and hyperpigmentation from hydroxyurea use
Spleen	• Acute splenic sequestration • Acute splenic infarction • Splenic abscesses • Traumatic spleen rupture	• Splenomegaly • Functional asplenia or hyposplenia due to auto-infarction of spleen leading to increased risk for infection with encapsulated organisms • Splenic infarction • Hypersplenism	• Risk of splenic rupture with contact sports in patients with splenomegaly • Impact of early and/or prolonged hydroxyurea therapy[b]

NOTE: CKD = chronic kidney disease; GERD = gastroesophageal reflux disease; NSAID = non-steroidal anti-inflammatory drug; SCT = sickle cell trait; VOE = vaso-occlusive episode.

[a] A prolonged QT interval is an electrical impulse that is measured by an electrocardiogram. The QT are the waves displayed on the paper results from the electrical impulses through the heart.

[b] Hemostatic activation refers to the hypercoagulable state that occurs downstream from the vaso-occlusive process in SCD (De Franceschi et al., 2011).

[c] Hydroxyurea, chronic transfusion therapy, and other disease-modifying therapies, when initiated early in life, may alter the natural history of SCD phenotype.

SOURCES: Adapted from Ballas et al., 2012b; Desai et al., 2014; Gale et al., 2015; Indik et al., 2016; Martins et al., 2012; Mehari and Klings, 2016; Osunkwo, 2011; Osunkwo et al., 2011; Powars et al., 1988; Wu et al., 2018.

with SCD. Among the chronic complications, cognitive impairment, particularly involving deficits in executive function, is highly prevalent in both children (Steen et al., 2005) and adults (Vichinsky et al., 2010).

Ninety percent of pediatric strokes can be prevented by transcranial Doppler (TCD) screening and prophylactic transfusion of children with high TCD velocities (Adams and Brambilla, 2005). However, screening and early interventions for other neurological complications in adults is not available.

Dental

It is well recognized that poor oral health is directly associated with increases in both cardiovascular and all-cause mortality (Jansson et al., 2002); this is also true for individuals with SCD. Individuals with SCD are prone to dental complications such as aseptic pulp necrosis, delay in dental eruption, mucosal damage due to anemia, dental nerve infarcts, and increased risk of caries and enamel erosion. Pain treatment with opioids contributes to these issues: gum and oral infection from poor dental hygiene and dry mouth from opioid use. The likelihood of hospitalization in adults with SCD increases with dental infections (Laurence et al., 2013). One study found that optimal dental care led to a statistically significant reduction in hospital admissions and total days hospitalized (Whiteman et al., 2016).

Endocrine System

Weight gain, metabolic syndrome, and obesity are increasingly recognized comorbidities in the SCD population, particularly in those with the compound heterozygous genotypes SC/SB+ (Mandese et al., 2019; Ogunsile et al., 2019). There is a high prevalence of vitamin D deficiency, osteopenia, and osteoporosis in SCD. Renal osteodystrophy in SCD may confer worsening chronic pain and is often unrecognized and nonresponsive to opioids (Elsurer et al., 2013; Seck et al., 2012). Similarly, vitamin D deficiency and osteoporosis or osteopenia can result in pain (Catalano et al., 2017; Glaser and Kaplan, 1997; Osunkwo, 2011).

Fat Embolism Syndrome

Fat embolism syndrome is a life-threatening complication of SCD that occurs due to VOE-induced ischemic bone marrow infarction and the release of fat globules into the venous circulation (Dang et al., 2005); it may lead to multi-organ failure syndrome and death (Gangaraju et al., 2016). Fat embolism syndrome in SCD has a high overall mortality rate of

64 percent in a recent report (Tsitsikas et al., 2014). Mortality was reduced to 29 percent with exchange transfusion, as compared with 61 percent in those receiving a simple transfusion and 91 percent in the untransfused group (Tsitsikas et al., 2014).

Gallbladder

Cholelithiasis (gallbladder stones) is common in SCD, and many patients undergo cholecystectomy at some point over their life span. However, there are limited data on whether elective cholecystectomy is warranted in people with SCD, particularly because patients with SCD are more susceptible to perioperative complications (Howard et al., 2013; Plummer et al., 2006; Solanki and McCurdy, 1979). Other hepatobiliary complications include acute intrahepatic cholestasis, sickle hepatopathy, and hepatic sequestration (the pooling of RBCs in the liver).

Gastrointestinal System

While there are limited reports of ischemia–reperfusion injury from sickling in the mesenteric vessels, chronic dyspepsia, decreased gastric and bowel motility, and gastroesophageal reflux disease are very common and may represent a form of autonomic dysfunction, particularly when coupled with the dysmotility side effect of opioids. NSAIDs for pain may also induce gastritis/esophagitis and upper and lower gastrointestinal bleeding (Gardner and Jaffe, 2015; Gardner and Jaffe, 2016).

Genitourinary and Reproductive System

The sexual and reproductive consequences of SCD are profound and poorly studied. There is an increased frequency of VOE during puberty, pregnancy, and menopause. Pregnancy remains high-risk and requires proactive co-management with high-risk obstetrics and attention to the risk of early fetal demise, pre- and post-eclampsia, preterm labor, deep vein thrombosis, and intrauterine growth restriction (IUGR). Women with SCD are at higher risk of maternal and fetal mortality and are more likely to undergo Cesarean sections than those without SCD (Hassell, 2005; Kuo and Caughey, 2016).

Fetal growth problems, such as IUGR and small for gestational age and prematurity, affect offspring with unclear long-term impacts (Oteng-Ntim et al., 2015). Women with RBC alloimmunization are at risk for having babies with hemolytic disease of the newborn, and those exposed to opioids are at increased risk for neonatal abstinence syndrome (Nnoli et al., 2018).

Up to 48 percent of male individuals with SCD experience recurrent episodes of priapism (sustained, undesired, painful erections); the peak incidence is during puberty and young adulthood with the hormonal surges in testosterone, but it may be seen as young as age 7 (Arduini and Trovo de Marqui, 2018). The long-term consequences of recurrent or stuttering priapism may include the early development of erectile dysfunction, penile fibrosis, and impotence (Mantadakis et al., 1999).

Hematopoietic System

Anemia, defined by a decreased hemoglobin concentration, is a hallmark of SCD and is almost invariably present in individuals with homozygous HbS (sickle cell anemia, or SCA). The symptoms of severe anemia include pallor, fatigue, decreased exercise tolerance, shortness of breath, and decreased cognitive function. The severity of anemia has been associated with serious complications such as stroke in children with SCD. Hemolysis (the premature destruction of RBCs) causes a cascade of downstream effects that cause chronic inflammation, as well as abnormalities in blood cells and the vessel wall function (Gordeuk et al., 2016). There is a large body of evidence that links the severity of hemolysis to severe complications, including pulmonary hypertension and chronic kidney disease (CKD) (Kato et al., 2017; Nouraie et al., 2013; Taylor et al., 2008).

Immune System and Spleen

Infarction of the spleen early in life causes autosplenectomy (i.e., the progressive transformation of the spleen into fibrous scar tissue) and functional asplenia (i.e., the absence of protection of the spleen from certain bacteria) (Brousse et al., 2014). Children who have undergone autosplenectomy are susceptible to infections from *S. pneumoniae* and other bacteria and may die from bacterial sepsis (Brousse et al., 2014). The institution of penicillin prophylaxis and immunizations against *H. influenzae* and *S. pneumoniae* early in life in children with SCD have proven to be very effective preventive strategies.

Musculoskeletal System

Most acute presentations of SCD involve bone pain, which may occur during acute hypoxic ischemic injury to a significant portion of a bone (Ballas et al., 2012b). If the injury persists over time, evolution to bony infarcts occurs. In the epiphysis, this is referred to as osteonecrosis (Vanderhave et al., 2018). Avascular necrosis is painful, may have significant function-limiting effects, and requires joint replacement in late stages

(Ballas et al., 2012b; Vanderhave et al., 2018). It may occasionally be difficult to distinguish bone infarcts from osteomyelitis in SCD.

Ophthalmic System

Ocular consequences of SCD include retinopathy (damage to the retina) that typically occurs in the peripheral retinal vascular bed, as compared with diabetic retinopathy, which is more likely to affect the central bed. Adequately diagnosing sickle retinopathy requires training; individuals with SCD are advised to get annual or biennial screening ophthalmological exams beginning at age 10 and to receive early timed intervention if retinopathy is identified (Yawn et al., 2014). Other ocular complications include bony infarcts of the orbital and facial bones and orbital hematomas, which can lead to vision-threatening complications.

Pulmonary Complications

Pulmonary complications are leading causes of death in SCD. Acute chest syndrome (ACS) is a major acute pulmonary complication that, without prompt intervention, carries high mortality (Novelli and Gladwin, 2016). Pulmonary hypertension is a chronic complication that affects predominantly adult individuals with homozygous HbS (prevalence of 6–10 percent) (Fonseca et al., 2012; Mehari et al., 2012; Parent et al., 2011). Pulmonary hypertension is an independent risk factor for death in SCD, with a 6-year mortality rate of approximately 40 percent (Mehari et al., 2012). Transthoracic echocardiography is an important screening tool for symptomatic individuals with SCD; abnormal blood flow across the tricuspid valve indicates an increased mortality risk in SCD (Gladwin et al., 2004) and risk-stratifies patients for additional pulmonary hypertension testing. Research is under way to determine the optimal screening strategies in individuals with SCD and the best therapeutic approaches for those with pulmonary hypertension confirmed by cardiac catheterization.

Asthma and airway hyperreactivity are significant comorbidities in SCD, particularly in children, and are associated with worse disease outcomes (Field et al., 2011). Finally, restrictive lung deficits are also more common in individuals with SCD.

Renal System

The kidney is compromised early in life with both glomerular and tubular damage. Individuals with SCD experience early mortality once end-stage renal disease ensues (McClellan et al., 2012) and may require renal replacement therapy. Kidney transplant has been successfully performed in patients with SCD (Boyle et al., 2016; Gérardin et al., 2019).

Renal medullary carcinoma is a rare, aggressive tumor that occurs in individuals with sickle cell trait (SCT) or SCD (less frequently) at a higher-than-average rate (Blas et al., 2019). Guidelines for diagnosis and management are needed, as well as an international registry and biorepository (Blas et al., 2019).

Screening for microalbuminuria identifies individuals with SCD at risk of developing CKD and is recommended by current guidelines.

Non-Organ-Specific Complications of SCD

Many SCD complications are not restricted to any one organ system, and the impact of the disease on QOL can be profound but hard to define and compartmentalize. Table 4-2 presents an overview of SCD complications that are not confined to one organ system and their related acute and chronic manifestations and comorbidities.

Behavioral Health in SCD

> *There were many days where I took the main medication*
> *just hoping that I would not wake up. I would not wake up*
> *to face another day of emotional pain. And the judgment*
> *that came from the community.*

—Jenn. N. (Open Session Panelist)

Researchers investigating the mental health impacts of living with SCD have focused primarily on the diagnoses of depression and anxiety as related to pain and pain coping behavior. Anie (2005) reported that the most common variables assessed included anxiety, depression, coping, neurological complications, and QOL. These studies are limited and allow for only correlative results as they differ in their sample size, the choice of a control group, and how each outcome was assessed. In individuals with SCD, pain affects psychological and behavioral health and creates challenges (Benton et al., 2011; Thomas et al., 1998).

Depression and anxiety As with other chronic diseases, depressive symptoms are frequently reported among youth and adults with SCD (Anie, 2005; Levenson, 2008; Lukoo et al., 2015). Jonassaint et al. (2016) found that across 12 SCD studies, the prevalence rates for depression were 2–57 percent. The PiSCES study also found high rates of depression, with 27.6 percent of 308 adults reporting depressive symptoms (Sogutlu et al., 2011).

TABLE 4-2 Summary of Non-Organ-Specific SCD Complications (Alphabetical Order)

SCD-Related Complications	Manifestations (Signs/Symptom Burden)			Comorbid Conditions
	Acute	Chronic		
Behavioral Health	• Acute psychosis due to pain • Opioid-induced psychosis	• Neurocognitive complications • PTSD • Depression • Anxiety • Pica • SUDs		• Poor socioeconomic status • Stigma/racism • Societal barriers • Catastrophizing • SUDs • School absenteeism • Unemployment
Constitutional	• Fatigue • Fever	• Fatigue • Exercise intolerance		• Poor exercise tolerance • Dehydration • General deconditioning
Growth	• Weight loss • Weight gain (particularly during prolonged admissions)	• Delayed puberty • Delayed linear growth • Obesity		• Overhydration, leading to anasarca
Malignancies	• Renal cell carcinoma	• Abnormal serum protein and urine electrophoresis, causing false alarms		• No evidence to support increased risk of malignancies in SCD on hydroxyurea
Nutrition	• Anorexia during acute VOE • Craving for salt/sugar	• Vitamin D, E, A deficiencies • Zinc deficiency • Increased caloric demand/hypermetabolism		• Renal tubular acidosis with electrolyte wasting • Adrenal insufficiency • Parasympathetic dysfunction

149

continued

TABLE 4-2 Continued

| SCD-Related Complications | Manifestations (Signs/Symptom Burden) | | Comorbid Conditions |
	Acute	Chronic	
Pain Syndromes	• Acute pain syndromes (dactylitis, extremities, back, chest, headache)	• Chronic pain syndromes • Neuropathic pain • CS • Opiate-induced hyperalgesia • Pain from avascular necrosis/skin ulcers, compression spine deformities (H-Fish-mouth vertebrae) • Osteopenia/osteoporosis from increased bone turnover • Vitamin D deficiency/rickets	• Hemorrhagic stroke, supraventricular tachycardia • DVT and prolonged exposure • Osteoarthritis • Degenerative disc disease • Rheumatoid arthritis • ROD • Osteopenia/osteoporosis • Vitamin D deficiency/rickets
Sleep	• Lethargy • Fatigue • Daytime somnolence	• Chronic insomnia • Hypersomnia	• Obstructive sleep apnea • Restless leg syndrome/periodic limb movements in sleep • Other sleep disorders • Poor sleep hygiene • Risk of motor vehicle accidents
Sudden Death Syndrome	• Within 24 hours of acute pain presentation • Within a few days after discharge from acute care	• Underlying chronic organ damage (e.g., pulmonary hypertension) predisposes to sudden death	• Thromboembolic disease • Infections • Arrhythmias

NOTE: CS = central sensitization; DVT = deep vein thrombosis; PTSD = posttraumatic stress disorder; ROD = renal osteodystrophy; SCD = sickle cell disease; SUD = substance use disorder; VOE = vaso-occlusive crisis.

SOURCES: Adapted from Ballas et al., 2012b; Field et al., 2019; Osunkwo, 2011; Osunkwo et al., 2011; While and Mullen, 2004; Wu et al., 2018.

One early study (Jenerette et al., 2005) used the Beck Depression Inventory (BDI) Fast Screen for 232 adults living with SCD. The SCD sample had higher levels of depression (26 percent) and depressive symptoms (32 percent) than the overall U.S. population (9.5 percent). The authors attributed their findings to the stigma of SCD.

Reports from the PiSCES project indicated that both adults and children with SCD experienced worse HRQOL than the general population, particularly in the domains of bodily pain, vitality, social function, and general health (Anie et al., 2002; Kater et al., 1999; McClish et al., 2005; Thomas and Taylor, 2002). In a prospective study using the BDI, involving 142 patients, results indicated that QOL scores were significantly but inversely related to depression, with high depression scores associated with worse QOL scores (Adam et al., 2017). Health care system usage and inpatient costs were also significantly higher for patients with high scores on the BDI; the adjusted total costs were nearly twice as high for the depressed group as for the non-depressed group.

Studies have found a reciprocal relationship between depressive symptoms and pain in SCD (Jonassaint et al., 2016). Depressed mood and negative thinking influence an individual's ability to cope with pain, and pain increases the risk of experiencing depression. People with SCD who report depressive symptoms also appear to have more frequent and severe pain. In the PiSCES study, depression was associated with increased reports of days with pain (71.1 versus 49.6 percent for the non-depressed group) and with increased pain impact during "non-crisis days" (judged according to distress, interference with normal activities, and overall mean pain scores) as compared with the non-depressed group (Levenson et al., 2008). Hasan et al. (2003) found that depressive symptoms were associated with more frequent ED visits and admissions for VOEs. In a systematic review of depression and health care use, Jonassaint et al. (2016) found that people with SCD who had depressive symptoms were more likely to have high health care use (2.8 times greater risk). This population also had more hospitalizations per year (Jonassaint et al., 2016).

The frequency of pain in a child and parent catastrophizing about that pain emerged as predictors of clinically significant depressive symptoms in children (Goldstein-Leever et al., 2018). Bakri et al. (2014) demonstrated the negative effects of repeated hospitalizations on the behavior of children with SCD, reporting increased rates of anxiety/depression, somatic complaint, withdrawn or aggressive behavior, and internalizing symptoms.

A similar relationship has been found between anxiety and pain in SCD. Adults with SCD have a prevalence rate of anxiety around 6.5 percent (Levenson et al., 2008). In the PiSCES study, people with SCD and anxiety symptoms also reported an increased use of opioids during crisis and non-crisis days (Levenson et al., 2008). This pattern is also present in children with SCD. A retrospective chart review found that children with SCD and anxiety symptoms had longer hospital stays and more hospitalizations for pain due to VOEs (Myrvik et al., 2012, 2013).

For some individuals, living with SCD is akin to experiencing recurrent episodes of psychological trauma. Individuals with SCD report experiencing a constant fear of death or feeling that the current trip to the ED will be their last because of the unpredictability of the acute exacerbations. Many people living with SCD settle into an "automatic survival mode," with hypervigilance and hyperreactivity to sound, speech, and movements, and this leads to a chronic fatigue and exhaustion similar to posttraumatic stress disorder (PTSD), which is caused by an intense, disturbing emotional response to a traumatic experience that involved actual or threatened death or serious injury or harm. PTSD has on occasion been reported in the SCD literature (Alao and Soderberg, 2002; Hofmann et al., 2007).

Although it seems intuitive that a relationship exists between SCD status and depression, it is difficult to confirm the etiology of that link. The existing research is imbalanced and has gaps and numerous associated methodological challenges, including the measurement of depression and the use of a control group. Clearly, this is an area in need of further research.

Insomnia and other sleep disorders People living with SCD commonly experience significant sleep problems. For instance, children have a higher prevalence of sleep-disordered breathing, which can contribute to learning difficulties, behavioral problems, higher blood pressure, and reduced growth (Valrie et al., 2007). Children also experience difficulty falling asleep, low blood oxygen levels at night, night awakenings, longer periods before rapid eye movement (REM) sleep, short REM sleep duration, urinary incontinence, and subsequent daytime sleepiness (Valrie et al., 2013). As adults, they are very likely to experience sleep-disordered breathing, with more than 70 percent reporting some sleep disturbance symptoms (Wallen et al., 2014). Additionally, adults with SCD have late sleep onset and decreased sleep duration and spend more time awake during the night (increased sleep fragmentation), with almost the entire sample (97 percent) reporting poor sleep (Wallen et al., 2014). Although sleep-disordered breathing is a significant health concern for individuals with SCD (Sharma et al., 2015), little physiological sleep research has been carried out, and the available interventions are limited.

Neurocognitive complications The physiologic effects of SCD increase the risk for a range of neurologic complications (e.g., stroke, silent cerebral infarct [SCI], microstructural white matter abnormalities), resulting in significant cognitive deficits (Kawadler et al., 2016; Prussien et al., 2019; Schatz et al., 2002). Children with SCD, with and without prior history of stroke or SCI, have higher rates of developmental disabilities. Specifically, among all African American children, 0.6 percent of the observed developmental disabilities (e.g., intellectual disabilities, cerebral palsy, and hearing and visual impairment) can be attributed to SCD. Furthermore, the increased risk for developmental disabilities in individuals with SCD is mostly due to stroke (Ashley-Koch et al., 2001).

Intelligence quotient (IQ) is the most commonly assessed aspect of cognition in the literature, and IQ is most often lower in people with SCD than in controls (e.g., siblings and peers) (Prussien et al., 2019). The most significant childhood IQ deficits are associated with stroke and SCI, but SCD patients with normal-appearing MRI tests may also have IQ deficits. Findings from a meta-regression of studies conducted in a pediatric SCD population indicated that there are significant differences of approximately 10, 6, and 7 points in IQ for children living with SCD with stroke (compared with those with SCI), SCI (compared with those with no SCI), and normal-appearing MRI (compared with children with no SCD and normal MRI), respectively (Kawadler et al., 2016). Cognitive deficits have been observed across a range of domains (e.g., memory, learning, language, visuospatial abilities) (Berkelhammer et al., 2007); however, the most significant and consistent deficits are in executive abilities (Hood et al., 2019), attention (Daly et al., 2012), and processing speed (Stotesbury et al., 2017).

The etiology, risk factors, and trajectory of cognitive impairment in individuals with SCD without a history of stroke or SCI is a major gap in knowledge.

Substance use disorders/opioid use disorders There is significant ambiguity and hesitancy surrounding the application of the terms SUD and "opioid use disorder" (OUD) in the context of SCD. This is partly due to the concerns about increasing stigma in an already stigmatized population and the fear that applying these terms will reduce access to optimal treatment for pain, which typically requires opioids. Nevertheless, it is important that appropriate terminology and diagnostic criteria be applied equally to all populations to avoid undertreatment, overtreatment, and inappropriate treatment; further worsen clinical outcomes; and reduce access to evidence-based care.

Unfortunately, there are relatively few publications that address the epidemiology of SUD or, more specifically, OUD in SCD. These are mostly case reports (Alao et al., 2003; Biedrzycki et al., 2009; Boulmay and Lottenberg, 2009; Kotila et al., 2015). In a large study on the epidemiology of pain in SCD, 31.4 percent of participants were identified as having an alcohol SUD (Levenson et al., 2007). Another study reported a 36 percent prevalence of cannabis use in SCD (Howard et al., 2005).

The assumption by providers and the general public is that the use of relatively high-dose opioids is universally associated with SUD in individuals with SCD. Because of this suspicion, the typical response of many clinicians is to withhold opioids, particularly in the acute setting, without a detailed assessment/evaluation of SUD. This response leads to significant conflict between patients and providers/health care systems, in addition to increased pain, suffering, complications from poorly treated pain, and the potential emergence of pseudo-addiction and related behaviors (Kotila et al., 2015).

In a disease where pain is characteristically severe and exposure to opioids is nearly universal, it is expected that some individuals with SCD will meet the criteria for SUD/OUD. Data from a large U.S. study show that 40 percent of SCD patients used opioids over a 12-month period (Han et al., 2018). However, opioid use has been constant and stable over time for the general population (2008–2013) (Ruta and Ballas, 2016). There was a 31.4 percent self-reported rate of SUD for alcohol in the PiSCES study (Levenson et al., 2007). Marijuana use is common in SCD, with one study finding that in a sample of 58 individuals living with SCD, 42 percent reported marijuana use in the past 2 years (Roberts et al., 2018). Deaths from opioid overdose in people living with SCD are markedly lower than in other non-cancer pain conditions, including low back pain, migraine, and fibromyalgia (Ruta and Ballas, 2016). All individuals should be assessed for the risk of SUD and provided access to optimal treatment for SUD and mental health disorders, if necessary.

Constitutional Symptoms

Fatigue Fatigue is described as "an overwhelming, debilitating, and sustained sense of exhaustion that decreases one's ability to carry out daily activities, including the ability to work effectively and to function at one's usual level in family or social roles" (Dantzer et al., 2014, p. 39) and is now recognized both in the general population and cancer literature as a significant morbidity. People with SCD frequently report chronic fatigue that is out of proportion to the degree of anemia and that can be debilitating, especially with older age. Fatigue negatively affects QOL and contributes to high rates of debilitation (Badawy et al., 2018a; Irvine et al., 1991). Fatigue in SCD causes poor vocation attainment, functional outcomes, relapses, and depression (Ameringer and Smith, 2011; Anderson et al., 2015).

There is limited understanding of the etiology of fatigue in SCD and no intervention studies that describe treatments to mitigate it.

Medical Comorbidities and SCD

Comorbidities compound SCD-related complications and adversely affect QOL. For example, asthma increases the risk of ACS, and obstructive sleep apnea increases the risk of stroke. Type 2 diabetes and hypertension are common comorbidities in adults (Zhou et al., 2019).

It is unclear whether children and adults with SCD have an increased risk of cancer. Recent data from California suggest that children and adults with SCD are at an increased risk for developing hematologic malignancies but may be at lower risk for solid tumors (Brunson et al., 2017). This study reported a more than two-fold increased risk of leukemia, but the influence of long-term therapies, such as hydroxyurea (HU), could not be investigated.

Sudden Death in SCD

VOE is the most common presentation associated with death in those with SCD (Rizio et al., 2020). Death can be sudden and unexpected, often occurring at home following a recent discharge from the hospital (approximately 40 percent) or within 24 hours of presentation to the hospital (28 percent) (Manci et al., 2003; Niraimathi et al., 2016). Infection is a leading cause of death (33–48 percent) (Manci et al., 2003). Other causes of death include overt organ failure, ACS, and stroke (Platt et al., 1994).

Evidence of bone marrow fat emboli is common in many autopsy cases of sudden death. In a large autopsy study, there was significantly more organ injury than recognized before death, so the clinical presentation often does not reflect the severity of hidden chronic end-organ damage (Manci et al., 2003).

MANAGEMENT OF SCD

Traditionally, SCD was considered a disease of childhood, and health care management approaches were focused on reducing the overwhelmingly high infant and child mortality from infections (Davis et al., 1997). The premise for the creation of Comprehensive Sickle Cell Centers of Excellence, which began with the National Sickle Cell Anemia Control Act of 1972, was the provision of early diagnosis and supportive care (Bonds, 2005; Manley, 1984; Scott, 1979). Embedded in the field of pediatrics, the centers focused primarily on newborn screening (NBS), preventing death from infection by implementing evidence-based penicillin prophylaxis guidelines, and administering vaccinations against pneumococcal infection. An additional focus was mitigating the pain and suffering associated with acute complications of the disease.

Now that more than 98 percent of children with SCD are surviving into adulthood (Quinn et al., 2010), a new model of care that addresses the underlying pathophysiology, its changes with age, and its concomitant medical and psychosocial comorbidities is critically needed (and will be discussed in Chapter 5).

Prevention of Complications of SCD

Pneumococcal and Infection Prophylaxis

Splenic dysfunction occurs early in childhood; 84 percent of infants develop asplenia by 12 months of age (Thompson, 2011) and 94 percent of children by 5 years of age. Asplenia increases the risk of infection, particularly with encapsulated organisms, such as *S. pneumoniae, H. influenzae* type b, and *Salmonella* species (Pearson, 1977).

In 1986 prophylactic oral penicillin therapy was evaluated in children with SCD and shown to decrease mortality and the number and frequency of infections during childhood (by 84 percent) (Gaston et al., 1986). Since then, penicillin prophylaxis by 4 months of age has been recommended as the standard of care. A 1995 study of 400 patients with SCD evaluated discontinuing penicillin therapy in children over 5 years old who had taken penicillin for at least 2 years and also received pneumococcal 23-valent vaccination (Falletta et al., 1995). The equivalency of infection rates on and off penicillin between the study groups led to the recommendations that some people with SCD may be able to discontinue penicillin therapy safely after age 5, while continuing to be monitored for infection (Falletta et al., 1995).

Immunizations with conjugate vaccines against *S. pneumoniae* and *H. influenza* type b have also been critically important at significantly reducing bacteremia in SCD (Gaston et al., 1986; John et al., 1984; Knight-Madden and Serjeant, 2001); the introduction of pneumococcal vaccines led to a drop of the incidence of invasive pneumococcal disease by 90.8 percent in children less than 2 years old and 93.4 percent in children older than 5 years (Halasa et al., 2007).

Transcranial Doppler and Stroke Prevention

Robust data also exist for primary stroke prevention using TCD as a high-quality screening tool (Krejza et al., 2010) and preventative chronic transfusions for persons identified as high risk (Bernaudin et al., 2011; Enninful-Eghan et al., 2010; Fullerton et al., 2004). Analysis of data from The Stroke Prevention Trial in Sickle Cell Anemia also showed that participants with normal internal carotid artery or middle cerebral artery velocity had a higher risk of stroke (10 times greater) if they had an elevated anterior cerebral artery velocity compared with those with normal anterior cerebral artery velocity (Kwiatkowski et al., 2006). Discontinuing chronic transfusion led to a resurgence of stroke risk and subsequent strokes within 1 year (Adams and Brambilla, 2005), so there remains a strong evidence-based recommendation of continuing transfusions to prevent stroke recurrence in children with SCD (NHLBI, 1997).

Disease-Modifying Agents

Hydroxyurea

HU, a drug originally developed to treat malignancies and myeloproliferative disorders, was tested for the treatment of SCD because of the discovery that patients on HU experienced increases in the production of fetal hemoglobin (HbF) (Charache et al., 1992; Platt et al., 1984). Higher HbF levels are partially protective against hemoglobin S polymerization, sickling, hemolysis, and their downstream effects. In addition, HU reduces leukocyte and platelet counts, thereby reducing cellular adhesion, and it acts as a nitric oxide donor. In 1995 the Multicenter Study of Hydroxyurea (MSH) found that HU led to a 44 percent reduction in the median number of VOEs and ACS episodes and also reduced transfusion requirements in patients with SCA (Charache et al., 1995). HU also reduced the number of severe VOEs requiring hospitalization and doubled both the time to first crisis and the time to second crisis (Charache et al., 1995). The MSH study led to the adoption of HU as a recommended therapeutic intervention for adults with SCA who have three or more moderate to severe VOEs in a 12-month period (Yawn et al., 2014). In the MSH trial there were no increased adverse effects compared with placebo, other than reversible myelosuppression (a decrease in bone marrow activity) (Charache et al., 1995). Longer-term data on HU in adults have confirmed its utility in mitigating acute SCD complications. A recent Cochrane review of 17 studies, including eight randomized controlled trials with 899 adults and children of all genotypes, found statistically significant improvements in VOE frequency, duration, and intensity and fewer hospital admissions, occurrences of ACS, and blood transfusions in the HU-treated groups (Nevitt et al., 2017). There remains insufficient evidence on the long-term benefits of HU in preventing chronic organ damage and on optimal dosing strategies, long-term risks (including effects on reproduction and fertility), and benefits in the hemoglobin SC genotype (Nevitt et al., 2017).

In 2011 the Pediatric Hydroxyurea Phase III Clinical Trial randomly assigned infants with HbSS or HbSβ^0-thalassemia, regardless of clinical severity, to receive placebo or HU for 2 years (McGann et al., 2012). The infants on HU had significant reductions in VOEs, dactylitis, and gastroenteritis as well as a reduced need for transfusions; HU was well tolerated, with no severe adverse events (Wang et al., 2011). The 12-month open label Hydroxyurea European Sickle Cell Disease Cohort study (ADDMEDICA SASA, 2015) assessed a new formulation of HU in pediatric patients. HU use increased HbF in the study population and reduced the percentage of patients with at least one VOE, one episode of ACS, and one hospitalization or transfusion after the 12-month period (FDA, 2017). In 2017 the U.S. Food and Drug Administration (FDA) approved the use of HU in pediatric patients (FDA, 2017).

No significant long-term toxicities have been detected in SCD cohorts followed for up to 15–20 years (Hankins et al., 2015; Steinberg et al., 2010), but concerns remain about more prolonged exposure, particularly in children; HU is a known carcinogen and teratogen in animals, albeit at higher doses than those used in patients (Sakano et al., 2001; Ziegler-Skylakakis et al., 1985). While women who have accidentally continued to take HU during pregnancy have not experienced embryonal toxicity and leukemogenesis has not been detected in SCD cohorts, continued surveillance for long-term toxicity remains important.

HU has been hailed as a "wonder drug" (Yurkiewicz, 2014) because of its multipronged mechanism of action and its efficacy and tolerable toxicity. Yet its adoption by the SCD community has proceeded at a slow pace, with providers under-prescribing the drug and patients remaining wary about its potential side effects, particularly with long-term use. Thus, the effectiveness of HU outside of clinical trials has been limited by poor adherence (Loiselle et al., 2016; Walsh et al., 2014). Research found that older adult individuals living with SCD are less likely to be using HU than individuals under age 30 (Sinha et al., 2018). Thus, HU education targeting older adults is clearly needed and may improve survival.

L-Glutamine and Other Emerging Therapies

FDA approved L-glutamine in 2017 to reduce acute complications in adults and children 5 years and older (Nevitt et al., 2017). L-glutamine is believed to enhance the capacity of the RBCs to handle oxidative stress. The Phase III study of L-glutamine in SCD involved 230 people 5–58 years old who received the treatment as a powder to be mixed with food or drink (Niihara et al., 2018). The outcomes demonstrated a 25 percent reduction in median VOEs compared with placebo and a 33 percent reduction in median hospitalizations compared with placebo. Adverse effects were minor and included low-grade nausea, noncardiac chest pain, fatigue, and musculoskeletal pain (Niihara et al., 2018). Approximately two-thirds of participants were also on HU, suggesting that L-glutamine may provide additional and potentially synergistic clinical benefits. L-glutamine is available in a powder formulation that needs to be mixed in with beverage or food, which may lead to poor adherence (Quinn, 2018). (Newly approved and emerging therapies are discussed in Chapter 7.)

Transfusion Therapy

RBC transfusions remain a cornerstone of supportive care for both acute and chronic life-threatening SCD complications. Transfusions provide non-sickle RBCs that correct the severe anemia from hemolysis and decrease the proportion of HbS-containing RBCs. Together, these effects improve oxygen-carrying capacity and reduce the hypoxic perfusion deficit from vaso-occlusion.

Exchange transfusion is an effective way to improve the total hemo-globin while rapidly reducing HbS. Exchange transfusions can be either manual (Porter and Huehns, 1987) or done with an automated cell sepa-rator (Janes et al., 1997; Kuo et al., 2012; Lawson et al., 1999; Tsitsikas et al., 2016). Exchange transfusions necessitate exposure to multiple blood units from different donors and often require a large-bore, double lumen central venous catheter.

Prophylactic transfusions are critically important in the prevention of stroke and post-operative complications in SCD, and they improve the out-comes of severe complications such as ACS (Emre et al., 1995; Velasquez et al., 2009) and multi-organ failure syndrome. An ongoing, multi-center, international clinical trial (NCT04084080) is exploring whether exchange transfusions improve morbidity and mortality in patients with high-risk disease (defined by high tricuspid regurgitant velocity [TRV], the combina-tion of moderately high TRV and high plasma N-terminal prohormone of brain natriuretic peptide, or the presence of CKD).

While potentially life-saving, transfusions in SCD patients may lead to significant complications, including iron overload, alloimmunization (the formation of antibodies against antigens present on the transfused RBCs) and hemolytic reactions, and infections. Iron overload is highly prevalent in SCD, with one study showing iron deposition in the liver, endocrine organs, cardiac muscle, and bones in 30 percent of 141 adults with SCD who died over a 25-year period; 7 percent of those deaths were attributed to iron overload (Darbari et al., 2006). In a larger cohort of 387 young adults with SCD, 45 percent of the 22 deaths were related to iron overload (Aduloju et al., 2008). Increased rates of alloimmunization have emerged (Rosse et al., 1990; Vichinsky et al., 1990) due to the wide genotypic variation in RBC phenotype among most blood donors, who are mostly Caucasian, and per-sons with SCD, who are predominantly of African American descent, caus-ing a high risk of hemolytic transfusion reactions (Vichinsky et al., 1990).

Current guidelines recommend transfusing donor RBCs that are pheno-typically antigen-matched to the patient for ABO, RhD, and the C, E, and K antigens in order to mitigate the risk of alloimmunization. For individuals with alloantibodies, blood group genotyping has helped decrease the risk of further alloimmunization (Ribeiro et al., 2009). Hemolytic transfusion reac-tions are harmful and potentially life-threatening complications of trans-fusions that occur in 4–10 percent of recipients (Mekontso Dessap et al., 2016; Narbey et al., 2017; Vidler et al., 2015). Occasionally, bystander hemolysis of native RBCs can also occur following transfusion, leading to a life-threatening hyperhemolytic crisis. This may present with severe anemia, severe hemolysis, and respiratory distress with ACS (50 percent of cases) (Habibi et al., 2016).

Person-Centered Management Approaches of SCD

SCD is a complex multi-system disorder, and its management requires a comprehensive, person-centric, multidisciplinary, and interdisciplinary approach, with disease self-management at its core. Unfortunately, this model of care remains out of reach for most persons affected by SCD.

Whole-Person Care

Whole-person SCD care includes both management of the effects of the disease—starting from primary, secondary, and tertiary prevention—and attention to psychosocial and QOL concerns. Whole-person care is critical to ensuring improved QOL, higher care quality (as reflected, for example, in the reduced use of acute care), increased patient satisfaction, and a reduced cost of care per patient. Okpala et al. (2002) recently suggested that to optimize clinical outcomes for individuals with SCD, care should be delivered by a multidisciplinary team that engages medical and nonmedical support services; care should include education for individuals living with SCD and their parents, genetic counseling, social services (e.g., vocational support provided by community-based organizations), infection prevention, dietary advice, psychotherapy, subspecialist medical care, maternal and child health, orthopedic and general surgery, pain control, physiotherapy, dental and eye care, drug dependency services, specialized nursing care, and the often-forgotten primary care. While the hematologist has historically been the primary driver of care coordination, given the current dearth of hematologists with SCD expertise, that role will need to be subsumed by any willing and committed provider who has received the proper training in SCD (Okpala et al., 2002).

Self-Management

Developing adequate self-management skills is essential for individuals to effectively manage a complex disease; disease self-management leads to increased medication adherence, improved pain management, and better health outcomes (Matthie et al., 2015; Nicholas et al., 2012). Recently, guidelines have been created with input from people living with SCD to improve disease knowledge in the SCD community (Cronin et al., 2018).

New tools for improving self-management and increasing health literacy can be found in the growing field of technology-based applications (mHealth or eHealth). Mobile or Internet-based methods allow for increased engagement and quick dissemination of knowledge remotely, without the need for face-to-face visits with health care providers. mHealth aims to increase coping skills and adherence while decreasing the stigma and bias that may result from direct provider interactions. Studies have shown that mobile technologies are effective not only in high-income countries such as the United States but also in low- and middle-income countries (Abaza and Marschollek, 2017).

Although the committee was unable to find any studies that have extensively examined mHealth for SCD, a recent review found that mHealth applications showed feasibility and moderate improvement of medication adherence and coping with pain (Badawy et al., 2018b). However, most of the studies in the review were small and lacked clearly defined clinical outcomes, so further work is needed to better adapt mHealth technology to different SCD populations. In addition, an in-depth review of mHealth tools is necessary to ensure that data security and patient confidentiality are preserved. CDC has developed the Living Well With Sickle Cell Disease Self-Care Toolkit to provide SCD education, prevention tips, and self-management tools (e.g., pain diaries) (CDC, 2019).

Lifestyle Modifications

While intense, episodic exercise may pose risks to patients with SCD (Campbell et al., 2009; Chirico et al., 2016), research has demonstrated that regular, moderate exercise training can be beneficial and may contribute to overall wellness and improved QOL. Data indicate that regular training reduces oxidative stress and thereby decreases the risks of developing chronic and acute complications (Connes et al., 2011). More and larger studies are needed to determine the best exercise training routines for providing functional benefits.

Another healthy lifestyle recommendation is to optimize water intake to maintain adequate hydration (NHLBI, 2002; Okomo and Meremikwu, 2017) because people living with SCD are more prone to dehydration. Westcott et al. (2017) found that only 31.8 percent of young adults with SCD were meeting fluid intake guidelines.

Optimizing nutritional intake is also paramount, although studies about the effects of specific micronutrients and macronutrients and dietary regimens in SCD are limited.

Cognitive Interventions

Screening for specific cognitive deficits in individuals with SCD may help predict later academic outcomes and stroke risk (Schatz et al., 2018) and may make it possible to deploy targeted cognitive interventions. Memory training programs are a non-pharmacological approach to improving academic outcomes. One study demonstrated that individuals with SCD who completed a working memory training program exhibited improved visual and working memory compared with non-completers (Hardy et al., 2016). Additionally, a small cohort of children with SCD with cerebral infarcts who completed weekly combined tutoring and memory/learning strategies had improved memory and academic achievement compared with controls at 2 years of age (King et al., 2004).

Attention is another cognitive domain of focus in SCD. Although the current literature is limited, children with SCD in the United States have rates of attention deficit hyperactivity disorder prevalence that are between 19 and 40 percent (Acquazzino et al., 2017; Benton et al., 2011; Lance et al., 2015), which are much higher than the general pediatric population (approximately 10 percent) (Xu et al., 2018). Thus, specific treatments to improve attention may also be beneficial in SCD.

SCT

One to 3 million Americans have SCT, with the prevalence of SCT in the United States being 8–10 percent in African Americans and lower in many other racial/ethnic groups, including Hispanics, South Asians, Southern Europeans, and Middle Easterners.

SCT is not considered a disease and does not typically cause the multiorgan complications associated with SCD (Naik and Haywood, 2015). Following certain extreme triggers, however, individuals with SCT may experience medical problems, including an increased risk for prevalent and incident chronic renal disease, pulmonary embolism, and rhabdomyolysis (Naik et al., 2018).

Recent epidemiological studies have identified three primary areas that require further research to understand the clinical implications of SCT. The first is exercise-related complications, which include exertional rhabdomyolysis, heat-associated collapse, and sudden death. A retrospective review of 2.1 million military personnel from 1977 to 1981 found that 12 of 28 unexplained sudden deaths were in individuals with SCT, with a relative risk (RR) of death that was 39.8 (95% confidence interval [CI], 17–90; $p < 0.001$) times higher among recruits with SCT than among peers without SCT (Kark et al., 1987). A more recent retrospective review of 273 deaths in the National Collegiate Athletic Association from 2004 to 2008 found 13 deaths categorized as exertion related, 5 in athletes with SCT, with an RR of 29 (Harmon et al., 2012). All exercise-related deaths in individuals with SCT were associated with extreme exertion and intense exercise, and both studies failed to adjust for confounders. Thus, prospective well-designed cohort studies to better elucidate the true RR of exertional death in SCT are urgently needed.

Individuals with SCD may develop renal abnormalities; rates of hematuria (blood in the urine) are higher than in the general population, and hyposthenuria (an impaired urine concentrating ability) is common. Epidemiological studies have lent support to the notion that SCT may predispose one to CKD. In a pooled analysis of 15,975 self-identified African Americans from five prospective population-based cohort studies—the Atherosclerosis Risk in Communities, Jackson Heart Study, Women's Health Initiative, Multi-Ethnic Study of Atherosclerosis, and Coronary Artery Risk Development in Young Adults—239 of the 2,233 individuals with CKD were found to have SCT, with a pooled adjusted odds ratio of 1.57 (95% CI 1.34–1.84) for CKD with SCT compared with those without SCT (Naik et al., 2014).

Further studies are required to better establish the relationship between SCT and CKD and the effect of SCT on the development of diabetic, hypertensive, and other risk-variant renal disease.

With universal NBS and mandatory screening of various adult populations for SCT, it is a moral obligation to conduct high-quality research to inform genetic counseling and personal and policy decisions, which must be conducted in a way that minimizes stigma. Robust, well-designed epidemiologic studies to answer critical questions about SCT are critical.

The American College of Obstetricians and Gynecologists recommends screening with a hemoglobin electrophoresis and complete blood count if there is suspicion for hemoglobinopathy based on ethnic background (ACOG, 2017). Some groups have recommended that, after screening, couples at risk for having a child with SCD should be offered genetic counseling and prenatal diagnosis testing (ACOG, 2007; Pecker and Naik, 2018).

In the United States, NBS for hemoglobinopathies was initiated in the 1990s to identify newborns with SCD and transfer them to SCD treatment centers for confirmatory testing and early interventions. Unfortunately, no national approach for informing families and providing information about the genetic and medical implications of SCT was in place at the time of NBS implementation and only limited progress has been made in this arena.

CONCLUSIONS AND RECOMMENDATIONS

Pain is the hallmark of SCD and is a predictor of mortality and QOL in individuals affected by the disease. The pathophysiology of acute and chronic pain in SCD is complex, which is the main reason why treatment remains suboptimal. The treatment of pain is further complicated by racial, cognitive, and socioeconomic factors.

In addition to pain, complications associated with SCD are numerous, as outlined in Tables 4-1 and 4-2. The disease affects almost every organ in the body and results in end-organ damage and symptoms that may be organ-related or constitutional, such as fatigue.

Individuals living with SCD may also experience various psychological symptoms, such as depression and anxiety, that often go undetected and therefore untreated. There is a strong link between psychological comorbidities and both acute and chronic pain. Neurocognitive deficits can also influence pain perception, ability to cope with pain, and response to treatment.

Evidence-based treatment strategies remain sparse for the prevention and management of the numerous complications of SCD. Current preventive strategies rest on infection prevention by vaccination and early penicillin prophylaxis and primary stroke prevention with chronic transfusion therapy. HU as a disease-modifying therapy has had a profound impact in reducing the rates of VOE and ACS. Transfusions also remain an important tool in the care of patients with SCD. Stem cell transplantation offers a cure, and new therapies have been recently approved or are under development (see Chapter 7). However, all treatments carry side effects, and poor medication adherence, partly stemming from mistrust of the medical environment, remains a significant concern.

A whole-person care approach has been proposed as the optimal means of providing care to individuals with SCD, with attention to lifestyle modification, behavioral interventions, and interventions aimed at alleviating cognitive deficits.

It is important that individuals with SCT receive the appropriate genetic counseling so that they understand the implications of their diagnosis. Further research is needed to fully understand the potential health-related complications associated with SCT.

Conclusion 4-1: Pain is the hallmark of SCD and is a predictor of mortality and quality of life in individuals affected by the disease. The pathophysiology of acute and chronic pain in SCD is complex and has not been completely elucidated, which has led to suboptimal care.

Conclusion 4-2: In addition to pain, complications associated with SCD are numerous. The disease affects almost every organ in the body and results in end-organ damage. Individuals living with SCD may experience various psychological symptoms, such as depression and anxiety, and most may go untreated. Therefore, it is critical to include a discussion of the critical role of addressing mental health in SCD.

Conclusion 4-3: There are limited data on the natural history of SCD and on how to address the growing disease burden in aging individuals with SCD.

Conclusion 4-4: There remains limited understanding of the health impact of SCT, particularly in certain high-risk groups, such as athletes and Army recruits. There are limited resources and no systematic strategies to track and counsel individuals who have been identified as SCT carriers at NBS.

Recommendation 4-1: Private and public funders and health professional associations should fund and conduct research to close the gaps in the existing evidence base for sickle cell disease care to inform the development of clinical practice guidelines and indicators of high-quality care.

Recommendation 4-2: The National Institutes of Health should fund research to elucidate the pathophysiology of sickle cell trait.

Recommendation 4-3: The Office of the Assistant Secretary for Health should partner with community-based organizations, the media, and other relevant stakeholders to disseminate information to promote awareness and education about the potential risks associated with sickle cell trait.

REFERENCES

Abaza, H., and M. Marschollek. 2017. mHealth application areas and technology combinations: A comparison of literature from high and low/middle income countries. *Methods of Information in Medicine* 56(7):e105–e122.

ACOG (American College of Obstetrics and Gynecology). 2007. ACOG practice bulletin no. 78: Hemoglobinopathies in pregnancy. *Obstetrics & Gynecology* 109(1):229–237.

ACOG. 2017. Carrier screening for genetic conditions. Committee opinion no. 691. *Obstetrics & Gynecology* 129:e41–e55.

Acquazzino, M. A., M. Miller, M. Myrvik, R. Newby, and J. P. Scott. 2017. Attention deficit hyperactivity disorder in children with sickle cell disease referred for an evaluation. *Journal of Pediatric Hematology/Oncology* 39(5):350–354.

Adam, S. S., C. M. Flahiff, S. Kamble, M. J. Telen, S. D. Reed, and L. M. De Castro. 2017. Depression, quality of life, and medical resource utilization in sickle cell disease. *Blood Advances* 1(23):1983–1992.

Adams, R. J., and D. Brambilla. 2005. Discontinuing prophylactic transfusions used to prevent stroke in sickle cell disease. *New England Journal of Medicine* 353(26):2769–2778.

ADDMEDICA SASA. 2015. *European Sickle Cell Disease Cohort—Hydroxyurea (ESCORT-HU).* https://clinicaltrials.gov/ct2/show/NCT02516579 (accessed April 4, 2019).

Aduloju, S., S. Palmer, and J. R. Eckman. 2008. Mortality in sickle cell patient transitioning from pediatric to adult program: 10 years Grady comprehensive sickle cell center experience. *Blood* 112(11):1426.

Alao, A. O., and M. Soderberg. 2002. Sickle cell disease and posttraumatic stress disorder. *International Journal of Psychiatry in Medicine* 32(1):97–101.

Alao, A. O., N. Westmoreland, and S. Jindal. 2003. Drug addiction in sickle cell disease: Case report. *International Journal of Psychiatry in Medicine* 33(1):97–101.

Ameringer, S., and W. R. Smith. 2011. Emerging biobehavioral factors of fatigue in sickle cell disease. *Journal of Nursing Scholarship* 43(1):22–29.

Anderson, L. M., T. M. Allen, C. D. Thornburg, and M. J. Bonner. 2015. Fatigue in children with sickle cell disease: Association with neurocognitive and social–emotional functioning and quality of life. *Journal of Pediatric Hematology/Oncology* 37(8):584–589.

Angst, M. S., and J. D. Clark. 2006. Opioid-induced hyperalgesia: A qualitative systematic review. *Anesthesiology* 104(3):570–587.

Anie, K. A. 2005. Psychological complications in sickle cell disease. *British Journal of Haematology* 129(6):723–729.

Anie, K. A., and J. Green. 2015. Psychological therapies for sickle cell disease and pain. *Cochrane Database of Systematic Reviews*(2):CD001916.

Anie, K. A., A. Steptoe, and D. H. Bevan. 2002. Sickle cell disease: Pain, coping and quality of life in a study of adults in the UK. *British Journal of Health Psychology* 7(Part 3):331–344.

Arduini, G. A. O., and A. B. Trovo de Marqui. 2018. Prevalence and characteristics of priapism in sickle cell disease. *Hemoglobin* 42(2):73–77.

ASH (American Society of Hematology). 2019. *CDC issues key clarification on guideline for prescribing opioids for chronic pain.* https://www.hematology.org/Newsroom/Press-Releases/2019/9537.aspx (accessed November 19, 2019).

Ashley-Koch, A., C. C. Murphy, M. J. Khoury, and C. A. Boyle. 2001. Contribution of sickle cell disease to the occurrence of developmental disabilities: A population-based study. *Genetics in Medicine* 3(3):181–186.

Badawy, S. M., L. Barrera, S. Cai, and A. A. Thompson. 2018a. Association between participants' characteristics, patient-reported outcomes, and clinical outcomes in youth with sickle cell disease. *BioMed Research International* 2018:8296139.

Badawy, S. M., R. M. Cronin, J. Hankins, L. Crosby, M. DeBaun, A. A. Thompson, and N. Shah. 2018b. Patient-centered eHealth interventions for children, adolescents, and adults with sickle cell disease: Systematic review. *Journal of Medical Internet Research* 20(7):e10940.

Baddam, S., I. Aban, L. Hilliard, T. Howard, D. Askenazi, and J. D. Lebensburger. 2017. Acute kidney injury during a pediatric sickle cell vaso-occlusive pain crisis. *Pediatric Nephrology* 32(8):1451–1456.

Baichoo, P., A. Asuncion, and G. El-Chaar. 2019. Intravenous acetaminophen for the management of pain during vaso-occlusive crises in pediatric patients. *Pharmacy and Therapeutics* 44(1):5–8.

Bakri, M. H., E. A. Ismail, G. O. Elsedfy, M. A. Amr, and A. Ibrahim. 2014. Behavioral impact of sickle cell disease in young children with repeated hospitalization. *Saudi Journal of Anaesthesia* 8(4):504–509.

Ballas, S. K. 2017. The use of cannabis by patients with sickle cell disease increased the frequency of hospitalization due to vaso-occlusive crises. *Cannabis Cannabinoid Research* 2(1):197–201.

Ballas, S. K. 2018. Comorbidities in aging patients with sickle cell disease. *Clinical Hemorheology and Microcirculation* 68(2–3):129–145.

Ballas, S. K., and E. D. Smith. 1992. Red blood cell changes during the evolution of the sickle cell painful crisis. *Blood* 79(8):2154–2163.

Ballas, S. K., K. Gupta, and P. Adams-Graves. 2012a. Sickle cell pain: A critical reappraisal. *Blood* 120(18):3647–3656.

Ballas, S. K., M. R. Kesen, M. F. Goldberg, G. A. Lutty, C. Dampier, I. Osunkwo, W. C. Wang, C. Hoppe, W. Hagar, D. S. Darbari, and P. Malik. 2012b. Beyond the definitions of the phenotypic complications of sickle cell disease: An update on management. *Scientific World Journal* 2012:949535.

Barabino, G. A., M. O. Platt, and D. K. Kaul. 2010. Sickle cell biomechanics. *Annual Review of Biomedical Engineering* 12:345–367.

Beiter, J. L., Jr., H. K. Simon, C. R. Chambliss, T. Adamkiewicz, and K. Sullivan. 2001. Intravenous ketorolac in the emergency department management of sickle cell pain and predictors of its effectiveness. *Archives of Pediatrics & Adolescent Medicine* 155(4):496–500.

Bellet, P. S., K. A. Kalinyak, R. Shukla, M. J. Gelfand, and D. L. Rucknagel. 1995. Incentive spirometry to prevent acute pulmonary complications in sickle cell diseases. *New England Journal of Medicine* 333(11):699–703.

Benton, T. D., R. Boyd, J. Ifeagwu, E. Feldtmose, and K. Smith-Whitley. 2011. Psychiatric diagnosis in adolescents with sickle cell disease: A preliminary report. *Current Psychiatry Reports* 13(2):111–115.

Benyamin, R., A. M. Trescot, S. Datta, R. Buenaventura, R. Adlaka, N. Sehgal, S. E. Glaser, and R. Vallejo. 2008. Opioid complications and side effects. *Pain Physician* 11(2 Suppl):S105–S120.

Berkelhammer, L. D., A. L. Williamson, S. D. Sanford, C. L. Dirksen, W. G. Sharp, A. S. Margulies, and R. A. Prengler. 2007. Neurocognitive sequelae of pediatric sickle cell disease: A review of the literature. *Child Neuropsychology* 13(2):120–131.

Bernaudin, F., S. Verlhac, C. Arnaud, A. Kamdem, S. Chevret, I. Hau, L. Coic, E. Leveille, E. Lemarchand, E. Lesprit, I. Abadie, N. Medejel, F. Madhi, S. Lemerle, S. Biscardi, J. Bardakdjian, F. Galacteros, M. Torres, M. Kuentz, C. Ferry, G. Socie, P. Reinert, and C. Delacourt. 2011. Impact of early transcranial Doppler screening and intensive therapy on cerebral vasculopathy outcome in a newborn sickle cell anemia cohort. *Blood* 117(4):1130–1140; quiz 1436.

Bhushan, D., K. Conner, J. M. Ellen, and E. M. S. Sibinga. 2015. Adjuvant acupuncture for youth with sickle cell pain: A proof of concept study. *Medical Acupuncture* 27(6):461–466.

Biedrzycki, O. J., D. Bevan, and S. Lucas. 2009. Fatal overdose due to prescription fentanyl patches in a patient with sickle cell/beta-thalassemia and acute chest syndrome: A case report and review of the literature. *American Journal of Forensic Medicine and Pathology* 30(2):188–190.

Blas, L., J. Roberti, J. Petroni, L. Reniero, and F. Cicora. 2019. Renal medullary carcinoma: A report of the current literature. *Current Urology Reports* 20(1):4.

Bodhise, P. B., M. Dejoie, Z. Brandon, S. Simpkins, and S. K. Ballas. 2004. Non-pharmacologic management of sickle cell pain. *Hematology* 9(3):235–237.

Bonds, D. R. 2005. Three decades of innovation in the management of sickle cell disease: The road to understanding the sickle cell disease clinical phenotype. *Blood Review* 19(2):99–110.

Borhade, M. B., and N. P. Kondamudi. 2019. *Sickle cell crisis.* StatPearls. https://www.ncbi.nlm.nih.gov/books/NBK526064 (accessed April 4, 2019).

Boulmay, B., and R. Lottenberg. 2009. Cocaine abuse complicating acute painful episodes in sickle cell disease. *Southern Medical Journal* 102(1):87–88.

Boyle, S. M., B. Jacobs, F. A. Sayani, and B. Hoffman. 2016. Management of the dialysis patient with sickle cell disease. *Seminars in Dialysis* 29(1):62–70.

Brandow, A. M., C. L. Stucky, C. A. Hillery, R. G. Hoffmann, and J. A. Panepinto. 2013. Patients with sickle cell disease have increased sensitivity to cold and heat. *American Journal of Hematology* 88(1):37–43.

Brandow, A. M., R. A. Farley, and J. A. Panepinto. 2014. Neuropathic pain in patients with sickle cell disease. *Pediatric Blood & Cancer* 61(3):512–517.

Brandow, A. M., R. A. Farley, M. Dasgupta, R. G. Hoffmann, and J. A. Panepinto. 2015. The use of neuropathic pain drugs in children with sickle cell disease is associated with older age, female sex, and longer length of hospital stay. *Journal of Pediatric Hematology and Oncology* 37(1):10–15.

Brousse, V., P. Buffet, and D. Rees. 2014. The spleen and sickle cell disease: The sick(led) spleen. *British Journal of Haematology* 166(2):165–176.

Brousseau, D. C., P. L. Owens, A. L. Mosso, J. A. Panepinto, and C. A. Steiner. 2010. Acute care utilization and rehospitalizations for sickle cell disease. *JAMA* 303(13):1288–1294.

Brunson, A., T. H. M. Keegan, H. Bang, A. Mahajan, S. Paulukonis, and T. Wun. 2017. Increased risk of leukemia among sickle cell disease patients in california. *Blood* 130(13):1597–1599.

Campbell, A., C. P. Minniti, M. Nouraie, M. Arteta, S. Rana, O. Onyekwere, C. Sable, G. Ensing, N. Dham, L. Luchtman-Jones, G. J. Kato, M. T. Gladwin, O. L. Castro, and V. R. Gordeuk. 2009. Prospective evaluation of haemoglobin oxygen saturation at rest and after exercise in paediatric sickle cell disease patients. *British Journal of Haematology* 147(3):352–359.

Campbell, C. M., G. Moscou-Jackson, C. P. Carroll, K. Kiley, C. Haywood, Jr., S. Lanzkron, M. Hand, R. R. Edwards, and J. A. Haythornthwaite. 2016. An evaluation of central sensitization in patients with sickle cell disease. *Journal of Pain* 17(5):617–627.

Carden, M. A., M. Fay, Y. Sakurai, B. McFarland, S. Blanche, C. DiPrete, C. H. Joiner, T. Sulchek, and W. A. Lam. 2017. Normal saline is associated with increased sickle red cell stiffness and prolonged transit times in a microfluidic model of the capillary system. *Microcirculation* 24(5):28106307.

Carden, M. A., D. C. Brousseau, F. A. Ahmad, J. Bennett, S. Bhatt, A. Bogie, K. Brown, T. C. Casper, L. L. Chapman, C. E. Chumpitazi, D. Cohen, C. Dampier, A. M. Ellison, H. Grasemann, R. W. Hickey, L. L. Hsu, S. Leibovich, E. Powell, R. Richards, S. Sarnaik, D. L. Weiner, and C. R. Morris. 2019. Normal saline bolus use in pediatric emergency departments is associated with poorer pain control in children with sickle cell anemia and vaso-occlusive pain. *American Journal of Hematology* 94(6):689–696.

Carroll, C. P. 2020. Opioid treatment for acute and chronic pain in patients with sickle cell disease. *Neuroscience Letters* 714:134534.

Carroll, C. P., S. Lanzkron, C. Haywood, Jr., K. Kiley, M. Pejsa, G. Moscou-Jackson, J. A. Haythornthwaite, and C. M. Campbell. 2016. Chronic opioid therapy and central sensitization in sickle cell disease. *American Journal of Preventive Medicine* 51(1 Suppl 1):S69–S77.

Catalano, A., G. Martino, N. Morabito, C. Scarcella, A. Gaudio, G. Basile, and A. Lasco. 2017. Pain in osteoporosis: From pathophysiology to therapeutic approach. *Drugs & Aging* 34(10):755–765.

Cataldo, G., S. Rajput, K. Gupta, and D. A. Simone. 2015. Sensitization of nociceptive spinal neurons contributes to pain in a transgenic model of sickle cell disease. *Pain* 156(4):722–730.

CDC (Centers for Disease Control and Prevention). 2019. *Living well with sickle cell disease self-care toolkit.* https://www.cdc.gov/ncbddd/sicklecell/documents/LivingWell-With-Sickle-Cell-Disease_Self-CareToolkit.pdf (accessed January 9, 2019).

Charache, S., and D. L. Page. 1967. Infarction of bone marrow in the sickle cell disorders. *Annals of Internal Medicine* 67(6):1195–1200.

Charache, S., G. J. Dover, R. D. Moore, S. Eckert, S. K. Ballas, M. Koshy, P. F. Milner, E. P. Orringer, G. Phillips, Jr., and O. S. Platt. 1992. Hydroxyurea: Effects on hemoglobin F production in patients with sickle cell anemia. *Blood* 79(10):2555–2565.

Charache, S., M. L. Terrin, R. D. Moore, G. J. Dover, F. B. Barton, S. V. Eckert, R. P. McMahon, and D. R. Bonds. 1995. Effect of hydroxyurea on the frequency of painful crises in sickle cell anemia. Investigators of the Multicenter Study of Hydroxyurea in Sickle Cell Anemia. *New England Journal of Medicine* 332(20):1317–1322.

Chirico, E. N., C. Faes, P. Connes, E. Canet-Soulas, C. Martin, and V. Pialoux. 2016. Role of exercise-induced oxidative stress in sickle cell trait and disease. *Sports Medicine* 46(5):629–639.

Citero, V. A., J. L. Levenson, D. K. McClish, V. E. Bovbjerg, P. L. Cole, B. A. Dahman, L. T. Penberthy, I. P. Aisiku, S. D. Roseff, and W. R. Smith. 2007. The role of catastrophizing in sickle cell disease—The PiSCES project. *Pain* 133(1–3):39–46.

Clark, R., N. B. Anderson, V. R. Clark, and D. R. Williams. 1999. Racism as a stressor for African Americans. A biopsychosocial model. *American Psychologist* 54(10):805–816.

Co, L. L., T. H. Schmitz, H. Havdala, A. Reyes, and M. P. Westerman. 1979. Acupuncture: An evaluation in the painful crises of sickle cell anaemia. *Pain* 7(2):181–185.

Cohen, S. P., P. J. Christo, S. Wang, L. Chen, M. P. Stojanovic, C. H. Shields, C. Brummett, and J. Mao. 2008. The effect of opioid dose and treatment duration on the perception of a painful standardized clinical stimulus. *Regional Anesthesia & Pain Medicine* 33(3):199–206.

Colloca, L., M. Flaten, and K. Meissner (eds.). 2013. *Placebo and pain*. New York: Academic Press.

Connes, P., R. Machado, O. Hue, and H. Reid. 2011. Exercise limitation, exercise testing and exercise recommendations in sickle cell anemia. *Clinical Hemorheology and Microcirculation* 49(1–4):151–163.

Conran, N., C. F. Franco-Penteado, and F. F. Costa. 2009. Newer aspects of the pathophysiology of sickle cell disease vaso-occlusion. *Hemoglobin* 33(1):1–16.

Cronin, R. M., T. L. Mayo-Gamble, S. J. Stimpson, S. M. Badawy, L. E. Crosby, J. Byrd, E. J. Volanakis, A. A. Kassim, J. L. Raphael, V. M. Murry, and M. R. DeBaun. 2018. Adapting medical guidelines to be patient-centered using a patient-driven process for individuals with sickle cell disease and their caregivers. *BMC Hematology* 18(1):12.

Cruz-Almeida, Y., C. D. King, B. R. Goodin, K. T. Sibille, T. L. Glover, J. L. Riley, A. Sotolongo, M. S. Herbert, J. Schmidt, B. J. Fessler, D. T. Redden, R. Staud, L. A. Bradley, and R. B. Fillingim. 2013. Psychological profiles and pain characteristics of older adults with knee osteoarthritis. *Arthritis Care & Research* 65(11):1786–1794.

Daly, B., M. C. Kral, R. T. Brown, D. Elkin, A. Madan-Swain, M. Mitchell, L. Crosby, D. Dematteo, A. Larosa, and S. Jackson. 2012. Ameliorating attention problems in children with sickle cell disease: A pilot study of methylphenidate. *Journal of Developmental and Behavioral Pediatrics* 33(3):244–251.

Dampier, C., P. LeBeau, S. Rhee, S. Lieff, K. Kesler, S. Ballas, Z. Rogers, W. Wang, and Comprehensive Sickle Cell Centers Clinical Trial Consortium site investigators. 2011. Health-related quality of life in adults with sickle cell disease (SCD): A report from the Comprehensive Sickle Cell Centers Clinical Trial Consortium. *American Journal of Hematology* 86(2):203–205.

Dampier, C., T. M. Palermo, D. S. Darbari, K. Hassell, W. Smith, and W. Zempsky. 2017. AAPT diagnostic criteria for chronic sickle cell disease pain. *Journal of Pain* 18(5):490–498.

Dang, N. C., C. Johnson, M. Eslami-Farsani, and L. J. Haywood. 2005. Bone marrow embolism in sickle cell disease: A review. *American Journal of Hematology* 79(1):61–67.

Dantzer, R., C. J. Heijnen, A. Kavelaars, S. Laye, and L. Capuron. 2014. The neuroimmune basis of fatigue. *Trends in Neuroscience* 37(1):39–46.

Darbari, D. S., and A. M. Brandow. 2017. Pain-measurement tools in sickle cell disease: Where are we now? *Hematology: American Society of Hematology Education Program* 2017(1):534–541.

Darbari, D. S., P. Kple-Faget, J. Kwagyan, S. Rana, V. R. Gordeuk, and O. Castro. 2006. Circumstances of death in adult sickle cell disease patients. *American Journal of Hematology* 81(11):858–863.

Darbari, D. S., Z. Wang, M. Kwak, M. Hildesheim, J. Nichols, D. Allen, C. Seamon, M. Peters-Lawrence, A. Conrey, M. K. Hall, G. J. Kato, and J. G. Taylor IV. 2013. Severe painful vaso-occlusive crises and mortality in a contemporary adult sickle cell anemia cohort study. *PLOS ONE* 8(11):e79923.

Davis, H., K. C. Schoendorf, P. J. Gergen, and R. M. Moore, Jr. 1997. National trends in the mortality of children with sickle cell disease, 1968 through 1992. *American Journal of Public Health* 87(8):1317–1322.

De Franceschi, L., M. D. Cappellini, and O. Olivieri. 2011. Thrombosis and sickle cell disease. *Seminars in Thrombosis and Hemostasis* 37(3):226–236.

DeBaun, M. R., D. L. Ghafuri, M. Rodeghier, P. Maitra, S. Chaturvedi, A. Kassim, and K. I. Ataga. 2019. Decreased median survival of adults with sickle cell disease after adjusting for left truncation bias: A pooled analysis. *Blood* 133(6):615–617.

Desai, A. A., A. R. Patel, H. Ahmad, J. V. Groth, T. Thiruvoipati, K. Turner, C. Yodwut, P. Czobor, N. Artz, R. F. Machado, J. G. N. Garcia, and R. M. Lang. 2014. Mechanistic insights and characterization of sickle cell disease-associated cardiomyopathy. *Circulation: Cardiovascular Imaging* 7(3):430–437.

Diggs, L. W. 1956. The crisis in sickle cell anemia: Hematologic studies. *American Journal of Clinical Pathology* 26(10):1109–1118.

Dinges, D. F., W. G. Whitehouse, E. C. Orne, P. B. Bloom, M. M. Carlin, N. K. Bauer, K. A. Gillen, B. S. Shapiro, K. Ohene-Frempong, C. Dampier, and M. T. Orne. 1997. Self-hypnosis training as an adjunctive treatment in the management of pain associated with sickle cell disease. *International Journal of Clinical and Experimental Hypnosis* 45(4):417–432.

Dobson, C. E., and M. W. Byrne. 2014. Original research: Using guided imagery to manage pain in young children with sickle cell disease. *American Journal of Nursing* 114(4):26–36; test 37, 47.

Dowell, D., T. M. Haegerich, and R. Chou. 2016. CDC guideline for prescribing opioids for chronic pain—United States, 2016. *MMWR Recommendations and Reports* 65(1):1–49.

Elmariah, H., M. E. Garrett, L. M. De Castro, J. C. Jonassaint, K. I. Ataga, J. R. Eckman, A. E. Ashley-Koch, and M. J. Telen. 2014. Factors associated with survival in a contemporary adult sickle cell disease cohort. *American Journal of Hematology* 89(5):530–535.

Elsurer, R., B. Afsar, and E. Mercanoglu. 2013. Bone pain assessment and relationship with parathyroid hormone and health-related quality of life in hemodialysis. *Renal Failure* 35(5):667–672.

Emre, U., S. T. Miller, M. Gutierez, P. Steiner, S. P. Rao, and M. Rao. 1995. Effect of transfusion in acute chest syndrome of sickle cell disease. *Journal of Pediatrics* 127(6):901–904.

Enninful-Eghan, H., R. H. Moore, R. Ichord, K. Smith-Whitley, and J. L. Kwiatkowski. 2010. Transcranial Doppler ultrasonography and prophylactic transfusion program is effective in preventing overt stroke in children with sickle cell disease. *Journal of Pediatrics* 157(3):479–484.

Ezenwa, M. O., R. E. Molokie, D. J. Wilkie, M. L. Suarez, and Y. Yao. 2015. Perceived injustice predicts stress and pain in adults with sickle cell disease. *Pain Management Nursing* 16(3):294–306.

Ezenwa, M. O., R. E. Molokie, Z. J. Wang, Y. Yao, M. L. Suarez, C. Pullum, J. M. Schlaeger, R. B. Fillingim, and D. J. Wilkie. 2016. Safety and utility of quantitative sensory testing among adults with sickle cell disease: Indicators of neuropathic pain? *Pain Practice* 16(3):282–293.

Ezenwa, M. O., Y. Yao, R. E. Molokie, Z. J. Wang, M. W. Mandernach, M. L. Suarez, and D. J. Wilkie. 2017. Coping with pain in the face of healthcare injustice in patients with sickle cell disease. *Journal of Immigrant and Minority Health* 19(6):1449–1456.

Ezenwa, M. O., R. E. Molokie, Z. J. Wang, Y. Yao, M. L. Suarez, B. Dyal, K. Abudawood, and D. J. Wilkie. 2018. Differences in sensory pain, expectation, and satisfaction reported by outpatients with cancer or sickle cell disease. *Pain Management Nursing* 19(4):322–332.

Falletta, J. M., G. M. Woods, J. I. Verter, G. R. Buchanan, C. H. Pegelow, R. V. Iyer, S. T. Miller, C. T. Holbrook, T. R. Kinney, E. Vichinsky, D. L. Becton, W. Wang, H. S. Johnstone, D. L. Wethers, G. H. Reaman, M. R. DeBaun, N. J. Grossman, K. Kalinyak, J. H. Jorgensen, A. Bjornson, M. D. Thomas, and C. Reid. 1995. Discontinuing penicillin prophylaxis in children with sickle cell anemia. Prophylactic penicillin study II. *Journal of Pediatrics* 127(5):685–690.

FDA (U.S. Food and Drug Administration). 2017. *FDA approves hydroxyurea for treatment of pediatric patients with sickle cell anemia.* https://www.fda.gov/drugs/resources-information-approved-drugs/fda-approves-hydroxyurea-treatment-pediatric-patients-sickle-cell-anemia (accessed April 4, 2019).

Field, J. J., J. Stocks, F. J. Kirkham, C. L. Rosen, D. J. Dietzen, T. Semon, J. Kirkby, P. Bates, S. Seicean, M. R. DeBaun, S. Redline, and R. C. Strunk. 2011. Airway hyperresponsiveness in children with sickle cell anemia. *Chest* 139(3):563–568.

Field, J. J., S. K. Ballas, C. M. Campbell, L. E. Crosby, C. Dampier, D. S. Darbari, D. K. McClish, W. R. Smith, and W. T. Zempsky. 2019. AAAPT diagnostic criteria for acute sickle cell disease pain. *Journal of Pain* 20(7):746–759.

Finan, P. H., B. R. Goodin, and M. T. Smith. 2013. The association of sleep and pain: An update and a path forward. *Journal of Pain* 14(12):1539–1552.

Fishbain, D. A., and A. Pulikal. 2019. Does opioid tapering in chronic pain patients result in improved pain or same pain vs increased pain at taper completion? A structured evidence-based systematic review. *Pain Medicine* 20(11):2179–2197.

Fonseca, G. H., R. Souza, V. M. Salemi, C. V. Jardim, and S. F. Gualandro. 2012. Pulmonary hypertension diagnosed by right heart catheterisation in sickle cell disease. *European Respiratory Journal* 39(1):112–118.

Franck, L. S., M. Treadwell, E. Jacob, and E. Vichinsky. 2002. Assessment of sickle cell pain in children and young adults using the adolescent pediatric pain tool. *Journal of Pain and Symptom Management* 23(2):114–120.

Fullerton, H. J., R. J. Adams, S. Zhao, and S. C. Johnston. 2004. Declining stroke rates in Californian children with sickle cell disease. *Blood* 104(2):336–339.

Gaartman, A., A. Sayedi, C. Van Tuijn, H. Heijboer, T. Netelenbos, B. Biemond, and E. Nur. 2019. *Complications of extra fluid therapy (hyperhydration) in sickle cell patients during vaso-occlusive painful crisis.* Paper presented at ASH Annual Meeting, December 7, Orange County Convention Center.

Gale, H. I., B. N. Setty, P. G. Sprinz, G. Doros, D. D. Williams, T. C. Morrison, T. A. Kalajian, P. Tu, S. N. Mundluru, M. N. Mehta, and I. Castro-Aragon. 2015. Implications of radiologic–pathologic correlation for gallbladder disease in children and young adults with sickle cell disease. *Emergency Radiology* 22(5):543–551.

Gangaraju, R., V. V. Reddy, and M. B. Marques. 2016. Fat embolism syndrome secondary to bone marrow necrosis in patients with hemoglobinopathies. *Southern Medical Journal* 109(9):549–553.

Gardner, C. S., and T. A. Jaffe. 2015. CT of gastrointestinal vasoocclusive crisis complicating sickle cell disease. *American Journal of Roentgenology* 204(5):994–999.

Gardner, C. S., and T. A. Jaffe. 2016. Acute gastrointestinal vaso-occlusive ischemia in sickle cell disease: CT imaging features and clinical outcome. *Abdominal Radiology* 41(3):466–475.

Gaston, M. H., J. I. Verter, G. Woods, C. Pegelow, J. Kelleher, G. Presbury, H. Zarkowsky, E. Vichinsky, R. Iyer, J. S. Lobel, S. Diamond, C. T. Holbrook, F. M. Gill, K. Ritchey, and J. M. Falletta. 1986. Prophylaxis with oral penicillin in children with sickle cell anemia. A randomized trial. *New England Journal of Medicine* 314(25):1593–1599.

Gérardin, C., A. Moktefi, C. Couchoud, A. Duquesne, N. Ouali, P. Gataut, A. Karras, D. Anglicheau, C. Lefaucheur, L. Figueres, L. Albano, A. Lionet, M. Novion, M.-J. Ziliotis, M. Louis, A. Del Bello, M. Matignon, K. Dahan, A. Habibi, F. Galacteros, P. Bartolucci, P. Grimbert, and V. Audard. 2019. Survival and specific outcome of sickle cell disease patients after renal transplantation. *British Journal of Haematology* 187(5):676–680.

Gladwin, M. T. 2017. Cardiovascular complications in patients with sickle cell disease. *Hematology: American Society of Hematology—Education Program* 2017(1):423–430.

Gladwin, M. T., V. Sachdev, M. L. Jison, Y. Shizukuda, J. F. Plehn, K. Minter, B. Brown, W. A. Coles, J. S. Nichols, I. Ernst, L. A. Hunter, W. C. Blackwelder, A. N. Schechter, G. P. Rodgers, O. Castro, and F. P. Ognibene. 2004. Pulmonary hypertension as a risk factor for death in patients with sickle cell disease. *New England Journal of Medicine* 350(9):886–895.

Glaser, D. L., and F. S. Kaplan. 1997. Osteoporosis. Definition and clinical presentation. *Spine* 22(24 Suppl):12s–16s.

Goldstein-Leever, A., L. L. Cohen, C. Dampier, and S. Sil. 2018. Parent pain catastrophizing predicts child depressive symptoms in youth with sickle cell disease. *Pediatric Blood & Cancer* 65(7):e27027.

Gordeuk, V. R., O. L. Castro, and R. F. Machado. 2016. Pathophysiology and treatment of pulmonary hypertension in sickle cell disease. *Blood* 127(7):820–828.

Habibi, A., A. Mekontso-Dessap, C. Guillaud, M. Michel, K. Razazi, M. Khellaf, B. Chami, D. Bachir, C. Rieux, G. Melica, B. Godeau, F. Galacteros, P. Bartolucci, and F. Pirenne. 2016. Delayed hemolytic transfusion reaction in adult sickle-cell disease: Presentations, outcomes, and treatments of 99 referral center episodes. *American Journal of Hematology* 91(10):989–994.

Halasa, N. B., S. M. Shankar, T. R. Talbot, P. G. Arbogast, E. F. Mitchel, W. C. Wang, W. Schaffner, A. S. Craig, and M. R. Griffin. 2007. Incidence of invasive pneumococcal disease among individuals with sickle cell disease before and after the introduction of the pneumococcal conjugate vaccine. *Clinical Infectious Diseases* 44(11):1428–1433.

Han, J., J. Zhou, S. L. Saraf, V. R. Gordeuk, and G. S. Calip. 2018. Characterization of opioid use in sickle cell disease. *Pharmacoepidemiology and Drug Safety* 27(5):479–486.

Hankins, J. S., M. B. McCarville, A. Rankine-Mullings, M. E. Reid, C. L. Lobo, P. G. Moura, S. Ali, D. P. Soares, K. Aldred, D. W. Jay, B. Aygun, J. Bennett, G. Kang, J. C. Goldsmith, M. P. Smeltzer, J. M. Boyett, and R. E. Ware. 2015. Prevention of conversion to abnormal transcranial Doppler with hydroxyurea in sickle cell anemia: A Phase III international randomized clinical trial. *American Journal of Hematology* 90(12):1099–1105.

Hardwick, W. E., Jr., T. G. Givens, K. W. Monroe, W. D. King, and D. Lawley. 1999. Effect of ketorolac in pediatric sickle cell vaso-occlusive pain crisis. *Pediatric Emergency Care* 15(3):179–182.

Hardy, S. J., K. K. Hardy, J. C. Schatz, A. L. Thompson, and E. R. Meier. 2016. Feasibility of home-based computerized working memory training with children and adolescents with sickle cell disease. *Pediatric Blood & Cancer* 63(9):1578–1585.

Harmon, K. G., J. A. Drezner, D. Klossner, and I. M. Asif. 2012. Sickle cell trait associated with a RR of death of 37 times in National Collegiate Athletic Association football athletes: A database with 2 million athlete-years as the denominator. *British Journal of Sports Medicine* 46(5):325–330.

Hasan, S. P., S. Hashmi, M. Alhassen, W. Lawson, and O. Castro. 2003. Depression in sickle cell disease. *Journal of the National Medical Association* 95(7):533–537.

Hassell, K. 2005. Pregnancy and sickle cell disease. *Hematology/Oncology Clinics of North America* 19(5):vii–viii, 903–916.

Hay, J. L., J. M. White, F. Bochner, A. A. Somogyi, T. J. Semple, and B. Rounsefell. 2009. Hyperalgesia in opioid-managed chronic pain and opioid-dependent patients. *Journal of Pain* 10(3):316–322.

Haywood, C., Jr., M. Diener-West, J. Strouse, C. P. Carroll, S. Bediako, S. Lanzkron, J. Haythornthwaite, G. Onojobi, and M. C. Beach. 2014. Perceived discrimination in health care is associated with a greater burden of pain in sickle cell disease. *Journal of Pain and Symptom Management* 48(5):934–943.

Haywood, L. J. 2009. Cardiovascular function and dysfunction in sickle cell anemia. *Journal of the National Medical Association* 101(1):24–30.

Helmerhorst, H. J., M. J. Schultz, P. H. van der Voort, E. de Jonge, and D. J. van Westerloo. 2015. Bench-to-bedside review: The effects of hyperoxia during critical illness. *Critical Care* 19:284.

Hofmann, M., M. de Montalembert, B. Beauquier-Maccotta, P. de Villartay, and B. Golse. 2007. Posttraumatic stress disorder in children affected by sickle-cell disease and their parents. *American Journal of Hematology* 82(2):171–172.

Hood, A. M., A. A. King, M. E. Fields, A. L. Ford, K. P. Guilliams, M. L. Hulbert, J. M. Lee, and D. A. White. 2019. Higher executive abilities following a blood transfusion in children and young adults with sickle cell disease. *Pediatric Blood & Cancer* 66(10):e27899.

Howard, J., K. A. Anie, A. Holdcroft, S. Korn, and S. C. Davies. 2005. Cannabis use in sickle cell disease: A questionnaire study. *British Journal of Haematology* 131(1):123–128.

Howard, J., M. Malfroy, C. Llewelyn, L. Choo, R. Hodge, T. Johnson, S. Purohit, D. C. Rees, L. Tillyer, I. Walker, K. Fijnvandraat, M. Kirby-Allen, E. Spackman, S. C. Davies, and L. M. Williamson. 2013. The Transfusion Alternatives Preoperatively in Sickle Cell Disease (TAPS) study: A randomised, controlled, multicentre clinical trial. *Lancet* 381(9870):930–938.

Indik, J. H., V. Nair, R. Rafikov, I. S. Nyotowidjojo, J. Bisla, M. Kansal, D. S. Parikh, M. Robinson, A. Desai, M. Oberoi, A. Gupta, T. Abbasi, Z. Khalpey, A. R. Patel, R. M. Lang, S. C. Dudley, B. R. Choi, J. G. Garcia, R. F. Machado, and A. A. Desai. 2016. Associations of prolonged QTC in sickle cell disease. *PLOS ONE* 11(10):e0164526.

Ingram, V. M. 2004. Sickle-cell anemia hemoglobin: The molecular biology of the first "molecular disease"—The crucial importance of serendipity. *Genetics* 167(1):1–7.

Irvine, D. M., L. Vincent, N. Bubela, L. Thompson, and J. Graydon. 1991. A critical appraisal of the research literature investigating fatigue in the individual with cancer. *Cancer Nursing* 14(4):188–199.

Janes, S., M. Pocock, E. Bishop, and D. Bevan. 1997. Automated red cell exchange in sickle cell disease. *British Journal of Haematology* 97:256–258.

Jansson, L., S. Lavstedt, and L. Frithiof. 2002. Relationship between oral health and mortality rate. *Journal of Clinical Periodontology* 29(11):1029–1034.

Jenerette, C., M. Funk, and C. Murdaugh. 2005. Sickle cell disease: A stigmatizing condition that may lead to depression. *Issues in Mental Health Nursing* 26(10):1081–1101.

John, A. B., A. Ramlal, H. Jackson, G. H. Maude, A. W. Sharma, and G. R. Serjeant. 1984. Prevention of pneumococcal infection in children with homozygous sickle cell disease. *BMJ* 288(6430):1567–1570.

Jonassaint, C. R., V. L. Jones, S. Leong, and G. M. Frierson. 2016. A systematic review of the association between depression and health care utilization in children and adults with sickle cell disease. *British Journal of Haematology* 174(1):136–147.

Kabat-Zinn, J. 2009. *Wherever you go, there you are: Mindfulness meditation in everyday life.* New York: Hachette Books.

Kalogeris, T., C. P. Baines, M. Krenz, and R. J. Korthuis. 2012. Cell biology of ischemia/reperfusion injury. *International Review of Cell and Molecular Biology* 298:229–317.

Kanter, J., and R. Kruse-Jarres. 2013. Management of sickle cell disease from childhood through adulthood. *Blood Reviews* 27(6):279–287.

Kark, J. A., D. M. Posey, H. R. Schumacher, and C. J. Ruehle. 1987. Sickle-cell trait as a risk factor for sudden death in physical training. *New England Journal of Medicine* 317(13):781–787.

Kassim, A. A., S. Pruthi, M. Day, M. Rodeghier, M. C. Gindville, M. A. Brodsky, M. R. DeBaun, and L. C. Jordan. 2016. Silent cerebral infarcts and cerebral aneurysms are prevalent in adults with sickle cell anemia. *Blood* 127(16):2038–2040.

Kater, A. P., H. Heijboer, M. Peters, T. Vogels, M. H. Prins, and H. S. Heymans. 1999. Quality of life in children with sickle cell disease in Amsterdam area. *Nederlands Tijdschrift voor Geneeskunde* 143(41):2049–2053.

Kato, G. J., M. H. Steinberg, and M. T. Gladwin. 2017. Intravascular hemolysis and the pathophysiology of sickle cell disease. *Journal of Clinical Investigation* 127(3):750–760.

Kauf, T. L., T. D. Coates, L. Huazhi, N. Mody-Patel, and A. G. Hartzema. 2009. The cost of health care for children and adults with sickle cell disease. *American Journal of Hematology* 84(6):323–327.

Kawadler, J. M., J. D. Clayden, C. A. Clark, and F. J. Kirkham. 2016. Intelligence quotient in paediatric sickle cell disease: A systematic review and meta-analysis. *Developmental Medicine and Child Neurology* 58(7):672–679.

King, A., D. White, M. Armstrong, R. McKinstry, M. Noetzel, and M. R. Debaun. 2004. An educational remediation program benefits children with sickle cell disease and cerebral infarcts. *Pediatric Research* 56(4):668.

Knight-Madden, J., and G. R. Serjeant. 2001. Invasive pneumococcal disease in homozygous sickle cell disease: Jamaican experience 1973–1997. *Journal of Pediatrics* 138(1):65–70.

Kotila, T. R., O. E. Busari, V. Makanjuola, and O. R. Eyelade. 2015. Addiction or pseudoaddiction in sickle cell disease patients: Time to decide—A case series. *Annals of Ibadan Postgraduate Medicine* 13(1):44–47.

Krejza, J., R. Chen, G. Romanowicz, J.L. Kwiatkowski, R. Ichord, M. Arkuszewski, R. Zimmerman, K. Ohene-Frempong, L. Desiderio, and E.R. Melhem. 2010. Sickle cell disease and transcranial Doppler imaging: Inter-hemispheric differences in blood flow Doppler parameters. *Stroke* 42:81–86.

Kuo, K., and A. B. Caughey. 2016. Contemporary outcomes of sickle cell disease in pregnancy. *American Journal of Obstetrics and Gynecology* 215(4):e501–e505.

Kuo, K. H. M., R. Ward, J. Howard, and P. Telfer. 2012. A comparison of chronic manual and automated red blood cell exchange transfusion in sickle cell disease patients from two comprehensive care centres in the United Kingdom. *Blood* 120(21):3430.

Kwiatkowski, J. L., S. Granger, D. J. Brambilla, R.C. Brown, S. T. Miller, R. J. Adams, and STOP Trial Investigators. 2006. Elevated blood flow velocity in the anterior cerebral artery and stroke risk in sickle cell disease: Extended analysis from the STOP trial. *British Journal of Haematology* 134(3):333–339.

Lance, E. I., A. M. Comi, M. V. Johnston, J. F. Casella, and B. K. Shapiro. 2015. Risk factors for attention and behavioral issues in pediatric sickle cell disease. *Clinical Pediatrics* 54(11):1087–1093.

Lanzkron, S., J. Little, J. Field, J. R. Shows, H. Wang, R. Seufert, J. Brooks, R. Varadhan, C. Haywood, Jr., M. Saheed, C. Y. Huang, B. Griffin, S. Frymark, A. Piehet, D. Robertson, M. Proudford, A. Kincaid, C. Green, L. Burgess, M. Wallace, and J. Segal. 2018. Increased acute care utilization in a prospective cohort of adults with sickle cell disease. *Blood Advances* 2(18):2412–2417.

Laurence, B., C. Haywood, Jr., and S. Lanzkron. 2013. Dental infections increase the likelihood of hospital admissions among adult patients with sickle cell disease. *Community Dental Health* 30(3):168–172.

Lawson, S., S. Oakley, N. A. Smith, and D. Bareford. 1999. Red cell exchange in sickle cell disease. *Clinical and Laboratory Haematology* 21:99–102.

Lee, M., S. M. Silverman, H. Hansen, V. B. Patel, and L. Manchikanti. 2011. A comprehensive review of opioid-induced hyperalgesia. *Pain Physician* 14(2):145–161.

Lemanek, K. L., M. Ranalli, and C. Lukens. 2009. A randomized controlled trial of massage therapy in children with sickle cell disease. *Journal of Pediatric Psychology* 34(10):1091–1096.

Levenson, J. L. 2008. Psychiatric issues in adults with sickle cell disease. *Primary Psychiatry* 15(5):45–49.

Levenson, J. L., D. K. McClish, B. A. Dahman, L. T. Penberthy, V. E. Bovbjerg, I. P. Aisiku, S. D. Roseff, and W. R. Smith. 2007. Alcohol abuse in sickle cell disease: The PiSCES project. *American Journal on Addiction* 16(5):383–388.

Levenson, J. L., D. K. McClish, B. A. Dahman, V. E. Bovbjerg, V. D. A. Citero, L. T. Penberthy, I. P. Aisiku, J. D. Roberts, S. D. Roseff, and W. R. Smith. 2008. Depression and anxiety in adults with sickle cell disease: The PiSCES project. *Psychosomatic Medicine* 70(2):192–196.

Loiselle, K., J. L. Lee, L. Szulczewski, S. Drake, L. E. Crosby, and A. L. Pai. 2016. Systematic and meta-analytic review: Medication adherence among pediatric patients with sickle cell disease. *Journal of Pediatric Psychology* 41(4):406–418.

Lu, K., M. C. Cheng, X. Ge, A. Berger, D. Xu, G. J. Kato, and C. P. Minniti. 2014. A retrospective review of acupuncture use for the treatment of pain in sickle cell disease patients: Descriptive analysis from a single institution. *Clinical Journal of Pain* 30(9):825–830.

Lubega, F. A., M. S. DeSilva, D. Munube, R. Nkwine, J. Tumukunde, P. K. Agaba, M. T. Nabukenya, F. Bulamba, and T. S. Luggya. 2018. Low dose ketamine versus morphine for acute severe vaso occlusive pain in children: A randomized controlled trial. *Scandinavian Journal of Pain* 18(1):19–27.

Lukoo, R. N., R. M. Ngiyulu, G. L. Mananga, J. L. Gini-Ehungu, P. M. Ekulu, P. M. Tshibassu, and M. N. Aloni. 2015. Depression in children suffering from sickle cell anemia. *Journal of Pediatric Hematology/Oncology* 37(1):20–24.

Manci, E. A., D. E. Culberson, Y. M. Yang, T. M. Gardner, R. Powell, J. Haynes, Jr., A. K. Shah, V. N. Mankad, and investigators of the Cooperative Study of Sickle Cell Disease. 2003. Causes of death in sickle cell disease: An autopsy study. *British Journal of Haematology* 123(2):359–365.

Mandese, V., E. Bigi, P. Bruzzi, G. Palazzi, B. Predieri, L. Lucaccioni, M. Cellini, and L. Iughetti. 2019. Endocrine and metabolic complications in children and adolescents with sickle cell disease: An Italian cohort study. *BMC Pediatrics* 19(1):56.

Manley, A. F. 1984. Legislation and funding for sickle cell services, 1972–1982. *American Journal of Pediatric Hematology/Oncology* 6(1):67–71.

Mantadakis, E., J. D. Cavender, Z. R. Rogers, D. H. Ewalt, and G. R. Buchanan. 1999. Prevalence of priapism in children and adolescents with sickle cell anemia. *Journal of Pediatric Hematology/Oncology* 21(6):518–522.

Martins, W. A., H. F. Lopes, F. M. Consolim-Colombo, F. Gualandro Sde, E. Arteaga-Fernandez, and C. Mady. 2012. Cardiovascular autonomic dysfunction in sickle cell anemia. *Autonomic Neuroscience* 166(1–2):54–59.

Matthie, N., C. Jenerette, and S. McMillan. 2015. Role of self-care in sickle cell disease. *Pain Management Nursing* 16(3):257–266.

McClellan, A. C., J. C. Luthi, J. R. Lynch, J. M. Soucie, R. Kulkarni, A. Guasch, E. D. Huff, D. Gilbertson, W. M. McClellan, and M. R. DeBaun. 2012. High one year mortality in adults with sickle cell disease and end-stage renal disease. *British Journal of Haematology* 159(3):360–367.

McClish, D. K., L. T. Penberthy, V. E. Bovbjerg, J. D. Roberts, I. P. Aisiku, J. L. Levenson, S. D. Roseff, and W. R. Smith. 2005. Health related quality of life in sickle cell patients: The PiSCES project. *Health and Quality of Life Outcomes* 3:50.

McGann, P. T., J. M. Flanagan, T. A. Howard, S. D. Derlinger, J. He, A. S. Kulharya, B. W. Thompson, and R. E. Ware. 2012. Genotoxicity associated with hydroxyurea exposure in infants with sickle cell anemia: Results from the BABY-HUG Phase III clinical trial. *Pediatric Blood Cancer* 59(2):254–257.

McMahon, S., M. Koltzenburg, I. Tracey, and D. Turk. 2013. *Wall & Melzack's textbook of pain, 6th ed.* Philadelphia, PA: Saunders.

Meghani, S. H., and N. Vapiwala. 2018. Bridging the critical divide in pain management guidelines from the CDC, NCCN, and ASCO for cancer survivors. *JAMA Oncology* 4(10):1323–1324.

Mehari, A., and E. S. Klings. 2016. Chronic pulmonary complications of sickle cell disease. *Chest* 149(5):1313–1324.

Mehari, A., M. T. Gladwin, X. Tian, R. F. Machado, and G. J. Kato. 2012. Mortality in adults with sickle cell disease and pulmonary hypertension. *JAMA* 307(12):1254–1256.

Mekontso Dessap, A., F. Pirenne, K. Razazi, S. Moutereau, S. Abid, C. Brun-Buisson, B. Maitre, M. Michel, F. Galacteros, P. Bartolucci, and A. Habibi. 2016. A diagnostic nomogram for delayed hemolytic transfusion reaction in sickle cell disease. *American Journal of Hematology* 91(12):1181–1184.

Moody, K., B. Abrahams, R. Baker, R. Santizo, D. Manwani, V. Carullo, D. Eugenio, and A. Carroll. 2017. A randomized trial of yoga for children hospitalized with sickle cell vaso-occlusive crisis. *Journal of Pain and Symptom Management* 53(6):1026–1034.

Myers, C. D., M. E. Robinson, T. H. Guthrie, S. P. Lamp, and R. Lottenberg. 1999. Adjunctive approaches for sickle cell chronic pain. *Alternative Health Practitioner* 5(3):203–212.

Myrvik, M. P., A. D. Campbell, M. M. Davis, and J. L. Butcher. 2012. Impact of psychiatric diagnoses on hospital length of stay in children with sickle cell anemia. *Pediatric Blood & Cancer* 58(2):239–243.

Myrvik, M. P., L. M. Burks, R. G. Hoffman, M. Dasgupta, and J. A. Panepinto. 2013. Mental health disorders influence admission rates for pain in children with sickle cell disease. *Pediatric Blood & Cancer* 60(7):1211–1214.

Naik, R. P., and C. Haywood, Jr. 2015. Sickle cell trait diagnosis: Clinical and social implications. *Hematology: American Society of Hematology—Education Program* 2015:160–167.

Naik, R. P., V. K. Derebail, M. E. Grams, N. Franceschini, P. L. Auer, G. M. Peloso, B. A. Young, G. Lettre, C. A. Peralta, R. Katz, H. I. Hyacinth, R. C. Quarells, M. L. Grove, A. G. Bick, P. Fontanillas, S. S. Rich, J. D. Smith, E. Boerwinkle, W. D. Rosamond, K. Ito, S. Lanzkron, J. Coresh, A. Correa, G. E. Sarto, N. S. Key, D. R. Jacobs, S. Kathiresan, K. Bibbins-Domingo, A. V. Kshirsagar, J. G. Wilson, and A. P. Reiner. 2014. Association of sickle cell trait with chronic kidney disease and albuminuria in African Americans. *JAMA* 312(20):2115–2125.

Naik, R. P., K. Smith-Whitley, K. L. Hassell, N. I. Umeh, M. de Montalembert, P. Sahota, C. Haywood, Jr., J. Jenkins, M. A. Lloyd-Puryear, C. H. Joiner, V. L. Bonham, and G. J. Kato. 2018. Clinical outcomes associated with sickle cell trait: A systematic review. *Annals of Internal Medicine* 169(9):619–627.

Narbey, D., A. Habibi, P. Chadebech, A. Mekontso-Dessap, M. Khellaf, J. D. Lelievre, B. Godeau, M. Michel, F. Galacteros, R. Djoudi, P. Bartolucci, and F. Pirenne. 2017. Incidence and predictive score for delayed hemolytic transfusion reaction in adult patients with sickle cell disease. *American Journal of Hematology* 92(12):1340–1348.

NASEM (National Academies of Sciences, Engineering, and Medicine). 2017. *The health effects of cannabis and cannabinoids: The current state of evidence and recommendations for research.* Washington, DC: The National Academies Press.

Nevitt, S. J., A. P. Jones, and J. Howard. 2017. Hydroxyurea (hydroxycarbamide) for sickle cell disease. *Cochrane Database of Systematic Reviews* 4:CD002202.

NHLBI (National Heart, Lung, and Blood Institute). 1997. *Clinical alert: Periodic transfusions lower stroke risk in children with sickle cell anemia.* https://www.nlm.nih.gov/databases/alerts/sickle97.html (accessed November 19, 2019).

NHLBI. 2002. *The management of sickle cell disease.* https://www.nhlbi.nih.gov/files/docs/guidelines/sc_mngt.pdf (accessed April 4, 2020).

NHLBI. 2014. *Evidence-based management of sickle cell disease: Expert panel report.* https://www.nhlbi.nih.gov/sites/default/files/media/docs/sickle-cell-disease-report%20020816_0.pdf (accessed June 18, 2019).

Nicholas, M. K., A. Asghari, M. Corbett, R. J. Smeets, B. M. Wood, S. Overton, C. Perry, L. E. Tonkin, and L. Beeston. 2012. Is adherence to pain self-management strategies associated with improved pain, depression and disability in those with disabling chronic pain? *European Journal of Pain* 16(1):93–104.

Niihara, Y., S. T. Miller, J. Kanter, S. Lanzkron, W. R. Smith, L. L. Hsu, V. R. Gordeuk, K. Viswanathan, S. Sarnaik, I. Osunkwo, E. Guillaume, S. Sadanandan, L. Sieger, J. L. Lasky, E. H. Panosyan, O. A. Blake, T. N. New, R. Bellevue, L. T. Tran, R. L. Razon, C. W. Stark, L. D. Neumayr, E. P. Vichinsky, for the investigators of the Phase 3 Trial of l-Glutamine in Sickle Cell Disease. 2018. A Phase 3 trial of L-glutamine in sickle cell disease. *New England Journal of Medicine* 379(3):226–235.

Niraimathi, M., R. Kar, S. E. Jacob, and D. Basu. 2016. Sudden death in sickle cell anaemia: Report of three cases with brief review of literature. *Indian Journal of Hematology & Blood Transfusion* 32(Suppl 1):258–261.

Niscola, P., F. Sorrentino, L. Scaramucci, P. de Fabritiis, and P. Cianciulli. 2009. Pain syndromes in sickle cell disease: An update. *Pain Medicine* 10(3):470–480.

Nnoli, A., N. S. Seligman, K. Dysart, J. K. Baxter, and S. K. Ballas. 2018. Opioid utilization by pregnant women with sickle cell disease and the risk of neonatal abstinence syndrome. *Journal of the National Medical Association* 110(2):163–168.

Nouraie, M., J. S. Lee, Y. Zhang, T. Kanias, X. Zhao, Z. Xiong, T. B. Oriss, Q. Zeng, G. J. Kato, J. S. Gibbs, M. E. Hildesheim, V. Sachdev, R. J. Barst, R. F. Machado, K. L. Hassell, J. A. Little, D. E. Schraufnagel, L. Krishnamurti, E. Novelli, R. E. Girgis, C. R. Morris, E. B. Rosenzweig, D. B. Badesch, S. Lanzkron, O. L. Castro, J. C. Goldsmith, V. R. Gordeuk, M. T. Gladwin, and Walk-PHASST investigators and patients. 2013. The relationship between the severity of hemolysis, clinical manifestations and risk of death in 415 patients with sickle cell anemia in the U.S. and Europe. *Haematologica* 98(3):464–472.

Novelli, E. M., and M. T. Gladwin. 2016. Crises in sickle cell disease. *Chest* 149(4):1082–1093.

Ogunsile, F. J., S. M. Bediako, J. Nelson, C. Cichowitz, T. Yu, C. Patrick Carroll, K. Stewart, R. Naik, C. Haywood, Jr., and S. Lanzkron. 2019. Metabolic syndrome among adults living with sickle cell disease. *Blood Cells, Molecules, and Disease* 74:25–29.

Ohene-Frempong, K., S. J. Weiner, L. A. Sleeper, S. T. Miller, S. Embury, J. W. Moohr, D. L. Wethers, C. H. Pegelow, and F. M. Gill. 1998. Cerebrovascular accidents in sickle cell disease: Rates and risk factors. *Blood* 91(1):288–294.

Okomo, U., and M. M. Meremikwu. 2007. Fluid replacement therapy for acute episodes of pain in people with sickle cell disease. *Cochrane Database of Systematic Reviews* 2:CD005406.

Okomo, U., and M. M. Meremikwu. 2017. Fluid replacement therapy for acute episodes of pain in people with sickle cell disease. *Cochrane Database of Systematic Reviews* 7:CD005406.

Okpala, I., V. Thomas, N. Westerdale, T. Jegede, K. Raj, S. Daley, H. Costello-Binger, J. Mullen, C. Rochester-Peart, S. Helps, E. Tulloch, M. Akpala, M. Dick, S. Bewley, M. Davies, and I. Abbs. 2002. The comprehensiveness care of sickle cell disease. *European Journal of Haematology* 68(3):157–162.

Okwerekwu, I., and J. A. Skirvin. 2018. Sickle cell disease pain management. *U.S. Pharmacist* 43(3):12–18.

O'Leary, J. D., M. W. Crawford, I. Odame, G. D. Shorten, and P. A. McGrath. 2014. Thermal pain and sensory processing in children with sickle cell disease. *Clinical Journal of Pain* 30(3):244–250.

Osunkwo, I. 2011. Complete resolution of sickle cell chronic pain with high dose vitamin D therapy: A case report and review of the literature. *Journal of Pediatric Hematology/Oncology* 33(7):549–551.

Osunkwo, I., E. I. Hodgman, K. Cherry, C. Dampier, J. Eckman, T. R. Ziegler, S. Ofori-Acquah, and V. Tangpricha. 2011. Vitamin D deficiency and chronic pain in sickle cell disease. *British Journal of Haematology* 153(4):538–540.

Osunkwo, I., P. Veeramreddy, J. Arnall, R. Crawford, J. Symanowski, R. Olaosebikan, S. Sanikommu, S. Newby, S. Wyatt, J. Sebaaly, and K. Rector. 2019. *Use of buprenorphine/ naloxone in ameliorating acute care utilization and chronic opioid use in adults with sickle cell disease.* Paper presented at ASH Annual Meeting, Valencia BC, Orange County Convention Center.

Oteng-Ntim, E., B. Ayensah, M. Knight, and J. Howard. 2015. Pregnancy outcome in patients with sickle cell disease in the UK—A national cohort study comparing sickle cell anaemia (HbSS) with HbSC disease. *British Journal of Haematology* 169(1):129–137.

Parent, F., D. Bachir, J. Inamo, F. Lionnet, F. Driss, G. Loko, A. Habibi, S. Bennani, L. Savale, S. Adnot, B. Maitre, A. Yaici, L. Hajji, D. S. O'Callaghan, P. Clerson, R. Girot, F. Galacteros, and G. Simonneau. 2011. A hemodynamic study of pulmonary hypertension in sickle cell disease. *New England Journal of Medicine* 365(1):44–53.

Pearson, H. A. 1977. Sickle cell anemia and severe infections due to encapsulated bacteria. *Journal of Infectious Diseases* 136 (Suppl 1):S25–S30.

Pecker, L. H., and R. P. Naik. 2018. The current state of sickle-cell trait: Implications for reproductive and genetic counseling. *Blood* 132(22):2331–2338.

Pegelow, C. H., E. A. Macklin, F. G. Moser, W. C. Wang, J. A. Bello, S. T. Miller, E. P. Vichinsky, M. R. DeBaun, L. Guarini, R. A. Zimmerman, D. P. Younkin, D. M. Gallagher, and T. R. Kinney. 2002. Longitudinal changes in brain magnetic resonance imaging findings in children with sickle cell disease. *Blood* 99(8):3014–3018.

Perlin, E., H. Finke, O. Castro, S. Rana, J. Pittman, R. Burt, C. Ruff, and D. McHugh. 1994. Enhancement of pain control with ketorolac tromethamine in patients with sickle cell vaso-occlusive crisis. *American Journal of Hematology* 46(1):43–47.

Platt, O. S., S. H. Orkin, G. Dover, G. P. Beardsley, B. Miller, and D. G. Nathan. 1984. Hydroxyurea enhances fetal hemoglobin production in sickle cell anemia. *Journal of Clinical Investigation* 74(2):652–656.

Platt, O. S., B. D. Thorington, D. J. Brambilla, P. F. Milner, W. F. Rosse, E. Vichinsky, and T. R. Kinney. 1991. Pain in sickle cell disease. Rates and risk factors. *New England Journal of Medicine* 325(1):11–16.

Platt, O. S., D. J. Brambilla, W. F. Rosse, P. F. Milner, O. Castro, M. H. Steinberg, and P. P. Klug. 1994. Mortality in sickle cell disease. Life expectancy and risk factors for early death. *New England Journal of Medicine* 330(23):1639–1644.

Plummer, J. M., N. D. Duncan, D. I. Mitchell, A. H. McDonald, M. Reid, and M. Arthurs. 2006. Laparoscopic cholecystectomy for chronic cholecystitis in Jamaican patients with sickle cell disease: Preliminary experience. *West Indian Medical Journal* 55(1):22–24.

Porter, J. B., and E. R. Huehns. 1987. Transfusion and exchange transfusion in sickle cell anaemias, with particular reference to iron metabolism. *Acta Haematologica* 78(2–3):198–205.

Powars, D., J. A. Weidman, T. Odom-Maryon, J. C. Niland, and C. Johnson. 1988. Sickle cell chronic lung disease: Prior morbidity and the risk of pulmonary failure. *Medicine* 67(1):66–76.

Procon.org. 2019. *Legal medical marijuana states and DC.* https://medicalmarijuana.procon. org/legal-medical-marijuana-states-and-dc (accessed November 19, 2019).

Prussien, K. V., L. C. Jordan, M. R. DeBaun, and B. E. Compas. 2019. Cognitive function in sickle cell disease across domains, cerebral infarct status, and the lifespan: A meta-analysis. *Journal of Pediatric Psychology* 44(8):948–958.

Puri, L., K. A. Nottage, J. S. Hankins, and D. L. Anghelescu. 2018. State of the art management of acute vaso-occlusive pain in sickle cell disease. *Paediatric Drugs* 20(1):29–42.

Puri, L., K. J. Morgan, and D. L. Anghelescu. 2019. Ketamine and lidocaine infusions decrease opioid consumption during vaso-occlusive crisis in adolescents with sickle cell disease. *Current Opinion in Supportive and Palliative Care* 13(4):402–407.

Quandt, S. A., J. C. Sandberg, J. G. Grzywacz, K. P. Altizer, and T. A. Arcury. 2015. Home remedy use among African American and white older adults. *Journal of the National Medical Association* 107(2):121–129.

Quinn, C. T. 2018. L-glutamine for sickle cell anemia: More questions than answers. *Blood* 132(7):689–693.

Quinn, C. T., Z. R. Rogers, T. L. McCavit, and G. R. Buchanan. 2010. Improved survival of children and adolescents with sickle cell disease. *Blood* 115(17):3447–3452.

Ramasubbu, C., and A. Gupta. 2011. Pharmacological treatment of opioid-induced hyperalgesia: A review of the evidence. *Journal of Pain and Palliative Care Pharmacotherapy* 25(3):219–230.

Rasolofo, J., M. Poncelet, V. Rousseau, and P. Marec-Berard. 2013. Analgesic efficacy of topical lidocaine for vaso-occlusive crisis in children with sickle cell disease. *Archives de Pédiatrie* 20(7):762–767.

Rayment, C., M. J. Hjermstad, N. Aass, S. Kaasa, A. Caraceni, F. Strasser, E. Heitzer, R. Fainsinger, and M. I. Bennett. 2013. Neuropathic cancer pain: Prevalence, severity, analgesics and impact from the European Palliative Care Research Collaborative Computerised Symptom Assessment Study. *Palliative Medicine* 27(8):714–721.

Reiner, K., L. Tibi, and J. D. Lipsitz. 2013. Do mindfulness-based interventions reduce pain intensity? A critical review of the literature. *Pain Medicine* 14(2):230–242.

Ribeiro, K. R., M. H. Guarnieri, D. C. da Costa, F. F. Costa, J. Pellegrino, Jr., and L. Castilho. 2009. DNA array analysis for red blood cell antigens facilitates the transfusion support with antigen-matched blood in patients with sickle cell disease. *Vox Sanguinis* 97(2):147–152.

Rizio, A. A., M. Bhor, X. Lin, K. L. McCausland, M. K. White, J. Paulose, S. Nandal, R. I. Halloway, and L. Bronte-Hall. 2020. The relationship between frequency and severity of vaso-occlusive crises and health-related quality of life and work productivity in adults with sickle cell disease. *Quality of Life Research*, January 13 [Epub ahead of print].

Roberts, J. D., J. Spodick, J. Cole, J. Bozzo, S. Curtis, and A. Forray. 2018. Marijuana use in adults living with sickle cell disease. *Cannabis and Cannabinoid Research* 3(1):162–165.

Rosse, W. F., D. Gallagher, T. R. Kinney, O. Castro, H. Dosik, J. Moohr, W. Wang, and P. S. Levy. 1990. Transfusion and alloimmunization in sickle cell disease. The cooperative study of sickle cell disease. *Blood* 76(7):1431–1437.

Ruta, N. S., and S. K. Ballas. 2016. The opioid drug epidemic and sickle cell disease: Guilt by association. *Pain Medicine* 17(10):1793–1798.

Sakano, K., S. Oikawa, K. Hasegawa, and S. Kawanishi. 2001. Hydroxyurea induces site-specific DNA damage via formation of hydrogen peroxide and nitric oxide. *Japanese Journal of Cancer Research* 92(11):1166–1174.

Schatz, J., R. L. Finke, J. M. Kellett, and J. H. Kramer. 2002. Cognitive functioning in children with sickle cell disease: A meta-analysis. *Journal of Pediatric Psychology* 27(8):739–748.

Schatz, J., A. M. Schlenz, K. E. Smith, and C. W. Roberts. 2018. Predictive validity of developmental screening in young children with sickle cell disease: A longitudinal follow-up study. *Developmental Medicine & Child Neurology* 60(5):520–526.

Schlaeger, J., M. Ezenwa, Y. Yao, M. Suarez, V. Angulo, D. Shuey, Z. Wang, R. Molokie, and D. Wikie. 2019. Association of pain, anxiety, depression, and fatigue with sensitization in outpatient adults with sickle cell disease. *Journal of Pain* 20(4):S24–S25.

Schliessbach, J., A. Siegenthaler, K. Streitberger, U. Eichenberger, E. Nuesch, P. Juni, L. Arendt-Nielsen, and M. Curatolo. 2013. The prevalence of widespread central hypersensitivity in chronic pain patients. *European Journal of Pain* 17(10):1502–1510.

Scott, R. B. 1979. Reflections on the current status of the national sickle cell disease program in the United States. *Journal of the National Medical Association* 71(7):679–681.

Seck, S. M., M. Dahaba, E. F. Ka, M. M. Cisse, S. Gueye, and A. O. Tal. 2012. Mineral and bone disease in black African hemodialysis patients: A report from Senegal. *Nephro-Urology Monthly* 4(4):613–616.

Shah, N., M. Bhor, L. Xie, S. Arcona, R. Halloway, J. Paulose, and H. Yuce. 2019. Evaluation of vaso-occlusive crises in United States sickle cell disease patients: A retrospective claims-based study. *Journal of Health Economics and Outcomes Research* 6(3):106–117.

Sharma, D., and A. M. Brandow. 2020. Neuropathic pain in individuals with sickle cell disease. *Neuroscience Letters* 714:134445.

Sharma, S., J. T. Efird, C. Knupp, R. Kadali, D. Liles, K. Shiue, P. Boettger, and S. F. Quan. 2015. Sleep disorders in adult sickle cell patients. *Journal of Clinical Sleep Medicine* 11(3):219–223.

Sil, S., C. Dampier, and L. L. Cohen. 2016. Pediatric sickle cell disease and parent and child catastrophizing. *Journal of Pain* 17(9):963–971.

Simckes, A. M., S. S. Chen, A. V. Osorio, R. E. Garola, and G. M. Woods. 1999. Ketorolac-induced irreversible renal failure in sickle cell disease: A case report. *Pediatric Nephrology* 13(1):63–67.

Simmons, L. A., H. Williams, S. Silva, F. Keefe, and P. Tanabe. 2019. Acceptability and feasibility of a mindfulness-based intervention for pain catastrophizing among persons with sickle cell disease. *Pain Management Nursing* 20(3):261–269.

Sinha, C. B., N. Bakshi, D. Ross, and L. Krishnamurti. 2018. From trust to skepticism: An in-depth analysis across age groups of adults with sickle cell disease on their perspectives regarding hydroxyurea. *PLOS ONE* 13(6):e0199375.

Sinha, C. B., N. Bakshi, D. Ross, and L. Krishnamurti. 2019. Management of chronic pain in adults living with sickle cell disease in the era of the opioid epidemic: A qualitative study. *JAMA Network Open* 2(5):e194410.

Smith, S. B., D. W. Maixner, R. B. Fillingim, G. Slade, R. H. Gracely, K. Ambrose, D. V. Zaykin, C. Hyde, S. John, K. Tan, W. Maixner, and L. Diatchenko. 2012. Large candidate gene association study reveals genetic risk factors and therapeutic targets for fibromyalgia. *Arthritis & Rheumatology* 64(2):584–593.

Smith, W. R., and M. Scherer. 2010. Sickle-cell pain: Advances in epidemiology and etiology. *Hematology: American Society of Hematology—Education Program* 2010:409–415.

Smith, W. R., L. T. Penberthy, V. E. Bovbjerg, D. K. McClish, J. D. Roberts, B. Dahman, I. P. Aisiku, J. L. Levenson, and S. D. Roseff. 2008. Daily assessment of pain in adults with sickle cell disease. *Annals of Internal Medicine* 148(2):94–101.

Sogutlu, A., J. L. Levenson, D. K. McClish, S. D. Rosef, and W. R. Smith. 2011. Somatic symptom burden in adults with sickle cell disease predicts pain, depression, anxiety, health care utilization, and quality of life: The PiSCES project. *Psychosomatics* 52(3):272–279.

Solanki, D. L., and P. R. McCurdy. 1979. Cholelithiasis in sickle cell anemia: A case for elective cholecystectomy. *American Journal of the Medical Sciences* 277(3):319–324.

Steen, R. G., C. Fineberg-Buchner, G. Hankins, L. Weiss, A. Prifitera, and R. K. Mulhern. 2005. Cognitive deficits in children with sickle cell disease. *Journal of Child Neurology* 20(2):102–107.

Steinberg, M. H., W. F. McCarthy, O. Castro, S. K. Ballas, F. D. Armstrong, W. Smith, K. Ataga, P. Swerdlow, A. Kutlar, L. DeCastro, M. A. Waclawiw, and investigators of the Multicenter Study of Hydroxyurea in Sickle Cell and MSH Patients' Follow-Up. 2010. The risks and benefits of long-term use of hydroxyurea in sickle cell anemia: A 17.5 year follow-up. *American Journal of Hematology* 85(6):403–408.

Stotesbury, H., J. Kawadler, P. Balfour, M. Koelbel, and F. J. Kirkham. 2017. *Cognitive deficits in sickle cell disease; links with nocturnal oxygen desaturation in adolescents, but not children.* Developmental Medicine and Child Neurology Conference: 43rd Annual Conference of the British Paediatric Neurology Association, BPNA 2017. United Kingdom. 2059(Suppl 2011):2037–2038.

Taylor, J. G., V. G. Nolan, L. Mendelsohn, G. J. Kato, M. T. Gladwin, and M. H. Steinberg. 2008. Chronic hyper-hemolysis in sickle cell anemia: Association of vascular complications and mortality with less frequent vasoocclusive pain. *PLOS ONE* 3(5):e2095.

Thomas, V. J., and L. M. Taylor. 2002. The psychosocial experience of people with sickle cell disease and its impact on quality of life: Qualitative findings from focus groups. *British Journal of Health Psychology* 7(Part 3):345–363.

Thomas, V. N., J. Wilson-Barnett, and F. Goodhart. 1998. The role of cognitive-behavioural therapy in the management of pain in patients with sickle cell disease. *Journal of Advanced Nursing* 27(5):1002–1009.

Thompson, A. A. 2011. Primary prophylaxis in sickle cell disease: Is it feasible? Is it effective? *Hematology: American Society of Hematology–Education Program* 2011:434–439.

Thompson, W. E., and I. Eriator. 2014. Pain control in sickle cell disease patients: Use of complementary and alternative medicine. *Pain Medicine* 15(2):241–246.

Tsai, S. L., E. Reynoso, D. W. Shin, and J. W. Tsung. 2018. Acupuncture as a nonpharmacologic treatment for pain in a pediatric emergency department. *Pediatric Emergency Care*, September 21 [Epub ahead of print].

Tsitsikas, D. A., G. Gallinella, S. Patel, H. Seligman, P. Greaves, and R. J. Amos. 2014. Bone marrow necrosis and fat embolism syndrome in sickle cell disease: Increased susceptibility of patients with non-SS genotypes and a possible association with human parvovirus B19 infection. *Blood Reviews* 28(1):23–30.

Tsitsikas, D. A., B. Sirigireddy, R. Nzouakou, A. Calvey, J. Quinn, J. Collins, F. Orebayo, N. Lewis, S. Todd, and R. J. Amos. 2016. Safety, tolerability, and outcomes of regular automated red cell exchange transfusion in the management of sickle cell disease. *Journal of Clinical Apheresis* 31(6):545–550.

Uwaezuoke, S. N., A. C. Ayuk, I. K. Ndu, C. I. Eneh, N. R. Mbanefo, and O. U. Ezenwosu. 2018. Vaso-occlusive crisis in sickle cell disease: Current paradigm on pain management. *Journal of Pain Research* 11:3141–3150.

Valrie, C. R., K. M. Gil, R. Redding-Lallinger, and C. Daeschner. 2007. Brief report: Sleep in children with sickle cell disease: An analysis of daily diaries utilizing multilevel models. *Journal of Pediatric Psychology* 32(7):857–861.

Valrie, C. R., M. H. Bromberg, T. Palermo, and L. E. Schanberg. 2013. A systematic review of sleep in pediatric pain populations. *Journal of Developmental and Behavioral Pediatrics* 34(2):120–128.

Van Damme, S., G. Crombez, P. Bijttebier, L. Goubert, and B. Van Houdenhove. 2002. A confirmatory factor analysis of the pain catastrophizing scale: Invariant factor structure across clinical and non-clinical populations. *Pain* 96(3):319–324.

Vanderhave, K. L., C. A. Perkins, B. Scannell, and B. K. Brighton. 2018. Orthopaedic manifestations of sickle cell disease. *Journal of the American Academy of Orthopaedic Surgeons* 26(3):94–101.

Velasquez, M. P., M. M. Mariscalco, S. L. Goldstein, and G. E. Airewele. 2009. Erythrocytapheresis in children with sickle cell disease and acute chest syndrome. *Pediatric Blood & Cancer* 53(6):1060–1063.

Vichinsky, E. P., A. Earles, R. A. Johnson, M. S. Hoag, A. Williams, and B. Lubin. 1990. Alloimmunization in sickle cell anemia and transfusion of racially unmatched blood. *New England Journal of Medicine* 322(23):1617–1621.

Vichinsky, E. P., L. D. Neumayr, J. I. Gold, M. W. Weiner, R. R. Rule, D. Truran, J. Kasten, B. Eggleston, K. Kesler, L. McMahon, E. P. Orringer, T. Harrington, K. Kalinyak, L. M. De Castro, A. Kutlar, C. J. Rutherford, C. Johnson, J. D. Bessman, L. B. Jordan, and F. D. Armstrong. 2010. Neuropsychological dysfunction and neuroimaging abnormalities in neurologically intact adults with sickle cell anemia. *JAMA* 303(18):1823–1831.

Vidler, J. B., K. Gardner, K. Amenyah, A. Mijovic, and S. L. Thein. 2015. Delayed haemolytic transfusion reaction in adults with sickle cell disease: A 5-year experience. *British Journal of Haematology* 169(5):746–753.

Vincent, L., D. Vang, J. Nguyen, B. Benson, J. Lei, and K. Gupta. 2016. Cannabinoid receptor-specific mechanisms to alleviate pain in sickle cell anemia via inhibition of mast cell activation and neurogenic inflammation. *Haematologica* 101(5):566–577.

Wallen, G. R., C. P. Minniti, M. Krumlauf, E. Eckes, D. Allen, A. Oguhebe, C. Seamon, D. S. Darbari, M. Hildesheim, L. Yang, J. D. Schulden, G. J. Kato, and J. G. Taylor 6th. 2014. Sleep disturbance, depression and pain in adults with sickle cell disease. *BMC Psychiatry* 14(207):207.

Walsh, K. E., S. L. Cutrona, P. L. Kavanagh, L. E. Crosby, C. Malone, K. Lobner, and D. G. Bundy. 2014. Medication adherence among pediatric patients with sickle cell disease: A systematic review. *Pediatrics* 134(6):1175–1183.

Wang, W. C., R. E. Ware, S. T. Miller, R. V. Iyer, J. F. Casella, C. P. Minniti, S. Rana, C. D. Thornburg, Z. R. Rogers, R. V. Kalpatthi, J. C. Barredo, R. C. Brown, S. A. Sarnaik, T. H. Howard, L. W. Wynn, A. Kutlar, F. D. Armstrong, B. A. Files, J. C. Goldsmith, M. A. Waclawiw, X. Huang, and B. W. Thompson. 2011. A multicenter randomised controlled trial of hydroxyurea (hydroxycarbamide) in very young children with sickle cell aneamia. *Lancet* 377(9778):1663–1672.

Westcott, E. 2017. *Healthy behaviors of adolescents and young adults with sickle cell disease.* Electronic Thesis or Dissertation. University of Cincinnati. https://etd.ohiolink.edu (accessed November 19, 2019).

While, A. E., and J. Mullen. 2004. Living with sickle cell disease: The perspective of young people. *British Journal of Nursing* 13(6):320–325.

Whiteman, L. N., C. Haywood, Jr., S. Lanzkron, J. J. Strouse, A. H. Batchelor, A. Schwartz, and R. W. Stewart. 2016. Effect of free dental services on individuals with sickle cell disease. *Southern Medical Journal* 109(9):576–578.

WHO (World Health Organization). 2018. WHO guidelines for the pharmacological and radiotherapeutic management of cancer pain in adults and adolescents. Geneva, Switzerland: World Health Organization.

Wilkie, D. J., R. Molokie, D. Boyd-Seal, M. L. Suarez, Y. O. Kim, S. Zong, H. Wittert, Z. Zhao, Y. Saunthararajah, and Z. J. Wang. 2010. Patient-reported outcomes: Descriptors of nociceptive and neuropathic pain and barriers to effective pain management in adult outpatients with sickle cell disease. *Journal of the National Medical Association* 102(1):18–27.

Williams, H., S. Silva, L. A. Simmons, and P. Tanabe. 2017. A telephonic mindfulness-based intervention for persons with sickle cell disease: Study protocol for a randomized controlled trial. *Trials* 18(1):218.

Woolf, C. J. 2011. Central sensitization: Implications for the diagnosis and treatment of pain. *Pain* 152(3 Suppl):S2–S15.

Wright, S. W., R. L. Norris, and T. R. Mitchell. 1992. Ketorolac for sickle cell vaso-occlusive crisis pain in the emergency department: Lack of a narcotic-sparing effect. *Annals of Emergency Medicine* 21(8):925–928.

Wu, Z., Z. Malihi, A. W. Stewart, C. M. Lawes, and R. Scragg. 2018. The association between vitamin D concentration and pain: A systematic review and meta-analysis. *Public Health Nutrition* 21(11):2022–2037.

Xu, G., L. Strathearn, B. Liu, B. Yang, and W. Bao. 2018. Twenty-year trends in diagnosed attention-deficit/hyperactivity disorder among U.S. children and adolescents, 1997–2016. *JAMA Network Open* 1(4):e181471.

Yale, S. H., N. Nagib, and T. Guthrie. 2000. Approach to the vaso-occlusive crisis in adults with sickle cell disease. *American Family Physician* 61(5):1349–1356.

Yawn, B. P., G. R. Buchanan, A. N. Afenyi-Annan, S. K. Ballas, K. L. Hassell, A. H. James, L. Jordan, S. M. Lanzkron, R. Lottenberg, W. J. Savage, P. J. Tanabe, R. E. Ware, M. H. Murad, J. C. Goldsmith, E. Ortiz, R. Fulwood, A. Horton, and J. John-Sowah. 2014. Management of sickle cell disease: Summary of the 2014 evidence-based report by expert panel members. *JAMA* 312(10):1033–1048.

Yurkiewicz, I. 2014. These agents prevent disease. Why aren't we using them? *Scientific American*. December 31. https://blogs.scientificamerican.com/unofficial-prognosis/these-agents-prevent-disease-why-aren-t-we-using-them (accessed April 4, 2020).

Zhang, D., C. Xu, D. Manwani, and P. S. Frenette. 2016. Neutrophils, platelets, and inflammatory pathways at the nexus of sickle cell disease pathophysiology. *Blood* 127(7):801–809.

Zhou, J., J. Han, E. A. Nutescu, W. L. Galanter, S. M. Walton, V. R. Gordeuk, S. L. Saraf, and G. S. Calip. 2019. Similar burden of type 2 diabetes among adult patients with sickle cell disease relative to African Americans in the U.S. population: A six-year population-based cohort analysis. *British Journal of Haematology* 185(1):116–127.

Ziegler-Skylakakis, K., L. R. Schwarz, and U. Andrae. 1985. Microsome- and hepatocyte-mediated mutagenicity of hydroxyurea and related aliphatic hydroxamic acids in V79 Chinese hamster cells. *Mutation Research* 152(2–3):225–231.

5

Health Care Organization and Use

Patients with sickle cell disease often feel like the ugly stepchildren in the health care setting.

—Tosin Ola (Open Session Panelist)

Chapter Summary

- Children and adults with sickle cell disease (SCD) require specialty and primary care services continuously across the life span.
- Efforts to improve care have focused on pediatric care, which has resulted in improved survival for children with SCD but little attention paid to care delivery and management for adults.
- Transition from pediatric to adult care is a defining moment for individuals with SCD; however, there is usually no formal process or structure for this transition.
- Adults with SCD tend to seek acute care, primarily for pain, in the emergency department.
- There is a need for a team-based comprehensive system/network of care that incorporates health and ancillary services to address the needs of children and adults with SCD.
- While it is not a disease, sickle cell trait (SCT) is associated with medical complications and should be further studied.
- Screening for SCT can be used for genetic counseling to inform the patient and to minimize unwanted outcomes.

INTRODUCTION

Chapter 4 described the complications and current management of sickle cell disease (SCD). This chapter discusses the health care system and the use of its services. As with other aspects of SCD, there are information gaps on health care use. Generally speaking, studies have been geared toward economic analyses related to cost rather than detailed descriptions of the services. Thus, it is often unclear what types of services were received, where they were delivered, who delivered them, and what models of delivery were employed.

Children and adults with SCD require both specialty and primary care services continuously across the life span. The unique aspects of care outlined in Chapter 4 often lead to an unpredictable need for urgent and emergency care to manage pain, fever, and neurologic symptoms as well as more predictable needs for care related to screening, early detection, and the management of chronic complications. A broad array of specialty services is required, including multidisciplinary expert providers, medical subspecialists, primary care providers (PCPs), surgeons, anesthesiologists, radiologists, social workers, behavioral health specialists, care coordinators, and community health workers (CHWs). Community-based organizations (CBOs) are essential to this care, as they support patient and community education, provide counseling, and address barriers to care by providing services ranging from transportation to care coordination. Provision of high-quality care that aligns with the six domains of health care quality (addressed in Chapter 6)[1] is critical. Furthermore, it is important that health care providers understand and consider the negative societal views of members of the SCD population, including stigma, racism, and various stereotypes, such as the assumption that someone coping with chronic pain is drug seeking (addressed in Chapter 2). Such views not only influence how care is provided but also who provides that care and where. The published literature often omits these subtleties, but the committee believes these aspects should be captured when considering how best to provide high-quality health care to individuals with SCD.

HEALTH CARE FOR CHILDREN WITH SCD

SCD affects children and adults in different ways. This is partly because children's bodies are progressing through developmental stages, while adult bodies change much less quickly and profoundly, and also simply a matter of time—adults with SCD have accumulated years of damage, which may result in a variety of consequences. Furthermore, children

---

[1] The six domains of health care quality are (1) safety, (2) effectiveness, (3) accessibility/timeliness, (4) person centeredness, (5) efficiency, and (6) equity (IOM, 2001b).

and adults have different capacities for understanding, making decisions about, and managing the disease. Thus, children require different types of care than adults.

Primary Care

Like all children, children with SCD should receive excellent primary care. According to the American Academy of Pediatrics (AAP), pediatric primary care encompasses:

> health supervision and anticipatory guidance; monitoring physical and psychosocial growth and development; age-appropriate screening; diagnosis and treatment of acute and chronic disorders; management of serious and life-threatening illness and, when appropriate, referral of more complex conditions; and provision of first contact care as well as coordinated management of health problems requiring multiple professional services. (AAP, 2011)

The content for well-child visits regarding health supervision, anticipatory guidance, monitoring physical and psychosocial development, and appropriate periodic screening and immunizations is delineated in Bright Futures publications.[2] The Early Periodic Screening, Diagnosis and Treatment (EPSDT) benefit also establishes requirements for children under age 21 on Medicaid to receive screening and treatment services. Although the two approaches certainly overlap, EPSDT emphasizes hearing, vision, and dental screening and treatment. In addition to routine well-child care, children with SCD must also receive specialized preventive care, as discussed in Chapter 4.

Providing the broad array of services needed by children with SCD requires a different model than that of routine pediatric health care. For children who are unable to access specialized sickle cell care centers, the medical home (discussed later in this chapter), a model formulated by AAP, is one model of care available for children with SCD. Ideally, a medical home provides care that is accessible, continuous, comprehensive, family-centered, coordinated, compassionate, and culturally effective to every child and adolescent. A pediatric medical home is a family-centered partnership within a community-based system that provides uninterrupted care with appropriate payment to support and sustain optimal health outcomes. Medical homes address preventative, acute, and chronic care from birth through transition to adulthood. "A medical home facilitates an integrated

---

[2] Bright Futures publications are geared toward health professionals and educators and cover topics such as health supervision, nutrition, and mental health for infants and children (Bright Futures, n.d.).

health system with an interdisciplinary team of patients and families, PCPs, specialists and subspecialists, hospitals and health care facilities, public health and the community" (AAP, n.d.).

In general, the literature supports the utility of the medical home model in improving health outcomes, reducing unneeded use of care, and improving family communication and functioning for children with chronic illness (Kuhlthau et al., 2011). Having a PCP, however, is not equivalent to a medical home for children with SCD, as the PCP may not offer many of the components needed (Liem et al., 2014; Raphael et al., 2013b) or provide the specific preventive services for optimal outcomes (Bundy et al., 2016). In these situations, it may be necessary for providers to create a "medical neighborhood" in which hematologists and PCPs closely collaborate to provide children with necessary care (Raphael and Oyeku, 2013).

Establishing the connections among providers necessary to assure more comprehensive care can be difficult due to the long wait times for available appointments (Martin et al., 2018) or inadequate referral patterns (Bundy et al., 2012; Martin et al., 2018). In a sample of children recruited in a sickle cell center or hospitalized for SCD, Raphael et al. (2013a) reported that children receiving comprehensive care from a medical home, as measured by specific, standardized questions eliciting parental report, had fewer emergency department (ED) visits and hospitalizations (Raphael et al., 2013a). However, the source of care was not further characterized. Rattler et al. (2016) conducted a study to examine the coordination of care and found that most caregivers reported having a PCP for their child, whereas only 25 percent of caregivers reported having access to coordinated care. The study also found that coordination of care resulted in 88.1 percent of caregivers feeling satisfied about the communication occurring between medical providers; however, only 67.3 percent of caregivers reported being satisfied with the communication occurring between doctors and non-medical service providers.

Other studies report that a comprehensive approach to care, especially an approach involving hematology, results in greater receipt of special preventive services for children with SCD (Bundy et al., 2016; Martin et al., 2018). Part of the association between more comprehensive care and reduced acute care use may reflect greater adherence to medication prescriptions among those with preventive visits (Walsh et al., 2014).

Another important factor in assessing the effectiveness of the medical home is the variation in the components that are implemented. In an evaluation of the medical homes for a sample of children with SCD, care coordination was more likely to be experienced than accessibility or comprehensiveness; however, the same study found that accessibility and coordination were associated with fewer ED visits (Liem et al., 2014).

Subspecialty Care

Children with SCD require a wide array of services for health maintenance, including (1) therapeutic interventions to prevent complications overall and in high-risk subpopulations, (2) screening for high-risk features and early detection of chronic complications, and (3) long-term disease-modifying therapies to decrease complications. Preventing infection, stroke, and acute pain and acute chest syndrome (ACS) episodes by starting hydroxyurea therapy early in life for children with the SS and $S\beta^0$ thalassemia types has been the mainstay of care. In addition, early treatment for acute febrile illness and acute pain has been the focus of acute complications. Detecting bacteremia and sepsis early leads to better outcomes by preventing morbidity and mortality. Aggressive treatment of acute pain and alleviating pain early may also decrease complications, such as ACS. Early assessment of pain and fever may detect other acute complications, such as ACS, splenic sequestration, and exacerbation of anemia. These services are provided in many settings but have traditionally developed in large, urban, academic hospitals. Emergency medicine teams are actively involved in managing these pediatric patients, but acute care by hematologists and other sickle cell experts has emerged as well. Infusion centers (discussed below) and acute care units staffed by experts allow for the rapid assessment and treatment of SCD complications without involving or with minimal support from emergency medicine.

The use of ambulatory subspecialty services has not been reported. In addition, the use of preventive care services unique to SCD, such as transcranial Doppler (TCD) screening, cannot always serve as a surrogate marker of subspecialty service use because children may be receiving care from a sickle cell expert but either the screening has not been ordered or appointments have not been kept. As an example, implementing TCD ultrasonography services to detect SCD-related stroke risk, specifically in children ages 2–16 years, started shortly after results of the multicenter trial recommended chronic transfusions for children at high risk for stroke based on TCD measurement of time-averaged mean of the maximum velocity in middle cerebral arterial circulation (Armstrong-Wells et al., 2009). However, recent data from six state Medicaid programs suggest that as few as 44 percent of children who require stroke risk screening actually receive it (Reeves et al., 2016).

Acute Care

As noted in Chapter 4, children with SCD experience repeated episodes of acute illness, such as pain, fevers, and aplastic crises, requiring ED visits or hospital admission. According to national estimates, children with SCD average about 0.6 ED admissions and at least one hospital admission per year (Brousseau et al., 2010). Approximately one-third of children with SCD will have neither an ED visit nor a hospital admission in any given year, whereas slightly more than 10 percent will have three or more such episodes. Data from a retrospective cross-sectional descriptive analysis of administrative medical claims found that in Texas, 37–43 percent of children with SCD have at least one ER visit per year, a figure that is consistent with the previous statement (Raphael et al., 2009).

A significant issue concerning acute care is that individuals with SCD often have repeat ED visits and admissions. For example, one study found that among children aged 1–9 years, 4.1 percent (95% confidence interval [CI] 3.6–4.6) of hospitalizations were followed by a return for a treat-and-release ED visit within 30 days after hospital admission and that 12.8 percent (95% CI 12.0–13.6) of hospitalized children had a second hospital admission within 30 days of the first admission. For all children with SCD between the ages of 10 and 17 years old, the corresponding rates were 6.9 percent (95% CI 6.4–7.4) and 23.4 percent (95% CI 22.5–24.3) (Brousseau et al., 2010). From 2009 to 2014, the most common diagnosis among children associated with a subsequent, unplanned readmission to the hospital was SCD, and SCD had the highest percentage of hospital readmissions overall. Thus, this study found that SCD was among the 10 most resource-intensive diagnoses for admission within the study population (Heslin et al., 2018). However, these results are from one study only, so care must be taken not to overstate these findings.

Dental Care[3]

As noted in Chapter 4, oral infections and gum disease are triggers for chronic inflammation and pain and are underlying factors for health care visits. Those with SCD may be more prone to dental problems due to hypoxia in the dentin following sickle crises, and individuals with SCD present with higher rates of dental caries than individuals in the general population (Laurence et al., 2006). Individuals with SCD may also present with delayed tooth eruption and pulpal necrosis that increase with age (Costa et al., 2013, 2016). In a population of 250 children and adolescents with SCD, 47 percent had caries and 14 percent had periodontal problems (Luna et al., 2018).

A retrospective analysis of 10 years (2000–2011) of dental records for 574 individuals with sickle cell anemia at the Center of Hematology and

---

[3] Because there are few data about dental care for individuals living with SCD at any age, research discussed in this section involves adolescents and adults.

Hemotherapy in Maranhao in Brazil was conducted to describe the use of dental services over time. The study population consisted primarily of children and young adults and a small number of adults. The study findings showed that teeth filling and extractions, periodontal treatment, and endodontic treatments were prevalent in the young adult and adult populations, signaling an increase in the need for these procedures as individuals with SCD age. The study authors speculate that the procedures could have been avoided with a care plan based on prevention and health promotion (Costa et al., 2016).

Importantly, the U.S. public insurance system does not universally provide dental coverage, even in Medicaid plans, for children or adults (Berdahl et al., 2016; Naavaal et al., 2017). Thus, there may be significant barriers to dental care access for patients with SCD. In one analysis of national data, Laurence et al. (2013) found that among patients having a sickle cell crisis, those with dental infections were 72 percent more likely to be admitted than were those not having dental infections (prevalence ratio [PR] = 1.72, 95% CI 1.58–1.87). One pilot study found that adults with SCD receiving free dental care demonstrated a significant reduction in the number of hospital admissions as well as in the total number of days spent in the hospital if dental work was completed; however, the study also found that there was an increase in the number of hospital days experienced by men in the study population (Whiteman et al., 2016). A recent Cochrane review did not identify any randomized controlled studies that evaluated interventions to treat dental complications in SCD, indicating a significant research gap and the need for randomized controlled studies in this area (Mulimani et al., 2016).

Educational Services

As discussed in Chapter 2, children and youth with SCD experience difficulties in school and may have poorer academic performance, as indicated by grade retention or lower academic grades. This increased risk for learning difficulties may make them eligible for special educational assistance.

Special Education System

Services for children with special educational needs are made available under the Individuals with Disabilities Education Act (IDEA), most recently reauthorized under the Every Student Succeeds Act in 2015. IDEA is meant to ensure that all children with disabilities have access to a free appropriate public education that emphasizes special education and related services designed to meet their unique needs and prepare them for further education, employment, and independent living (ED, n.d.). Services for children ages 0–2 are provided under Part C of the act (often referred to as early intervention), and older children are covered under Part B. Services provided through the educational system end at 21 years old. Thereafter, youth and young adults with significant disabilities may be eligible for vocational and rehabilitation services if these may improve their ability to obtain employment (Linebaugh, n.d.). In higher education, Section 504 and Title II of the Americans with Disabilities Act prohibit discrimination due to disabilities and require reasonable accommodations (ED, 2020). However, services available to individuals who are more than 21 years old are not as plentiful as those offered to individuals with SCD while they are in the primary and secondary education school system.

Early Intervention (Part C of IDEA)

This is a state-run program with funding from the federal government. To be eligible, children

1. should be experiencing developmental delays, as measured by appropriate diagnostic instruments and procedures, in one or more of the following five areas: cognitive development, physical development, communication development, social or emotional development, or adaptive development; or
2. have a diagnosed physical or mental condition that has a high probability of resulting in developmental delay (ED, 2016).

Services under Part C must meet certain minimal criteria and can be delivered through a variety of state agencies. However, the minimal criteria refer primarily to the processes that the state must implement and do not specify quality. States also have leeway to specify what conditions qualify for early intervention, especially under the "at-risk" rubric.

Children with SCD could clearly qualify for early intervention under "at-risk" criteria. SCD falls under the general category of genetic conditions but is not specified as a qualifying condition (Office of Special Education Programs, 2011). Access to early intervention would require a developmental assessment by the PCP or other provider and referral to early intervention services if developmental problems were noted. This strategy requires a problem, is not necessarily preventive, and places an additional burden of proof on the family, further reducing access to services. The committee found no literature examining early intervention for children with SCD. In general, for special needs populations, such access depends on the restrictiveness of the state criteria and the severity of dysfunction (McManus et al., 2009, 2019). Having a medical home does not improve referrals to Part C of IDEA (Ross et al., 2018).

Special Education Schools (Part B)

As with early intervention, to be eligible for a special education school, a child must have a disability that falls in 1 of 13 categories and need special services to succeed in school. Federal funding is provided to states to pay for the estimated increased cost of special education. The funding is primarily distributed to public schools except for when a private school provides the required services, thus making it eligible for funding. An additional requirement is that the child have a free and appropriate public education.

During their primary and secondary educational careers, children and youth with SCD are more likely to exhibit lower academic attainment, performances (as measured by receipt of special education services), and retention rates than the reported national averages, as well as lower attainment, performances, and retention rates than those reported for healthy African American children (Crosby et al., 2015; Epping et al., 2013; Fowler et al., 1988). Some of these trends are a reflection of the direct impact of SCD on academic attainment, performance, and retention due to frequent hospitalizations, SCD-related neurocognitive complications, and medical visits. Socioeconomic adversity also plays a role, as do the characteristics of the educational support available to the child while at home (Ladd et al., 2014). As with early intervention, however, a child receiving special education services does not mean that those services are adequate to the child's needs. One study found that a multidisciplinary intervention to improve school performance in children with SCD succeeded in increasing the proportion with an individualized education program, a requirement of special education, but did not affect grade retention or absenteeism 2 years after the intervention (King et al., 2006). The major driver of the results was the child's intelligence quotient, suggesting that improving academic performance may require preventing brain injury.

Evidence from Children with Special Health Care Needs and with Medical Complexity

Because of the sparsity of literature directly related to SCD, the committee reviewed evidence from the general literature on children with chronic or complex conditions to inform their understanding of the medical needs of children with serious chronic conditions. Children with SCD fall under the rubric of children with special health care needs (CSHCN), who are defined as "having or being at increased risk for chronic physical, developmental, behavioral, or emotional conditions and who also require health and related services of a type or amount beyond that required by children generally" (McPherson et al., 1998, p. 138). Systems of care for

CSHCN are dependent on ensuring that families are partners in care; that there is early and continuous screening; access to a medical home to provide community-based, coordinated care; adequate insurance and funding to cover services; and a plan for families and providers to help patients transition to adult care and services (HRSA, 2019). For children and youth with SCD, such systems would include the routine primary care necessary for all children but also access to the special preventive services needed for SCD, emergency and hospital services for acute complications, and the specialists and rehabilitative services required to improve functioning.

Children with SCD may also qualify as children with medical complexity (CMC). Within the pediatric population this group is important because of the high costs of care, unmet health needs, variability in the quality of care received, and potentially poorer health outcomes, all of which are associated with their diagnosis. Children with SCD can be identified at a population level through the use of administrative data, and survey data may help characterize any confounding that may occur as the result of the presence of one or more chronic conditions (Berry et al., 2015).

The impetus behind CMC and CSHCN classification schemes is that chronic conditions in children tend to be relatively rare illnesses. While the management of the individual conditions may be quite specific, chronic conditions share a number of common characteristics. For example, they may require coordinating several types of services and specialty providers, place substantial burden on caregivers to organize and actually provide care in the home, incur increased cost depending on insurance and other sources of support, and require a specific plan to transition to adult care. Information is lacking on some of these issues for SCD, so the committee relied on the more general literature to illustrate concerns.

Data about the use of services by CSHCN and CMC can be obtained from national surveys. The National Survey of Children's Health (Data Resource Center for Child and Adolescent Health, n.d.) and its predecessors use a specific algorithm to identify CSHCN, whereas other national datasets may rely on parental report of "fair or poor health." In addition to national surveys, data on health care use may also be obtained from other administrative or medical records databases such as hospital discharge records (Grosse et al., 2010).

The research on CSHCN supports the importance of a medical home arrangement in improving physical and mental health outcomes, satisfaction with care, accessibility, efficiency in health services use, access, systems, and communication. The effects of a medical home arrangement on family functioning and family costs were less consistent (Kuhlthau et al., 2011). When coordinated care is provided through state insurance plans (e.g., Medicaid and State Children's Health Insurance Program managed care), the results are mixed (Huffman et al., 2010). One study found that those with managed care plans experienced fewer unmet needs (including dental care) than those without managed care plans, but health care use was similar between the two groups. However, the study also found that plans that provided specialty services through carve-outs had decreased access to such services. Parental satisfaction was also less because of the limitations in the providers who were in the plans (Huffman et al., 2010).

Despite the potential advantages of a medical home, there are variations in access to this type of coordinated care. While access to coordinated care is similar between those with and without special needs (about 43 percent versus 53 percent, respectively), only 23 percent to 36 percent of children had a medical home if they were from a home where English was not the primary language or where parents exhibited low educational attainment or had low income (Lichstein et al., 2018). CSHCN with private insurance were more likely to have a medical home than CSHCN with any public insurance (about 52 percent versus 36 percent, respectively) (Lichstein et al., 2018).

In terms of access to health services, the literature generally supports an independent association between minority status and Medicaid insurance, with minority children having lower rates of established PCPs and preventive well-child or dental care visits (Berdahl et al., 2016; Elixhauser et al., 2002). While children who are reported to be in fair or poor health have higher outpatient use and more prescriptions, it is unclear whether this is in proportion to their medical needs (Elixhauser et al., 2002). Minority children are also less likely to receive early educational interventions, regardless of the strictness of the eligibility criteria in the state. The literature also provides evidence that the earlier and more intense the early intervention, the better the outcomes (Litt et al., 2018; McManus et al., 2019); unfortunately, some studies found that children from minority groups or children whose mothers did not speak English received less intensive early intervention services (McManus et al., 2019; Richardson et al., 2019).

Access to subspecialty services is dependent on the availability of subspecialists in the community, which varies substantially across the United States. Subspecialty service availability is one area in which African American children have a slight advantage over non-African American children, as the concentration of African American children in urban areas aligns with the high concentration of specialty services in corresponding areas (Ray et al., 2014). Ray et al. (2014) found that children in areas of low to moderate concentrations of specialists report more mental health problems. Unmet needs in the low specialty areas often reflected a lack of providers and the need for transportation (Ray et al., 2014).

Enabling Services[4]

Enabling services are defined as

> non-clinical services that do not include direct patient services that enable individuals to access health care and improve health outcomes. Enabling services include case management, referrals, translation/interpretation, transportation, eligibility assistance, health education, environmental health risk reduction, health literacy, and outreach. (HRSA, n.d., p. 2)

Case Management and Care Coordination

Among the most frequently cited enabling services are studies and descriptions of care coordination/case management. Pordes et al. (2018) provide a useful framework for coordination in medical complexity. They postulate three basic care models: the primary care-centered (PCC), consultative- or co-management-centered (CC), and episode-based (EB) models. PCC is analogous to the medical home. CC is the familiar reliance on specialty clinics to coordinate care with an individual's PCP; this model acts as a bridge between primary and tertiary care. EB is dependent on coordination around a specific episode of care (e.g., hospitalization) to facilitate transitioning the child to the home. Case management services may improve acute pain and chronic pain management, but their use is under-reported (Brennan-Cook et al., 2018).

The CC model would appear more appropriate for SCD, as Pordes et al. (2018) note that the target population for this model would include those with rare disorders, novel treatments, or high dependence on medical technology, especially those who may live at a distance from the tertiary center. In one study of medically fragile children, such a model reduced hospitalizations and hospital days and resulted in decreased tertiary center costs (Gordon et al., 2007).

As noted above, the PCC model or medical home for children with SCD has produced mixed results. In more general CMC populations, the PCC model is associated with fewer unmet care needs (Boudreau et al., 2014), less functional disability (Litt and McCormick, 2015), and lower out-of-pocket costs (Porterfield and DeRigne, 2011). Part of the difficulty in obtaining replicable results for researchers examining outcomes associated with the PCC model may be a reflection of the methodological gaps in this research (Pordes et al., 2018) and the complexity of implementing an effective model that may require a number of stakeholders and substantial investment (Berry et al., 2017).

---

[4] It is important to note that adults as well as children are eligible for enabling services.

While it was not their focus, Pordes et al. (2018) acknowledge that care coordination may involve stand-alone case management services provided by an insurance company or community agency. As noted above, the evidence is mixed as to the effect of the medical home on parents' experience of coordination and reduced use of acute care. In at least one study, the stand-alone model proved less effective (Wood et al., 2009). The committee found no studies comparing different types of case management in the care of children with SCD.

Community Health Workers and Community Educator Counselors

Services provided by CHWs include support for medication adherence, support through transition from pediatric- to adult-focused care services, and care coordination (Green et al., 2017; Wood et al., 2009). The Patient Navigator to Reduce Readmissions study is a single-site, multi-diagnoses pragmatic clinical effectiveness trial that compares a multifaceted, stakeholder-supported navigator intervention with usual care processes for hospital-to-home transitions for individuals hospitalized with various conditions, including SCD (Prieto-Centurion et al., 2019). The study uses trained CHWs to conduct in-person visits in the hospital and after discharge, in addition to telephone-based coaching, and compared the results with those from usual care in order to improve the experience of hospital-to-home transition of care and reduce the 30-day readmission rate. While it is still ongoing, this study includes early and continuous patient and caregiver engagement with clinicians and health system administrators in an iterative process to determine the behavioral components that are critical to success (Prieto-Centurion et al., 2019). Additional information on the role that CHWs play in SCD care can be found in Chapter 8.

Transportation Services

A lack of transportation services is a significant barrier to health care use in patients with chronic health conditions (Syed et al., 2013). The use of transportation services is reported to state funding authorities for individuals living with SCD; however, this information is not published. Access to information about the need for transportation services and the type of services used would be useful in improving our understanding of barriers to care and developing funding sources. The need for transportation to and from medical appointments and following hospitalizations is expected, but further investigation is warranted into whether transportation to pharmacies, dental visits, and behavioral health appointments could benefit this population.

Telehealth Services

Telehealth comprises the broader consumer-facing methods or means of support provided to patients to enhance health care delivery and clinical outcomes (Ray and Kahn, 2020). Telemedicine, a type of telehealth, is the use of technology to provide clinical care from a provider to a patient. Telehealth support helps improve access to care by filling a gap that traditional models of health care delivery have exposed (Ray and Kahn, 2020).

Telehealth can also prove vital in addressing the psychosocial needs of people living with SCD. An interactive mobile monitoring system using text messaging via a web-based platform to deliver acceptance and commitment therapy,[5] a form of cognitive behavioral therapy (CBT), has been shown to provide real-time psychotherapy intervention to adolescents living with SCD (Cheng et al., 2013). The final results of this study have not been released, but a similar intervention showed significant favorable effects for depression, mindfulness, and other psychological symptoms in individuals with chronic pain (Yang et al., 2017), suggesting the need for more definitive studies in SCD.

Two recently funded clinical trials leveraging telehealth among transition-age individuals with SCD are currently ongoing. One study compares the effectiveness of two self-management support interventions (by CHWs and the mobile health iManage app) versus enhanced usual care[6] (Children's Hospital of Philadelphia et al., 2018). The second study compares the effectiveness of a structured, education-based transition model with or without virtual peer mentoring through a web-based platform (Osunkwo and PCORI, 2018). Both studies will evaluate the role of the interventions in improving health-related quality of life (HRQOL) and acute care use.

A recent meta-analysis of the literature on telehealth in SCD management over the past two decades describes interventions for 747 participants, including older children and adolescents (69 percent) and adults older than 18 years of age (31 percent), via text messaging (25 percent), native mobile (19 percent), or web-based apps (31 percent) in addition to mobile direct observation (13 percent) and Internet-delivered CBT therapy (13 percent), interactive gamification (13 percent), and electronic pill bottles (6 percent) (Badawy et al., 2018a). Telehealth interventions targeted mostly medication adherence (31 percent); self-management, pain reporting, and symptom reporting (44 percent); stress, coping, sleep, and daily

---

[5] The focus is on enabling patients to accept troublesome thoughts instead of fighting to reduce them (Guarna, 2009).

[6] Usual care is a condition in which health care personnel determine a patient's care independent of a research team; enhanced usual care is when usual care is improved (enhanced) by using research protocols (Freedland et al., 2011).

activities reporting (25 percent); cognitive training for memory (6 percent); SCD and reproductive health knowledge (31 percent); CBT (13 percent); and guided relaxation interventions (6 percent) (Badawy et al., 2018a). While various telehealth modalities are being used in SCD management with demonstrated feasibility and acceptability, outcomes data on efficacy are modest, as study sample sizes have been small (Anderson et al., 2018; Cady et al., 2009). Future research should particularly be directed toward enhancing disease education, health literacy, and facilitating positive health behavior changes (Issom et al., 2015).

The concept of "telementoring" refers to virtual, case-based peer learning in a hub-and-spoke model by bringing together teams of disease experts and other health care professionals who manage the individuals locally, increasing provider knowledge and comfort, and equipping providers with disease-specific expertise. The telementoring model has been applied through the Health Resources and Services Administration (HRSA), which funded the Sickle Cell Disease Treatment Demonstration Regional Collaborative Program (SCDTDRCP) to expand access to care by providing the local care team with access to expert consultation and peer dialogue around disease management questions (Shook et al., 2016; Stewart et al., 2016). While it is too early to evaluate its impact on health outcomes for SCD, the educational impact of telementoring models has been demonstrated to be feasible and effective in educating providers on delivering specialty care from a distance and improving health care delivery (Salgia et al., 2014).

Translation Services

While the committee found no publications addressing access to language translation services for SCD management, the population of interest consists of racial and ethnic groups whose first language is not necessarily English. There are increasing numbers of Spanish-speaking individuals living with SCD in the United States. Most states also have a high proportion of African and European immigrants with SCD who do not speak English as their first language. Being in a home where English is not the primary language does not necessarily result in language delay; the child may be up to date in the other languages. However, children may be slower to speak if toggling between English and another language, but eventually they become fluent in both. Furthermore, one study found that parents with limited English proficiency were more likely to report that their CSHCN were uninsured and had no usual source of care or medical home (Eneriz-Wiemer et al., 2014).

It is well known that children with language and cognitive delays have early-onset school difficulties (Cheng et al., 2014) and that these complications are common in children with SCD (Crosby et al., 2015). Therefore, it is important that there is an assessment for language proficiency in the family of those with SCD, as a failure to recognize this as a barrier may lead to suboptimal care. Health care systems, providers, and public health departments continue to be cognizant of and responsive to the growing diversity of the patients in their catchment area by providing educational materials in multiple languages to meet patients' needs. For example, the Massachusetts Department of Public Health's website provides information in at least 12 languages (Commonwealth of Massachusetts, 2020). Providers serving the SCD population can leverage existing translated health care materials prepared for the general patient population. Finally, hearing loss is a known complication of SCD and may be the result of ischemic insults to the cochlea or as a consequence of common SCD medications, transfusional iron overload, and infections (Stuart and Smith, 2019). Alternative forms of language support, such as sign language, may also be needed in this population.

Health Literacy Services

Understanding English does not assure that materials for and communications with those with SCD will be equally well understood and acted on. Educational information provided to persons living with SCD should reflect Centers for Disease Control and Prevention (CDC) recommendations for actionability and understandability as measured by the Clear Communication Index[7] to ensure that the information is accessible to individuals with low health literacy (McClure et al., 2016). Clinical experience demonstrates low health literacy among caregivers of children with SCD and adolescents and adults living with SCD (Perry et al., 2017; Yee et al., 2019). Someone with low health literacy can be presumed to have low adherence to clinical care recommendations and low understanding of the disease. However, the committee found few studies that have explored the relationship between health literacy and health care use in people living with SCD. One study suggests that there is no relationship between health literacy and acute care service use (Caldwell, 2019). Large studies with representative samples of individuals living with SCD are needed.

Home Health Care Services

Home health care has been available for children living with chronic conditions since the 1990s. It is rarely covered by private insurance, so enrollment in Medicaid is required. As with many aspects of Medicaid,

---

[7] The Clear Communication Index is a research-based tool developed by the Centers for Disease Control and Prevention to assess public communication materials (CDC, 2019a).

substantial variation exists among states regarding the implementation of the necessary waivers and other mechanisms. Moreover, the low levels of payment for services and the scarcity of skilled workers further limits access to such services. Suggestions for changes include integrating home health services into a child-focused health care system and greater reliance on telehealth support (Foster et al., 2019). The committee found no literature regarding home care services for children with SCD.

TRANSITION FROM PEDIATRIC TO ADULT CARE

More than 95 percent of children with SCD will survive into adulthood due to successes associated with early diagnosis, innovative preventative therapies, and improved comprehensive care (Hassell, 2010; Lanzkron et al., 2013; NHLBI, 2014; Quinn et al., 2010). However, transition to adulthood with SCD is often associated with a loss in the gains made during the childhood period. Changes in the course and consequences of the disease shift from adolescence to adulthood. This is most evident in adult mortality rates and in the patterns of health care usage, particularly in the use of acute care. A major issue for health care providers is to maintain therapeutic continuity across this transition. However, there is limited research to support evidence-based interventions that effectively reduce the high mortality and morbidity associated with the transition period (Hamideh and Alvarez, 2013).

Impact of Transition

Mortality

Mortality rates among children with SCD have declined significantly. A study by Hamideh and Alvarez (2013), using data from U.S. death certificates from the periods 1999–2009 and 1979–1998, found that mortality rates were significantly decreased in the 1999–2009 period. Compared with the 1979–1998 period, mortality rates had decreased by 61 percent in infants less than 1 year of age, 67 percent in children aged 1–4 years, and 22 to 35 percent in children aged 5–19 years. However, mortality rates for individuals more than 19 years of age were seen to increase from 0.6 in the 15- to 19-year group to 1.4/100,000 in the 20- to 24-year group (Hamideh and Alvarez, 2013). This period corresponds to the transition period from pediatric to adult medical care. Paulukonis et al. (2016) also found increases in mortality rates during the transition period. Based on surveillance data from California and Georgia, they reported a tripling of all-cause mortality among 15- to 24-year-olds compared with those under age 14.

Health Care Use

Where young adults with SCD receive care is another noticeable change during the transition period. The ED becomes a primary site of care for young adults with SCD. An examination of data from 4,636 patients with SCD from the California Registry and Surveillance System for Hemoglobinopathies project found a higher use of acute care services among young adults with SCD. From 2005 to 2014 the average number of annual ED visits for patients with SCD was 2.1; ED use was highest among young adults (2.8 visits for individuals aged 20–29.9 years) (Paulukonis et al., 2017).

Hospitalizations and readmissions are also higher in young adults. Data from the Healthcare Cost and Utilization Project 2000–2016 Nationwide Inpatient Sample showed that hospitalizations and readmissions are also higher in young adults. Adults ages 18–34 with SCD had the highest number of hospital inpatient stays (67,900 stays in 2016) compared with individuals with SCD in any other age groups (less than 26,000 stays for each of the other age groups in 2016) (Fingar et al., 2019). Furthermore, in 2016 the all-cause 30-day readmission rates following initial inpatient stays among patients with SCD were highest among those ages 18–44 (39.4 percent) and lowest among those younger than 18 (20.1 percent) (Fingar et al., 2019).

Continuity of Care

The disparities in health outcomes during transition for young adults with SCD result from a complex interplay of factors related to the patients, their families and social networks, communities, health care providers and health care systems, practice settings, and government policies. The main challenge with transition for any chronic condition of childhood is the loss of continuity in medical care and psychosocial support, which can have a negative impact on short- and long-term outcomes. The committee was unable to find accepted standards for how best to transition young adults with SCD to adult care. However, there have been requests from the SCD community and stakeholders (including providers, health care systems, insurance payers, CBOs, patients, and family members) for a standardized process. There are models and indicators of successful transition, discussed further in this chapter and in Chapter 6, for the general population that could form the basis for an approach for the SCD population.

Barriers to Transition

Several patient, provider, and health system factors contribute to the poor health outcomes of young adults with SCD during transition (Bemrich-Stolz et al., 2015; Sobota et al., 2015; Treadwell et al., 2016). Some young adults with SCD struggle emotionally with adjusting from a more paternalistic pediatric model to the adult "individualistic" model of care. Adherence to disease-modifying treatment drops significantly as they cope with the developmental maturation process (Blum et al., 1993). Some young adults with SCD report having inadequate information about adult care and a poor understanding of their disease and how it becomes more complex with age (Sobota et al., 2015). Knowledge gaps and poor communication also exist among pediatric and adult providers, compounding issues created by a lack of a standardized patient education curriculum for young adults with SCD (Sobota et al., 2015). Changes or lapses in insurance lead to gaps in comprehensive care—specialized and primary—during transition, amplifying the existing barriers to accessing crucial services as the disease burden is increasing (Crowley et al., 2011).

Models of Transition

In 2011 AAP, in partnership with the American Academy of Family Physicians and the American College of Physicians, co-authored an expert opinion and consensus statement that provided clear guidance and a supportive decision algorithm to describe practice-based recommendations and six core elements for the health care transition of adolescents into adulthood, to maximize their lifelong functioning (AAP et al., 2011). These six elements include transition policy, transition tracking, transition readiness, transition planning, transition and transfer of care, and transition completion (AAP et al., 2011; White and Cooley, 2018). In 2018 the two authors updated their guidance to provide more practice-based quality improvement specificity for the six core elements (White and Cooley, 2018). Further expansion of the six core elements of optimal transition was refined by the Got Transition™/Center for Health Care Transition Improvement, which resulted in an open access comprehensive toolkit for clinicians (ACP, 2019). A time-series comparative study at five large pediatric and adult academic primary care practices in the District of Columbia found that quality improvement activities based on the Got Transition core elements resulted in improvements in transition from pediatric to adult care, as measured with the Health Care Transition Index (pediatric and adult versions) (McManus et al., 2015a). Another pediatric-to-adult managed care transition pilot project for young adults with chronic mental health challenges used the quality improvement process to incorporate the Six Core Elements of Health Care Transition (2.0) into routine care, showing significant improvement in the transition index and all six elements over an 18-month period (McManus et al., 2015b).

Young adults with SCD transitioning to adult care have specific needs. The critical components of transition readiness for patients include an increase in disease knowledge, independence with self-care skills, and improved pediatric and adult provider transition support (Monaghan et al., 2013). Structured patient education increases disease knowledge, provides self-management skills, and is effective at increasing autonomy, self-efficacy, and disease self-management, which reduces acute complications in juvenile diabetes (Monaghan et al., 2013).

While most transition coordination models use education to address specific patient-level barriers to care (e.g., medication adherence, disease knowledge, transition readiness), it is also important to address the more complex societal ecosystems (e.g., family, school, culture, laws) within which the young adults with SCD must navigate independently in adulthood (Griffin et al., 2013). Health system–based interventions alone are inadequate to address all their needs during transition. Researchers recommend a holistic transition framework that is multifaceted and incorporates the medical, psychosocial, education, vocational, and other needs of young adults as well as the involvement of the primary care and specialty care teams (DeBaun and Telfair, 2012; Treadwell et al., 2011). The impact of CBOs and urgent care teams needs to be explored. Best practices, particularly around transition readiness, optimizing transition success across various care delivery sites, and models of care require further investigation.

Young adults with SCD have also identified isolation as a key challenge during the transition process, and learning from someone who has been through the process is a desirable component of transition (Sobota et al., 2015). The importance of peer mentoring, where an older peer with experience provides support and guidance, was repeatedly mentioned as a desired approach by patient panelists who participated in the National Academies of Sciences, Engineering, and Medicine's SCD committee's open sessions. A pilot project on peer mentoring for 40 mentees with SCD demonstrated that peer mentoring can effectively sustain support for young adults with SCD by reducing isolation and improving community engagement and self-efficacy while modeling independent life skills without the high cost of professional support systems (Okochi et al., 2019).

A comparative effectiveness study sponsored by the Patient-Centered Outcomes Research Initiative is currently under way at 14 clinical sites across the eastern United States to examine the effect of a structured education-based transition program with or without peer mentoring (PCORI, 2020). The program was modeled after the six core elements in Got Transition and tailored specifically for pediatric and adult SCD clinics (PCORI, 2020). Sites received coaching using the model for improvement methodology and participated in monthly quality improvement coaching calls. All sites have systematically improved their transition processes, indicated by their scores on an SCD transition process measurement tool that measures adherence to the six core elements. This model has also proven feasible within large health systems (Jones et al., 2019) and a Medicaid managed care plan (McManus et al., 2015b). The 2016 National Survey of Children's Health of 20,708 adolescents, aged 12–17 years, found that only 17 percent of CSHCN met the overall transition measure that was calculated based on three elements: whether a health care provider discussed the fact that health care will shift eventually to an adult health care provider, whether a health care provider actively worked with youth to gain self-care skills or to understand that health care will change at age 18, and whether the youth had time alone with a health care provider during the last preventive visit (Lebrun-Harris et al., 2018). Efforts need to be intensified to ensure that all CSHCN, including those with SCD, receive adequate transition planning support (Lebrun-Harris et al., 2018).

In an effort to develop a transition model that works for young adults with SCD, researchers stress that the process must begin early, perhaps even as early as birth, and incorporate the whole life perspective. Areas of emphasis for transitioning should include "preparing pediatric patients for the culture of adult medicine, promoting self-advocacy in obtaining support from schools and employers, and addressing issues of funding of health care services" (Treadwell et al., 2011, p. 119).

HEALTH CARE FOR ADULTS WITH SCD

Just a few decades ago SCD was characterized as a childhood disease because relatively few individuals with the disease lived far into their adult years. However, advances in treatment have led to SCD being characterized as a lifelong, chronic condition. Subsequently, adults with SCD in the United States and other countries require health care that manages and responds to disease-related symptoms. One major factor that distinguishes adults with SCD from children is that adults' bodies bear the history of years of SCD's effects. One study found that by the time individuals with SCD reached adulthood, the majority (59.3 percent) had accumulated end-organ damage involving at least one organ and 24.0 percent had multiple organs involved. The number of end organs affected is positively correlated with mortality (Chaturvedi et al., 2018). This makes adults' health care requirements different in various ways.

Primary Care

Individuals with SCD are at high risk for developing multi-system acute and chronic conditions associated with significant morbidity and mortality (Mainous et al., 2019; NHLBI, 2014). They can also develop the usual medical comorbidities seen in the general population. Therefore, health care for adults with SCD should consist of frequent routine visits with a sickle cell expert to monitor for end-organ damage and develop an individualized plan of care for pain and overall disease management and routine preventative care visits with PCPs, dentists, and obstetrician/gynecologists. Primary care should encompass health promotion, disease prevention, health maintenance counseling, patient education, and diagnosis and treatment of acute and chronic illness in a variety of health care settings supported by different health care personnel (IOM, 1996). The PCP's role is to advocate for the patient within the health care system to accomplish cost-effective care by coordinating services and promoting communication that encourages patients to be fully engaged as active partners (IOM, 1996).

While most children with SCD are cared for by specialists (e.g., pediatric hematologists), most adults transition to PCPs due to the lack of a comprehensive nationwide network of adult SCD providers (Grosse et al., 2009). A recent analysis of data on 1,147 adults with SCD from eight health systems in Florida found that 30.4 percent were cared for by a PCP, while 18.7 percent were cared for by an adult hematologist, 27.5 percent by both a PCP and a hematologist, and 23.3 percent by neither a PCP nor a hematologist (Mainous et al., 2019). Individuals receiving care from both a PCP and a hematologist were less likely to have frequent hospitalizations than those cared for by a single specialist, leading the researchers to conclude that individuals with SCD will benefit from care from both a hematologist and PCP. It is important to establish management strategies between primary care and adult or pediatric sickle cell subspecialists to enhance PCPs' knowledge of overall SCD care and improve its outcomes.

There are various reasons why very few adults with SCD receive appropriate care in the primary care setting. The challenges of dealing with chronic pain as well as managing opioid therapy, implicit bias and stigma, assumptions around opioid use in SCD reflecting addiction, and provider knowledge deficits about SCD all contribute to reduced access to evidence-based primary care services (Brennan-Cook et al., 2018; Gomes et al., 2015). Many adults with SCD do not consider their PCP as a gateway for accessing more specialized health care services and, therefore, do not make use of specialized services even when they are available. PCPs see a myriad of rare disorders and have significant challenges maintaining expertise and keeping abreast of improvements and new treatments for managing complex conditions (Mehta et al., 2006). A survey of more than 1,000 family physicians found that only 15.7 percent of physicians under the age of 50 and 25.1 percent of physicians over the age of 50 felt comfortable treating individuals with SCD (Mainous et al., 2015). In another study, among 1,288 general internists and pediatricians surveyed, only 32 percent of general internists reported being comfortable providing primary care for adults with SCD (Okumura et al., 2008).

In response to the poor rates of co-management between PCPs and hematologists, one state has established a management model to optimize SCD outcomes and mitigate the high cost of care, particularly for adults. Community Care of North Carolina (CCNC) established a population health model for managing the approximately 3,000 individuals living with SCD in the state in 2017 who were publicly insured under the Medicaid managed care organization. CCNC identified, through multi-stakeholder conversations, barriers to accessing care that led to poor outcomes and increased the cost of care, including irregular/poor follow-up with both PCPs and hematologists, a lack of insurance, and the distance from the specialty SCD centers in the state (Steiner et al., 2008). Through partnerships between the North Carolina Department of Public Health and the six specialty centers, CCNC established a framework to facilitate the implementation of best practices in primary care and co-management between PCPs, specialists, and EDs, leveraging the role of payer-deployed case managers and establishing communication pathways to disseminate provider support tools (CCNC, n.d.; Lunyera et al., 2017; Rushton et al., 2019). The case manager is a member of the health care team who develops a longitudinal relationship with the individuals living with SCD and acquires robust knowledge of their medical experiences and psychosocial and behavioral health needs. The case manager can then tailor care coordination support for each individual based on lived experience to help improve overall QOL and health outcomes (Brennan-Cook et al., 2018).

Implementing clinical decision support tools embedded in the electronic health record (EHR) is another way to support PCPs by providing examples of evidence-based care for individuals living with SCD. One study used a best-practice alert educational information for the provider (implemented in the EHR) about screening for transfusional iron overload using a simple blood test (serum ferritin) (Mainous et al., 2018). Elevated serum ferritin is well established in population studies as increasing the risk for all-cause mortality (Mainous et al., 2004) among adults with SCD (Darbari et al., 2006). Results from one study showed that clinician decision support paired with provider education was particularly effective in helping PCPs address this frequently unrecognized but potentially lethal complication (Peterson et al., 2015). Because the intervention was also cost effective and did not increase the burden on the PCP, it was recommended as a feasible practice change (Peterson et al., 2015).

Like children with SCD, adults with SCD often do not receive the routine preventive care recommended by the U.S. Preventive Services Task Force or the immunizations recommended by the Advisory Committee on Immunization Practices. SCD falls under the category of "additional risk factors," which includes anatomical or functional asplenia and may include chronic lung, liver, or kidney disease, particularly as adults age and develop

end-organ damage (CDC, 2019b). Asplenia in SCD is often underappreci-
ated by providers and affected individuals. It is also recommended that
women of childbearing age regularly use contraception to reduce the risks
of unintended pregnancy, with the nuance that the progestin-only and barrier methods are preferred (CDC, 2010; Smith-Whitley, 2014).

Specialty Care[8]

There is a significant dearth of high-quality, evidence-based research
to guide the ambulatory management of adults with SCD, with even fewer
descriptive reports on adult SCD programs (Andemariam and Jones, 2016;
Grosse et al., 2009). The lack of evidence poses a challenge for managing
these individuals outside of SCD centers. Access to high-quality care is
limited further by the limited supply of providers with specific SCD expertise, even within specialty care centers. The committee loosely defines
an adult SCD expert as a clinician with both the necessary willingness and
prerequisite experience. Unlike in pediatric care, where SCD management
is a core component of hematology/oncology fellowship training, an adult
SCD specialist may or may not have done a fellowship to become a trained
hematologists/oncologist. Many adult hematologists and oncologists are
also uncomfortable managing adults with SCD or may prefer to practice
oncology, which is perceived to be more lucrative than hematology.

Most adults with SCD will have acute pain episodes, and many more
will experience chronic pain, the management of which is nuanced, expe-
riential, and unstandardized. In an ongoing prospective study, Examining Sickle Cell Acute Pain in the Emergency Versus Day Hospital, which
examines baseline characteristics of adults with SCD within 60 miles of
four cities in the United States, 54 percent of individuals with hemoglobin
SS disease and 46 percent with hemoglobin SC disease had three or more
acute visits over a 12-month period, and 68 percent of the study cohort
reported having chronic pain (Lanzkron et al., 2018a). Therefore, SCD specialists must develop expertise with acute and chronic pain in the context
of SCD, a skill that is not often acquired during subspecialty training but
rather gained by immersive experience. As will be addressed in Chapter 6
on workforce development, the pool of adult SCD experts in the United
States has a diverse training background, including hematology, oncology,
pulmonology, critical care, emergency medicine, internal medicine, family
medicine, pediatrics, pediatric hematology/oncology, and psychiatry.

---

[8] Due to the lack of documentation of these workforce issues in the literature, some of the
discussion in this section is informed by the committee's expert opinion as practitioners and
presentations by invited speakers at committee open session meetings.

Unlike pediatrics, the majority of health care use by adults living with SCD is acute; this reflects the decline in ambulatory care monitoring, especially around the time of transition from pediatric to adult care (Blinder et al., 2015). Medicaid claims data from 8 states on 3,208 individuals showed that access to targeted disease therapies (chronic transfusions, iron chelation, and hydroxyurea [HU]) significantly dropped after age 16, with increased rates of complications and increased health care costs (Blinder et al., 2013).

Ambulatory care for adults with SCD is often not shared or coordinated among providers with the appropriate expertise to manage both SCD and non-SCD comorbidities. A shared care model in which the PCP comanages a patient with complex specialized medical needs alongside a specialist with expertise in the condition of interest has been proposed for adults with SCD, like the models described for children above (Treadwell et al., 2011). This model was evaluated across eight health systems in Florida, and the results suggest that there is a benefit in reducing acute care use; in particular, the model appears to better address total health care needs because individuals benefit from the complementary expertise of the providers (Mainous et al., 2019). This model has been well received, and it is believed to better capture comorbidities and prevent complications (Smith et al., 2008a), leading to successful clinical outcomes among patients with cancer (Klabunde et al., 2013), chronic kidney disease (Scherpbier-de Haan et al., 2013), and mental health issues (Lester, 2005), and it would likely produce similar results for patients with other chronic diseases such as SCD. Research evaluating the comparative effectiveness of various models of co-management will be essential to ensuring improved outcomes for individuals with SCD, particularly as they transition from pediatric to adult care (Grosse et al., 2009).

There is a lack of standardization and clear descriptions of what should be done at each specialty clinic visit and how frequent these visits should be for adults living with SCD. Current trends still assume that "milder" forms of SCD require less frequent medical touch points, despite evidence that these genotypes (SC, SB+ thalassemia) suffer similar burdens of pain and specific organ comorbidities (avascular necrosis, retinopathy) that require more frequent monitoring and attention. Outpatient follow-up with a provider shortly following an acute care visit has been associated with reduced rates of rehospitalization (Leschke et al., 2012).

Missed appointments are a significant challenge and another barrier to care; patients can be dismissed from care if they miss more than two to three appointments with a specific provider (Cronin et al., 2019). It is important that the care team identifies and proactively addresses risk factors for poor adherence to both scheduled appointments and prescribed therapies. These risk factors include social determinants, psychosocial variables, social support, health literacy, and spirituality (Cronin et al., 2018).

Subspecialty Care

Adults with SCD need access to various subspecialists to support the management of their multi-organ comorbidities that are specific to SCD. The most common subspecialists are radiologists, pharmacists, ophthalmologists, orthopedics, obstetrician/gynecologists, pulmonologists, cardiologists, nephrologists, and surgeons (see Table 6-1 in Chapter 6). The committee found no literature on the rates at which adults with SCD are seen by these subspecialty providers, nor did the committee find any literature assessing the experiences of subspecialists in the care of adults with SCD; these areas represent a significant research gap.

Acute Care

Acute pain is the most common reason that individuals with SCD seek health care, even though the vast majority of acute pain episodes are managed at home (Dampier et al., 2002b; McClish et al., 2006; Smith et al., 2008b). Such episodes are particularly an issue for adults (Yale et al., 2000). Children and adolescents also experience acute pain episodes. For example, one study conducted in children and adolescents, which required participants to keep daily diary entries to record their pain history, found that daily pain and acute pain exacerbations are relatively infrequent in childhood but increase in adolescence (Dampier et al., 2002a).

There are long-term consequences associated with poorly treated acute pain in individuals with SCD, including progression to chronic pain syndromes, adverse effects of chronic opioid usage, psychological maladjustment, poor QOL, and excessive use of health care (Telfer and Kaya, 2017). When acute pain is left untreated, there is the potential for acute neurohumoral changes, neuronal remodeling, and long-lasting psychological, emotional, and economic distress, which may ultimately lead to prolonged chronic pain states (Dunwoody et al., 2008; Gjeilo et al., 2014; Polomano et al., 2008).

Regardless of the approach, adequately managing acute pain is the only known way to prevent the development of chronic pain, which has been well described and appreciated in the literature concerning post-operative pain. Nevertheless, this method to address acute pain has been poorly applied in the SCD context, even though SCD has a well-known pathophysiological mechanism that results in recurrent episodes of acute pain. Unfortunately, for nearly a century these consequences of poorly treated acute pain have not been considered in the development of standardized home-based SCD pain management protocols, nor have they been considered in the education and communication about SCD pain and its management for patients and providers. There remains a major research gap in this area that has been heightened by the emotional response of providers and the community to the widely publicized opioid crisis.

Home-Based SCD Pain Management

Currently, the home management of acute SCD pain in adults typically starts with physical rest and oral hydration, followed by as-needed oral analgesics with or without muscle relaxants. The oral analgesics include acetaminophen, non-steroidal anti-inflammatory drugs (NSAIDs), and various opioid preparations. Many adults, however, are on daily, long-acting opioids for chronic pain and are advised to continue taking these and to add short-acting preparations for pain management. Ideally, this regimen would be developed using shared decision making with the SCD provider to establish an individualized pain management plan (Ballas, 2005; Balsamo et al., 2019).

For adults with SCD, chronic pain is often the norm rather than the exception. One study found that 51 percent of participants reported pain on at least half of the days during the study period (Smith et al., 2008b). Any pain was 10 times more likely to be managed at home than in the acute care setting, whereas crisis pain was only 4 times more likely to be managed at home (Smith et al., 2008b). Interestingly, home opioid use was variable and was related to having more pain, more crises, and higher acute care use. This offers a broad research opportunity to help individuals with SCD establish a structured regimen for managing their various types of pain (e.g., chronic pain, acute pain exacerbation, acute pain crisis) logically and systematically, using opioids when appropriate (Smith et al., 2008b).

Systematic efforts to help individuals living with SCD understand their personal pain experience and adopt optimal evidence-based strategies for acute SCD pain self-management are scarce, perhaps because of the difficulty these individuals encounter in describing their pain (Jenerette et al., 2014; Matthie and Jenerette, 2017). Especially starting in adolescence, when pain experiences start to peak, individuals report having significant barriers to effectively describing and characterizing their pain (Lee et al., 2012). Individuals may also seek pain relief through complementary and alternative methods, such as prayer, relaxation techniques, massage, exercise, and spiritual healing; however, these methods have not been well studied and are not well understood by the health care establishment (Clayton-Jones and Haglund, 2016; Thompson and Eriator, 2014). While the research on the efficacy of these approaches is limited, providers need to be aware of them in developing patient-centered approaches for care management (Mongiovi et al., 2016).

Institutional Acute Care

Home-based pain management and health system–based acute SCD pain management (acute care use) occur at the opposite ends of a wide spectrum of SCD pain frequency and severity (Smith et al., 2008b). When pain management is attempted at home and fails, individuals will seek acute care. Acute SCD pain that requires health care use is addressed either in the ED or in a separate hospital-based location designed to avoid the delays in access to pain management that are often inherent in busy urban EDs. If the pain is not controlled at home, patients may elect to go to a day infusion center, an ED, or a hospital clinical decision unit (CDU). Chapter 2 detailed some of the challenges for getting care even in the ED.

Day Hospitals and Infusion Centers

There are several day hospitals or infusion centers around the country, some of which are solely for the use of adults presenting with acute vaso-occlusive crisis (VOC) and others that function as shared facilities for SCD and other hematological diagnoses. These facilities are commonly available for limited times and provide analgesic and supportive therapy for those not requiring an extended stay to manage an uncomplicated acute SCD pain episode (Lanzkron et al., 2015). This approach to care is resource intensive and requires dedicated physical space along with specialty-trained multi-disciplinary personnel. However, these facilities offer a viable strategy for managing acute VOC pain due to their effectiveness in reducing admission rates and length of stay and overall health care costs compared with care in the ED (Adewoye et al., 2007; Benjamin et al., 2000; Han et al., 2018).

Effective treatment of an acute SCD pain episode follows three main principles: (1) provide prompt pain control using analgesics with high bio-availability; (2) use supportive care strategies that include intracellular re-hydration with hypotonic fluid (oral or intravenous), correction of hypoxia and acidosis, and other supportive care, including rest; and (3) use targeted treatment of the underlying trigger, such as infection or other complications (Platt et al., 2002). Often the third component is overlooked, not investigated, or ignored, and individuals with SCD suffer needless progression of complications and high morbidity and mortality. The Georgia Comprehensive Sickle Cell Center established the first 24-hour acute care center for SCD with a philosophy of prompt access to pain relief and engagement in ongoing comprehensive care to improve disease outcomes for its large SCD population (see Appendix F). There are algorithms for treating an acute pain episode using a combination of opioids and NSAIDs, with guidance on optimal dosing based on the half-life of each medication and frequent close monitoring for response and toxicity (Platt et al., 2002; Raphael et al., 2008). According to these recommendations, oral or parenteral analgesia should be supplied as promptly as possible, with current guidelines recommending within 30 minutes of triage or within 60 minutes of registration (NHLBI, 2014). This promptness is now considered a measure of quality of care for SCD. It is appropriate to re-evaluate the individual after the first dose of analgesia. This evaluation is important in determining the efficacy of the treatment and in identifying any untoward toxicity, such as the oversedation, itching, and nausea that commonly occur with opiates. A frequent objective reassessment of the individual for pain and other symptoms is recommended every 15 to 30 minutes, with redosing of the analgesic in the case of poor pain control. These actions are associated with fewer hospital admissions, reduced length of stay, and increased patient satisfaction (Brandow et al., 2016; Inoue et al., 2016; Kavanagh et al., 2015; Tanabe et al., 2017).

Unfortunately, while re-evaluating pain status and redosing analgesia within the recommended 15–30 minutes may occur in an SCD day hospital or CDU, as discussed below, it is rare in most EDs, for variety of reasons. Additional evidence-based strategies for optimizing ED acute pain management are needed (Glassberg, 2017).

Clinical Decision Unit

A CDU is a newer care option for evaluating and treating acute VOC pain. It allows for the evaluation of pain and high-dose analgesic therapy over an extended period in an inpatient-like setting. CDUs are typically open for longer periods than infusion centers but follow similar protocol-based algorithms for delivering optimal pain management and investigating the reasons or triggers for acute pain exacerbation.

While CDUs are not dedicated to SCD patients (they address a wide variety of illnesses for which patients may require up to 24 hours of care), uncomplicated VOC is a diagnosis that, with proper entry criteria and an individualized treatment plan, can be successfully treated with a short stay in a CDU (Cline et al., 2018). There are robust data on the pharmacoeconomic and clinical superiority of managing acute VOC using these specialized/targeted facilities with the right staffing and infrastructure.

A recent study comparing the care received by 370 children seeking care for acute VOC in either a CDU or the ED showed that the 140 children with SCD who were managed in the CDU were given the choice of an initial analgesic that was adherent to pain management guidelines (84 percent versus 45 percent), had less time to first analgesia (32 minutes versus 70 minutes), and had a lower admission rate (29 percent versus 57 percent [odds ratio (OR) = 3.82; 95% CI 1.87–7.82]) than children receiving care in the ED (Karkoska et al., 2019). While an ED-based dedicated observation unit has strong potential to affect the quality of the pain treatment, individuals with SCD continue to report negative experiences with provider attitudes, implicit bias, and stigma during their encounters with the ED and acute care in general. The committee was unable to find studies that investigated CDUs for adults, but there is no reason to assume it would not also be effective for adults living with SCD.

Emergency Department

The ED is the most commonly used resource to evaluate and treat acute VOC pain and SCD complications in adults. In eight geographically disparate states in the United States containing 21,112 individuals with SCD, there was a mean of 2.59 acute care encounters per person per year, with the highest rates observed among publicly insured 18- to 30-year-olds (4.8 acute care encounters per person year) (Brousseau et al., 2010). EDs are open 24 hours per day, 7 days per week and have the resources to provide comprehensive evaluation and treatment. The ED has the advantage of being able to provide parenteral analgesic that may not available in the outpatient setting.

In addition, the ED is the optimal place to address unusual pain presentations or additional symptoms, such as shortness of breath and mental status changes that may herald a severe complication rather than an uncomplicated pain crisis (Telfer and Kaya, 2017). For a person who does not have readily available transportation to a CDU or SCD day hospital, access to the ED is often possible by calling 911. Thus, it is possible that individuals with SCD whose health care needs could be managed at a CDU or SCD day hospital may end up in the ED. The disadvantage of seeking care for acute SCD pain in the ED is the lack of familiarity between patient and provider, delayed care due to ED overcrowding, and the lack of provider familiarity with SCD. ED care is also quite expensive. According to 2009 estimates for approximately 70,000 individuals with SCD in the United States, the cumulative health care costs for individuals living with SCD exceed $1.1 billion per annum, representing mostly acute care use or ED and hospital admissions (Kauf et al., 2009). There is a nationwide trend to implement ED observational units to manage overcrowding and contain costs (Wiler et al., 2011). To standardize acute SCD pain management and optimize care outcomes in EDs, some EDs have implemented an observation unit as an alternative to a separate CDU or day hospital (Gowhari et al., 2015; Lyon et al., 2014). Regardless of the location of care, providers and health care teams should follow the tenets outlined in Table 5-1.

One major issue concerning individuals, particularly adults, with SCD is the extensive use of EDs for acute pain management. Paulukonis et al. (2017) performed the largest epidemiologic study on ED use by SCD patients, following a cohort of 4,636 California SCD patients over a 10-year period (2005–2014). The study found that nearly all (93 percent) of those individuals had visited an ED at least once (for any diagnosis) and 4,100 (88 percent) of the study participants had at least one treat-and-release ED encounter during that time (Paulukonis et al., 2017). The average number of ED visits was 2.1 visits per person per year. In a single year

TABLE 5-1 The ABCs for Managing Acute Sickle Cell Pain

A	Assess pain using a universal pain assessment tool.
B	Believe the patient's pain level.
C	Look for complications and causes, such as infection, gallstones, and splenomegaly.
D	Implement drugs and distraction, using • pain medications (e.g., opioids, NSAIDs if no contraindication, adjuvants); • standardized dosing regimens or individualized plans when available (see NHLBI expert report guidelines for pain management); and • distraction with music, TV, and relaxation techniques to reduce anxiety and anticipatory pain.
E	Ensure that the environment is conducive to rest. The area should be quiet, with privacy.
F	Provide fluids (hypotonic D5W or D5 1/4 NS). Give a fixed dosing of analgesia—on a time schedule, not as needed or PRN.

NOTE: NHLBI = National Heart, Lung, and Blood Institute; NSAID = non-steroidal anti-inflammatory drug; PRN = pro re nata ("when necessary").
SOURCE: Adapted from Platt et al., 2002, with permission.

(2005), 53 percent of those in the cohort had no treat-and-release ED visits, 35 percent had 1–3 visits, 9 percent had 4–10 visits, and 3 percent had 11 or more visits; individuals in the highest-use group accounted for 45 percent of all of the ED visits during the study period. ED use was highest among young adults and higher among older adults than children (Paulukonis et al., 2017). Other studies have estimated an acute care use rate of 2.59 to 3.0 visits per patient per year (Brousseau et al., 2010; Lanzkron et al., 2018a). In two studies, adults accounted for the majority of all ED visits and hospitalizations (Lanzkron et al., 2010; Yusuf et al., 2010).

The information the committee found regarding ED visits by patients with SCD is the result of analyses of data collected from either a single clinical institution, a consortium of institutions, or a dataset based on a single source of administrative data (i.e., hospital discharge or Medicaid); each dataset has strengths and weaknesses associated with data quality. Data solely from clinical care centers may not accurately reflect the general SCD population. By contrast, administrative data rely on *International Classification of Diseases* (ICD) codes to identify patients with SCD, and these data include a larger number of patients, including those who receive care outside of SCD clinical centers. However, the correlation between SCD ICD codes and a laboratory-confirmed diagnosis of SCD has been deemed unsatisfactory (Paulukonis et al., 2017). Thus, larger-scale epidemiologic studies are needed to develop an accurate measure of acute care use by SCD patients to guide treatment protocols (Lanzkron et al., 2015).

Inpatient Admissions

Pain is one of the most common reasons for hospitalization and re-admission in individuals with SCD (Ho et al., 2019); however, the complications leading to readmission may also include pain and fever. Annual hospitalization rates for patients with SCD are 178 to 216 per 100,000 (Okam et al., 2014). Hospitalization rates did not decrease after the U.S. Food and Drug Administration approval of HU (Okam et al., 2014). One possible explanation for this may be limited access to or poor adherence to HU, per a study conducted in adolescents (Badawy et al., 2018b).

As noted in Chapter 4, SCD is one of the 10 most common reasons for pediatric hospital readmissions (Heslin et al., 2018). Readmission rates for adults with SCD are high as well. Risk factors for readmission vary, but lack of a PCP and a recent missed appointment are important indicators in the adult population (Brodsky et al., 2017; Cronin et al., 2019).

Unplanned readmission rates were highest for 18- to 30-year-olds (Brousseau et al., 2010). Readmission is also higher among those with public insurance (Brousseau et al., 2010). The percentage of readmissions that are medically necessary versus those that are not has not been determined.

High-Use Acute Care

A small subpopulation of individuals living with SCD accesses acute care at rates significantly more than two standard deviations above the mean of the population. These individuals are often referred to as "super-users" and may present to sickle cell day units and hospital EDs much more frequently than others with a similar disease and comorbidity burden (Carroll et al., 2011). One study found that approximately 20 percent of the SCD population accounts for 54 percent of all ED visits (Epstein et al., 2006).

Super-users may have a more severe level of disease, have a higher psychosocial and behavioral health burden with less social support, or lack coordinated care resources (Aisiku et al., 2009). While the data are limited, Simpson et al. (2017) found that instituting comprehensive coordinated health care plans involving a multitude of support services (physicians, advanced practice providers, pharmacists, social workers, psychologists, and psychiatrists) was beneficial for a small sample of super-user adults. The intervention was also beneficial in reducing annualized acute care use across all measured indexes (Simpson et al., 2017). Compared with preintervention, the authors found statistically significant reductions in the annualized number of ED visits (decrease of 16.5 visits per patient-year). They also found lower annualized ED length of stay (decreased by 115.3 hours per patient-year), inpatient admissions (decreased by 4.20 admissions per patient-year), inpatient length of stay (decreased by 35.8 hours per patient-year), and visits where the patient left before treatment (decreased by 13.7 visits per patient-year) (Simpson et al., 2017).

Post-Acute Care

The transition from inpatient hospitalization or ED visits to home provides an opportunity to decrease hospital readmission or return visits to the ED. The transitional care strategies from the hospital to home for patients with SCD during this process are not reported. This may represent a missed opportunity for case management by nurses and CHWs (Logan, 2019).

A novel program, Aiming to Improve Readmissions Through Integrated Hospital Transitions, was established by a regional health care system to smooth the transition from acute care to community residence by reducing the 30-day readmission rate for a population with a high risk for readmission (McWilliams et al., 2019). This unblinded pragmatic randomized controlled trial included 1,876 patients under the care of a hospitalist for their inpatient admission to receive either usual care after discharge or care in a dedicated post-acute care multidisciplinary transition services clinic run by hospitalists. The clinic offered close follow-up for 30 days with access to a free-standing clinic that included a transition-dedicated internist, a pharmacist, and paramedicine, behavioral health, and social work providers, with scheduling frequency and provider type matched to patient needs (McWilliams et al., 2019). The hospital follow-up could occur either in person or virtually in patients' homes (facilitated by paramedicine) and included a comprehensive medication reconciliation by a pharmacist and, at a minimum, weekly contact with a transition services team member with coordinated support to transition to the next appropriate care location after 30 days. While the 30-day readmission rate did not change in the group receiving transition services, those readmitted were less likely to require intensive care compared with the usual care group (15.5 percent versus 26.8 percent) ($p < 0.02$) (McWilliams et al., 2019). These transition services were later made available to adults with SCD as a non-randomized cohort with targeted efforts to increase community acceptance and engagement and strong collaboration between the SCD provider and the transition services provider team. Early indications show that there has been a positive impact on reducing readmission rates for adults with SCD who use transition services.

Rehabilitation Services

Rehabilitation services are needed for multiple reasons in the SCD population. Physical disability (Swanson et al., 2011) is not uncommon and occurs after complications, such as stroke, avascular necrosis of the hips and shoulders, and leg ulcers, or after a prolonged hospitalization with extremely limited physical activity, such as those hospitalizations that occur with pain episodes. Historically, physical medicine and rehabilitation inpatient stays occurred after stroke in order to address the motor deficits associated with cerebral infarction and hemorrhage. For many children and adults with SCD and avascular necrosis of the hips and shoulders, physical and occupational therapy are used to improve pain and address mobility after surgical interventions. Patients with shoulder avascular necrosis require occupational therapy, but their use of these services is underreported. Many require surgical management of avascular necrosis, which includes core decompression and hip replacement (Mallet et al., 2018). Physical therapy after hip replacement is essential for recovery, but where these services occur varies widely in the general population. Inpatient and outpatient services to improve mobility after surgery are limited by access to local services, transportation, and insurance (Clarke et al., 2017). The use of these services needs to be addressed in children and adults with SCD.

Kinesiotherapy, aquatic rehabilitation, and physical therapy may all be effective for managing acute and chronic pain (Alcorn et al., 1984). The use of physical therapy is not reported but seems to be prescribed particularly during or following prolonged inpatient stays for pain.

Palliative Care

Palliative care services are a holistic approach that includes advance care planning, disease management, pain relief, and support for bereavement and grief using open and supportive communication strategies among the health care team, patients, and their families (Wilkie et al., 2010). Palliative care services to improve the QOL for people with serious illness, such as SCD, have been explored as a method to improve pain management and to support end of life, which typically occurs two to three decades earlier in individuals with SCD than in the general population (Ajayi et al., 2016). More than 78 percent of adults with SCD die in the ED or hospital at an average age of 45 (±16 years).

Palliative services are, however, underused during end-of-life care for individuals with SCD (Johnston et al., 2019). Referral patterns for palliative care for non-cancer patients often reflect the need for support with symptom management, particularly for pain (Ghanem et al., 2011). The factors influencing patterns of palliative care service use require further exploration.

Transfusion Medicine Services

Children and adults with SCD require intermittent and long-term red blood cell (RBC) transfusions across the life span to decrease the proportion of sickle hemoglobin (HbS) relative to hemoglobin A and to increase the oxygen-carrying capacity of RBCs, as discussed in Chapter 4. Transfusions may be administered as simple or exchange transfusions. Exchange transfusions may be manual or automated, both of which are equally effective, but patients and providers may prefer the ease of automated exchange. However, access to automated exchange transfusion may be limited in some hospitals and in the outpatient setting for several reasons, including equipment cost and maintenance and prior inability to bill at an increased level for the procedure.

Behavioral Health

Published data on behavioral or mental health service use in children and adults with SCD suggest that children with mental health conditions use health services–related pain management at higher rates than those without such conditions, citing higher annual admission rates and longer lengths of stay (Myrvik et al., 2013) (see Chapter 4 for a more detailed discussion on behavioral and mental health). However, other studies imply that poor physical functioning rather than poor mental functioning increases health care use in adults with SCD (Artz et al., 2009). Few data are published on health care use that does not involve pain management. However, in other chronic illnesses, such as obesity, adults with both obesity and mental illness use health services more than those with just obesity (Shen et al., 2008).

Facilitating Employment for Individuals Living with SCD

The Office of Disability Employment Policy in the U.S. Department of Labor offers guidelines for workplace accommodations for individuals living with SCD (JAN, 2019). Eligibility for accommodations is outlined under the Americans with Disabilities Act. These accommodations may include allowing for a flexible schedule in order for the individual to receive necessary medical treatment, the provision of an adjustable workstation, and the use of an aide if needed.

Facilitating employment for individuals living with SCD can be a positive factor in managing health care use. Williams et al. (2018) followed 95 individuals living with SCD prospectively and found that having employment was significantly associated with decreased health care interactions. More information about employment outcomes for individuals living with SCD can be found in Chapter 2.

COMPREHENSIVE SCD CARE DELIVERY MODEL

Ultimately, enabling the delivery of effective treatment to all individuals living with SCD at all stages of the disease will require developing and implementing a comprehensive SCD care delivery model. There have been efforts toward this end, but the resulting models fall short of ideal in various ways. This section examines the current state of comprehensive SCD care, its strengths and weaknesses, and systems of comprehensive care for other diseases that could serve as models for SCD.

Overview of Historical, Federally Funded SCD Comprehensive Care Centers

Historically, the terminology "comprehensive sickle cell centers" was applied to those receiving funding through the National Institutes of Health's comprehensive sickle cell centers program from 1972 to 2013 (NHLBI, 2006). These programs were funded for SCD basic, translational, and clinical research and had strong clinical services at the core by providing activities such as diagnosis, counseling, and education concerning SCD and related disorders. This philosophy of strong clinical care as the backbone of research initiatives stemmed from the early comprehensive sickle cell centers, created by the 1972 National Sickle Cell Anemia Control Act, which provided the authority to establish treatment programs. Funding was limited, and no more than 10 centers were funded (Howard University, n.d.). When federal support for these centers ended, many sickle cell programs that were not federally funded had adopted the terminology "comprehensive sickle cell center" for their clinical care programs but without the assurance that they had all the required components.

Although there is little published on the history of the comprehensive sickle cell centers, their influence set the stage for the infrastructure of sickle cell programs. In 2008 the National Heart, Lung, and Blood Institute research program was restructured to focus on basic and translational research, specific grants, an expansion of the trials network to attract a broader array of participants, enhanced genomic research, and guidelines (NHLBI, 2008). This shift also led to the genesis of the concept of a clinical "center" for the care of children and adults with SCD that was termed the "comprehensive sickle cell center."

Defining a Model for Comprehensive SCD Care

As with many rare conditions with early childhood mortality, the focus of SCD care in the 1960s and 1970s was on curtailing mortality by preventing infections. The splenic dysfunction that leads to an increased risk for infection was well established by the time that the 1972 Sickle Cell Disease Control Act was implemented. One of the first efforts of the comprehensive sickle cell centers was the Prophylactic Penicillin Study in 1983 (Gaston et al., 1986). This randomized controlled trial demonstrated an 84 percent decreased rate of infection in the penicillin group (Gaston et al., 1986). Initiating oral penicillin early in life, before splenic dysfunction, became the goal for a national newborn screening (NBS) program (Therrell et al., 2015).

The success of the NBS program and improved access to comprehensive care for children with SCD increased the proportion of children living to their third decade (Quinn et al., 2010). Comprehensive care was bolstered by implementing evidence-based care for infection and stroke prevention and by fostering widespread use of HU and protocol-driven pediatric care. Unfortunately, the resources adopted to support pediatric care did not evolve to include the adult care setting. Currently, sickle cell experts for adult-focused care are in short supply but increasingly high demand (see Chapter 6).

Key components of "comprehensive sickle cell centers" include a system of care for children and adults with SCD across the life span. Services include health maintenance and preventive care in outpatient settings, where patient education, anticipatory guidance, and behavioral health are managed by a multidisciplinary team. Individuals with SCD have psychosocial needs that should be addressed along with their medical needs. Centers often understand patients' challenges relating to stigma and health disparities, although this was not mandated in the funding requirements. These centers were embedded within health care systems that provided for the unique health care needs of SCD and were geared to ensure coordinated care. Below is a brief description of the desirable components, identified by the committee, of a team-based, comprehensive care delivery model:

- *Health maintenance and prevention.* These are services aimed at establishing a disease steady state across the life span, including genetic testing for hemoglobin variants and RBC antigens and the management of long-term therapies, including HU, chronic transfusions, and stem cell therapies.
- *Medical subspecialty care.* This was initially focused on support for stroke and neurocognitive disorder management and pulmonology for asthma, ACS, and chronic lung disease management. It has since evolved to include a myriad of specialists targeting the multi-system complications of SCD discussed in Chapter 4.
- *Neuropsychiatric and neurology services.* These services include evaluation for neurocognitive deficits, executive function, cerebral ischemia ("silent" and "overt" manifestations), and cerebral vasculopathy. Neuroimaging to assess Chiari malformations and aneurysms is a component of care, coupled with radiology services.
- *Behavioral health.* These services address depression, posttraumatic stress, anxiety, pica, opioid use disorders, and other behavioral health issues in an environment of care that acknowledges poverty, racism, and its associated behavioral health management strategies.

- *Radiology.* These are specialized services for TCD ultrasonography for the accurate assessment of TCD velocities to assess stroke risk, echocardiology techniques to accurately assess tricuspid regurgitation jet velocities, imaging scans to assess pulmonary hypertension, magnetic resonance imaging for stroke management, and imaging tests to detect avascular necrosis.
- *Blood bank and transfusion medicine.* These appropriately provide RBC units with extended antigen matching, the administration of RBC quantities that avoid hyperviscosity, automated and manual erythrocytapheresis to rapidly decrease HbS without increasing overall hemoglobin values, and the minimization of transfusional iron overload.
- *Surgical care.* These surgical subspecialty services are familiar with common indications for surgery, such as cholecystectomy, splenectomy, hip replacement, adenotonsillectomy, C-section, and ophthalmologic procedures, and the risk of surgical complications unique to SCD peri-operatively and long term.
- *Anesthesia and sedation services.* These are specialized services to assess risk for the development of post-operative ACS.
- *Genetic counseling.* These activities provide genetic counseling services to individuals diagnosed by NBS or other screening modalities, with accurate anticipatory guidance provided concerning sickle cell trait (SCT) diagnosis, pregnancy planning, and other issues.
- *Education and vocational services.* These activities provide training and information about SCD to health care professionals at the center and in the community or region that the center serves and to patients, their families, and communities, with linkages to community support to optimize patient education and vocation.
- *Research.* The comprehensive sickle cell centers conducted research to improve the treatment and prevention of complications, enhance the transfer of these new findings to the clinical setting, and identify new research directions. While research was a core component of the original design, centers were also required to provide supportive activities in diagnosis, management education, and counseling and to spread the research agenda across basic, translational, clinical, and outcomes topics.
- *Data management core.* Each center was supported by a central data coordinating point as a shared resource for data management, statistical support, and the standardization and development of research protocols, data element definitions, and staff training.
- *Physical and occupational therapy.* These are ambulatory services in physical therapy, occupational therapy, and physical medicine and rehabilitation for avascular necrosis, reconditioning following

prolonged hospitalizations, and weight management for healthy weight.

- *Community outreach.* This involved establishing communication channels between the comprehensive sickle cell center and the community via liaisons, who would inform the community about programs and provide community input into programmatic development and priorities. Traditionally, these liaisons were members of a formally established SCD CBO with a close affiliation via formal membership to the national advocacy agency (the Sickle Cell Disease Association of America) and a broad scope of supportive services (see Chapter 8 for more information). One step in improving services in the community might be to tap into the experiences of these groups to identify and disseminate best practices.

The comprehensive centers model was an excellent attempt to operationalize a care delivery model for infants and children, who had an exorbitantly high childhood mortality rate at that time. The next iteration of comprehensive centers should include attention to the morbidities that affect the aging population along with formalized tracking and measurement of both the research and clinical and supportive care components. There are various models through which this care may be provided, and the following section outlines one.

Redesigning the Care Delivery Model

After the release of the Institute of Medicine (IOM) report *Crossing the Quality Chasm* (IOM, 2001b), which highlighted the highly fragmented nature and poorly designed care processes of the American health system, new models for health care delivery were developed and implemented, such as the patient-centered medical home (PCMH) and comprehensive primary care plus (CPC+). These models were designed in response to challenges identified in that report (IOM, 2001b):

- Redesign care processes to effectively meet the needs of the chronically ill.
- Improve information technologies to support chronic care.
- Manage the growing knowledge base with training, workforce development, and clinical decision support.
- Coordinate patient care across time, specialty, and location/ intensity of service (outpatient and inpatient).
- Advance effectiveness of teams and multidisciplinary training.
- Incorporate process and outcome measurement into daily work.

The findings from the 2014–2017 SCDTDRCP and its precursor, the Working to Improve Sickle Cell Healthcare project (2011–2015), recommended that developing a system of care for individuals with SCD should include the main tenets of the PCMH such as a PCP for comprehensive care and continuous relationship, a multidisciplinary team, and specialists and community providers (Adams et al., 2017). These recommendations and proposed operational elements have been incorporated into specific care delivery models, such as the PCMH and CPC+. Other disease-specific models, such as the cystic fibrosis (CF) care center accreditation standards, address these recommendations in way that are similar to how they are addressed by the PCMH and CPC+. However, such recommendations should take into consideration that health systems are complex, adaptive, and governed by shared goals and simple rules (IOM, 2001b). The current standard of SCD care in the United States does not follow the new rules for a 21st-century health care system (IOM, 2001b) (see Table 5-2). This will need to be changed in order to deliver team-based comprehensive care to individuals with SCD.

The PCMH is a model for delivering care with a core focus on advancing primary care and the health care home (Rich et al., 2012). The PCMH focuses on comprehensive, patient-centered, coordinated care with accessible services and commitment to quality and safety (Rich et al., 2012). Comprehensive care involves using a team-based approach to provide mental and physical health care. Patient-centered care is oriented around the

TABLE 5-2 Simple Rules for the 21st-Century Health Care System

Current Approach	New Rule
Care is based primarily on visits.	Care is based on a continuous healing relationship.
Professional autonomy drives variability.	Care is customized according to patient needs.
Professionals control care.	The patient is the source of control.
Information is a record.	Knowledge is shared and information flows.
Decision making is based on training and experience.	Decision making is evidence based.
Do no harm is an individual responsibility.	Safety is a system property.
Secrecy is necessary.	Transparency is necessary.
The system reacts to needs.	Needs are anticipated.
Cost reduction is sought.	Waste is continuously decreased.
Preference is given to professional roles over the system.	Cooperation among clinicians is a priority.

SOURCE: IOM, 2001b.

patient's needs, values, and preferences. Coordinated care provides the patient with acute and chronic care resources across a continuum. Accessible services include telehealth and after-hour health services to ensure that patients' needs and preferences are met. Finally, the PCMH's commitment to quality and safety involves using patient data for quality improvement purposes.

CPC+ is a primary care medical home model with a focus on advancing primary care through regionally based multi-payer payment reform and care delivery transformation (CMS, 2019). By 2019, 2,851 primary care practices and 55 payers across 18 regions in the United States were participating in CPC+ (CMS, 2019). Key functions of CPC+ include access and continuity, care management, comprehensiveness and coordination, patient and caregiver engagement, and planned care and population health. The three payment elements of CPC+ include a care management fee, performance-based incentive payment, and payment under the Medicare physician fee schedule.

The committee reviewed the PCMH, CPC+, CF care centers, and the hemophilia model of care and identified the following examples of how those care models operationalized the structural elements of an ideal care model (see Box 5-1).

Comparison with Cystic Fibrosis

The Cystic Fibrosis Foundation (CFF) accreditation rules maximize the learning of the complex, adaptive, health care system. The lack of these guidelines for SCD leaves care unimproved. While there is more than one method to accomplish good-quality care delivery for SCD, the absence of standards, expectations, and funding creates disparities within health care and between SCD care and that of other rare diseases, such as CF (recognized as one of the best examples of system design for a chronic disease of childhood). At a minimum, a single health professional could coordinate care for a population of patients with SCD, coordinating appointments, providing specialty-specific checklists, maintaining transition registries and disease registries, providing disease-specific education for patients and families, and connecting PCPs and specialty providers (Bodenheimer et al., 2002b).

As a model for excellent outcomes in childhood chronic illness, CFF requires accredited centers to prepare the workforce, with all specialties demonstrating teaching medical students, residents, and other workers in the health care field the highest standards of care. Such a requirement would also help SCD and other rare and childhood chronic illnesses. Additionally, educational materials and even "certification" pathways for health professionals to become proficient in SCD management would be a mechanism

---

BOX 5-1
Key Elements for an Ideal Care Model

Team-Based Care
- Clinician-led, multidisciplinary team that includes patient and family involvement for shared decision making
- Pre-visit planning
- Alternative appointment types

Patient-Centered Care
- Multidisciplinary medical and behavioral health assessments
- Program priorities match patient priorities and needs
- Cultural appropriateness
- Outreach
- Clinical decision support
- Self-management
- Shared decision making

Patient Access to Care
- Access to monitoring and evaluation
- Access to outpatient services
- Access to medical records and continuous care

Case Management
- Risk assessment and mitigation through care management
- Person-centered care plan and care management

Care Coordination and Transitions
- Newborn screening
- Transitions of care

Quality Improvement Initiatives
- Transparency in methods for measuring and reporting clinical outcomes
- Patient needs assessment
- Qualitative and quantitative evaluation
- Benchmarking
- Continuous improvement for data-driven quality improvement

---

for increasing payment for practices that perform population management and high-quality care across all domains of care.

Comparison with Hemophilia

Like SCD and CF, hemophilia is a rare hereditary disorder whose treatment uses significant resources for the health care system (Tarantino and Pindolia, 2017). In 2016 the National Hemophilia Foundation in collaboration with McMaster University created a guideline on the use of care models for managing hemophilia. This guidance proposes the use of an integrated care model, including an integrated care team (NHF, 2016).

The evidence on the impact of the integrated care model for the hemophilia population is limited but positive; two separate research reviews cited the lack of rigorous research on the impact of hemophilia care models. Young et al. (2016) conducted a systematic review and found some evidence (described as low- to very low-quality) that, in comparison with other models of care, the integrated care model for hemophilia produces better outcomes (decreased mortality and fewer hospitalizations, fewer ED visits, fewer missed school and work days). Stoffman et al. (2019) reviewed research regarding hemophilia care according to the World Federation of Hemophilia guidelines and described four aspects of care models that are recommended: global guidelines and protocols, collaboration with other countries, patient registries to track resource use, and the provision of personal care to optimize treatment outcomes. The CF model and hemophilia are further described in Chapter 8.

Sickle Cell Disease Treatment Demonstration Regional Collaborative Program

The SCDTDRCP, which began in 2004 and was funded by HRSA, serves as a good model for organizing the delivery of comprehensive SCD care. Currently the SCDTDRCP provides grants to five regional networks consisting of sickle cell treatment centers, federally qualified health centers, and CBOs in 43 states across the United States to provide coordinated, comprehensive, culturally competent, and family-centered care to people with SCD and SCT[9] (Adams et al., 2017). The goals of the SCDTDRCP are to improve care delivery and access for people with SCD and SCT, increase the number of providers with SCD expertise and knowledge of SCD treatment methods, and increase the use of HU for people with SCD. To improve access to medical care and educational services, teams in the SCDTDRCP have implemented Project Extension for Community Healthcare Outcomes (ECHO), which uses telementoring to connect local clinicians to experts from sickle cell centers and allows hematologists to share knowledge with PCPs via real-time, virtual provider-to-provider education and mentoring for sickle cell care and webinars on relevant SCD topics (Adams et al.,

---

[9] The five regional grantees in the SCDTDRCP are Johns Hopkins in the Northeast region, Charlotte Mecklenburg Hospital in the Southeast region, Cincinnati Children's Hospital in the Midwest region, Washington University in the Heartland and Southwest region, and the Center for Inherited Blood Disorders in the Pacific region (Adams et al., 2017).

2017). The SCDTDRCP also improves the patient–provider interaction by using the Chronic Care Model (CCM) approach. The goal of the CCM is to improve health outcomes for patients with chronic illnesses by changing care delivery (Bodenheimer et al., 2002a). In order to provide patient-centered, evidence-based care, the CCM focuses on six components: community resources and policies, health care organization, self-management support, delivery system design, decision support, and clinical information systems (Bodenheimer et al., 2002a). The SCDTDRCP also offers a framework for continuous improvement; information collected from the SCDTDRCP, through a national collaborative website, was analyzed using core metrics to identify best practices for care delivery, educational materials for SCD treatment, and the efficacy of the SCDTDRCP (Adams et al., 2017). An evaluation of the SCDTDRCP showed demonstrable results in improving access to care, HU use, and provider education (see Appendix H). The geographic organization and reach of the program as well as the existing networks could form the basis of comprehensive models of care throughout the country.

Hemoglobinopathy Learning Collaborative

The Hemoglobinopathy Learning Collaborative, which was created under the auspices of the SCDTDRCP, has been implementing continuous quality improvement principles in the management and outcomes of SCD and other hemoglobinopathies (Oyeku et al., 2012). In a Delphi study, five drivers of quality improvement were identified: a strong community network; knowledgeable individuals, families, and providers; reliable identification and follow-up; seamless co-management between primary and specialty care; and the appropriate treatment of acute episodes (Oyeku et al., 2012). These five themes are consistent with PCMH, CPC+, and CF structural elements and should be included in SCD care.

BARRIERS TO COMPREHENSIVE CARE

There are various barriers to developing a system of comprehensive care for SCD; this section describes several such barriers and possible ways to overcome them.

Geographic Barriers

Few individuals living with SCD are seen by or have access to a comprehensive sickle cell center with specialized providers (Grosse et al., 2009). One barrier to comprehensive care for the chronically ill is geographic distance from specialized care, especially in rural areas (Kimmel et al., 2018).

In addition, individuals with SCD may have difficulty finding appropriate primary care for several reasons, including the discomfort of providers with ambulatory care or managing disease-specific conditions (Whiteman et al., 2015). A lack of familiarity with SCD may also result in clinician attitudes that further limit care (Haywood et al., 2009). The CDC Sickle Cell Data Collection Project is collecting data on the geographic location of the sickle cell population in California and Georgia. This information combined with health care usage data will inform unmet health needs. Models such as Project ECHO should be explored to improve provider access to sickle cell expertise to improve patient outcomes (Zhou et al., 2016).

Innovative Care Models to Overcome Geographic Barriers

To overcome geographic barriers, newly available technologies may prove useful. These innovative approaches may focus on the individual with SCD and on providers. E-mail and text messaging have allowed patients far greater ease of connecting with providers (Raphael and Oyeku, 2013). For providers, telemedicine with videos has been used to enhance the delivery of primary care (Woods et al., 1998). A more sophisticated approach, Project ECHO, is an interactive model of training hospital and acute care providers in high-quality, culturally sensitive care for individuals with SCD (Arora et al., 2007). Project ECHO uses telementoring through a hub-and-spoke model, in which the expert providers are the academic "hub" and the clinicians in the local communities are the "spokes" who provide the knowledge and guidance needed to provide SCD patients with proper care (Project ECHO, 2020).

Models Incorporating Community-Based Organizations

Another innovative model is the CDC-designed collaborative approach for addressing chronic care, which involves CBOs. This model uses four strategies: (1) epidemiology and surveillance, (2) environmental approaches that support health, (3) health system interventions to improve the use of clinical and preventive services, and (4) community resources linked to clinical services (Bauer et al., 2014). Employing similar models for SCD alongside an integration of behavioral and integrative health should be considered.

Financial and Socioeconomic Barriers

Insurance Coverage

In a series of reports (IOM, 2001a, 2002a,b, 2003a,b, 2004), the IOM laid out the importance of health insurance to individual and community health. It corrected the myths about the uninsured; delineated the effects of a lack of insurance on treatment for various serious conditions; emphasized the influence of the family on access to insurance and the effect of changes in family formation on insurance; delineated the effect of a lack of insurance on the health and well-being of individuals, families, and communities; and presented principles for reducing lack of coverage. Of particular importance to the current report, the reports emphasize the disproportionate burden on minority and low-income families and the changes in insurance coverage that can emerge with changes in employment or family composition, such the loss of family coverage for young adults. Although the reports do not examine SCD specifically, they do emphasize the importance of insurance in obtaining primary care and care for chronic illnesses. A later report found that there was an increase in the uninsured, especially low-wage earners, and an increase in restrictive policies for those with insurance (IOM, 2009). Thus, it would be expected that the type and content of health insurance would be a major influence on the ability of SCD patients to access medical care.

Private insurance is also variable. Until the Patient Protection and Affordable Care Act, private health insurance companies could use a pre-existing condition as a basis for denying individual insurance coverage (KFF, 2019). Evidence from the CF population suggests that extending parental coverage for young adults to the age of 26 resulted in greater access to care, even though it does not automatically guarantee better health (Lanzkron et al., 2018b). Even with private insurance, coverage may vary due to changes in jobs or other reasons. Insurance may not be adequate for the individual's needs, particularly durable medical equipment (NASEM, 2017), behavioral health care (IOM, 2003c), and dental care (Berdahl et al., 2016).

Finally, not all types of insurance may be considered equivalent. Anand et al. (2017) reported that among children undergoing hematopoietic stem cell transplant, those with private insurance were more likely to receive it. Previous sections of this chapter have also noted the variation in state Medicaid plans for both general services and CSHCN.

Other Barriers

As suggested by the enabling services, other factors influence access to care, including specialist availability, transportation needs, the availability of comprehensible patient materials, and, potentially, the need for translation services. As noted in Chapter 2, a number of social factors influence access to care, including stigma, bias, and lack of public awareness.

SERVICES FOR SCT

Screening in the United States occurs in newborns, during pregnancy, and before participation in National Collegiate Athletic Association Division I, II, and III sports. Other opportunities for screening should occur for immigrants. The purpose of screening is two-fold: (1) to detect SCD and establish appropriate referrals for those with it and (2) to detect those at risk for having children with SCD.

SCT is associated with medical complications. Individuals with SCT have an increased risk for chronic renal disease, pulmonary embolism, and rhabdomyolysis (Naik et al., 2018). Recent data support the possibility of an association between SCT and atrial fibrillation (Douce et al., 2019).

Genetic counseling for families with children with SCT and for individuals with SCT improves the understanding of the risk of having offspring with SCD. In this context, rapid screening tests that use chemical reactions to determine the presence of HbS are not sufficient to provide accurate information for genetic counseling. The best test for hemoglobinopathies is a hemoglobin electrophoresis that quantifies the proportion of normal and variant hemoglobins. When accompanied by a complete blood count, better evaluations regarding the beta thalassemia trait are possible.

Screening for SCT and other hemoglobinopathy traits should be performed with genetic counseling before and during pregnancy. The American College of Obstetricians and Gynecologists (ACOG) recommends screening with a hemoglobin electrophoresis and complete blood count if there is a suspicion of hemoglobinopathy based on ethnic background (ACOG, 2017). A 2007 ACOG bulletin recommended that parents who are determined to be SCT carriers be provided genetic counseling to better inform their decisions regarding reproduction and prenatal genetic testing (ACOG, 2007). More research is needed on the use of genetic counseling for individuals with SCT (Pecker and Naik, 2018).

CONCLUSIONS AND RECOMMENDATIONS

There is a paucity of data concerning access to and the use of health care by children and adults with SCD. The impact of socioeconomic and psychosocial factors, including comorbid conditions and mental health condition needs, should be addressed in this population. The lack of such information will make it difficult to plan needed services and assess their impact. Thus, one part of a strategic plan would be to define and implement systems to gather the information related to health care use and the organizational health care infrastructure and the CBO infrastructure needed to provide high-quality care. One suggestion, as described in Chapter 3 and this chapter, would be to develop registry and surveillance systems that collect information on not only patient demographics and metrics but also providers, services, and organizational infrastructure. Another might be to leverage existing national surveys to focus on SCD by combining years of data to obtain a sufficient sample. A third would be to exploit administrative datasets (e.g., insurance, Medicaid) to obtain a clearer picture of existing health care use among people with SCD (Grosse et al., 2010). Models of care should be explored to determine whether any seem superior for addressing SCD, given the barriers to care and the need to take into account health worker shortages (see Chapter 6). However, the benefit of pre-existing relationships among the SCD community, hospitals, and CBOs should be exploited. CDC's strategic model for chronic illness delivery that incorporates community resources linked to clinical services should be explored further. These concepts must be explored in the context of increasing access to high-quality health care.

> *Conclusion 5-1: The available evidence suggests that the receipt of comprehensive care from a medical home is associated with fewer emergency department visits and hospitalizations for children with SCD. The receipt of comprehensive care involving a hematologist is also associated with greater receipt of preventive services for children with SCD. While children with SCD are cared for by a pediatric hematologist, they transition to adult health care providers who may or may not have experience with providing care for SCD.*

> *Conclusion 5-2: There are no publications on the status of dental health among individuals with SCD. Considering that a substantial portion of the SCD population is covered by public insurance, it is important to note that the U.S. public insurance system does not universally provide dental coverage, so there are significant barriers to access to dental care for individuals with SCD.*

> *Conclusion 5-3: By the time individuals with SCD reach adulthood, the majority (59 percent) of them have developed end-organ damage involving at least one organ, thus necessitating care delivery from a primary care and adult sickle cell specialist and other providers to ensure comprehensive SCD care delivery and to improve outcomes.*

> *Conclusion 5-4: Individuals with pain are more likely to manage their pain at home for a variety of reasons. However, home opioid use is variable and related to having more pain, more crises, and higher acute care use, thus offering an opportunity for research to help individuals with SCD establish structured regimens for managing care at home.*

Conclusion 5-5: The transition from pediatric to adult care is a critical time for individuals with SCD. Young adults experience increased disease complications and end-organ damage, face loss of health insurance and of the usual source of care, and feel inadequately prepared to manage their disease. There are models of transition for other diseases that can inform coordinated transitions for individuals with SCD.

Conclusion 5-6: Mental health care is significantly compromised in SCD partly due to the chronic burden of disease and the impact of pain and pain treatments on the brain. There is a lack of good evidence regarding the natural history of mental health in SCD and detailed information on the psychological and psychosocial effect on patients as they age into adults.

Recommendation 5-1: The Office of the Assistant Secretary for Health, through the Office of Minority Health, should convene a panel of relevant stakeholders to delineate the elements of a comprehensive system of sickle cell disease (SCD) care, including community supports to improve health outcomes, quality of life, and health inequalities. Relevant stakeholders may include the National Minority Quality Forum, National Medical Association, American Society of Pediatric Hematology/Oncology, American Academy of Pediatrics, American Board of Pediatrics, American College of Physicians, American Society of Hematology, Sickle Cell Disease Association of America Inc., Sickle Cell Adult Provider Network, and other key clinical disciplines and stakeholders engaged in SCD care; health systems; and individuals living with SCD and their families.

Recommendation 5-2: The Centers for Medicare & Medicaid Services should work with state Medicaid programs to develop and pilot reimbursement models for the delivery of coordinated sickle cell disease health care and support services.

Recommendation 5-3: The U.S. Department of Education should collaborate with state departments of health and education and local school boards to develop educational materials to provide guidance for teachers, school nurses, school administrators, and primary care providers to support the medical and academic needs of students with sickle cell disease.

Recommendation 5-4: The National Heart, Lung, and Blood Institute; Health Resources and Services Administration; Centers for Disease

Control and Prevention; and U.S. Food and Drug Administration should collaborate with the American Society for Hematology, Pediatric Emergency Care Applied Research Network, Patient-Centered Outcomes Research Institute, and private funders of quality improvement initiatives to foster the development of quality improvement collaboratives.

REFERENCES

AAP (American Academy of Pediatrics). 2011. Reaffirmed policy statement—Pediatric primary health care. *Pediatrics* 127(2):397.

AAP, AAFP (American Academy of Family Physicians), ACP (American College of Physicians), and Transitions Clinical Report Authoring Group. 2011. Supporting the health care transition from adolescence to adulthood in the medical home. *Pediatrics* 128(1):182–200.

ACOG (American College of Obstetricians and Gynecologists). 2007. ACOG practice bulletin number 78: Hemoglobinopathies in pregnancy. *Obstetrics and Gynecology* 109(1):229–238.

ACOG. 2017. Carrier screening for genetic conditions. Committee opinion no. 691. *Obstetrics and Gynecology* 129:e41–e55.

ACP (American College of Physicians). 2019. *Pediatric to Adult Care Transitions Initiative.* https://www.acponline.org/clinical-information/high-value-care/resources-for-clinicians/pediatric-to-adult-care-transitions-initiative (accessed January 17, 2020).

Adams, B., C. Berardi, S. Berns, K. Devlin, L. Forbush, B. Lambiaso, S. Lawrence, S. Oyeku, and S. Selk. 2017. *Sickle cell disease treatment demonstration program: Congressional report.* https://www.nichq.org/sites/default/files/resource-file/SCDTDP-Congressional-Report-2017_0.pdf (accessed January 30, 2020).

Adewoye, A. H., V. Nolan, L. McMahon, Q. Ma, and M. H. Steinberg. 2007. Effectiveness of a dedicated day hospital for management of acute sickle cell pain. *Haematologica* 92(6):854–855.

Aisiku, I. P., W. R. Smith, D. K. McClish, J. L. Levenson, L. T. Penberthy, S. D. Roseff, V. E. Bovbjerg, and J. D. Roberts. 2009. Comparisons of high versus low emergency department utilizers in sickle cell disease. *Annals of Emergency Medicine* 53(5):587–593.

Ajayi, T. A., K. P. Edmonds, K. Thornberry, and R. A. Atayee. 2016. Palliative care teams as advocates for adults with sickle cell disease. *Journal of Palliative Medicine* 19(2):195–201.

Alcorn, R., B. Bowser, E. J. Henley, and V. Holloway. 1984. Fluidotherapy and exercise in the management of sickle cell anemia. A clinical report. *Physical Therapy* 64(10):1520–1522.

Anand, S., R. Theodore, A. Mertens, P. A. Lane, and L. Krishnamurti. 2017. Health disparity in hematopoietic cell transplantation for sickle cell disease: Analyzing the association of insurance and socioeconomic status among children undergoing hematopoietic cell transplantation. *Blood* 130(Suppl 1):4636.

Andemariam, B., and S. Jones. 2016. Development of a new adult sickle cell disease center within an academic cancer center: Impact on hospital utilization patterns and care quality. *Journal of Racial and Ethnic Health Disparities* 3(1):176–182.

Anderson, L. M., S. Leonard, J. Jonassaint, J. Lunyera, M. Bonner, and N. Shah. 2018. Mobile health intervention for youth with sickle cell disease: Impact on adherence, disease knowledge, and quality of life. *Pediatric Blood & Cancer* 65(8):e27081.

Armstrong-Wells, J., B. Grimes, S. Sidney, D. Kronish, S. C. Shiboski, R. J. Adams, H. J. Fullerton. 2009. Utilization of TCD screening for primary stroke prevention in children with sickle cell disease. *Neurology* 72(15):1316–1321.

Arora, S., C. M. Geppert, S. Kalishman, D. Dion, F. Pullara, B. Bjeletich, G. Simpson, D. C. Alverson, L. B. Moore, D. Kuhl, and J. V. Scaletti. 2007. Academic health center management of chronic diseases through knowledge networks: Project ECHO. *Academic Medicine* 82(2):154–160.

Artz, N., J. Zhang, and D. Meltzer. 2009. Physical and mental health in adults hospitalized with sickle cell disease: Impact on resource use. *Journal of the National Medical Association* 101(2):139–144.

Badawy, S. M., R. M. Cronin, J. Hankins, L. Crosby, M. DeBaun, A. A. Thompson, and N. Shah. 2018a. Patient-centered eHealth interventions for children, adolescents, and adults with sickle cell disease: Systematic review. *Journal of Medical Internet Research* 20(7):e10940.

Badawy, S. M., A. A. Thompson, J. L. Holl, F. J. Penedo, and R. I. Liem. 2018b. Healthcare utilization and hydroxyurea adherence in youth with sickle cell disease. *Pediatric Hematology and Oncology* 35(5–6):297–308.

Ballas, S. K. 2005. Pain management of sickle cell disease. *Hematology/Oncology Clinics of North America* 19(5):v, 785–802.

Balsamo, L., V. Shabanova, J. Carbonella, M. V. Szondy, K. Kalbfeld, D. A. Thomas, K. Santucci, M. Grossman, and F. Pashankar. 2019. Improving care for sickle cell pain crisis using a multidisciplinary approach. *Pediatrics* 143(5):e20182218.

Bauer, U. E., P. A. Briss, R. A. Goodman, and B. A. Bowman. 2014. Prevention of chronic disease in the 21st century: Elimination of the leading preventable causes of premature death and disability in the USA. *Lancet* 384(9937):45–52.

Bemrich-Stolz, C. J., J. H. Halanych, T. H. Howard, L. M. Hilliard, and J. D. Lebensburger. 2015. Exploring adult care experiences and barriers to transition in adult patients with sickle cell disease. *International Journal of Hematology and Therapy* 1(1):PMC475676.

Benjamin, L. J., G. I. Swinson, and R. L. Nagel. 2000. Sickle cell anemia day hospital: An approach for the management of uncomplicated painful crises. *Blood* 95(4):1130–1136.

Berdahl, T., J. Hudson, L. Simpson, and M. C. McCormick. 2016. Annual report on children's health care: Dental and orthodontic utilization and expenditures for children, 2010–2012. *Academic Pediatrics* 16(4):314–326.

Berry, J. G., M. Hall, E. Cohen, M. O'Neill, and C. Feudtner. 2015. Ways to identify children with medical complexity and the importance of why. *Journal of Pediatrics* 167(2):229–237.

Berry, S., P. Barovechio, E. Mabile, and T. Tran. 2017. Enhancing state medical home capacity through a care coordination technical assistance model. *Maternal and Child Health Journal* 21(10):1949–1960.

Blinder, M. A., F. Vekeman, M. Sasane, A. Trahey, C. Paley, and M. S. Duh. 2013. Age-related treatment patterns in sickle cell disease patients and the associated sickle cell complications and healthcare costs. *Pediatric Blood & Cancer* 60(5):828–835.

Blinder, M. A., M. S. Duh, M. Sasane, A. Trahey, C. Paley, and F. Vekeman. 2015. Age-related emergency department reliance in patients with sickle cell disease. *Journal of Emergency Medicine* 49(4):513–522.

Blum, R. W., D. Garell, C. H. Hodgman, T. W. Jorissen, N. A. Okinow, D. P. Orr, and G. B. Slap. 1993. Transition from child-centered to adult health-care systems for adolescents with chronic conditions. A position paper of the Society for Adolescent Medicine. *Journal of Adolescent Health* 14(7):570–576.

Bodenheimer, T., E. H. Wagner, and K. Grumbach. 2002a. Improving primary care for patients with chronic illness. *JAMA* 288(14):1775–1779.

Bodenheimer, T., E. H. Wagner, and K. Grumbach. 2002b. Improving primary care for patients with chronic illness: The Chronic Care Model, part 2. *JAMA* 288(15):1909–1914.

Boudreau, A. A., J. M. Perrin, E. Goodman, D. Kurowski, W. C. Cooley, and K. Kuhlthau. 2014. Care coordination and unmet specialty care among children with special health care needs. *Pediatrics* 133(6):1046–1053.

Brandow, A. M., M. Nimmer, T. Simmons, T. Charles Casper, L. J. Cook, C. E. Chumpitazi, J. Paul Scott, J. A. Panepinto, and D. C. Brousseau. 2016. Impact of emergency department care on outcomes of acute pain events in children with sickle cell disease. *American Journal of Hematology* 91(12):1175–1180.

Brennan-Cook, J., E. Bonnabeau, R. Aponte, C. Augustin, and P. Tanabe. 2018. Barriers to care for persons with sickle cell disease: The case manager's opportunity to improve patient outcomes. *Professional Case Management* 23(4):213–219.

Bright Futures. n.d. *Publications.* https://www.brightfutures.org/publications/TMP3ss42k9eat.htm (accessed January 23, 2020).

Brodsky, M. A., M. Rodeghier, M. Sanger, J. Byrd, B. McClain, B. Covert, D. O. Roberts, K. Wilkerson, M. R. DeBaun, and A. A. Kassim. 2017. Risk factors for 30-day readmission in adults with sickle cell disease. *American Journal of Medicine* 130(5):e601.e609–e601.e615.

Brousseau, D. C., P. L. Owens, A. L. Mosso, J. A. Panepinto, and C. A. Steiner. 2010. Acute care utilization and rehospitalizations for sickle cell disease. *JAMA* 303(13):1288–1294.

Bundy, D. G., J. Muschelli, G. D. Clemens, J. J. Strouse, R. E. Thompson, J. F. Casella, and M. R. Miller. 2012. Ambulatory care connections of Medicaid-insured children with sickle cell disease. *Pediatric Blood & Cancer* 59(5):888–894.

Bundy, D. G., J. Muschelli, G. D. Clemens, J. J. Strouse, R. E. Thompson, J. F. Casella, and M. R. Miller. 2016. Preventive care delivery to young children with sickle cell disease. *Journal of Pediatric Hematology/Oncology* 38(4):294–300.

Cady, R., S. Finkelstein, and A. Kelly. 2009. A telehealth nursing intervention reduces hospitalizations in children with complex health conditions. *Journal of Telemedicine and Telecare* 15(6):317–320.

Caldwell, E. P. 2019. The influence of health literacy on emergency department utilization and hospitalizations in adolescents with sickle cell disease. *Public Health Nursing* 36(6):765–771.

Carroll, C. P., C. Haywood, Jr., and S. Lanzkron. 2011. Prediction of onset and course of high hospital utilization in sickle cell disease. *Journal of Hospital Medicine* 6(5):248–255.

CCNC (Community Care of North Carolina). n.d. *Sickle cell program.* https://www.communitycarenc.org/what-we-do/care-management/population-health-outreach-and-care-coordination/sickle-cell-program (accessed January 23, 2020).

CDC (Centers for Disease Control and Prevention). 2010. U.S. medical eligibility criteria for contraceptive use, 2010: Adapted from the *World Health Organization medical eligibility criteria for contraceptive use, 4th edition. Morbidity and Mortality Weekly Report* 59(RR04):1–6.

CDC. 2019a. *The CDC Clear Communication Index.* https://www.cdc.gov/ccindex/index.html (accessed January 23, 2020).

CDC. 2019b. *Immunization schedules.* https://www.cdc.gov/vaccines/schedules/index.html (accessed January 23, 2020).

Chaturvedi, S., D. L. Ghafuri, N. Jordan, A. Kassim, M. Rodeghier, and M. R. DeBaun. 2018. Clustering of end-organ disease and earlier mortality in adults with sickle cell disease: A retrospective-prospective cohort study. *American Journal of Hematology* 93(9):1153–1160.

Cheng, C., R. C. Brown, L. L. Cohen, J. Venugopalan, T. H. Stokes, and M. D. Wang. 2013. IACT—An interactive mHealth monitoring system to enhance psychotherapy for adolescents with sickle cell disease. *Conference Proceedings of the Annual International Conference of the IEEE Engineering in Medicine and Biology Society* 2013:2279–2282.

Cheng, E. R., M. Palta, M. Kotelchuck, J. Poehlmann, and W. P. Witt. 2014. Cognitive delay and behavior problems prior to school age. *Pediatrics* 134(3):e749.

Children's Hospital of Philadelphia, Children's Hospital Medical Center Cincinnati, Steven and Alexandra Cohen Children's Medical Center of Northwell Health, Connecticut Children's Medical Center, and Patient-Centered Outcomes Research Institute. 2018. *Community health workers and mHealth for sickle cell disease care.* https://clinicaltrials.gov/ct2/show/NCT03648710 (accessed January 23, 2020).

Clarke, J. L., S. Bourn, A. Skoufalos, E. H. Beck, and D. J. Castillo. 2017. An innovative approach to health care delivery for patients with chronic conditions. *Population Health Management* 20(1):23–30.

Clayton-Jones, D., and K. Haglund. 2016. The role of spirituality and religiosity in persons living with sickle cell disease: A review of the literature. *Journal of Holistic Nursing* 34(4):351–360.

Cline, D. M., S. Silva, C. E. Freiermuth, V. Thornton, and P. Tanabe. 2018. Emergency department (ED), ED observation, day hospital, and hospital admissions for adults with sickle cell disease. *Western Journal of Emergency Medicine* 19(2):311–318.

CMS (Centers for Medicare & Medicaid Services). 2019. *Comprehensive primary care plus.* https://innovation.cms.gov/initiatives/Comprehensive-Primary-Care-Plus (accessed January 30, 2020).

Commonwealth of Massachusetts. 2020. *Department of Public Health.* https://www.mass.gov/orgs/department-of-public-health (accessed January 17, 2020).

Costa, C. P., E. B. Thomaz, and F. Souza Sde. 2013. Association between sickle cell anemia and pulp necrosis. *Journal of Endodontics* 39(2):177–181.

Costa, C. P. S., B. T. C. Aires, E. Thomaz, and S. F. C. Souza. 2016. Dental care provided to sickle cell anemia patients stratified by age: A population-based study in northeastern Brazil. *European Journal of Dentistry* 10(3):356–360.

Cronin, R. M., J. S. Hankins, J. Byrd, B. M. Pernell, A. Kassim, P. Adams-Graves, A. A. Thompson, K. Kalinyak, M. R. DeBaun, and M. Treadwell. 2018. Modifying factors of the health belief model associated with missed clinic appointments among individuals with sickle cell disease. *Hematology (Amsterdam, Netherlands)* 23(9):683–691.

Cronin, R. M., J. S. Hankins, J. Byrd, B. M. Pernell, A. Kassim, P. Adams-Graves, A. Thompson, K. Kalinyak, M. DeBaun, and M. Treadwell. 2019. Risk factors for hospitalizations and readmissions among individuals with sickle cell disease: Results of a U.S. survey study. *Hematology (Amsterdam, Netherlands)* 24(1):189–198.

Crosby, L. E., N. E. Joffe, M. K. Irwin, H. Strong, J. Peugh, L. Shook, K. A. Kalinyak, and M. J. Mitchell. 2015. School performance and disease interference in adolescents with sickle cell disease. *Journal of Development and Physical Disabilities* 34(1):14–30.

Crowley, R., I. Wolfe, K. Lock, and M. McKee. 2011. Improving the transition between paediatric and adult healthcare: A systematic review. *Archives of Disease in Childhood* 96(6):548–553.

Dampier, C., B. Ely, D. Brodecki, and P. O'Neal. 2002a. Characteristics of pain managed at home in children and adolescents with sickle cell disease by using diary self-reports. *Journal of Pain* 3(6):461–470.

Dampier, C., E. Ely, D. Brodecki, and P. O'Neal. 2002b. Home management of pain in sickle cell disease: A daily diary study in children and adolescents. *Journal of Pediatric Hematology/Oncology* 24(8):643–647.

Darbari, D. S., P. Kple-Faget, J. Kwagyan, S. Rana, V. R. Gordeuk, and O. Castro. 2006. Circumstances of death in adult sickle cell disease patients. *American Journal of Hematology* 81(11):858–863.

Data Resource Center for Child and Adolescent Health. n.d. *About the National Survey of Children's Health.* https://www.childhealthdata.org/learn-about-the-nsch/NSCH (accessed May 15, 2019).

DeBaun, M. R., and J. Telfair. 2012. Transition and sickle cell disease. *Pediatrics* 130(5):926–935.

Douce, D. R., E. Z. Soliman, R. Naik, H. I. Hyacinth, M. Cushman, C. A. Winkler, G. Howard, E. M. Lange, L. A. Lange, M. R. Irvin, and N. A. Zakai. 2019. Association of sickle cell trait with atrial fibrillation: The REGARDS cohort. *Journal of Electrocardiology* 55:1–5.

Dunwoody, C. J., D. A. Krenzischek, C. Pasero, J. P. Rathmell, and R. C. Polomano. 2008. Assessment, physiological monitoring, and consequences of inadequately treated acute pain. *Pain Management Nursing* 9(1 Suppl):S11–S21.

ED (U.S. Department of Education). 2016. *Early intervention program for infants and toddlers with disabilities.* https://www2.ed.gov/programs/osepeip/index.html (accessed May 15, 2019).

ED. 2020. *Disability discrimination: Frequently asked questions.* https://www2.ed.gov/about/offices/list/ocr/frontpage/faq/disability.html (accessed January 17, 2020).

ED. n.d. *About IDEA (Individuals with Disabilities Act).* https://sites.ed.gov/idea/about-idea/#IDEA-Purpose (accessed May 15, 2019).

Elixhauser, A., S. R. Machlin, M. W. Zodet, F. M. Chevarley, N. Patel, M. C. McCormick, and L. Simpson. 2002. Health care for children and youth in the United States: 2001 annual report on access, utilization, quality, and expenditures. *Ambulatory Pediatrics* 2(6):419–437.

Eneriz-Wiemer, M., L. M. Sanders, D. A. Barr, and F. S. Mendoza. 2014. Parental limited English proficiency and health outcomes for children with special health care needs: A systematic review. *Academic Pediatrics* 14(2):128–136.

Epping, A. S., M. P. Myrvik, R. F. Newby, J. A. Panepinto, A. M. Brandow, and J. P. Scott. 2013. Academic attainment findings in children with sickle cell disease. *Journal of School Health* 83(8):548–553.

Epstein, K., E. Yuen, J. M. Riggio, S. K. Ballas, and S. M. Moleski. 2006. Utilization of the office, hospital and emergency department for adult sickle cell patients: A five-year study. *Journal of the National Medical Association* 98(7):1109–1113.

Fingar, K. R., P. L. Owens, L. D. Reid, K. Mistry, and M. L. Barrett. 2019. Characteristics of inpatient hospital stays involving sickle cell disease, 2000–2016. *Healthcare Cost Utilization Project Statistical Brief* 251.

Foster, C. C., R. K. Agrawal, and M. M. Davis. 2019. Home health care for children with medical complexity: Workforce gaps, policy, and future directions. *Health Affairs* 38(6):987–993.

Fowler, M. G., J. K. Whitt, R. R. Lallinger, K. B. Nash, S. S. Atkinson, R. J. Wells, and C. McMillan. 1988. Neuropsychologic and academic functioning of children with sickle cell anemia. *Journal of Developmental and Behavioral Pediatrics* 9(4):213–220.

Freedland, K. E., D. C. Mohr, K. W. Davidson, and J. E. Schwartz. 2011. Usual and unusual care: Existing practice control groups in randomized controlled trials of behavioral interventions. *Psychosomatic Medicine* 73(4):323–335.

Gaston, M. H., J. I. Verter, G. Woods, C. Pegelow, J. Kelleher, G. Presbury, H. Zarkowsky, E. Vichinsky, R. Iyer, J. S. Lobel, S. Diamond, C. T. Holbrook, F. M. Gill, K. Ritchey, and J. M. Falletta. 1986. Prophylaxis with oral penicillin in children with sickle cell anemia. *New England Journal of Medicine* 314(25):1593–1599.

Ghanem, H. M., R. M. Shaikh, A. M. Alia, A. S. Al-Zayir, and S. A. Alsirafy. 2011. Pattern of referral of noncancer patients to palliative care in the eastern province of Saudi Arabia. *Indian Journal of Palliative Care* 17(3):235–237.

Gjeilo, K. H., R. Stenseth, and P. Klepstad. 2014. Risk factors and early pharmacological interventions to prevent chronic postsurgical pain following cardiac surgery. *American Journal of Cardiovascular Drugs* 14(5):335–342.

Glassberg, J. A. 2017. Improving emergency department-based care of sickle cell pain. *Hematology: American Society of Hematology—Education Program* 2017(1):412–417.

Gomes, L. M. X., T. L. de Andrade Barbosa, E. D. S. Vieira, A. P. Caldeira, H. de Carvalho Torres, and M. B. Viana. 2015. Perception of primary care doctors and nurses about care provided to sickle cell disease patients. *Revista Brasileira de Hematologia e Hemoterapia* 37(4):247–251.

Gordon, J. B., H. H. Colby, T. Bartelt, D. Jablonski, M. L. Krauthoefer, and P. Havens. 2007. A tertiary care-primary care partnership model for medically complex and fragile children and youth with special health care needs. *Archives of Pediatrics and Adolescent Medicine* 161(10):937–944.

Gowhari, M., L. Kavoliunaite, J. Bonnye, S. Brown, R. E. Molokie, L. L. Hsu, and V. R. Gordeuk. 2015. Impact of a dedicated sickle cell acute care observation unit on rate of hospital admission for acute pain crisis. *Blood* 126(23):4584.

Green, N. S., D. Manwani, S. Matos, A. Hicks, L. Soto, Y. Castillo, K. Ireland, Y. Stennett, S. Findley, H. Jia, and A. Smaldone. 2017. Randomized feasibility trial to improve hydroxyurea adherence in youth ages 10–18 years through community health workers: The HABIT study. *Pediatric Blood & Cancer* 64(12):26689.

Griffin, A., J. Gilleland, A. Johnson, L. Cummings, T. New, T. Brailey, J. Eckman, and I. Osunkwo. 2013. Applying a developmental–ecological framework to sickle cell disease transition. *Clinical Practice in Pediatric Psychology* 1(3):250–263.

Grosse, S. D., M. S. Schechter, R. Kulkarni, M. A. Lloyd-Puryear, B. Strickland, and E. Trevathan. 2009. Models of comprehensive multidisciplinary care for individuals in the United States with genetic disorders. *Pediatrics* 123(1):407–412.

Grosse, S. D., S. L. Boulet, D. D. Amendah, and S. O. Oyeku. 2010. Administrative data sets and health services research on hemoglobinopathies: A review of the literature. *American Journal of Preventive Medicine* 38(4 Suppl):S557–S567.

Guarna, J. 2009. *Comparing ACT and CBT.* https://contextualscience.org/comparing_act_and_cbt (accessed January 23, 2020).

Hamideh, D., and O. Alvarez. 2013. Sickle cell disease related mortality in the United States (1999–2009). *Pediatric Blood & Cancer* 60(9):1482–1486.

Han, J., S. L. Saraf, L. Kavoliunaite, S. Jain, J. Hassan, L. L. Hsu, R. E. Molokie, V. R. Gordeuk, and M. Gowhari. 2018. Program expansion of a day hospital dedicated to manage sickle cell pain. *American Journal of Hematology* 93(1):E20–E21.

Hassell, K. L. 2010. Population estimates of sickle cell disease in the U.S. *American Journal of Preventive Medicine* 38(4 Suppl):S512–S521.

Haywood, C., Jr., M. C. Beach, S. Lanzkron, J. J. Strouse, R. Wilson, H. Park, C. Witkop, E. B. Bass, and J. B. Segal. 2009. A systematic review of barriers and interventions to improve appropriate use of therapies for sickle cell disease. *Journal of the National Medical Association* 101(10):1022–1033.

Heslin, K. C., P. L. Owens, L. A. Simpson, J. P. Guevara, and M. C. McCormick. 2018. Annual report on health care for children and youth in the United States: Focus on 30-day unplanned inpatient readmissions, 2009 to 2014. *Academic Pediatrics* 18(8):857–872.

Ho, T. N., A. A. Shmelev, A. Joshi, and N. Ho. 2019. Trends in hospitalizations for sickle cell disease related-complications in USA 2004–2012. *Journal of Hematology* 8(1):11–16.

Howard University. n.d. *About the Center For Sickle Cell Disease.* http://www.sicklecell.howard.edu/about.htm (accessed January 29, 2020).

HRSA (Health Resources and Services Administration). 2019. *Children with special health care needs.* https://mchb.hrsa.gov/maternal-child-health-topics/children-and-youth-special-health-needs (accessed May 1, 2019).

HRSA. n.d. *Health center program terms and definitions.* https://www.hrsa.gov/sites/default/files/grants/apply/assistance/Buckets/definitions.pdf (accessed January 23, 2020).

Huffman, L. C., G. A. Brat, L. J. Chamberlain, and P. H. Wise. 2010. Impact of managed care on publicly insured children with special health care needs. *Academic Pediatrics* 10(1):48–55.

Inoue, S., I. Khan, R. Mushtaq, S. R. Sanikommu, C. Mbeumo, J. LaChance, and M. Roebuck. 2016. Pain management trend of vaso-occulsive crisis (VOC) at a community hospital emergency department (ED) for patients with sickle cell disease. *Annals of Hematology* 95(2):221–225.

IOM (Institute of Medicine). 1996. *Primary care: America's health in a new era.* Washington, DC: National Academy Press.

IOM. 2001a. *Coverage matters: Insurance and health care.* Washington, DC: National Academy Press.

IOM. 2001b. *Crossing the quality chasm: A new health system for the 21st century.* Washington, DC: National Academy Press.

IOM. 2002a. *Health insurance is a family matter.* Washington, DC: The National Academies Press.

IOM. 2002b. *Care without coverage: Too little, too late.* Washington, DC: The National Academies Press.

IOM. 2003a. *Hidden costs, values lost: Uninsurance in America.* Washington, DC: The National Academies Press.

IOM. 2003b. *A shared destiny: Community effects of uninsurance.* Washington, DC: The National Academies Press.

IOM. 2003c. *The future of the public's health in the 21st century.* Washington, DC: The National Academies Press.

IOM. 2004. *Insuring America's health: Principles and recommendations.* Washington, DC: The National Academies Press.

IOM. 2009. *America's uninsured crisis: Consequences for health and health care.* Washington, DC: The National Academies Press.

Issom, D. Z., A. Zosso, F. Ehrler, R. Wipfli, C. Lovis, and S. Koch. 2015. Exploring the challenges and opportunities of eHealth tools for patients with sickle cell disease. *Studies in Health Technology and Informatics* 216:898.

JAN (Job Accommodation Network). 2019. *Accommodation and compliance series: Employees with sickle cell anemia.* Morgantown, WV: Job Accommodation Network.

Jenerette, C. M., C. A. Brewer, and K. I. Ataga. 2014. Care seeking for pain in young adults with sickle cell disease. *Pain Management Nursing* 15(1):324–330.

Johnston, E. E., O. O. Adesina, E. Alvarez, H. Amato, S. Paulukonis, A. Nichols, L. J. Chamberlain, and S. Bhatia. 2019. Acute care utilization at end of life in sickle cell disease: Highlighting the need for a palliative approach. *Journal of Palliative Medicine* 23(1):24–32.

Jones, M. R., T. J. Hooper, C. Cuomo, G. Crouch, T. Hickam, L. Lestishock, S. Mennito, and P. H. White. 2019. Evaluation of a health care transition improvement process in seven large health care systems. *Journal of Pediatric Nursing* 47:44–50.

Karkoska, K., A. Appiah-Kubi, J. Rocker, G. Stoffels, and B. Aygun. 2019. Management of vaso-occlusive episodes in the day hospital decreases admissions in children with sickle cell disease. *British Journal of Haematology* 186(6):855–860.

Kauf, T. L., T. D. Coates, L. Huazhi, N. Mody-Patel, and A. G. Hartzema. 2009. The cost of health care for children and adults with sickle cell disease. *American Journal of Hematology* 84(6):323–327.

Kavanagh, P. L., P. G. Sprinz, T. L. Wolfgang, K. Killius, M. Champigny, A. Sobota, D. Dorfman, K. Barry, R. Miner, and J. M. Moses. 2015. Improving the management of vaso-occlusive episodes in the pediatric emergency department. *Pediatrics* 136(4):e1016.

KFF (Kaiser Family Foundation). 2019. *Nearly 54 million Americans have pre-existing conditions that would make them uninsurable in the individual market without the ACA.* https://www.kff.org/health-reform/press-release/nearly-54-million-americans-have-pre-existing-conditions-that-would-make-them-uninsurable-in-the-individual-market-without-the-aca (accessed August 28, 2020).

Kimmel, A. D., S. P. Masiano, R. S. Bono, E. G. Martin, F. Z. Belgrave, A. A. Adimora, B. Dahman, H. Galadima, and L. M. Sabik. 2018. Structural barriers to comprehensive, coordinated HIV care: Geographic accessibility in the U.S. South. *AIDS Care* 30(11):1459–1468.

King, A., S. Herron, R. McKinstry, S. Bacak, M. Armstrong, D. White, and M. DeBaun. 2006. A multidisciplinary health care team's efforts to improve educational attainment in children with sickle-cell anemia and cerebral infarcts. *Journal of School Health* 76(1):33–37.

Klabunde, C. N., P. K. Han, C. C. Earle, T. Smith, J. Z. Ayanian, R. Lee, A. Ambs, J. H. Rowland, and A. L. Potosky. 2013. Physician roles in the cancer-related follow-up care of cancer survivors. *Family Medicine* 45(7):463–474.

Kuhlthau, K. A., S. Bloom, J. Van Cleave, A. A. Knapp, D. Romm, K. Klatka, C. J. Homer, P. W. Newacheck, and J. M. Perrin. 2011. Evidence for family-centered care for children with special health care needs: A systematic review. *Academic Pediatrics* 11(2):136–143.

Ladd, R. J., C. R. Valrie, and C. M. Walcott. 2014. Risk and resilience factors for grade retention in youth with sickle cell disease. *Pediatric Blood & Cancer* 61(7):1252–1256.

Lanzkron, S., C. P. Carroll, and C. Haywood, Jr. 2010. The burden of emergency department use for sickle-cell disease: An analysis of the National Emergency Department Sample Database. *American Journal of Hematology* 85(10):797–799.

Lanzkron, S., C. P. Carroll, and C. Haywood, Jr. 2013. Mortality rates and age at death from sickle cell disease: U.S., 1979–2005. *Public Health Reports* 128(2):110–116.

Lanzkron, S., C. P. Carroll, P. Hill, M. David, N. Paul, and C. Haywood, Jr. 2015. Impact of a dedicated infusion clinic for acute management of adults with sickle cell pain crisis. *American Journal of Hematology* 90(5):376–380.

Lanzkron, S., J. Little, J. Field, J. R. Shows, H. Wang, R. Seufert, J. Brooks, R. Varadhan, C. Haywood, Jr., M. Saheed, C. Y. Huang, B. Griffin, S. Frymark, A. Piehet, D. Robertson, M. Proudford, A. Kincaid, C. Green, L. Burgess, M. Wallace, and J. Segal. 2018a. Increased acute care utilization in a prospective cohort of adults with sickle cell disease. *Blood Advances* 2(18):2412–2417.

Lanzkron, S., G. S. Sawicki, K. L. Hassell, M. W. Konstan, R. I. Liem, and S. A. McColley. 2018b. Transition to adulthood and adult health care for patients with sickle cell disease or cystic fibrosis: Current practices and research priorities. *Journal of Clinical and Translational Science* 2(5):334–342.

Laurence, B., D. George, D. Woods, A. Shosanya, R. V. Katz, S. Lanzkron, M. Diener-West, and N. Powe. 2006. The association between sickle cell disease and dental caries in African Americans. *Special Care in Dentistry* 26(3):95–100.

Laurence, B., C. Haywood, Jr., and S. Lanzkron. 2013. Dental infections increase the likelihood of hospital admissions among adult patients with sickle cell disease. *Community Dental Health Journal* 30(3):168–172.

Lebrun-Harris, L. A., M. A. McManus, S. M. Ilango, M. Cyr, S. B. McLellan, M. Y. Mann, and P. H. White. 2018. Transition planning among U.S. youth with and without special health care needs. *Pediatrics* 142(4):e20180194.

Lee, L., R. Askew, J. Walker, J. Stephen, and A. Robertson-Artwork. 2012. Adults with sickle cell disease: An interdisciplinary approach to home care and self-care management with a case study. *Home Healthcare Nurse* 30(3):172–183; quiz 183–185.

Leschke, J., J. A. Panepinto, M. Nimmer, R. G. Hoffmann, K. Yan, and D. C. Brousseau. 2012. Outpatient follow-up and rehospitalizations for sickle cell disease patients. *Pediatric Blood & Cancer* 58(3):406–409.

Lester, H. 2005. Shared care for people with mental illness: A GP's perspective. *Advances in Psychiatric Treatment* 1(1):133–141.

Lichstein, J. C., R. M. Ghandour, and M. Y. Mann. 2018. Access to the medical home among children with and without special health care needs. *Pediatrics* 142(6):e20181795.

Liem, R. I., C. O'Suoji, P. S. Kingsberry, S. A. Pelligra, S. Kwon, M. Mason, and A. A. Thompson. 2014. Access to patient-centered medical homes in children with sickle cell disease. *Maternal and Child Health Journal* 18(8):1854–1862.

Linebaugh, M. n.d. *Vocational rehabilitation for individuals with disabilities.* https://www.nolo.com/legal-encyclopedia/vocational-rehabilitation-individuals-with-disabilities.html (accessed May 15, 2019).

Litt, J. S., and M. C. McCormick. 2015. Care coordination, the family-centered medical home, and functional disability among children with special health care needs. *Academic Pediatrics* 15(2):185–190.

Litt, J. S., M. M. Glymour, P. Hauser-Cram, T. Hehir, and M. C. McCormick. 2018. Early intervention services improve school-age functional outcome among neonatal intensive care unit graduates. *Academic Pediatrics* 18(4):468–474.

Logan, D. R. 2019. Transition from hospital to home: The role of the nurse case manager in promoting medication adherence in the Medicare population. *Creative Nursing* 25(2):126–132.

Luna, A., M. Gomes, A. Granville-Garcia, and V. Menezes. 2018. Perception of treatment needs and use of dental services for children and adolescents with sickle cell disease. *Oral Health Preventive Dentistry* 16(1):51–57.

Lunyera, J., C. Jonassaint, J. Jonassaint, and N. Shah. 2017. Attitudes of primary care physicians toward sickle cell disease care, guidelines, and comanaging hydroxyurea with a specialist. *Journal of Primary Care & Community Health* 8(1):37–40.

Lyon, M., L. C. Sturgis, A. Kutlar, M. Gibson, R. Lottenberg, and R. Gibson. 2014. Admission rates for an observation unit clinical pathway for the treatment of uncomplicated sickle cell disease vasoocclusive crisis. *Annals of Emergency Medicine* 64(4, Suppl):S65–S66.

Mainous, A. G., 3rd, J. M. Gill, and P. J. Carek. 2004. Elevated serum transferrin saturation and mortality. *Annals of Family Medicine* 2(2):133–138.

Mainous, A. G., 3rd, R. J. Tanner, C. A. Harle, R. Baker, N. K. Shokar, and M. M. Hulihan. 2015. Attitudes toward management of sickle cell disease and its complications: A national survey of academic family physicians. *Anemia* 2015:853835.

Mainous, A. G., 3rd, P. J. Carek, K. Lynch, R. J. Tanner, M. M. Hulihan, J. Baskin, and T. D. Coates. 2018. Effectiveness of clinical decision support based intervention in the improvement of care for adult sickle cell disease patients in primary care. *Journal of the American Board of Family Medicine* 31(5):812–816.

Mainous, A. G., 3rd, B. Rooks, R. J. Tanner, P. J. Carek, V. Black, and T. D. Coates. 2019. Shared care for adults with sickle cell disease: An analysis of care from eight health systems. *Journal of Clinical Medicine* 8(8):1154.

Mallet, C., A. Abitan, C. Vidal, L. Holvoet, K. Mazda, A. L. Simon, and B. Ilharreborde. 2018. Management of osteonecrosis of the femoral head in children with sickle cell disease: Results of conservative and operative treatments at skeletal maturity. *Journal of Children's Orthopaedics* 12(1):47–54.

Martin, B. M., L. N. Thaniel, B. J. Speller-Brown, and D. S. Darbari. 2018. Comprehensive infant clinic for sickle cell disease: Outcomes and parental perspective. *Journal of Pediatric Health Care* 32(5):485–489.

Matthie, N., and C. Jenerette. 2017. Understanding the self-management practices of young adults with sickle cell disease. *Journal of Sickle Cell Disease and Hemoglobinopathies* 2017:76–87.

McClish, D. K., J. L. Levenson, L. T. Penberthy, S. D. Roseff, V. E. Bovbjerg, J. D. Roberts, I. P. Aisiku, and W. R. Smith. 2006. Gender differences in pain and healthcare utilization for adult sickle cell patients: The PiSCES project. *Journal of Women's Health (Larchmt)* 15(2):146–154.

McClure, E., J. Ng, K. Vitzthum, and R. Rudd. 2016. A mismatch between patient education materials about sickle cell disease and the literacy level of their intended audience. *Preventing Chronic Disease* 13:E64.

McManus, B., M. C. McCormick, D. Acevedo-Garcia, M. Ganz, and P. Hauser-Cram. 2009. The effect of state early intervention eligibility policy on participation among a cohort of young CSHCN. *Pediatrics* 124(Suppl 4):S368–S374.

McManus, M., P. White, A. Barbour, B. Downing, K. Hawkins, N. Quion, L. Tuchman, W. C. Cooley, and J. W. McAllister. 2015a. Pediatric to adult transition: A quality improvement model for primary care. *Journal of Adolescent Health* 56(1):73–78.

McManus, M., P. White, R. Pirtle, C. Hancock, M. Ablan, and R. Corona-Parra. 2015b. Incorporating the six core elements of health care transition into a Medicaid managed care plan: Lessons learned from a pilot project. *Journal of Pediatric Nursing* 30(5):700–713.

McManus, B. M., Z. Richardson, M. Schenkman, N. Murphy, and E. H. Morrato. 2019. Timing and intensity of early intervention service use and outcomes among a safety-net population of children. *JAMA Network Open* 2(1):e187529.

McPherson, M., P. Arango, H. Fox, C. Lauver, M. McManus, P. W. Newacheck, J. M. Perrin, J. P. Shonkoff, and B. Strickland. 1998. A new definition of children with special health care needs. *Pediatrics* 102(1 Pt 1):137–140.

McWilliams, A., J. Roberge, W. E. Anderson, C. G. Moore, W. Rossman, S. Murphy, S. McCall, R. Brown, S. Carpenter, S. Rissmiller, and S. Furney. 2019. Aiming to Improve Readmissions Through Integrated Hospital Transitions (AIRTIGHT): A pragmatic randomized controlled trial. *Journal of General Internal Medicine* 34(1):58–64.

Mehta, S. R., A. Afenyi-Annan, P. J. Byrns, and R. Lottenberg. 2006. Opportunities to improve outcomes in sickle cell disease. *American Family Physician* 74(2):303–310.

Monaghan, M., M. Hilliard, R. Sweenie, and K. Riekert. 2013. Transition readiness in adolescents and emerging adults with diabetes: The role of patient–provider communication. *Current Diabetes Reports* 13(6):900–908.

Mongiovi, J., Z. Shi, and H. Greenlee. 2016. Complementary and alternative medicine use and absenteeism among individuals with chronic disease. *BMC Complementary and Alternative Medicine* 16:248.

Mulimani, P., S. K. Ballas, A. B. Abas, and L. Karanth. 2016. Treatment of dental complications in sickle cell disease. *Cochrane Database of Systematic Reviews* 4:CD011633.

Myrvik, M. P., L. M. Burks, R. G. Hoffman, M. Dasgupta, and J. A. Panepinto. 2013. Mental health disorders influence admission rates for pain in children with sickle cell disease. *Pediatric Blood & Cancer* 60(7):1211–1214.

Naavaal, S., L. K. Barker, and S. O. Griffin. 2017. The effect of health and dental insurance on U.S. children's dental care utilization for urgent and non-urgent dental problems—2008. *Journal of Public Health Dentistry* 77(1):54–62.

Naik, R. P., K. Smith-Whitley, K. L. Hassell, N. I. Umeh, M. de Montalembert, P. Sahota, C. Haywood, Jr., J. Jenkins, M. A. Lloyd-Puryear, C. H. Joiner, V. L. Bonham, and G. J. Kato. 2018. Clinical outcomes associated with sickle cell trait: A systematic review. *Annals of Internal Medicine* 169(9):619–627.

NASEM (National Academies of Sciences, Engineering, and Medicine). 2017. *The promise of assistive technology to enhance activity and work participation.* Washington, DC: The National Academies Press.

NHF (National Hemophilia Foundation). 2016. National Hemophilia Foundation–McMaster University guideline on care models for hemophilia management. www.hemophilia.org/researchers-healthcare-providers/guideline-on-care-models-for-hemophilia-management (accessed March 11, 2020).

NHLBI (National Heart, Lung, and Blood Institute). 2006. *Comprehensive sickle cell centers (U54).* https://grants.nih.gov/grants/guide/rfa-files/rfa-hl-06-008.html (accessed January 30, 2020).

NHLBI. 2008. *Report of the National Heart, Lung, and Blood Advisory Council subcommittee review of the NHLBI sickle cell disease program.* https://www.nhlbi.nih.gov/events/2008/report-national-heart-lung-and-blood-advisory-council-subcommittee-review-nhlbi-sickle (accessed June 18, 2019).

NHLBI. 2014. *Evidence-based management of sickle cell disease: Expert panel report.* https://www.nhlbi.nih.gov/sites/default/files/media/docs/sickle-cell-disease-report%20020816_0.pdf (accessed June 18, 2019).

Office of Special Education Programs. 2011. Part C of the Individuals with Disabilities Education Act: Final regulations: Nonregulatory guidance. Place Published: U.S. Department of Education. https://sites.ed.gov/idea/files/Final_Regulations_Part_C_Guidance.pdf (accessed November 19, 2019).

Okam, M. M., S. Shaykevich, B. L. Ebert, A. M. Zaslavsky, and J. Z. Ayanian. 2014. National trends in hospitalizations for sickle cell disease in the United States following the FDA approval of hydroxyurea, 1998–2008. *Medical Care* 52(7):612–618.

Okochi, J., M. Tsiagbe, W. Joseph, J. James, K. Osmond-Joseph, P. Telfer, F. Barroso, and B. Kaya. 2019. Peer to peer mentoring for patients with sickle cell disease—Interim analysis of results from a pilot programme in east London. *British Journal of Haematology* 185(S1):116.

Okumura, M. J., M. Heisler, M. M. Davis, M. D. Cabana, S. Demonner, and E. A. Kerr. 2008. Comfort of general internists and general pediatricians in providing care for young adults with chronic illnesses of childhood. *Journal of General Internal Medicine* 23(10):1621–1627.

Osunkwo, I., and PCORI (Patient-Centered Outcomes Research Institute). 2018. *LCI-HEM-SCD-ST3P-UP-001: The sickle cell Trevor Thompson transition project (STt3P-UP study) (ST3P-UP).* https://clinicaltrials.gov/ct2/show/NCT03593395 (accessed January 23, 2020).

Oyeku, S. O., C. J. Wang, R. Scoville, R. Vanderkruik, E. Clermont, M. E. McPherson, W. G. Adams, and C. J. Homer. 2012. Hemoglobinopathy learning collaborative: Using quality improvement (QI) to achieve equity in health care quality, coordination, and outcomes for sickle cell disease. *Journal of Health Care for the Poor and Underserved* 23(3 Suppl):34–48.

Paulukonis, S. T., J. R. Eckman, A. B. Snyder, W. Hagar, L. B. Feuchtbaum, M. Zhou, A. M. Grant, and M. M. Hulihan. 2016. Defining sickle cell disease mortality using a population-based surveillance system, 2004 through 2008. *Public Health Reports* 131(2):367–375.

Paulukonis, S. T., L. B. Feuchtbaum, T. D. Coates, L. D. Neumayr, M. J. Treadwell, E. P. Vichinsky, and M. M. Hulihan. 2017. Emergency department utilization by Californians with sickle cell disease, 2005–2014. *Pediatric Blood & Cancer* 64(6).

PCORI (Patient-Centered Outcomes Research Institute). 2020. *Comparing transitional care for teens and young adults with sickle cell disease with and without peer mentoring* https://www.pcori.org/research-results/2017/comparing-transitional-care-teens-and-young-adults-sickle-cell-disease-and (accessed January 16, 2020).

Pecker, L. H., and R. P. Naik. 2018. The current state of sickle cell trait: Implications for reproductive and genetic counseling. *Hematology: American Society of Hematology— Education Program* 2018(1):474–481.

Perry, E. L., P. A. Carter, H. A. Becker, A. A. Garcia, M. Mackert, and K. E. Johnson. 2017. Health literacy in adolescents with sickle cell disease. *Journal of Pediatric Nursing* 36:191–196.

Peterson, L. E., B. Blackburn, R. L. Phillips, Jr., and A. G. Mainous, 3rd. 2015. Family medicine department chairs' opinions regarding scope of practice. *Academic Medicine* 90(12):1691–1697.

Platt, A., J. R. Eckman, J. Beasley, and G. Miller. 2002. Treating sickle cell pain: An update from the Georgia Comprehensive Sickle Cell Center. *Journal of Emergency Nursing* 28(4):297–303.

Polomano, R. C., C. J. Dunwoody, D. A. Krenzischek, and J. P. Rathmell. 2008. Perspective on pain management in the 21st century. *Pain Management Nursing* 9(1 Suppl):S3–S10.

Pordes, E., J. Gordon, L. M. Sanders, and E. Cohen. 2018. Models of care delivery for children with medical complexity. *Pediatrics* 141(Suppl 3):S212–S223.

Porterfield, S. L., and L. DeRigne. 2011. Medical home and out-of-pocket medical costs for children with special health care needs. *Pediatrics* 128(5):892–900.

Prieto-Centurion, V., S. Basu, N. Bracken, E. Calhoun, C. Dickens, R. J. DiDomenico, R. Gallardo, V. Gordeuk, M. Gutierrez-Kapheim, L. L. Hsu, S. Illendula, M. Joo, U. Kazmi, A. Mutso, A. S. Pickard, B. Pittendrigh, J. L. Sullivan, M. Williams, and J. A. Krishnan. 2019. Design of the patient navigator to reduce readmissions (PArTNER) study: A pragmatic clinical effectiveness trial. *Contemporary Clinical Trials Communications* 15:100420.

Project ECHO. 2020. *Model.* https://echo.unm.edu/about-echo/model (accessed January 30, 2020).

Quinn, C. T., Z. R. Rogers, T. L. McCavit, and G. R. Buchanan. 2010. Improved survival of children and adolescents with sickle cell disease. *Blood* 115(17):3447–3452.

Raphael, J. L., and S. O. Oyeku. 2013. Sickle cell disease pain management and the medical home. *Hematology: American Society of Hematology—Education Program* 2013:433–438.

Raphael, J. L., A. Kamdar, T. Wang, H. Liu, D. H. Mahoney, and B. U. Mueller. 2008. Day hospital versus inpatient management of uncomplicated vaso-occlusive crises in children with sickle cell disease. *Pediatric Blood & Cancer* 51(3):398–401.

Raphael, J. L., C. L. Dietrich, D. Whitmire, D. H. Mahoney, B. U. Mueller, and A. P. Giardino. 2009. Healthcare utilization and expenditures for low income children with sickle cell disease. *Pediatric Blood & Cancer* 52(2):263–267.

Raphael, J. L., T. L. Rattler, M. A. Kowalkowski, D. C. Brousseau, B. U. Mueller, and T. P. Giordano. 2013a. Association of care in a medical home and health care utilization among children with sickle cell disease. *Journal of the National Medical Association* 105(2):157–165.

Raphael, J. L., T. L. Rattler, M. A. Kowalkowski, B. U. Mueller, and T. P. Giordano. 2013b. The medical home experience among children with sickle cell disease. *Pediatric Blood & Cancer* 60(2):275–280.

Rattler, T. L., A. M. Walder, H. Feng, and J. L. Raphael. 2016. Care coordination for children with sickle cell disease: A longitudinal study of parent perspectives and acute care utilization. *American Journal of Preventive Medicine* 51(1 Suppl 1):S55–S61.

Ray, K. N., and J. M. Kahn. 2020. Connected subspecialty care: Applying telehealth strategies to specific referral barriers. *Academic Pediatrics* 20(1):16–22.

Ray, K. N., D. L. Bogen, M. Bertolet, C. B. Forrest, and A. Mehrotra. 2014. Supply and utilization of pediatric subspecialists in the United States. *Pediatrics* 133(6):1061–1069.

Reeves, S. L., B. Madden, G. L. Freed, and K. J. Dombkowski. 2016. Transcranial Doppler screening among children and adolescents with sickle cell anemia. *JAMA Pediatrics* 170(6):550–556.

Rich, E., D. Lipson, J. Libersky, and M. Parchman. 2012. *Coordinating care for adults with complex care needs in the patient-centered medical home: Challenges and solutions.* https://pcmh.ahrq.gov/sites/default/files/attachments/coordinating-care-for-adults-with-complex-care-needs-white-paper.pdf (accessed February 3, 2020).

Richardson, Z. S., M. A. Khetani, E. Scully, J. Dooling-Litfin, N. J. Murphy, and B. M. McManus. 2019. Social and functional characteristics of receipt and service use intensity of core early intervention services. *Academic Pediatrics* 19(7):722–732.

Ross, S. M., E. Smit, E. Twardzik, S. W. Logan, and B. M. McManus. 2018. Patient-centered medical home and receipt of Part C early intervention among young CSHCN and developmental disabilities versus delays: NS-CSHCN 2009–2010. *Maternal and Child Health Journal* 22(10):1451–1461.

Rushton, S., D. Murray, C. Talley, S. Boyd, K. Eason, M. Earls, and P. Tanabe. 2019. Implementation of an emergency department screening and care management referral process for patients with sickle cell disease. *Professional Case Management* 24(5):240–248.

Salgia, R. J., P. B. Mullan, H. McCurdy, A. Sales, R. H. Moseley, and G. L. Su. 2014. The educational impact of the specialty care access network-extension of community healthcare outcomes program. *Telemedicine Journal and e-Health* 20(11):1004–1008.

Scherpbier-de Haan, N. D., G. M. Vervoort, C. van Weel, J. C. Braspenning, J. Mulder, J. F. Wetzels, and W. J. de Grauw. 2013. Effect of shared care on blood pressure in patients with chronic kidney disease: A cluster randomised controlled trial. *British Journal of General Practice* 63(617):e798–e806.

Shen, C., U. Sambamoorthi, and G. Rust. 2008. Co-occurring mental illness and health care utilization and expenditures in adults with obesity and chronic physical illness. *Disease Management* 11(3):153–160.

Shook, L. M., C. B. Farrell, K. A. Kalinyak, S. C. Nelson, B. M. Hardesty, A. G. Rampersad, K. L. Saving, W. J. Whitten-Shurney, J. A. Panepinto, R. E. Ware, and L. E. Crosby. 2016. Translating sickle cell guidelines into practice for primary care providers with Project ECHO. *Medical Education Online* 21:33616.

Simpson, G. G., H. R. Hahn, A. A. Powel, R. R. Leverence, L. A. Morris, L. G. Thompson, M. S. Zumberg, D. J. Borde, J. A. Tyndall, J. J. Shuster, D. M. Yealy, and B. R. Allen. 2017. A patient-centered emergency department management strategy for sickle-cell disease super-utilizers. *Western Journal of Emergency Medicine* 18(3):335–339.

Smith, S. M., S. Allwright, and T. O'Dowd. 2008a. Does sharing care across the primary-specialty interface improve outcomes in chronic disease? A systematic review. *American Journal of Managed Care* 14(4):213–224.

Smith, W. R., L. T. Penberthy, V. E. Bovbjerg, D. K. McClish, J. D. Roberts, B. Dahman, I. P. Aisiku, J. L. Levenson, and S. D. Roseff. 2008b. Daily assessment of pain in adults with sickle cell disease. *Annals of Internal Medicine* 148(2):94–101.

Smith-Whitley, K. 2014. Reproductive issues in sickle cell disease. *Blood* 124(24):3538–3543.

Sobota, A. E., E. Umeh, and J. W. Mack. 2015. Young adult perspectives on a successful transition from pediatric to adult care in sickle cell disease. *International Journal of Hematology Research* 2(1):17–24.

Steiner, B. D., A. C. Denham, E. Ashkin, W. P. Newton, T. Wroth, and L. A. Dobson, Jr. 2008. Community Care of North Carolina: Improving care through community health networks. *Annals of Family Medicine* 6(4):361–367.

Stewart, R. W., L. N. Whiteman, J. J. Strouse, C. P. Carroll, and S. Lanzkron. 2016. Improving inpatient care for individuals with sickle cell disease using the Project ECHO model. *Southern Medical Journal* 109(9):568–569.

Stoffman, J., N. G. Andersson, B. Branchford, K. Batt, R. D'Orion, C. Escuriola Ettinghausen, D. P. Hart, V. Jimenez Yuste, K. Kavakli, M. E. Mauso, K. Nogami, C. Ramirez, and R. Wu. 2019. Common themes and challenges in hemophilia care: A multinational perspective. *Hematology* 24(1):39–48.

Stuart, A., and M. R. Smith. 2019. The emergence and prevalence of hearing loss in children with homozygous sickle cell disease. *International Journal of Pediatric Otorhinolaryngology* 123:69–74.

Swanson, M. E., S. D. Grosse, and R. Kulkarni. 2011. Disability among individuals with sickle cell disease: Literature review from a public health perspective. *American Journal of Preventive Medicine* 41(6 Suppl 4):S390–S397.

Syed, S. T., B. S. Gerber, and L. K. Sharp. 2013. Traveling towards disease: Transportation barriers to health care access. *Journal of Community Health* 38(5):976–993.

Tanabe, P., C. E. Freiermuth, D. M. Cline, and S. Silva. 2017. A prospective emergency department quality improvement project to improve the treatment of vaso-occlusive crisis in sickle cell disease: Lessons learned. *Joint Commission Journal on Quality and Patient Safety* 43(3):116–126.

Tarantino, M. D., and V. K. Pindolia. 2017. Hemophilia management via data collection and reporting: Initial findings from the Comprehensive Care Sustainability Collaborative. *Journal of Managed Care and Specialty Pharmacy* 23(1):51–56.

Telfer, P., and B. Kaya. 2017. Optimizing the care model for an uncomplicated acute pain episode in sickle cell disease. *Hematology: American Society of Hematology—Education Program* 2017(1):525–533.

Therrell, B. L., Jr., M. A. Lloyd-Puryear, J. R. Eckman, and M. Y. Mann. 2015. Newborn screening for sickle cell diseases in the United States: A review of data spanning 2 decades. *Seminars in Perinatology* 39(3):238–251.

Thompson, W. E., and I. Eriator. 2014. Pain control in sickle cell disease patients: Use of complementary and alternative medicine. *Pain Medicine* 15(2):241–246.

Treadwell, M., J. Telfair, R. W. Gibson, S. Johnson, and I. Osunkwo. 2011. Transition from pediatric to adult care in sickle cell disease: Establishing evidence-based practice and directions for research. *American Journal of Hematology* 86(1):116–120.

Treadwell, M., S. Johnson, I. Sisler, M. Bitsko, G. Gildengorin, R. Medina, F. Barreda, K. Major, J. Telfair, and W. R. Smith. 2016. Self-efficacy and readiness for transition from pediatric to adult care in sickle cell disease. *International Journal of Adolescent Medicine and Health* 28(4):381–388.

Walsh, K. E., S. L. Cutrona, P. L. Kavanagh, L. E. Crosby, C. Malone, K. Lobner, and D. G. Bundy. 2014. Medication adherence among pediatric patients with sickle cell disease: A systematic review. *Pediatrics* 134(6):1175–1183.

White, P. H., and W. C. Cooley. 2018. Supporting the health care transition from adolescence to adulthood in the medical home. *Pediatrics* 142(5):e20182587.

Whiteman, L. N., C. Haywood, Jr., S. Lanzkron, J. J. Strouse, L. Feldman, and R. W. Stewart. 2015. Primary care providers' comfort levels in caring for patients with sickle cell disease. *Southern Medical Journal* 108(9):531–536.

Whiteman, L. N., C. Haywood, Jr., S. Lanzkron, J. J. Strouse, A. H. Batchelor, A. Schwartz, and R. W. Stewart. 2016. Effect of free dental services on individuals with sickle cell disease. *Southern Medical Journal* 109(9):576–578.

Wiler, J. L., M. A. Ross, and A. A. Ginde. 2011. National study of emergency department observation services. *Academic Emergency Medicine* 18(9):959–965.

Wilkie, D. J., B. Johnson, A. K. Mack, R. Labotka, and R. E. Molokie. 2010. Sickle cell disease: An opportunity for palliative care across the life span. *Nursing Clinics of North America* 45(3):375–397.

Williams, H., R. N. S. Silva, D. Cline, C. Freiermuth, and P. Tanabe. 2018. Social and behavioral factors in sickle cell disease: Employment predicts decreased health care utilization. *Journal of Health Care for the Poor and Underserved* 29(2):814–829.

Wood, D., N. Winterbauer, P. Sloyer, E. Jobli, T. Hou, Q. McCaskill, and W. C. Livingood. 2009. A longitudinal study of a pediatric practice-based versus an agency-based model of care coordination for children and youth with special health care needs. *Maternal and Child Health Journal* 13(5):667–676.

Woods, K., A. Kutlar, R. K. Grigsby, L. Adams, and M. E. Stachura. 1998. Primary-care delivery for sickle cell patients in rural Georgia using telemedicine. *Telemedicine Journal* 4(4):353–361.

Yale, S. H., N. Nagib, and T. Guthrie. 2000. Approach to the vaso-occlusive crisis in adults with sickle cell disease. *American Family Physician* 61(5):1349–1356.

Yang, S. Y., R. Moss-Morris, and L. M. McCracken. 2017. iACT-CEL: A feasibility trial of a face-to-face and Internet-based acceptance and commitment therapy intervention for chronic pain in Singapore. *Pain Research and Treatment* 2017:6916915.

Yee, M. E. M., E. K. Meyer, R. M. Fasano, P. A. Lane, C. D. Josephson, and A. G. Brega. 2019. Health literacy and knowledge of chronic transfusion therapy in adolescents with sickle cell disease and caregivers. *Pediatric Blood & Cancer* 66(7):e27733.

Young, C. H. T., N. Santesso, M. Pai, C. Kessler, N. S. Key, M. Makris, T. Navarro-Ruan, J. M. Soucie, H. J. Schunemann, and A. Iorio. 2016. Care models in the management of haemophilia: A systematic review. *Haemophilia* 22(Suppl 3):31–40.

Yusuf, H. R., H. K. Atrash, S. D. Grosse, C. S. Parker, and A. M. Grant. 2010. Emergency department visits made by patients with sickle cell disease: A descriptive study, 1999-2007. *American Journal of Preventive Medicine* 38(4 Suppl):S536–S541.

Zhou, C., A. Crawford, E. Serhal, P. Kurdyak, and S. Sockalingam. 2016. The impact of Project ECHO on participant and patient outcomes: A systematic review. *Academic Medicine* 91(10):1439–1461.

6

Delivering High-Quality
Sickle Cell Disease Care with a
Prepared Workforce

*There needs to be a concise way of capturing that information
and understanding what the implications are of different
treatments and different delivery systems on different people,
capture that somehow, and be able to feed that back to
the clinician and the patient that are in the midst of trying
to make a really important treatment decision.*

—Sara van G. (Open Session Panelist)

Chapter Summary

- Providing high-quality care for sickle cell disease (SCD) requires identifying evidence-based services for individuals with SCD and the availability of a trained and willing multidisciplinary workforce.
- More evidence is needed to establish clinical guidelines and quality indicators for the management of SCD.
- Adherence to the two National Quality Forum–endorsed measures (i.e., high-quality, evidence-based measures) is poor.
- There are significant workforce training needs to achieve high-quality care in SCD.
- Although a multidisciplinary team approach is recommended, there is little or no evidence that this is occurring consistently across the institutions providing care for individuals living with SCD.

High-quality care for individuals living with sickle cell disease (SCD) should be evidence-based and accompanied by clear, measurable metrics that assess quality and improve performance. Care should be delivered by a well-trained workforce that is willing and able to provide the necessary services. Chapter 4 discussed the myriad acute and chronic complications that individuals living with SCD experience, and Chapter 5 detailed the comprehensive health care and health-related services that individuals living with SCD and sickle cell trait (SCT) need for optimal health outcomes. This chapter examines the state of evidence associated with clinical practice guidelines for managing the care of children and adults with SCD and the current state of health system performance assessment in delivering those services. This chapter also discusses strategies for addressing the obstacles to developing a cadre of health professionals who are prepared to deliver high-quality care. As discussed in Chapter 5, the committee recommends the use of a multidisciplinary team of providers to address the complex care needs of individuals living with SCD.

Some health care providers may be uncomfortable with providing SCD care because of a lack of knowledge and understanding about the clinical condition and the affected population. Clinical practice guidelines are an effective way of standardizing care and informing health care providers (especially non-experts) of the appropriate services that individuals living with SCD need. Commensurate endorsed quality metrics allow individual providers and systems to measure how well they adhere to available guidelines in providing such care and the consistency of this application to "every patient, every time."

GUIDELINES FOR HIGH-QUALITY SCD CARE

Introduction

The discussion in this section is guided by the quality framework from two prior National Academies of Sciences, Engineering, and Medicine (the National Academies) publications, *Crossing the Quality Chasm: A New Health System for the 21st Century* (IOM, 2001) and *Crossing the Global Quality Chasm: Improving Health Care Worldwide* (NASEM, 2018). As noted in Figure 6-1, achieving quality requires ongoing attention by the health care system to provide care that is safe, effective, accessible/timely, efficient, equitable, and person-centered (NASEM, 2018).

Health care organizations and clinicians assess how well they are achieving these quality aims by assessing performance on metrics indicative of high-quality care. To foster the delivery of high-quality SCD care, health care providers need information and tools that synthesize available knowledge into clinical practice, and clinicians, organizations, and payers

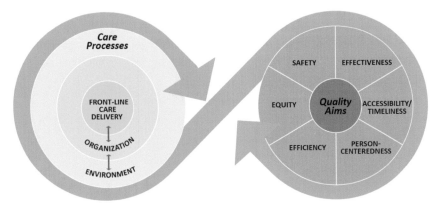

FIGURE 6-1 Guiding framework for the transformation of care delivery.
SOURCE: NASEM, 2018.

need to be able to measure, reward, and identify opportunities for improving quality. Quality measures, performance indicators, and clinical practice guidelines are all relevant tools. Where there is a strong evidence base, defined as well-conducted randomized controlled trials and robust data to support performance tracking, these evidence-based SCD services can be defined as quality measures.

> Quality measures are tools that help us measure or quantify health care processes, outcomes, patient perceptions, and organizational structure and/or systems that are associated with the ability to provide high-quality health care and/or that relate to one or more quality goals for health care. (CMS, 2020)

There are currently two measures for SCD care that have been endorsed by the National Quality Forum (NQF) (discussed in this chapter). Quality or performance indicators are "standardized evidence-based measures of health care quality that can be used … to measure and track clinical performance and outcomes" (AHRQ, n.d.). Quality indicators are used to benchmark actual performance against recommended practices; these are collected for reporting purposes and may be tied to payment. When the evidence base is insufficiently robust or still being gathered for services that the expert consensus sees as beneficial, clinical practice guidelines can be developed to guide care delivery. "Clinical practice guidelines are statements that include recommendations intended to optimize patient care that are informed by a systematic review of evidence [and expert opinion] and an assessment of the benefits and harms of alternative care options" (IOM, 2011a, p. 15). These guidelines help to standardize care by translating the existing research into recommendations for clinicians on the most beneficial services for different patient populations.

The structural aspects of health system design, such as the availability of a trained workforce and the use of data collection systems, are critical to adopting, measuring, and implementing quality measures and performance indicators.

Development of SCD-Specific Clinical Guidelines

As early as 1972 there were efforts to provide treatment guidelines for SCD, which were led by the National Heart, Lung, and Blood Institute (NHLBI) and a group of funded investigators who were aligned with the establishment of the SCD comprehensive care centers (Prabhakar et al., 2010; Smith et al., 2006). In 1984 NHLBI published the first set of national guidelines for SCD management, which were subsequently updated in 1989, 1995, 1999, and 2002 (NHLBI, 2002). In 2002 the American Academy of Pediatrics' (AAP's) Section on Hematology/Oncology and its Committee on Genetics published guidelines specific to SCD management for children with SCD (AAP, 2002).

In 2009 NHLBI convened an expert panel to develop guidelines for SCD management, which included health care professionals in areas such as pediatric and adult hematology, family medicine, and evidence-based medicine (Yawn et al., 2014). The expert panel, along with an independent methodology committee, reviewed the literature, rated the quality of evidence, and evaluated the strength of the recommendations. The quality of evidence was assessed using a modified Grading of Recommendations Assessment, Development and Evaluation (GRADE) framework (Balshem et al., 2011). The NHLBI expert panel's process adapts the GRADE process and rates the quality of recommendations as "strong," "moderate," or "weak." The panel therefore added the "moderate" category to the regular GRADE framework of "strong" or "weak" recommendations to capture research that is from either low-quality randomized controlled trials or large, well-conducted observational studies. The expert panel also made consensus recommendations based on evidence-based practice guidelines from other entities, such as the U.S. Preventive Services Task Force (USPSTF) and the Advisory Committee on Immunization Practices (Yawn et al., 2014).

Before finalizing its recommendations, the expert panel sought input from a number of associations with expertise in SCD, including AAP, the American Society of Hematology (ASH), and the American Society of Pediatric Hematology/Oncology (ASPHO). The resulting guidelines, *Evidence-Based Management of Sickle Cell Disease*, were published in 2014 (Yawn et al., 2014). Highlights of the NHLBI clinical guidelines covering health maintenance, the management of acute and chronic complications associated with SCD, and the use of hydroxyurea (HU) and transfusion therapy is included in Box 6-1.

BOX 6-1
Highlights of the National Heart, Lung, and Blood Institute
Expert Panel Recommendations for SCD, 2014

Highlights of the Sickle Cell Disease Expert Panel Report[a]

Health Maintenance
- Penicillin prophylaxis at least through age 5 years and vaccination against *Streptococcus pneumoniae* for all ages
- Screen children annually from age 2–16 years with transcranial Doppler for stroke risk
- Screen all individuals beginning at age 10 years for microalbuminuria and proteinuria with spot urine to estimate protein/creatinine ratio
- No restrictions on progestin-only contraceptives (pills, injections, and implants), levonorgestrel, intrauterine devices, or barrier methods for women with sickle cell disease (SCD)

Management of Acute Complications
- Use an individualized prescribing and monitoring protocol for SCD pain episodes or an SCD-specific protocol whenever possible
- For severe pain, rapidly initiate around-the-clock parenteral analgesics, reassess frequently, titrate to relief
- Immediate evaluation of all fevers > 101.3°F (38.5°C) and prompt administration of antibiotics in the case of affected children
- Do not give transfusions to treat priapism or acute renal failure unless there are other indications for transfusions
- Evaluate for acute chest syndrome in the setting of acute onset of respiratory symptoms irrespective of the absence of fever; hospitalize for further management if an infiltrate is seen on chest X-ray or if oxygenation is subnormal

Management of Chronic Complications
- Use a combination of patient-reported pain relief, adverse effects, and functional outcomes to guide the use of long-term opioids for chronic pain
- Treat avascular osteonecrosis with analgesics and consult physical therapy and orthopedics for assessment and follow-up
- Obtain echocardiogram only in patients with signs or symptoms suggestive of pulmonary hypertension
- Initiate angiotensin-converting enzyme inhibitor therapy for adults with microalbuminuria or proteinuria and no other apparent cause

Hydroxyurea and Transfusion Therapies
- Treat all adults with hydroxyurea who have a history of three or more moderate to severe pain episodes in a 12-month period
- Treat adults with severe or recurrent acute chest syndrome with hydroxyurea

continued

BOX 6-1 Continued

- Consult an established prescribing and monitoring protocol to ensure proper use of hydroxyurea and maximize benefits and safety
- In infants 9 months of age or older, children, and adolescents with sickle cell anemia, offer treatment with hydroxyurea regardless of clinical severity to reduce complications (e.g., pain, dactylitis, acute chest syndrome, anemia) related to SCD
- In adults with sicckle cell anemia who have sickle cell–associated pain that interferes with daily activities and quality of life, initiate treatment with hydroxyurea
- Transfuse with red blood cells to bring the hemoglobin up to 10 grams per deciliter prior to operative procedures
- When transfusion is indicated, always use an extended red blood cell cross-matching protocol to include matching for C, E, and K antigens

---

[a] The complete set of clinical practice guidelines, quality of the evidence, and strength of the recommendations are available at https://www.nhlbi.nih.gov/health-topics/evidence-based-management-sickle-cell-disease (accessed January 30, 2020).
SOURCES: Yawn and John-Sowah, 2015; republished and adapted with permission of the American Society of Hematology from Thompson, 2014; permission conveyed through Copyright Clearance Center, Inc.

Only a few of the strongly recommended NHLBI guidelines are supported by high-quality evidence. The majority of the recommended health care services had moderate or low evidence, indicating a huge gap in the evidence base for SCD interventions. Despite these gaps, the expert panel indicated that moderate-strength recommendations can be used to develop protocols to guide care delivery (Yawn et al., 2014). Recommended services with low-quality evidence represent areas where some variation in care may be acceptable because the services may be appropriate for only a subset of the SCD population. There is a need to generate research to fill in the evidence gaps for strongly recommended services where the supporting evidence base was moderate or weak or for services with moderate or weak recommendations.

Despite the NHLBI guidelines being a considerable contribution to improving the quality of care delivered, experts have noted that they have shortcomings, which offer valuable lessons for developing the next round of clinical guidelines for SCD. Citing recommendations from the Institute of Medicine (IOM) report *Clinical Practice Guidelines We Can Trust*, which offers criteria by which guidelines should be assessed, experts note that the NHLBI panel did not include patient representation, thus missing the opportunity to solicit patient perspective and preferences. Additionally, the perspective of health professional associations representing clinical specialties that have expertise in the management of some of the clinical complications associated with SCD (e.g., chronic kidney disease [CKD], pulmonary hypertension, obstructive lung disease, and stroke) was not solicited in the development of the guidelines (DeBaun, 2014; Thompson, 2014). Also, there are prevalent SCD complications that are notably missing from the NHLBI guidelines, such as asthma, screening for and management of pulmonary hypertension, and hematopoietic stem cell transplant (DeBaun, 2014; Thompson, 2014).

In addition to the 2014 NHLBI guidelines, ASH initiated an effort in 2016 to develop guidelines for screening, diagnosis, and management for five SCD-related areas: transfusion support, cardiopulmonary and kidney disease, cerebrovascular disease, pain, and stem cell transplantation. The Mayo Clinic Evidence-Based Practice Research Center led the systematic review of evidence for the ASH work. At the time of the development of this report, ASH had released guidelines for the screening, diagnosis, and management of SCD-related cardiopulmonary and renal complications (Liem et al., 2019) and transfusion support (Chou et al., 2020). Final guidelines are in development from ASH for cerebrovascular disease, transplantation, and the management of acute and chronic pain (ASH, n.d.).

National Quality Forum–Endorsed SCD-Specific Measures

NQF was created in 1999 in response to the report of the President's Advisory Commission on Consumer Protection and Quality in the Healthcare Industry (NQF, n.d.c). The commission concluded that an organization like NQF should be created to improve the measurement and reporting of quality health care indicators. An NQF endorsement of quality measures signifies a rigorous review of the science and evidence base supporting the measure and input from key stakeholders, including patients and families, to develop consensus about measures that warrant a "best in class" designation (NQF, n.d.a).

NQF-endorsed measures are used widely at the federal, state, and local levels for payment and reporting. Currently, NQF has endorsed two measures related to SCD for measuring high-quality care for children (NQF, 2018):

1. NQF measure #2797, "Transcranial Doppler Ultrasonography Screening among Children with Sickle Cell Anemia: The percentage of children ages 2 through 15 years old with sickle cell anemia (Hemoglobin SS) who received at least one transcranial Doppler (TCD) screening within a year."

2. NQF measure #3166, "Antibiotic Prophylaxis Among Children with Sickle Cell Anemia: The percentage of children ages 3 months to 5 years old with sickle cell anemia (SCA, hemoglobin [Hb] SS) who were dispensed appropriate antibiotic prophylaxis for at least 300 days within the measurement year."

The evidence on adherence to NQF-endorsed measures in SCD care is not robust. The following section discusses the available information on adherence to these measures.

Transcranial Doppler Screening

TCD screening is a significant advance in identifying and preventing stroke in children and adolescents with SCD. However, studies have consistently demonstrated that fewer than half of all eligible patients have received proper TCD screening. Raphael et al. (2008) found that the average yearly TCD screening rate for eligible pediatric patients (207 in the evaluation) was 45 percent. Eckrich et al. (2013) found that among a cohort of 338 children with SCD who were publicly insured, the cumulative incidence rates of annual TCD screening increased from 2.5 percent in 1997 to 68.3 percent in 2008. While screening increased significantly over the study period, 31 percent of children did not receive TCD screening over the entire study period. Reeves et al. (2016) conducted a retrospective cross-sectional study using Medicaid claims data from 2005 to 2010 and found that among 4,775 children and adolescents (2–16 years old), TCD screening rates increased over the 6-year study period from 22 percent to 44 percent ($p < 0.001$). The authors also found that screening rates varied substantially across states and that the receipt of well-child visits was associated with higher odds of a TCD screening. In a retrospective chart review of 195 children ages 2–16 years who were eligible for TCD screening, Hussain et al. (2015) found that only 41 percent had achieved the standard of care. Bundy et al. (2016) conducted a retrospective cohort study of children aged 2–5 years and found that only 25 percent of the children had received one or more TCD screenings during the 14-month study period. The children who were most likely to receive a TCD (42 percent) were those with two or more hematologist visits.

A lack of knowledge about TCD guidelines has been identified as a barrier to TCD screening among some physicians. Reeves et al. (2015) conducted a survey of primary care, neurology, and hematology physicians to explore the factors that influence physician adherence to TCD screening guidelines for children with SCD. They found variation in the degree to which physicians felt well informed about screening guidelines. Of the 276 survey respondents, more primary care providers (PCPs) reported not feeling well informed (66 percent) than neurologists (25 percent) and hematologists (6 percent). Bollinger et al. (2011) found that a lack of knowledge in caregivers may also be a barrier that prevents children with SCD from receiving annual TCD screening.

Penicillin Prophylaxis

Infants and young children with SCD are susceptible to bacteremia and meningitis due to *Streptococcus pneumonia*; penicillin prophylaxis decreases episodes of pneumococcal bacteremia. Kanter et al. (2017) evaluated commercial and Medicaid claims data for children with SCD and found that more than 80 percent of insured children aged 1–5 received a prescription for penicillin prophylaxis. However, other studies suggest that a prescription does not guarantee receipt of or optimal adherence to the medication, so the rates of adherence are much lower. For example, Beverung et al. (2014) conducted a retrospective cohort study using Wisconsin Medicaid claims data and found that only 18 percent of eligible children 5 years or older were adherent, as defined by a medication possession ratio[1] of greater than 80 percent (18.18%, 95% confidence interval [CI] 11.31–25.05). Bundy et al. (2016) conducted a retrospective cohort study (using Maryland Medicaid claims data) of 266 children aged 2–5 years and found that 30 percent had consistently filled prophylactic antibiotic prescriptions. Having more than two hematologist visits or generalist visits that were not for well-child care was associated with more consistent antibiotic prophylaxis. Finally, Reeves et al. (2018) evaluated Medicaid claims data from six states for children aged 3 months to 5 years with SCA (2005–2012) and found that only 18 percent received at least 300 days of antibiotics. Furthermore, well-child visits were found to be associated with increased odds of receiving at least 300 days of antibiotics (odds ratio [OR] 1.08, 95% CI 1.02–1.13).

These findings indicate that there is a need to promote adherence to NQF-endorsed measures. Some strategies for promoting uptake of measures are discussed later in the chapter.

Recommendations Adapted from Other Stakeholder Groups

Several other associations for health professionals have developed evidence-based recommendations for managing care for adults and children that are relevant for the SCD population. Organizations whose recommendations appear in the 2014 NHLBI guidelines include USPSTF, the Advisory Committee on Immunization Practices, the World Health Organization, the

---

[1] The medication possession ratio is calculated as follows: (sum of days supplied) / [(number of days from first encounter) – (number of days hospitalized)] (Beverung et al., 2014).

Centers for Disease Control and Prevention (CDC), and the American Pain Society. The consensus-adapted recommendations for SCD care pertain primarily to beneficial preventive services and include immunizations, screening for hepatitis C virus (HCV) and retinopathy, contraception use, reproductive counseling, and opioid use during pregnancy, as shown in Table 6-1. The NHLBI guidelines also included adapted consensus guidelines for chronic pain management. As with other recommended services, the National Academies SCD committee's literature review identified very little data on adherence to recommended vaccinations and preventive services in the SCD population. The next section briefly reviews the available information.

Immunizations

Pneumococcal vaccination Individuals with SCD are at extremely high risk of fatal pneumococcal infection and therefore are routinely immunized with pneumococcal conjugate vaccine (PCV) and pneumococcal polysaccharide vaccine (PPSV, sometimes referred to as PPV). Neunert et al. (2016) examined retrospective medical record and claims data to identify eligible children with SCA aged 24–36 months between January 1, 2004, and December 31, 2008; they found that of 125 children, 73.6 percent received PPV as recommended. Similarly, Beverung et al. (2014) found that 77 percent of eligible children received PCV7,[2] and 50 percent of children less than 18 years of age received PPSV23 at least once in a 4-year period, whereas 38 percent of adults over 18 years of age had received PPSV23 at least once in a 4-year period. Ter-Minassian et al. (2019) reviewed the medical records of all persons with SCD seen at Kaiser Permanente Mid-Atlantic States (KPMAS) and the Adult Sickle Cell Disease Program at Johns Hopkins Hospital (JHH) from January 1, 2014, to December 31, 2015, to assess quality of care. Among 146 KPMAS patients, 85 percent had documentation of ever receiving PCV13 or PPSV23, but only 52 percent had received both. Among 308 JHH patients, 87 percent had documentation of receipt of either PCV13 or PPSV23, but only 30 percent had both.

Influenza vaccine Influenza vaccination is recommended in the United States for everyone 6 months and older and may be even more important for people with SCD, for whom infections can be more serious and associated with additional SCD-related complications. There are several studies evaluating the rates of influenza vaccination for persons with SCD.

---

[2] PCV7 was the first pneumococcal conjugate vaccine licensed by the U.S. Food and Drug Administration. The pneumococcal conjugate vaccine recommended currently is PCV13, which offers protection against an increased number of types of pneumococcal infection. For more information, see https://www.cdc.gov/vaccines/vpd/pneumo/public/index.html (accessed December 23, 2019).

Beverung et al. (2014) found that only 30.3 percent of children and 11.6 percent of adults were considered adherent[3] over a 5-year period. The percent of non-adherence (zero vaccinations per influenza season) among children was 17.5 percent and 38.2 percent in adults (Beverung et al., 2014). Bundy et al. (2016) conducted a retrospective cohort study of children aged 2–5 years and found that 41 percent received at least one influenza immunization during the study period. Children with two or more hematologist visits were most likely to be immunized (62 percent versus 35 percent for children without a hematologist visit).

Ter-Minassian et al. (2019) reviewed the medical records of persons with SCD seen at KPMAS and JHH for adherence to seasonal influenza vaccination. They found documentation of influenza vaccination in 75 percent of KPMAS participants and 51 percent of JHH participants.

Meningococcal vaccination Ter-Minassian et al. (2019) also reviewed the medical records of persons with SCD seen at KPMAS and JHH to assess meningococcal vaccination rates. Vaccination rates were low prior to 2016, with only 24 percent of KPMAS and 17 percent of JHH patients having had documentation of meningococcal vaccination.

The little evidence available on adherence to immunization guidelines suggests that there is room to promote adherence to recommended immunizations for individuals with SCD. At least one of the consensus-adapted recommendations—influenza vaccination—is NQF endorsed, meaning that it can be included in reporting and payment programs to promote accountability and adherence. The National Academies SCD committee was able to identify only limited evidence on adherence to the other strongly recommended services for SCD.

PATIENT-CENTERED DIMENSIONS OF
HIGH-QUALITY CARE

The available guidelines for management of SCD focus primarily on managing the disease and associated complications and thus miss other important dimensions of high-quality care that pertain to the impact of the disease on an individual's health-related quality of life (HRQOL) or their experience with the health care system, especially in care transitions for children from pediatric care into adult care.

---

[3] "Adherence rate was calculated by dividing the number of influenza vaccines received by the number of eligible influenza seasons.... Individuals were considered adherent if their vaccination rate was greater or equal to 0.80 per influenza season." Other categories of adherence were moderate (vaccination rate of 0.05–0.79 per season) and low (vaccination rate of 0.01–0.49 per season) (Beverung et al., 2014).

Health-Related Quality of Life

HRQOL refers to the effects of health, illness, and treatment on an individual's quality of life (QOL) (Ferrans et al., 2005; Wilson and Cleary, 1995). Seminal work on HRQOL proposed measuring patient outcomes in five areas: biological function, symptoms, functional status, general health perceptions, and overall QOL (Ferrans et al., 2005; Wilson and Cleary, 1995).

Tools for measuring HRQOL have been adapted over time to assess the health effects of specific illnesses or conditions. In 2002 stakeholders participating in NHLBI gatherings that were focused on the treatment needs of individuals living with SCD identified the need to document patient-reported outcomes (PROs) (Treadwell et al., 2014). In response to this need, efforts began to develop SCD-specific tools as part of an NHLBI-sponsored Adult Sickle Cell Quality of Life Measurement Information System (ASCQ-Me) project (Treadwell et al., 2014). ASCQ-Me was developed as a set of self-administered items that assess the impact of SCD on adult functioning (Keller et al., 2017; Treadwell et al., 2014). The health domains assessed by the ASCQ-Me include emotional impact, pain impact, sleep impact, social functioning impact, stiffness impact, pain episodes, and an SCD medical history checklist (Keller et al., 2017; Treadwell et al., 2014).[4] In a recent systematic literature review of PRO instruments used in SCD, the ASCQ-Me was considered to have strong content validity and internal reliability and good construct validity with respect to psychometric properties (Sarri et al., 2018). The tool was recently validated in a UK population (Cooper et al., 2019).

In addition, to assess the experiences of adults living with SCD in accessing care and the quality of care received, the ASCQ-Me Quality of Care (ASCQ-Me QOC) tool was developed. The tool has four domains focusing on access, provider communication, emergency department (ED) care, and ED pain treatment. Results based on the ASCQ-Me QOC indicate that adults with SCD report deficiencies in ED care related to race and their disease condition (Evensen et al., 2016).

It should be noted that in the design of the ASCQ-Me QOC a number of domain questions (access and provider communication) are very similar to or identical to those found in the Consumer Assessment of Healthcare Providers and Systems (CAHPS)[5] surveys (Evensen et al., 2016). These surveys were designed to understand patient experiences with health care. There are a number of surveys; some surveys ask about a patient's experience with

---

[4] For more information on the tool, see www.HealthMeasures.net/ASCQ-Me (accessed January 6, 2020).

[5] For more information on the CAHPS surveys, see https://www.ahrq.gov/cahps/about-cahps/cahps-program/index.html (accessed January 6, 2020).

providers (clinician and groups), while others ask about experiences with care delivered in facilities (e.g., adult and child hospitals). Supplements to these surveys have been developed, such as one that provides questions specific to children with chronic conditions. While a CAHPS survey specific to SCD has not been developed (e.g., parallel to the CAHPS Cancer Care Survey[6]), items from the various surveys could be helpful in understanding the patient experience of care for individuals with SCD.

Efforts to develop a tool to assess the HRQOL of children living with SCD resulted in the development of the Pediatric QOL™—Sickle Cell Disease Module (PedsQL™ SCD Module). The module is a self- or parent proxy-administered survey that assesses HRQOL in children aged 2–18 years (Panepinto et al., 2013). The PedsQL™ SCD Module comprises nine scales: (1) pain and hurt, (2) pain impact, (3) pain management and control, (4) worry I, (5) worry II, (6) emotions, (7) treatment, (8) communication I, and (9) communication II (Panepinto et al., 2013). In the systematic review of PRO instruments, the PedsQL™ SCD Module was found to have strong internal reliability, but its other psychometric properties were unclear (Sarri et al., 2018). The SCD module complements other non-SCD-specific PRO instruments such as the PedsQL™ 4.0 Generic Core Scales (Varni et al., 2001) and the PedsQL™ Multidimensional Fatigue Scale (Panepinto et al., 2014), which assess other aspects of HRQOL in children.

A number of other tools specific to the SCD population have been developed with a focus on pain and self-efficacy. With respect to pain assessment, Zempsky et al. (2013) developed the Sickle Cell Disease Pain Burden Interview–Youth for use in youth and young adults aged 7–21 years. The brief tool, which consists of seven items, is administered by interview and inquires about days of pain and the impact of pain in the past month. Questions assess the impact of pain on mood, functional ability, and QOL. The tool has strong internal reliability and good content validity, construct validity, and test-retest reliability (Sarri et al., 2018).

According to Edwards et al. (2001), disease self-efficacy refers to an individual's beliefs about his or her ability to achieve a desired health outcome. With respect to SCD and self-efficacy, Clay and Telfair (2007) and Edwards et al. (2000) used a nine-item scale focusing on the ability of adults and adolescents living with SCD to engage in daily functional activities. They found that high levels of self-efficacy were related to fewer physical, psychological, and total SCD symptoms (Clay and Telfair, 2007; Edwards et al., 2000). The instrument was assessed as having strong internal reliability in the recent systematic review (Sarri et al., 2018).

---

[6] For information on the CAHPS Cancer Care Survey, see https://www.ahrq.gov/cahps/surveys-guidance/cancer/index.html (accessed January 6, 2020).

The above-cited SCD-specific tools provide an opportunity to develop a better understanding of the burden that SCD imposes on the QOL of individuals living with SCD and their experiences with providers and health systems. HRQOL outcomes also point to areas of clinical practice that may need improvement, such as deficiencies in how patients are assessed and treated for pain in EDs as well as non-clinical interventions and strategies to better support individuals in developing self-efficacy, carrying out activities of daily living, and social functioning.

Patient Engagement in Care Through Shared Decision Making

Shared decision making (SDM) is defined as "a process of communication in which clinicians and patients work together to make informed health care decisions that align with what matters most to patients and their individual concerns, preferences, goals, and values" (NQF, n.d.b).[7] NQF issued a national call to action to ensure that SDM in clinical practice is a standard of care for all patients (NQF, n.d.b). SDM in SCD care is critical but evolving.

Decisions about disease-modifying therapies for SCD often require patient adherence in order to be optimally effective (e.g., HU) or involve significant risks (e.g., bone marrow transplant, CRISPR gene editing). These decisions are complex and preference sensitive, and patients/families should be informed and involved in making them. This requires an effective partnership between patients and families and clinicians based on trust and clear communication.

Results from a study of physicians' perceptions of patient decisional needs and physicians' approaches to decision making showed that physicians tended to use two approaches to treatment-related decision making (Bakshi et al., 2017). One approach was characterized by the physician advocating for a specific treatment plan with the objective of convincing the patient to accept that plan. The second approach was characterized by the physician emphasizing the need to discuss all treatment approaches. Bakshi et al. (2017) found that which approach a physician used was influenced by a number of factors, including the characteristics of the patient, disease severity, the nature of the therapies, institutional frameworks, and other decision characteristics. Another study that directly observed dialogue about initiation of HU between patients and clinicians found that clinicians did not uniformly present the risks of HU and that patient concerns about

---

[7] For more information on NQF shared decision making, see http://www.qualityforum.org/National_Quality_Partners_Shared_Decision_Making_Action_Team_.aspx (accessed January 6, 2020).

HU were not always raised and discussed (Lee et al., 2018). A recent qualitative study of patients' perspectives on the process of deciding whether to take HU and physician communication found that providers who involved patients in SDM empowered those patients to start HU treatment (Jabour et al., 2019). However, patients who perceived that their providers were not attentive to their concerns reported having disengaged from HU treatment (Jabour et al., 2019).

Researchers are exploring ways to develop decision aids to assist in SDM. Crosby et al. (2015, 2019) developed an HU decision aid that increased HU knowledge and decreased decisional conflict. Other decision aids for transplant and non-transplant treatments exist for SCD (Sullivan et al., 2018). For example, Sickle Options is a website that provides information on treatment options, risks, and benefits and relates them to personal values.[8] A Cochrane review of 105 studies on decision aids for a variety of clinical decisions found that when the aids are used, people improve their knowledge of options, feel better informed, and have a better understanding of what matters most to them (high-quality evidence), and they probably have more accurate expectations of the benefits and harms of options and participate more in decision making (moderate-quality evidence) (Stacey et al., 2017). Given the paucity of research in this area specific to SCD, there are ample research opportunities to examine SDM and the effectiveness of decision aids in improving patient knowledge and decision making in SCD care.

Pain Management

Pain management is a source of frustration for both patients and providers and an impetus for discrimination, confusion, and dissatisfaction; as noted by Anie et al. (2012, p. 1), "sickle cell pain assessment is a crucial and difficult task." There are some best practices for pain control, but these have not been disseminated widely or implemented outside of institutions serving high numbers of patients with SCD. ASH is creating guidelines for treating SCD-related pain, but the recommendations are still in draft form (ASH, 2019).

There are a number of reasons that pain management for individuals living with SCD is difficult. For example, a number of researchers and health care professionals have noted the difficulty in treating the pain episodes of individuals living with SCD because of the subjectivity associated with the experience of pain (Okwerekwu and Skirvin, 2018). Many providers

---

[8] For more information on Sickle Options, see http://sickleoptions.org/en_US (accessed January 6, 2020).

underestimate the severity of these pain episodes in spite of the fact that "pain management should be based on patient-reported severity," according to the 2014 NHLBI sickle cell management guidelines (Yawn and John-Sowah, 2015).

There is also a great deal of variability in the intensity, duration, and frequency of pain episodes, as discussed in Chapter 4 (Geller and O'Connor, 2008). Given the challenges with defining, measuring, and treating pain episodes, it is not surprising that there is little in the quality improvement literature about effective pain management. Added to this is that clinician attitudes and race- and disease-based discrimination significantly affect the implementation of evidence-based guidelines (e.g., administering pain medication in the ED within 30 minutes) and clinical outcomes for individuals living with SCD.

Pain management for individuals living with SCD must be seen in the context of the current opioid crisis. Sinha et al. (2019), for example, collected qualitative data from 15 interview subjects about their perceptions of pain management from 2017 to 2018, after the 2016 CDC guidelines for chronic pain management were published. Interviewees reported that their opioid prescriptions were managed more closely by their health care providers and that their opioid use was monitored more closely than previously. This stigmatization of opioid use in managing SCD pain in light of the opioid crisis has negatively affected the care that these individuals are receiving (Sinha et al., 2019).

The National Academies has published several reports that can be used with this current report to create an effective system of care for people living with SCD and SCT, including *Crossing the Quality Chasm* (IOM, 2001), *Unequal Treatment: Confronting Racial and Ethnic Disparities in Health Care* (IOM, 2003), *Relieving Pain in America: A Blueprint for Transforming Prevention, Care, Education, and Research* (IOM, 2011b), and *The Role of Nonpharmacological Approaches to Pain Management* (NASEM, 2019), and Telfer and Kaya (2017) suggest an integrated approach to treating sickle cell pain in the absence of a standard protocol.

Transition from Pediatric to Adult Care

As described in Chapter 5, adolescents and young adults who transfer from pediatric to adult care encounter many challenges that affect their care. Individuals may lack the knowledge (e.g., SCD complication history) and skills (e.g., decision making, communication) needed to take an active role in their care and successfully navigate the adult health care system (Jordan et al., 2013). Compounding the transition to adult health care are the many other life transitions that young adults experience (e.g., emotional—establishing new friendships; social—living independently;

academic—graduating from high school/college/vocational program) (de Montalembert and Guitton, 2014). Despite the complexity of the transition to adult care, the field has identified several indicators of a successful transition for young adults living with SCD.

> *When I was in peds, I got amazing care. I was really encouraged to know … what worked for me. And then when I transition[ed] to adult, it was totally different. I started being accused of drug seeking just because I knew what dose of Dilaudid I needed in the ER.*
>
> —Teonna W. (Open Session Panelist)

Indicators of a Successful Transition

National organizations have developed position statements, guidance, and white papers defining a high-quality transition process for youth with chronic conditions and individuals with SCD. One available source of guidance, for example, is Got Transition™, discussed in Chapter 5. NHLBI provides guidance on adolescent health care and transitions in its report *The Management of Sickle Cell Disease*. That guidance, developed by a multidisciplinary group of experts, highlights transition readiness based on developmental age, transition discussions before transfer, the introduction of adult providers in the pediatric setting, and a focus on the coordination of care (NHLBI, 2002). In 2015, ASPHO and the Association of Pediatric Hematology/Oncology Nurses developed a policy statement for the transition of individuals living with SCD from pediatric to adult health, which identifies the following elements as essential: transition planning, multidisciplinary transition team, transfer process, and confirmation of transfer. In 2017 an expert panel from the Sickle Cell Adult Provider network used a modified Delphi process to identify nine quality indicators for transition, including five that were identified by Oyeku and Faro (2017) in their review of SCD quality improvement indicators for transition from pediatric to adult care: (1) communication between pediatric and adult providers, (2) time to first visit at the adult provider, (3) patient self-efficacy, (4) QOL, and (5) trust with the adult provider (Oyeku and Faro, 2017; Sobota et al., 2017).

The efforts mentioned above to provide guidance and indicators for the transition from adolescent to adult care share common elements, suggesting agreement across the field and a strong foundation for the development of SCD transition quality indicators. Despite this agreement, transition metrics are not routinely collected and tracked across programs, which has resulted in variations in the quality of care in the United States and other countries (Treadwell et al., 2018). The next section briefly reviews some additional outcomes and process indicators identified through the work of various organizations that can be measured and tracked to improve the quality of transitions.

Insurance coverage and access to adult providers Young adults with SCD may have limited access to health insurance (de Montalembert and Guitton, 2014). They may lose their health insurance coverage as they move from their parents' plan to their own. Enrolling in and maintaining health insurance, particularly public health insurance, can be a challenging and time-consuming process, as discussed in Chapter 2. This lack of or delay in obtaining insurance coverage is a significant obstacle in accessing care and may seriously affect quality and continuity of care as young adults may avoid regular care and become more reliant on urgent or emergency care.

Transition education and readiness assessment There is a need to assess the quality of transition planning and preparation, as individuals with SCD are generally unprepared for transition. The implementation of the transition core elements appears to be challenging. Okumura et al. (2008) found that 89 percent of providers in the survey supported a systematic transition process, but Telfair et al. (2004a,b) found that only 67 percent reported integrating transition core elements in their practice.

It has been shown that young adults may have a poor understanding of their medical history (Williams et al., 2015). DeBaun and Telfair (2012) identified educational milestones for the transition period to improve the transition process. Milestones include the adolescent having knowledge about his or her SCD phenotype, having the ability to articulate the most important components of his or her medical history, being able to manage pain according to a pain plan, and being aware of preventive measures for SCD complication, to name a few (DeBaun and Telfair, 2012). Additional research is needed to describe the interplay between cognition and disease knowledge in pediatric SCD (Hood et al., 2019). Young adults are able to identify specific health topics and barriers (e.g., mistrust, maintaining health insurance, employment difficulties, and managing stress) to be addressed in an individualized transition program (Bemrich-Stolz et al., 2015). Despite high interest in learning about transition (Williams et al., 2015), young adults may not attend transition-specific activities (Sivaguru et al., 2015). Lebensburger et al. (2012) supports starting the transition process early to better meet the needs of the patients from the beginning.

Routine assessment of transition readiness is variable across the United States; only certain SCD clinics and centers have integrated this into usual care. Several tools for measuring transition readiness exist, including the Transition Readiness Assessment Questionnaire and the Transition Intervention Program—Readiness for Transition assessment (Treadwell et al., 2016).

Communication/coordination of adult and pediatric providers Inadequate communication between adult and pediatric providers may cause poor continuity of care (Treadwell et al., 2011), which sets the stage for recurrent hospitalizations, mistrust, and poorer health outcomes (Hunt and Sharma, 2010). Interventions targeting care coordination have led to improvements in the transfer of care and in overall quality. Hankins et al. (2012) piloted a transition program that helped adolescents identify an adult medical home. Data indicated that the program was feasible and showed promise for improving the transfer process. A patient-centered medical home may be another approach to improving coordination of transition care. In this model the pediatric provider conducts regular monitoring, documents complications and treatments, and communicates with an adult provider during and immediately after transition (Kelly et al., 2002).

Time to first visit with adult provider Centers with well-established SCD transition programs use a registry to track eligibility, participation, and transfer completion. For example, the Duke University Medical Center conducted a retrospective chart review of individuals with SCD aged 18–23 years to identify care gaps (e.g., time to transfer), successful transition rates (completed appointment at an adult clinic 1 year post-transition), and associated factors (Hill et al., 2014). The data showed that only one-third of patients transitioned successfully and that a care gap exists for 18- to 20-year-olds (Hill et al., 2014). This study supports the importance of tracking individuals with SCD to improve the quality of care pre- and post-transition.

Quality of life In the transition period, QOL indicators such as Pediatric QOL and Adult Sickle Cell QOL can help identify and prioritize health problems, facilitate discussions between the adolescent and providers, and identify areas needing greater medical, emotional, or social support.

Patient self-efficacy Self-efficacy (the individual's confidence in his or her ability to manage SCD on a daily basis) affects transition readiness (Treadwell et al., 2016). A 2015 review and 2016 multisite study found that youth with higher self-efficacy were more ready for transition (Molter and Abrahamson, 2015; Treadwell et al., 2016). Another 2015 study found that adults living with SCD reported improvements in autonomy and self-efficacy after transition (Bemrich-Stolz et al., 2015). Consequently, many transition programs target increasing patient self-management skills as a way of increasing self-efficacy. Moreover, 50 percent of SCD clinics responding to a survey about transition services and needs reported that they had a written list of desirable self-management skills (Sobota et al., 2011).

To better prepare young adults with SCD for the transfer to adult care, there is a need to help them develop increased confidence in their life skills.

In an effort to overcome neurocognitive or health literacy challenges that may interfere with attaining self-management skills (e.g., medication adherence), some programs have begun to integrate technology (e.g., videos, apps) into their care. Additional research is needed to understand essential components for increasing self-management skills and the most effective modalities (e.g., groups, in person, online, mobile apps) (Matthie et al., 2015).

PROMOTING UPTAKE OF RECOMMENDATIONS FOR SCD CARE

There are a number of beneficial and effective services recommended for SCD care; two of these recommended services are endorsed by NQF as quality measures. Several other specialty organizations (ASH, ASPHO, American College of Emergency Physicians (ACEP), AAP, American Academy of Family Physicians, American College of Physicians) and non-specialty organizations and governmental entities (CDC, USPSTF, NHLBI) have also developed consensus guidelines/recommendations to support quality metrics for the general population and SCD that should be applied consistently to the SCD population. In 2011 a panel of experts recommended 41 indicators for managing SCD care for children, including a subset of eight indicators[9] that they believe will result in considerable improvement on QOL and health outcomes for children with SCD (Wang et al., 2011). The 41 indicators covered 18 topic areas, including some of the areas identified throughout this report as having opportunity for improvement, such as genetic counseling, transition to adult care, hematopoietic stem cell transplant, and comprehensive planning (Wang et al., 2011). These prior efforts can inform future attempts to expand indicators for high-quality SCD care. Internationally, standards of SCD care developed by the National Health Service and the Sickle Cell Society in the United Kingdom are valuable resources for SCD care management in the United States (Public Health England, 2019; Sickle Cell Society, 2018).

Clinical guidelines and metrics that are supported by evidence are, however, not widely applied because there is a lack of systematic efforts to foster the development of evidence-based learnings from iterative quality improvement in the SCD management. As a result, the quality and outcomes for SCD lag behind those of other rare, inheritable, and chronic diseases, such as cystic fibrosis (CF), hemophilia, and juvenile idiopathic arthritis. There is a need to implement and measure these underused guidelines and metrics.

The two NQF-endorsed measures can be immediately measured for public reporting and tied to payment. For 2019 the Centers for Medicare &

---

[9] The eight indicators cover the following topics: timely assessment and treatment of pain and fever, comprehensive planning, penicillin prophylaxis, transfusion, and the transition to adult care (Wang et al., 2011).

Medicaid Services (CMS) announced that it would be maintaining the current core set of pediatric quality measures that states use for reporting the performance of Medicaid programs (CMS, 2018). Freed (2019) said CMS had "missed a historic opportunity to definitively address a national shame, the poor state of care provided to children with sickle cell disease," because the Pediatric Measure Application Partnership (P-MAP) had recommended certain changes, such as to include the two NQF-endorsed measures in the core measure set. P-MAP is a multi-stakeholder panel that guides the U.S. Department of Health and Human Services (HHS) in selecting performance measurements for federal health programs.

QUALITY INDICATORS FOR SCT AND GENETIC COUNSELING FOR SCD AND SCT

Although SCT may be considered clinically benign, it affects nearly 300 million individuals worldwide (Grant et al., 2011). As stated in Chapter 3, all U.S. newborn screening (NBS) programs are state-based, so there are no requirements for them to report data to a national source. There are also no federal standards or consensus definitions for reporting or governing NBS data (Therrell et al., 2015). In 2009, CDC hosted a meeting on SCT and invited key stakeholders to engage in discussions to identify gaps in public health, health care delivery, epidemiologic research,[10] and community-based outreach and to develop an agenda for the future for SCT. The meeting deliberations culminated in recommendations for community awareness and education, screening practices, ethical and legal issues, prevention of negative health outcomes, and epidemiological and clinical research (Grant et al., 2011). The National Academies SCD committee was unable to find any data on adherence to these guidelines other than efforts referenced in Chapters 3 and 5 and found no studies specifically examining quality.

Many individuals with SCT are identified through state NBS programs. Notification of NBS results varies widely by state. No best practices have yet been established for notifying families of results that improve a family's ability to inform their child about his or her SCT and educate him or her about the implications. Programs that inform families of NBS results in person should be explored (Salm et al., 2012).

There are no guidelines or best practices for genetic counseling for individuals with SCT during adolescence or young adulthood, yet this is typically the time when family planning and decisions about contraception occur. When providing genetic counseling to women about their risk for having a child with SCD, it is important that the correct test is used

---

[10] For more information on epidemiological research, see https://www.sciencedirect.com/topics/medicine-and-dentistry/cohort-effect (accessed August 3, 2020).

to assess hemoglobinopathy trait status. Hemoglobin electrophoresis and other hemoglobin quantitative separation methods are best (Naik and Haywood, 2015). Solubility tests, such as Sickledex and Sickle Cell Screen, are misleading. These tests do not distinguish SCD from SCT, nor do they detect the presence of other hemoglobin variants that may place a couple at risk for having a child with SCD, and false negatives and false positives are common. These tests should not be used for genetic counseling. Protocols for screening children and adults for SCD or SCT should use hemoglobin electrophoresis or other reliable hemoglobin separation methods, and organizations such as the National Collegiate Athletic Association and others should adopt this screening approach (Tubman and Field, 2015). Other tests such as a complete blood count may be necessary to detect beta thalassemia carriers, who also need genetic counseling. Quality indicators should be developed and tracked to ensure that appropriate tests are used, particularly for pregnant women (ACOG, 2017). In addition, individuals should be screened once in their lifetime, with confirmatory testing when appropriate. Repeated testing for a genetic state is not cost effective. Methods to store information about SCT and other hemoglobinopathy traits should be part of the health record, and NBS results should be stored and available to individuals when requested.

The National Library of Medicine developed a Newborn Screening Coding and Terminology Guide to standardize NBS test results (NLM, 2018). Another effort to standardize definition and data collection is the Hemoglobinopathy Uniform Medical Language Ontology (HUMLO) Project (NIH, 2008). The goal of HUMLO was to create an ontology for researchers and federal programs. Similarly, the PhenX Project sought to identify consensus measures for genetics that could be used in large-scale genomic studies (Hamilton et al., 2011).

There are no consensus guidelines on when or how to screen (e.g., methods, specific tests) individuals living with SCT for clinical complications (see Chapter 4). This is a notable gap in the literature, particularly because there is strong evidence for some clinical complications (e.g., CKD) (Naik et al., 2018b).

An NQF-like endorsement mechanism is needed for all indicators of high-quality SCD services across the life span, similar to what has been done for asthma, children from low-income families, and other groups. This will require developing measure sets, similar to the ones in Figure 6-2, that incorporate core metrics relevant for all adults and children in addition to core metrics specifically relevant for individuals with SCD and SCT.

Developing and accrediting comprehensive care centers will facilitate adherence to quality indicators and existing and future quality measures, because these centers' accreditation and performance can be tied to providing recommended services for SCD.

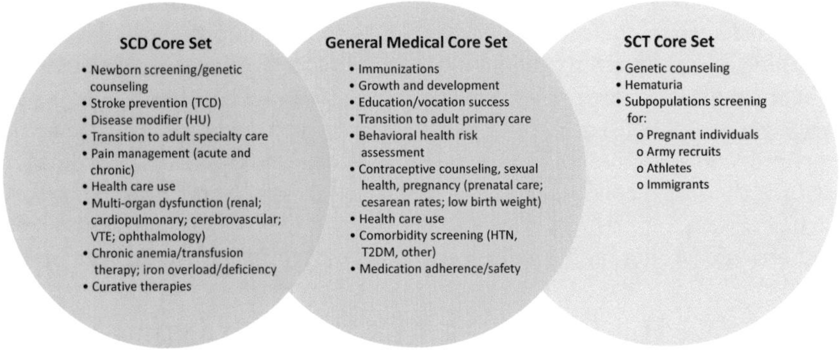

FIGURE 6-2 Core measure sets for SCD care.
NOTE: HTN = hypertension; HU = hydroxyurea; T2DM = type 2 diabetes mellitus; TCD = transcranial Doppler screening; VTE = venous thromboembolism.

SUMMARY

The evidence supporting the guidelines for SCD care is highly variable, relying on expert consensus but highlighting research gaps. The evidence for a comprehensive, systematic approach to quality care delivery for SCD is lacking, and the science of quality in SCD care appears to lag behind other diseases in several areas:

- The majority of SCD quality indicators are supported with poor-quality evidence, often with consensus expert recommendation as the highest level of evidence available.
- There are multiple sets of quality indicators, but none are comprehensive or universally accepted or applied.
- There is a lack of data streams to measure adherence to quality indicators, requirements for centers to report their adherence to quality metrics, incentives to promote reporting, and public transparency of reports when available.
- There is neither funding nor a priority established for quality metrics in SCD, even in the face of poor performance of clinical systems. Furthermore, there has been no formal, systematic quality improvement of training programs.

There is no metric to support compassionate care in the health care system, particularly in light of the outright mistreatment of individuals with SCD presenting with pain—the most notable feature of SCD outside of death. Continued inaction over the past 18 years and a lack of required certifications has set back quality in SCD care, perpetuated mistrust of the health care system, and delayed the development of life-saving treatments and standards of care. In the absence of robust evidence from randomized controlled trials, the quality of health care can be improved by leveraging learning collaboratives across health systems to foster the consistent application of available evidence-based guidelines and to obtain data on the effectiveness of consensus guidelines in improving outcomes. The disparities in applying available guideline-based care, the lack of care coordination within the delivery system and across the life span, and other structural deficiencies all contribute to poor outcomes in the SCD population. Defining and measuring high-quality care is a key step to improving outcomes.

THE AVAILABILITY OF A TRAINED AND PREPARED WORKFORCE

The committee believes that achieving the goal of delivering high-quality SCD health care to all will rest in part on the availability of an active, highly trained workforce. This section will describe the challenges associated with accessing such a workforce.

Multidisciplinary Teams

Treatment for people with SCD is best managed by a multidisciplinary team of professionals delivering comprehensive care. Traditionally, hematologists coordinate the management of care and liaise with other specialties, as they generally have the most familiarity with the multiple SCD complications and presentations (Grosse et al., 2009). In addition to medical providers, the members of the comprehensive care team should include behavioral health providers (e.g., psychologists, neuropsychologists, and psychiatrists), social workers, dietitians, physiotherapists, massage therapists, community health workers (CHWs), care coordinators, and school liaison officers. Furthermore, strong partnerships with community health services and voluntary agencies enhance the likelihood of the multidisciplinary team's success (Okpala et al., 2002). Comprehensive care has several beneficial effects, such as improved QOL, reduced ED visits, and shorter hospital admissions (Okpala et al., 2002; Vichinsky, 1991).

The importance of social services and psychological support should not be underestimated. Services that may be needed include psychological treatment (e.g., mindfulness techniques and cognitive behavioral therapy), neuropsychological testing, general information and advice, disability assistance, transportation, financial allowances, practical help in the home or school, and assistance with care transition. However, access to these services is often institution dependent and further reduced in adult care. Such services often require specialized clinical experience and technical expertise and are harder to access outside of comprehensive care centers.

Although SCD is more common than CF in the United States, only a minority of individuals with SCD are seen at specialized centers (Smith et al., 2006). In stark contrast, there are more than 115 comprehensive, multidisciplinary CF care centers in the United States that are accredited and funded by the Cystic Fibrosis Foundation (CFF). CFF also maintains a national registry of CF patients who attend accredited centers (CFF, 2019). Using expert panels made up of physicians and scientists, it published consensus guidelines for best practices in CF care (e.g., guidelines for the management of infants with CF) (CFF et al., 2009; Conway et al., 2014). CFF also supports quality improvement activities to improve medical and care process at CF centers (Godfrey and Oliver, 2014; Grosse et al., 2009). A comprehensive network of care that can surveil health outcomes, develop best practices, and monitor the quality of care for SCD does not exist.

Strategies recommended in the IOM report *Retooling for an Aging America: Building the Healthcare Workforce* (IOM, 2008) to increase health workers for the geriatric population may be applicable to SCD. These strategies include the following:

- Congress should allocate money in the budget to monitor the workforce.
- Hospitals should encourage resident training across all settings.
- All licensure, renewal, and maintenance of certification activities should measure competence in areas relevant to the topic.
- States and the federal government should increase minimum training standards in this topic.
- Public and private payers should include financial incentives to increase the number of topic specialists in all professions.
- Payers should promote and reward models of care shown to be effective.
- Federal agencies should promote advances in technology to increase the efficiency and safety of caregiving.
- Public, private, and community organizations should provide funding and ensure that adequate training opportunities are available in the community for informal caregivers.

Table 6-1 presents the essential care team members (core team) required to provide high-quality care for individuals with SCD, the specific roles for care team members, the level of training/experience necessary, and potential barriers to an available and well-prepared workforce. The committee employed a variety of methods in determining team members. First, the committee identified specialists and clinical services historically involved in SCD care. Next, the committee identified providers and specialists essential for addressing the routine, acute, and subacute care needs of individuals

TABLE 6-1 Multidisciplinary Team of Medical Providers and Specialists Necessary to Provide Comprehensive SCD Care

SCD Team Member or Service	Guideline for Provider Training	Team Member Role	Workforce Barrier
Hematologist/physician with expertise in SCD	*Expertise* in the evidence-based management of individuals with SCD	Provide core treatment for individuals with SCD; coordinate overall management and liaise with other specialties.	There is a workforce shortage because older hematologists are retiring and fewer new physicians are entering the field.
Emergency medicine	*Knowledge* of evidence-based management of individuals with SCD	Recognize the acute manifestations of SCD, provide early pain management and resuscitation, and quickly determine patient disposition.	Negative provider attitudes toward individuals with SCD are a barrier to the delivery of guideline-adherent pain care.
PCP	*Knowledge* of evidence-based management of individuals with SCD	Recognize manifestations of SCD and implement clinical advances in treatment in clinical practice; assist with patient education, medication/transfusion monitoring, and disease complication screening follow-up.	There are not enough PCPs with the comprehensive knowledge and expertise to care for individuals with SCD. There is a reluctance to devote time and effort to support a rarely seen population.
Nurse practitioner/physician assistants	*Knowledge* of evidence-based management of individuals with SCD	Assist with patient education, medication/transfusion monitoring, and disease complication screening follow-up.	There is no formal training with the SCD population.
Nurse care coordinator and nurses with SCD expertise	*Knowledge* of evidence-based management of individuals with SCD	Conduct initial assessment in clinics, assist with appointment scheduling, address patient-specific insurance issues, administer infusions in cooperation with the pharmacist, and perform exchange blood transfusions.	There is no formal training with the SCD population (negative provider biases and attitudes can influence care). Nurse care coordinators are only available at larger institutions.

First Level Core Team Members

Blood bank and transfusion medicine services	*Knowledge* of evidence-based management of individuals with SCD	Provide testing for extended RBC antigens and RBC alloimmunization. Exchange transfusion services.	Individuals with SCD commonly become alloimmunized to RBC antigens—a contributing factor is that the donor base is predominantly Caucasian.
Psychologist/psychiatrist	*Comfortable discussing* evidence-based management of individuals with SCD	Provide psychological support for mental issues, such as depression, anxiety, pain management, grief counseling, transition to adult care, and pharmacological treatment.	Knowledge gaps about SCD and negative provider attitudes contribute to poor communication.
Neuropsychologist	*Comfortable discussing* evidence-based management of individuals with SCD	Assess for cognitive challenges, as individuals with SCD are at high risk of neuropsychological problems (i.e., cognitive, emotional, social, or behavioral).	Social, cultural, linguistic/communication, and financial issues interfere with making and keeping appointments for traditionally scheduled neuropsychological evaluations.
Social worker	*Comfortable discussing* evidence-based management of individuals with SCD	Assess the specific needs to ensure that services are provided to meet the identified needs; address social determinants of health and barriers to care.	Available options for social services are often inadequate for the specific needs of individuals with SCD.

continued

TABLE 6-1 Continued

SCD Team Member or Service	Guideline for Provider Training	Team Member Role	Workforce Barrier
Second Level Core Team Members			
Pulmonologist	*Knowledge* of evidence-based management of individuals with SCD	Assess and provide treatment recommendations for pulmonary complications, which include ACS, asthma, lower airway obstruction, and airway hyper-responsiveness/bronchodilator response.	There is limited formal training with the SCD population.
Neurologist	*Knowledge* of evidence-based management of individuals with SCD	Assess and provide treatment recommendations for neurologic complications, which include stroke, silent cerebral infarct, moyamoya syndrome, posterior reversible encephalopathy syndrome, cerebral fat embolism, and cerebral venous sinus thrombosis.	There is limited formal training with the SCD population.
Dentist/dental hygienist	*Knowledge* of evidence-based management of individuals with SCD	Assess and provide treatment for dental complications, which include caries or cavities, tooth hypomineralization, orofacial pain, neuropathy, facial swelling, pallor of oral mucosa, malocclusions, infections, pulpal necrosis, cortical erosions, medullary hyperplasia, and abnormal trabecular spacing.	There is limited formal training with the SCD population.
Ophthalmologist	*Knowledge* of evidence-based management of individuals with SCD	Screen and provide treatment recommendations on vision complications. Every part of the eye can be affected by microvascular occlusions in SCD. The major cause of vision loss is proliferative sickle cell retinopathy. Screening before age 10 is recommended.	There is limited formal training with the SCD population and a lack of evidence regarding the optimal management of sickle retinopathy.

Role	Knowledge	Responsibilities	Notes
Nephrologist	*Knowledge* of evidence-based management of individuals with SCD	Assess and provide treatment for renal manifestations, which include hyperfiltration, hypertrophy, impaired urinary concentration, microalbuminuria, macroalbuminuria, hematuria, acute and chronic kidney injury, and end-stage renal disease.	SCD presents unique challenges in the marked heterogeneity of renal involvement. Current therapeutic approaches are largely adopted from other kidney diseases.
Obstetrician/ gynecologist	*Knowledge* of evidence-based management of individuals with SCD	Perform SCD screening and adult patient care through prenatal screening, folic acid supplementation, and pregnancy management.	Many OB/GYNs who care for individuals with SCD are not consistent with the College Practice Guidelines on the screening of certain target groups and folic acid supplementation.
Pharmacist	*Knowledge* of evidence-based management of individuals with SCD	Provide pharmacologic management of SCD pain, which may involve the use of non-opioid medications, opioids, and adjuvants; HU monitoring; patient education and health maintenance counseling.	The focus of training is oncology rather than benign hematology.
Genetic counselor	*Knowledge* of evidence-based management of individuals with SCD	Provide premarital and prenatal counseling and testing.	This role requires additional sensitivity when working with a majority black population.
Transition coordinator	*Knowledge* of evidence-based management of individuals with SCD	Evaluate patients for transfer readiness; prepare for transition and undertake an ongoing discussion about the transition process when patients reach their early teens; coordinate transfer to adult providers.	This will often be a part-time position shared with nursing or social work and only available at larger institutions.
Community health worker	*Basic knowledge* of evidence-based management of individuals with SCD	Assist with medication adherence, transitions of care, patient education, and education/vocation assistance.	There are no national standards for training, which is designed by the organizations that employ CHWs.

continued

278

TABLE 6-1 Continued

SCD Team Member or Service	Guideline for Provider Training	Team Member Role	Workforce Barrier
Patient and family advisory group(s)	*Basic knowledge of evidence-based management of individuals with SCD*	Identify and drive projects important to individuals with SCD. Engage in decisions that affect quality of care. Promote patient- and family-centered care. Advise and advocate for children and their families.	This is only available at larger institutions.
Data quality analyst	*Knowledge of evidence-based management of individuals with SCD*	Develop and implement databases, identify trends, and interpret data from SCD clinical research.	There is no formal training with the SCD population. This position is only available at larger institutions conducting clinical research.
Palliative care /integrative medicine	*Basic knowledge of evidence-based management of individuals with SCD*	Provide therapies, including non-pharmacological approaches to improve QOL. Integrative medicine may also include herbal remedies, diet and exercise interventions, acupuncture, acupressure, and aromatherapy.	Palliative care model has limited use with SCD population. There is no formal training with the SCD population. This position is only available at larger institutions.
Physical therapist	*Basic knowledge of evidence-based management of individuals with SCD*	Provide therapies to reduce stress and pain and improve range of motion, which can include aerobic and breathing exercises, massages, or transcutaneous electrical nerve stimulation to disrupt pain sensors and relax muscles.	There is no formal training with the SCD population.

Ancillary Team Members

Education/ vocational rehabilitation services	*Basic knowledge of* evidence-based management of individuals with SCD	Assist with obtaining special education services for youth (school intervention); provide counseling and assistance related to educational attainment, vocational counseling, job training opportunities, and academic and employment accommodations.	There is no formal training with the SCD population. This position is only available at larger institutions.
Financial advisor/ counselor	*Basic knowledge of* evidence-based management of individuals with SCD	Assist with completing insurance applications and paying medical bills.	There is no formal training with the SCD population. This position is only available at larger institutions.
Pastoral care	*Basic knowledge of* evidence-based management of individuals with SCD	Provide emotional and spiritual support; explore spiritual questions and concerns.	There is no formal training with the SCD population. This position is only available at larger institutions.

NOTE: ACS = acute chest syndrome; CHW = community health worker; HU = hydroxyurea; OB/GYNs = obstetricians and gynecologists; PCP = primary care provider; QOL = quality of life; RBC = red blood cell; SCD = sickle cell disease.

SOURCES: Informed by Agrawal et al., 2019; CFF, n.d.; Farooq and Testai, 2019; McIntosh, 2016; Mulimani et al., 2016; Okpala et al., 2002; Scott, 2016; Simon et al., 2016; Wilkie et al., 2010; and National Academies SCD committee judgment.

with SCD, as discussed in Chapter 4. Finally, the committee considered multidisciplinary care team models from other chronic, inheritable diseases, such as CF (CFF, n.d.).

The SCD care team members are classified as core or supplementary based on their level of involvement in managing the clinical and psychosocial complications of SCD (see Chapter 4) or in decreasing disparities in care (e.g., CHWs). The committee also considered disciplines currently providing care that are perceived as beneficial by clinicians or patients (e.g., financial counselors). Some members of the core team, such as hematologists and ED physicians, currently treat children and adults with SCD in the United States. However, the committee determined that PCPs, nurses, and other advanced practice practitioners, with the right level of preparation, could manage the care of patients with SCD as needed. Second-level core team members assist with managing SCD complications but are designated as level 2 because they may not serve the entire SCD population and instead focus on individuals with a specific complication or need (e.g., a pulmonologist may work with patients with pulmonary hypertension, but not all patients with SCD will have pulmonary complications). Ancillary team members may provide services on an ad hoc basis or may provide enabling services but influence the way that care is delivered or managed by addressing key social contributors (determinants) of health.

TRAINING THE NEXT GENERATION OF SCD CARE PROVIDERS

There have been some efforts by national organizations and health care systems to recruit and retain the SCD workforce of the future. For example, ASH offers a training series for hematologists and internists to guide them in starting an adult SCD clinic. However, additional programming and resources are needed to foster the development of a well-trained multidisciplinary SCD workforce. In addition, a lack of diversity among health care providers may contribute to disparities in health care service. Having providers who are similar to the patients in important dimensions, such as race, ethnicity, and language, promotes effective communication and can improve patient–provider relationships. Diversity among faculty, staff, and trainees enhances creative problem solving and fosters robust decision making, innovation, and productivity both in the health care setting and the workplace in general (Alsan et al., 2018; Cohen et al., 2002; Forbes Insights, 2011; Hunt et al., 2015). Thus, to identify the best and brightest, national organizations and the health care system should implement specific recruitment and retention strategies that address identified gaps in training and professional development; this is essential for achieving and maintaining high-quality care. The next section summarizes current efforts in workforce development and identifies gaps and opportunities for training in hematology, emergency medicine, primary care, and non-hematologic disciplines.

Hematology[11]

The growing need for greater clinical and research training in benign hematology has long been recognized. The number of physicians entering the field is decreasing, and many are not engaged in research (Hoots et al., 2015; Soffer and Hoots, 2018). Minorities are also under-represented in hematology/medical oncology, with only about 6 percent of individuals identifying as black/African American and about 8 percent as Hispanic (Santhosh and Babik, 2020). Further exacerbating the problem, hematology/medical oncology trainees receive little early clinical exposure to non-malignant hematology (Marshall et al., 2018).

Curriculums in combined programs of hematology/medical oncology have been hypothesized to contribute to a shortage of researchers in benign hematology (Naik et al., 2018a). Of the 134 fellowship programs in the United States, 132 are combined double-board programs for hematology/medical oncology; only two institutions currently offer hematology-only programs (Naik et al., 2018a). Further reducing opportunities for training, the Accreditation Council for Graduate Medical Education no longer mandates the number of months required for nonmalignant hematology instruction in fellowships. Traditionally, one-third of a fellow's time used to be spent in nonmalignant hematology training (Wallace et al., 2015). These difficulties are mirrored outside of the United States. For example, in UK medical schools, rotations are offered in cardiology, surgery, and psychiatry, but there is no dedicated rotation in hematology. Instead, exposure to hematology is largely tested as part of a syllabus focused on pathology (Mandan et al., 2016).

Intellectual curiosity and stimulation are significant determining factors for medical students and internal medicine residents when choosing a focus (Marshall et al., 2018). Hematology covers a wide breadth of topics that relate to both malignant and nonmalignant diseases, which makes hematologists important in advancing the research and treatment of many diseases. Third-year fellows have described benign hematology as more "complicated" and "overwhelming" than malignant hematology or medical oncology (Bernstein et al., 2017). Currently, there is little early clinical exposure to benign hematology that highlights its intellectual excitement (Marshall et al., 2018). Less than 6 percent of graduates plan to practice primarily in nonmalignant hematology (Todd et al., 2004). Importantly,

---

[11] See Appendix J for additional training models for hematologists.

even at programs where exposure to benign hematology is mandatory, such as the University of Pennsylvania, only around one out of seven or eight fellows is training in benign hematology (Loren, 2009).

Additionally, there are generally fewer available mentors than in other specialties. A lack of or ineffective mentorship has been observed for potential hematology fellows, which can contribute to difficulty in hiring and retaining junior faculty, disillusionment with academia, and reduced grant funding (Straus et al., 2013). Fellows in hematology/oncology training programs have reported that mentorship opportunities tend to happen "randomly," rather than individuals being able to actively seek out a relationship. Additionally, there are generally more available mentors in oncology, which can play a decisive role in the career decision process (Wallace et al., 2016). Without effective mentorship, it is difficult to generate excitement and inspire the same enthusiasm, and there are fewer networking opportunities to develop other productive relationships (Sambunjak et al., 2010).

Medical students and fellows have a misconception that there are fewer jobs available in hematology than in oncology. Instead, projections indicate a shortage in both hematology and oncology. Overall the demand for hematology/oncology services is projected to grow 40 percent, whereas the supply may grow only 25 percent (Yang et al., 2014). In 2013, a survey of practice-based hematology was sent to 36 percent of ASH's membership (5,081 physicians) (ASH, 2015). One-quarter of respondents indicated that they were considering retirement in the next 5 years (ASH, 2015; Tejaswini, 2015). Compounding the problem, many of these physicians specialize in benign hematology, and there is no pool of new fellows to replenish them. Patient loads are already so high that several cancer centers are searching for hematologists to join their faculty (Hoots et al., 2015; Sharma et al., 2019).

Starting salaries for hematology providers tend to be lower than other hematology and oncology specialties; pediatric hematologists/oncologists are among the 20 specialties with the lowest annual earnings (approximately $223,000) according to the Doximity 2019 physician compensation report, which includes responses from 90,000 U.S. physicians (Doximity, 2019). Compounding this comparatively low earning rate, according to a survey of 236 hematology–oncology fellows training at 56 participating cancer centers, 37 of them graduated with more than $100,000 in debt (Horn et al., 2011). Higher debt levels have been shown to increase stress and influence the likelihood of considering income potential when choosing a specialty (Rohlfing et al., 2014). For those seeking grant funding in hematological research, the outlook is no better. A National Institutes of Health (NIH) physician–scientist workgroup found that the number of investigators submitting and receiving NIH grants in the field declined by about 70 percent over the past 13 years (Hoots et al., 2015). Because of these challenges, basic science advances in hematology await translation into clinical practice, and the care of nonmalignant hematology patients is suffering (Sharma et al., 2019; Soffer and Hoots, 2018).

The Division of Blood Diseases and Resources of NHLBI collaborated with ASH to convene a series of two overlapping working groups in 2012 and 2013 to identify potential strategies to address the declining clinical and research workforce in hematology (Hoots et al., 2015). They identified the following strategies:

- Early identification of future young physician–scholars as high school students and undergraduates and provision of summer internships and travel awards to conferences, particularly targeting students from diverse backgrounds. Introduction to hematologic practice and discovery should also start early through the Internet, television (e.g., documentaries), and science-based programming.
- During medical school, the introduction to hematology course could be moved to the first rather than second year of instruction to increase interest. Demonstrations for medical students in the classroom and hospital and clinic settings can illustrate the wide range of hematologic practice and the high impact of hematologic discoveries. If possible, it would also be beneficial for medical students to attend a comprehensive sickle cell clinic either on site or at an affiliated institution. Supplemental training could include rotation in the blood bank or attendance at a local blood center education program.
- Partnerships with the pharmaceutical industry may provide teaching and learning opportunities through translational and clinical trials.
- Grant funding mechanisms are needed for early career investigators. NHLBI and the National Institute of Diabetes and Digestive and Kidney Diseases have a short-term pilot program that funds hematologic laboratory programs for up to 6 months of mentored experiences for pre- and post-doctoral trainees. The ASH Alternative Training Pathway Grant also funds innovative training experiences that combine hematology with another field, such as pharmacology, or in combined pediatric/adult hematology.

Easing the financial burden from student loans and offering financial incentives for research on and treatment of the SCD population is another way to attract health care professionals to specialize in SCD care. The current federal loan repayment programs (LRPs) offered through NIH and the Health Resources and Services Administration (HRSA) can be further enhanced to attract more providers to the SCD workforce. The National Health Service Corps (NHSC) LRP

> offers primary care medical, dental, and mental and behavioral health care providers the opportunity to have their student loans repaid, while earning a competitive salary, in exchange for providing health care in urban, rural, or tribal communities with limited access to care. (HHS, 2019)

The current program offers $30,000–$50,000 to eligible applicants, depending on the health professional shortage area (HPSA) they work in, for 2 years of full-time service; applicants also have a half-time service option. Similarly, medical and dental students and other allied health providers seeking to enter primary care careers may be eligible for NHSC scholarships if they commit to providing service in a designated HPSA (HHS, 2020a). These opportunities need to be disseminated to students and health professionals who may be interested in providing care to the SCD population but who have concerns regarding student loan debt. Recently in response to the opioid epidemic, Congress directed HRSA to establish the NHSC Substance Use Disorder Workforce LRP to attract a workforce to provide the comprehensive care needed to effectively treat substance use disorders (HHS, 2020b). The committee believes that due to the dire need to develop and sustain the SCD workforce, establishing an LRP specifically for the SCD workforce could help to achieve this goal.

NIH also offers intramural and extramural LRPs of up to $50,000 annually for researchers in return for a commitment to conduct research relevant to the mission of NIH (NIH Division of Loan Repayment, n.d.). These programs are, however, limited (eight LRPs total) and competitive, which means that SCD clinicians and researchers are competing with those working with much larger disease populations. Considering the multitude of research gaps identified for SCD and SCT, NIH is encouraged to expand these LRPs, including designating SCD as a health disparity to incentivize early career SCD researchers.

Emergency Medicine

Individuals with SCD often require care in the ED, which may sometimes act as a safety net for those who have no other option or no access to a medical home (Yusuf et al., 2010). Emergency medicine care providers are often suspicious of SCD patients who have frequent ED visits (Shapiro et al., 1997) and may view patients with high ED use as addicts and label them "drug-seeking." These inaccurate beliefs can lead to some individuals with SCD avoiding the ED for fear of being perceived as malingering or opioid dependent. Negative provider attitudes can affect redosing of pain medication (Glassberg et al., 2013) and result in longer wait times at the ED (Haywood et al., 2013) (see Chapter 5).

Glassberg (2017), an emergency medicine physician at the Mount Sinai Comprehensive Sickle Cell Program at the Icahn School of Medicine at Mount Sinai, has developed four tenets for improving ED care for patients with SCD (see Figure 6-3): reducing negative provider attitudes, reducing the time to first dose of analgesic medication, improving ED pain care beyond the first dose, and improving ED patient safety.

Supplemental education about SCD disease-related processes for emergency providers has proved successful. Examples include a workshop led by six SCD experts to improve provider knowledge of common acute and chronic physiologic complications, pain pathophysiology, and best practices for analgesic management in the ED setting. The workshop assessed pre- and post-workshop knowledge and had its greatest impact on shifting

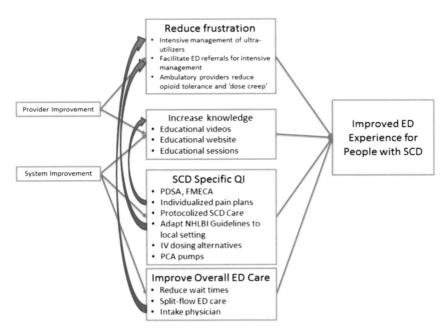

FIGURE 6-3 Elements of improving the emergency department experience.
NOTE: ED = emergency department; FMECA = failure mode, effects, and criticality analysis; IV = intravenous; NHLBI = National Heart, Lung, and Blood Institute; PCA = patient-controlled analgesia; PDSA = plan-do-study-act; QI = quality improvement; SCD = sickle cell disease.
SOURCE: Glassberg, 2017. Republished with permission of the American Society of Hematology; permission conveyed through Copyright Clearance Center, Inc.

the perception of ED providers regarding addiction in the SCD population (Tanabe et al., 2013). Similarly, a short video intervention that included an adult hematologist discussing challenges about seeking treatment for pain with SCD patients reduced negative provider attitudes (Haywood et al., 2011). More recently, another short online video intervention was delivered by e-mail to emergency providers; it included both provider and patient perspectives regarding the challenges in managing in ED care for patients with SCD pain and resulted in improved provider attitudes about SCD (Singh et al., 2016).

Other models to improve care in the ED include a multidisciplinary SCD committee, such as the program at Jefferson University Hospitals (JUH). Aside from internists, who provide both inpatient and outpatient care, this multidisciplinary team includes an outpatient sickle cell nurse, a sickle cell social worker, a psychiatrist, specialized sickle cell hematologists, and nurse practitioners (JUH, n.d.). The program focuses on long-term care for patients with SCD. Patients can attend monthly self-support group meetings coordinated by a JUH social worker who teaches techniques to reduce stress and teaches the patients about their disease and its complications. The program also offers a 24/7 observation unit (JUH, n.d.).

Improving ED Management for Individuals with SCD is another innovative program that warrants replication on a larger scale. The program has advanced the treatment of SCD-related pain in the ED, leading to more rapid pain relief. The multidisciplinary team of physicians, nurses, social workers, and individuals living with SCD works to increase awareness and decrease negative provider attitudes about SCD patients. The team has also created a user-friendly treatment algorithm to help guide ED treatment (CCNC Sickle Cell Task Force, n.d.), a webpage devoted the care of patients with SCD in the ED that is an educational resource for providers (Duke University School of Medicine, 2012), and an SCD toolbox app that offers providers access to the latest evidence-based guidelines and to an SCD specialist (Improving Sickle Cell Care in North Carolina and Community Care of North Carolina, n.d.). In addition, the program holds an annual educational conference aimed at improving knowledge and open communication among providers, patients, and families.

The Emergency Department of Sickle Cell Care Coalition (EDSC[3]) is a national forum whose goal is to improve the emergency care of patients with SCD in the United States. ACEP created the coalition in collaboration with multiple public, private, and professional partners. EDSC[3] primarily focuses on disseminating research findings to local and national stakeholders, supporting the education of ED providers and patients regarding the appropriate management of SCD-related pain and other complications, supporting advocacy and community outreach efforts, and supporting the development of appropriate metrics to improve the emergency care of patients with SCD. EDSC[3] is an excellent resource for training-related issues for emergency medicine providers working with SCD patients in the ED; it also includes links to podcasts with SCD experts and a blog supporting conversations regarding equity, fact sheets, training modules, pain consortium materials, and protocols (EDSC[3], n.d.).

Primary Care

High-quality primary care treatment can limit preventable and costly interactions with the health care system. Currently, however, there are insufficient PCPs with the comprehensive knowledge and expertise to care for people with SCD (Mainous et al., 2015), and PCPs' greatest challenge is adequate pain management (Utuama et al., 2015). Parents of children with SCD feel that current care from PCPs is inadequate (Raphael et al., 2013). Additionally, when children with SCD experience more health care barriers (i.e., experience of marginalization), it is more challenging to receive high-quality care that is accessible, comprehensive, and well coordinated (Jacob et al., 2016).

Project Extension for Community Healthcare Outcomes (ECHO) is a rapidly growing national network of telementoring hubs for training and knowledge sharing, with the goal of improving capacity and access to specialty care for rural and underserved populations. SCD ECHO hubs are regionally based and managed by a designated regional coordinating center. Their virtual learning teleECHO™ programs are open to community providers, PCPs, and SCD stakeholders in the United States and across the world. HRSA funds and manages this program, which is a relatively low-cost option that can mentor and train PCPs, offer feedback on difficult cases, and share knowledge and expertise through monthly didactics and clinical case presentations. The program is a proven way to increase knowledgeable PCPs (Shook et al., 2016). In 2020, HRSA, in collaboration with the Office of Minority Health at HHS, launched a 6-month pilot of a national SCD ECHO, the Sickle Cell Disease Training and Mentoring Program (HHS, n.d.). The program, which is targeted at PCPs, offers a telehealth series taught by a hematologist covering topics such as pain management, HU, and preventive services (HHS, n.d.). Regional hubs have been successful in increasing PCP knowledge about SCD (Shook et al., 2016); the committee recommends an evaluation of the program at the end of the pilot to determine its effectiveness and opportunities for scaling.

"The Department of Health and Human Services has given grants to nine facilities to develop programs to improve services for patients with SCD" (Butterfield, 2013). For the Johns Hopkins University School of Medicine, this grant led to the development of the Improving Health Outcomes and Medical Education for Sickle Cell Disease (iHOMES) Network.

The iHOMES team found that 40 percent of community physicians surveyed were uncomfortable with their ability to provide ambulatory care or manage comorbidities for SCD patients. More than half felt uncomfortable managing SCD pain and medications. The aims of the network are twofold (Butterfield, 2013). First, it has expanded physician training by having internal medicine residents at JHH provide primary care to SCD patients. Second, it offers community providers a number of support mechanisms (JHM, n.d.).

Non-Hematologic Medical Providers

The complex nature of SCD creates care needs that require medical and allied health expertise from providers other than hematologists, emergency medicine providers, and PCPs (Okpala et al., 2002). Other members of the SCD medical treatment team include, but are not limited to, nurses and nurse practitioners, physician assistants, blood bank and transfusion specialists, neurologists, radiologists, dentists, ophthalmologists, obstetrician/gynecologists, genetic counselors, integrative medicine specialists, nephrologists, orthopedists, pulmonologists, psychologists, and social workers (see Table 6-1). Training related to SCD-related complications varies widely, with most providers receiving little to no specific training (Hanik et al., 2014). There are currently no uniform practices or standardized protocols, which can make it challenging for providers to administer care. Provider racial or cultural biases also affect clinical care and treatment decisions (Bulgin et al., 2018) (see Chapter 2).

Knowledge gaps about SCD and the best standard of care contribute to poor communication between patients and SCD specialists (Azonobi et al., 2014) and to poor patient satisfaction and outcomes. The most difficult hurdle is that most providers serve very few SCD patients (Mainous et al., 2015). Because interactions are so infrequent, providers may be somewhat reluctant to devote time and effort to support a rarely seen population. Furthermore, the unpredictable and often persistent nature of the pain and other complications associated with SCD pose a difficult challenge for providers (Utuama et al., 2015). There are no known objective measures that indicate the presence or severity of this pain, which introduces a great deal of clinical uncertainty into the patient–provider relationship (Matthias et al., 2010) (see Chapter 5).

It may be challenging for some providers to improve patient outcomes because they do not have a sufficient volume of cases. In the quality literature, higher volumes generally correlate with improved outcomes. The exact reasons are not known, but they are suspected to follow from the opportunity to develop increased provider skill, multidisciplinary teams, and access to specialized resources. Other fields have overcome this barrier using distance learning and consultation and telementoring (e.g., TeleECHO for HCV).

In addition to the challenge of prevailing health care professionals' workforce shortages in the United States, which is not specific to the SCD population, most of the care team members identified in Table 6-1 have limited or no formal training in the SCD population and so would need to be prepared to effectively deliver care. Yet, there are systemic challenges (e.g., reimbursement models) that also contribute to the workforce challenges. There are a few models that offer strategies for preparing disease-specific specialists, including the HIV specialist model, conferred through the American Academy of HIV Medicine (AAHIVM).

The American Academy of HIV Medicine's HIV Specialist Model

AAHIVM convened a group of individuals who had been offering HIV care in order to establish standards for delivering high-quality care. Several types of health care providers, including physicians, nurse practitioners, physician assistants, and pharmacists, can receive a professional credential (e.g., HIV specialist, expert, or pharmacist) if they actively care for more than 25 HIV patients (AAHIVM, 2020). The goals of the credentialing process are to (1) improve the quality of HIV care, (2) broaden patient access to quality care, and (3) expand the number of HIV-specialized medical care providers (AAHIVM, 2020; Sweet, n.d.). AAHIVM offers a core curriculum and training program that provides basic knowledge on HIV for new providers and information about clinical advances and complex topics for experienced providers (AAHIVM, 2020; Sweet, n.d.). This credentialing model could be applied to health professionals who are interested in treating the SCD population.

CONCLUSIONS AND RECOMMENDATIONS

Despite national efforts to improve quality in SCD care, that quality remains poor for most individuals in the United States. National quality metrics have not been developed, resulting in significant variations. Some SCD programs track and perform well on consensus-based quality indicators (e.g., transition readiness assessment); however, data suggest that the overall performance on the few evidence-based quality metrics identified (e.g., penicillin, stroke prevention) is poor. This overall inadequate state of care hinders the advancement of comprehensive, multidisciplinary, effective, data-driven programs for individuals living with SCD and SCT. Pain management is also an area where there is a lack of quality measures.

Routine preventive care is necessary for both pediatric and adult patients with SCD, and some routine indicators, such as developmental assessment in pediatrics, need to be performed more frequently due to SCD-related complications. Quality indicators for SCD acute, subacute, and chronic care have been identified in the literature but are not endorsed or tracked by any national entity. For example, NHLBI guidelines recommend offering HU at 9 months of age, yet uptake ranges from 14 to 28 percent for clinical samples. Similarly, TCD is known to detect the risk of stroke, but patients receive it about 23–45 percent of the time. Barriers to the implementation of evidence-based or consensus guidelines need to be quantified, defined, measured, and tracked to improve the system of care.

Adolescents and young adults who transfer from pediatric to adult care encounter many challenges that affect their quality of care. Several national organizations and quality initiatives have developed transition metrics. Data indicate that although these individuals may be participating in programs to prepare them for transition, a high number do not successfully transfer to an adult provider. These youth also tend to use the ED more than other individuals with SCD, which is another indicator that the quality of care during this time may be inadequate. New SCD transition programs and initiatives using quality improvement methods to improve the transition process hold promise for decreasing disparities in care experienced during this time.

To develop a body of endorsed relevant quality metrics that can be adequately disseminated and tracked to measure their impact, there needs to be an NQF-like entity that formulates, tracks, and transparently reports on the adherence of systems to these metrics for SCD, similar to what has been done for asthma, children from low-income families, and other groups. There should also be a parallel organization that monitors performance and provides guidance on mitigating poor performance, with an appropriate accountability that could be tied to payment/reimbursement.

Access to providers and the availability of a trained, prepared workforce are key issues that have not been adequately addressed in SCD care. The lack of adult hematologists and other providers further contributes to variations in care. Some individuals receive treatment from multidisciplinary teams with experience managing SCD, while others have providers with limited awareness of SCD and its many complications. There are limited educational and training opportunities for providers and trainees who wish to specialize in SCD care. Along with the lack of diversity in the workforce, there is a need for competency training in the sociocultural factors in the patient experience of care in order to improve relationships between patients and health care teams. This chapter identifies the team members needed to provide high-quality care for all SCD patients, the team members needed to care for individuals who experience specific complications (e.g., pulmonary hypertension, stroke), and training gaps and opportunities. Individuals with SCD may also experience sociodemographic challenges that can affect their receipt of high-quality care. Ancillary team members, such as financial counselors, can help to mitigate sociodemographic barriers or increase resilience factors (e.g., pastoral care), thereby improving access to and delivery of care. Provider certification models (e.g., HIV expert) and hub-and-spoke models, such as Project ECHO, can help to build and maintain a well-prepared SCD workforce.

SCT is even less well understood, and little is known about the relevant quality of care. There is also a need to develop national reporting guidelines. Instituting the best practices of SCT notification and genetic counseling would vastly improve the care provided and allow for the examination of clinical outcomes.

> Conclusion 6-1: Many of the approaches to SCD management lack a good evidence base, particularly to support current treatment strategies. The lack of evidence-based guidelines results in inconsistent treatment approaches across centers and providers, reduced access to care, and poor outcomes. Strategies are needed to enhance the evidence base to support the treatment of SCD.

> Conclusion 6-2: The evidence for a comprehensive, systematic approach to the delivery of high-quality care for SCD is lacking, and the science of quality in SCD care lags behind other diseases in several areas: SCD clinical guidelines are supported with poor quality evidence; there are multiple sets of guidelines, but none are universally accepted or cover the services needed for comprehensive care; adherence to clinical guidelines and quality indicators is not measured, reported, required, incentivized, or included in public transparency reports; and there is evidence of a lack of funding and priority for the development of quality metrics in SCD. There is ample evidence from other disease areas that can be leveraged for SCD care while research is generated to fill in the gaps in the evidence base.

> Conclusion 6-3: There is a need for provider- and patient-focused strategies to increase the uptake of guidelines and metrics for SCD that have a strong evidence base.

> Conclusion 6-4: Optimal treatment for people with SCD is best managed by a multidisciplinary team of professionals delivering comprehensive high-quality care. Traditionally, hematologists have coordinated the management of care and liaised with other specialties. Comprehensive, high-quality care delivery for SCD requires the availability and preparedness of a multidisciplinary

team of providers—behavioral health providers (e.g., psychologists, neuropsychologists, and psychiatrists), social workers, dietitians, physiotherapists, massage therapists, community health workers, care coordinators, and school liaison officers. Substantial barriers, such as an aging workforce, workforce shortages, negative provider attitudes, and a lack of training, have contributed to a limited workforce for SCD care.

Recommendation 6-1: Federal agencies including the Agency for Healthcare Research and Quality; National Heart, Lung, and Blood Institute; Health Resources and Services Administration; Centers for Disease Control and Prevention; and U.S. Food and Drug Administration should work together with and fund researchers and professional associations to develop and track a series of indicators to assess the quality of sickle cell disease care, including the patient experience, the prevention of disease complications, and health outcomes.

Recommendation 6-2: The Centers for Medicare & Medicaid Services and private payers should require the reporting of expert consensus-driven sickle cell disease (SCD) quality measures and other metrics of high-quality health care for persons with SCD.

Recommendation 6-3: The U.S. Department of Health and Human Services should fund efforts to identify and mitigate potentially modifiable disparities in mortality and health outcomes. Specific subgroups to consider include young adults in transition from pediatric to adult care, pregnant women, and older adults.

Recommendation 6-4: The National Institutes of Health should disseminate information on loan repayment opportunities to incentivize health care professionals interested in conducting research on sickle cell disease (SCD). The Health Resources and Services Administration should add populations with SCD as a designated population health professional shortage area under the National Health Service Corps program and create a loan repayment program for health care professionals working with SCD populations.

Recommendation 6-5: Health professional associations (American Society of Hematology, American College of Obstetricians and Gynecologists, American College of Emergency Physicians, American Academy of Family Physicians,[12] American Academy of Pediatrics, American

---

[12] This text was revised since the prepublication release of this report to correct American Association of Family Practitioners to American Academy of Family Physicians.

College of Physicians, National Medical Association) and organizations for other relevant health professionals such as advanced practice providers, nurses, and community health workers should convene an Academy of Sickle Cell Disease (SCD) Medicine to support SCD providers through education, credentialing, networking, and advocacy.

Recommendation 6-6: Health professional associations and graduate and professional schools should develop early and effective mentoring programs to link early career health professionals with seasoned providers to generate interest in sickle cell disease care.

REFERENCES

AAHIVM (American Academy of HIV Medicine). 2020. *American Academy of HIV Medicine credentialing handbook*. Washington, DC: American Academy of HIV Medicine.

AAP (American Academy of Pediatrics). 2002. Health supervision for children with sickle cell disease. *Pediatrics* 109(3):526.

ACOG (American College of Obstetricians and Gynecologists). 2017. Carrier screening for genetic conditions. Committee opinion no. 691. *Obstetrics and Gynecology* 129:e41–e55.

Agrawal, S., W. B. Burton, D. Manwani, D. Rastogi, and A. De. 2019. A physicians survey assessing management of pulmonary airway involvement in sickle cell disease. *Pediatric Pulmonology* 54(7):993–1001.

AHRQ (Agency for Healthcare Research and Quality). n.d. *AHRQ quality indicators*. https://www.qualityindicators.ahrq.gov (accessed April 9, 2020).

Alsan, M., O. Garrick, and G. C. Graziani. 2018. Does diversity matter for health? Experimental evidence from Oakland. *NBER Working Paper No. 24787*. https://www.nber.org/papers/w24787.pdf (accessed July 1, 2020).

Anie, K. A., H. Grocott, L. White, M. Dzingina, G. Rogers, and G. Cho. 2012. Patient self-assessment of hospital pain, mood and health-related quality of life in adults with sickle cell disease. *BMJ Open* 2(4):1–6.

ASH (American Society of Hematology). 2015. Adapting to changes in practice-based hematology. *ASH Clinical News*, May 15. https://www.ashclinicalnews.org/spotlight/adapting-to-changes-in-practice-based-hematology (accessed April 12, 2020).

ASH. 2019. *ASH draft recommendations on sickle cell disease-related pain*. https://www.hematology.org/Clinicians/Guidelines-Quality/Documents/9558.aspx (accessed February 28, 2020).

ASH. n.d. *ASH clinical practice guidelines on sickle cell disease*. https://www.hematology.org/SCDguidelines (accessed February 28, 2020).

Azonobi, I. C., B. L. Anderson, V. R. Byams, A. M. Grant, and J. Schulkin. 2014. Obstetrician-gynecologists' knowledge of sickle cell disease screening and management. *BMC Pregnancy and Childbirth* 14(1):356.

Bakshi, N., C. B. Sinha, D. Ross, K. Khemani, G. Loewenstein, and L. Krishnamurti. 2017. Proponent or collaborative: Physician perspectives and approaches to disease modifying therapies in sickle cell disease. *PLOS ONE* 12(7):e0178413.

Balshem, H., M. Helfand, H. J. Schunemann, A. D. Oxman, R. Kunz, J. Brozek, G. E. Vist, Y. Falck-Ytter, J. Meerpohl, S. Norris, and G. H. Guyatt. 2011. Grade guidelines: 3. Rating the quality of evidence. *Journal of Clinical Epidemiology* 64(4):401–406.

Bemrich-Stolz, C. J., J. H. Halanych, T. H. Howard, L. M. Hilliard, and J. D. Lebensburger. 2015. Exploring adult care experiences and barriers to transition in adult patients with sickle cell disease. *International Journal of Hematology and Therapy* 1(1):PMC4756764.

Bernstein, E., N. A. Podoltsev, and A. Lee. 2017. Teaching hematology to fellows: A qualitative study. *Blood* 130(Suppl 1):5641.

Beverung, L. M., D. Brousseau, R. G. Hoffmann, K. Yan, and J. A. Panepinto. 2014. Ambulatory quality indicators to prevent infection in sickle cell disease. *American Journal of Hematology* 89(3):256–260.

Bollinger, L. M., K. G. Nire, M. M. Rhodes, D. J. Chisolm, and S. H. O'Brien. 2011. Caregivers' perspectives on barriers to transcranial Doppler screening in children with sickle-cell disease. *Pediatric Blood & Cancer* 56(1):99–102.

Bulgin, D., P. Tanabe, and C. Jenerette. 2018. Stigma of sickle cell disease: A systematic review. *Issues in Mental Health Nursing* 39(8):675–686.

Bundy, D. G., J. Muschelli, G. D. Clemens, J. J. Strouse, R. E. Thompson, J. F. Casella, and M. R. Miller. 2016. Preventive care delivery to young children with sickle cell disease. *Journal of Pediatric Hematology and Oncology* 38(4):294–300.

Butterfield, S. 2013. *"Sic"ing primary care physicians on sickle cell disease.* https://acpinternist. org/archives/2013/04/sickle-cell.htm (accessed December 15, 2019).

CCNC (Community Care of North Carolina) Sickle Cell Task Force. n.d. *Emergency department vaso-occlusive crisis management: Adults and children.* https://sickleemergency. duke.edu/sites/default/files/ccnc-voc-protocol.pdf (accessed December 15, 2019).

CFF (Cystic Fibrosis Foundation). 2019. *2018 patient registry: Annual data report.* https:// www.cff.org/Research/Researcher-Resources/Patient-Registry/2018-Patient-Registry-Annual-Data-Report.pdf (accessed March 6, 2019).

CFF. n.d. *Your CF care team.* https://www.cff.org/Care/Your-CF-Care-Team (accessed December 15, 2019).

CFF, D. Borowitz, K. A. Robinson, M. Rosenfeld, S. D. Davis, K. A. Sabadosa, S. L. Spear, S. H. Michel, R. B. Parad, T. B. White, P. M. Farrell, B. C. Marshall, and F. J. Accurso. 2009. Cystic Fibrosis Foundation evidence-based guidelines for management of infants with cystic fibrosis. *Journal of Pediatrics* 155(6 Suppl):S73–S93.

Chou, S. T., M. Alsawas, R. M. Fasano, J. J. Field, J. E. Hendrickson, J. Howard, M. Kameka, J. L. Kwiatkowski, F. Pirenne, P. A. Shi, S. R. Stowell, S. L. Thein, C. M. Westhoff, T. E. Wong, and E. A. Akl. 2020. American Society of Hematology 2020 guidelines for sickle cell disease: Transfusion support. *Blood Advances* 4(2):327–355.

Clay, O. J., and J. Telfair. 2007. Evaluation of a disease-specific self-efficacy instrument in adolescents with sickle cell disease and its relationship to adjustment. *Child Neuropsychology* 13(2):188–203.

CMS (Centers for Medicare & Medicaid Services). 2018. 2019 updates to the child and adult core health care quality measurement sets. https://www.medicaid.gov/sites/default/files/ federal-policy-guidance/downloads/cib112018.pdf (accessed March 5, 2020).

CMS. 2020. *Quality measures.* https://www.cms.gov/Medicare/Quality-Initiatives-Patient-Assessment-Instruments/QualityMeasures/index.html (accessed February 27, 2020).

Cohen, J. J., B. A. Gabriel, and C. Terrell. 2002. The case for diversity in the health care workforce. *Health Affairs* 21(5):90–102.

Conway, S., I. M. Balfour-Lynn, K. De Rijcke, P. Drevinek, J. Foweraker, T. Havermans, H. Heijerman, L. Lannefors, A. Lindblad, M. Macek, S. Madge, M. Moran, L. Morrison, A. Morton, J. Noordhoek, D. Sands, A. Vertommen, and D. Peckham. 2014. European Cystic Fibrosis Society standards of care: Framework for the cystic fibrosis centre. *Journal of Cystic Fibrosis* 13:S3–S22.

Cooper, O., H. McBain, S. Tangayi, P. Telfer, D. Tsitsikas, A. Yardumian, and K. Mulligan. 2019. Psychometric analysis of the Adult Sickle Cell Quality of Life Measurement Information System (ACSQ-ME) in a UK population. *Health and Quality of Life Outcomes* 17(1):74.

Crosby, L. E., L. M. Shook, R. E. Ware, and W. B. Brinkman. 2015. Shared decision making for hydroxyurea treatment initiation in children with sickle cell anemia. *Pediatric Blood & Cancer* 62(2):184–185.

Crosby, L. E., A. Walton, L. M. Shook, R. E. Ware, M. Treadwell, K. L. Saving, M. Britto, J. Peugh, E. McTate, S. Oyeku, C. Nwankwo, and W. B. Brinkman. 2019. Development of a hydroxyurea decision aid for parents of children with sickle cell anemia. *Journal of Pediatrics Hematology and Oncology* 41(1):56–63.

de Montalembert, M., and C. Guitton. 2014. Transition from paediatric to adult care for patients with sickle cell disease. *British Journal of Haematology* 164(5):630–635.

DeBaun, M. R. 2014. The challenge of creating an evidence-based guideline for sickle cell disease. *JAMA* 312(10):1004–1005.

DeBaun, M. R., and J. Telfair. 2012. Transition and sickle cell disease. *Pediatrics* 130(5):926–935.

Doximity. 2019. *2019 physician compensation report: Third annual study.* https://s3.amazonaws.com/s3.doximity.com/press/doximity_third_annual_physician_compensation_report_round4.pdf (accessed March 6, 2020).

Duke University School of Medicine. 2012. *Emergency department sickle cell disease: Crisis management and beyond.* https://sickleemergency.duke.edu (accessed December 15, 2019).

Eckrich, M. J., W. C. Wang, E. Yang, P. G. Arbogast, A. Morrow, J. A. Dudley, W. A. Ray, and W. O. Cooper. 2013. Adherence to transcranial Doppler screening guidelines among children with sickle cell disease. *Pediatric Blood & Cancer* 60(2):270–274.

EDSC[3] (Emergency Department Sickle Cell Care Coalition). n.d. About the EDSC[3]. https://www.acep.org/by-medical-focus/hematology/sickle-cell (accessed November 19, 2019).

Edwards, R., J. Telfair, H. Cecil, and J. Lenoci. 2000. Reliability and validity of a self-efficacy instrument specific to sickle cell disease. *Behaviour Research and Therapy* 38(9):951–963.

Edwards, R., J. Telfair, H. Cecil, and J. Lenoci. 2001. Self-efficacy as a predictor of adult adjustment to sickle cell disease: One-year outcomes. *Psychosomatic Medicine* 63(5):850–858.

Evensen, C. T., M. J. Treadwell, S. Keller, R. Levine, K. L. Hassell, E. M. Werner, and W. R. Smith. 2016. Quality of care in sickle cell disease: Cross-sectional study and development of a measure for adults reporting on ambulatory and emergency department care. *Medicine (Baltimore)* 95(35):e4528.

Farooq, S., and F. D. Testai. 2019. Neurologic complications of sickle cell disease. *Current Neurology and Neuroscience Reports* 19(4):17.

Ferrans, C. E., J. J. Zerwic, J. E. Wilbur, and J. L. Larson. 2005. Conceptual model of health-related quality of life. *Journal of Nursing Scholarship* 37(4):336–342.

Forbes Insights. 2011. *Global diversity and inclusion: Fostering innovation through a diverse workforce.* New York: Forbes.

Freed, G. L. 2019. A missed opportunity to address a national shame: The case of sickle cell disease in the United States. *JAMA Pediatric* 173(8):715–716.

Geller, A. K., and M. K. O'Connor. 2008. The sickle cell crisis: A dilemma in pain relief. *Mayo Clinic Proceedings* 83(3):320–323.

Glassberg, J. A. 2017. Improving emergency department-based care of sickle cell pain. *Hematology: American Society of Hematology—Education Program* 2017(1):412–417.

Glassberg, J. A., P. Tanabe, A. Chow, K. Harper, C. Haywood Jr., M. R. DeBaun, and L. D. Richardson. 2013. Emergency provider analgesic practices and attitudes toward patients with sickle cell disease. *Annals of Emergency Medicine* 62(4):293–302.

Godfrey, M. M., and B. J. Oliver. 2014. Accelerating the rate of improvement in cystic fibrosis care: Contributions and insights of the Learning and Leadership Collaborative. *BMJ Quality & Safety* 23(Suppl 1):i23–i32.

Grant, A. M., C. S. Parker, L. B. Jordan, M. M. Hulihan, M. S. Creary, M. A. Lloyd-Puryear, J. C. Goldsmith, and H. K. Atrash. 2011. Public health implications of sickle cell trait: A report of the CDC meeting. *American Journal of Preventive Medicine* 41(6 Suppl 4):S435–S439.

Grosse, S. D., M. S. Schechter, R. Kulkarni, M. A. Lloyd-Puryear, B. Strickland, and E. Trevathan. 2009. Models of comprehensive multidisciplinary care for individuals in the United States with genetic disorders. *Pediatrics* 123(1):407–412.

Hamilton, C. M., L. C. Strader, J. G. Pratt, D. Maiese, T. Hendershot, R. K. Kwok, J. A. Hammond, W. Huggins, D. Jackman, H. Pan, D. S. Nettles, T. H. Beaty, L. A. Farrer, P. Kraft, M. L. Marazita, J. M. Ordovas, C. N. Pato, M. R. Spitz, D. Wagener, M. Williams, H. A. Junkins, W. R. Harlan, E. M. Ramos, and J. Haines. 2011. The PhenX toolkit: Get the most from your measures. *American Journal of Epidemiology* 174(3):253–260.

Hanik, M., K. M. Sackett, and L. L. Hartman. 2014. An educational module to improve healthcare staffs' attitudes toward sickle cell disease patients. *Journal for Nurses in Professional Development* 30(5):231–236.

Hankins, J. S., R. Osarogiagbon, P. Adams-Graves, L. McHugh, V. Steele, M. P. Smeltzer, and S. M. Anderson. 2012. A transition pilot program for adolescents with sickle cell disease. *Journal of Pediatric Health Care* 26(6):e45–e49.

Haywood, C., S. Lanzkron, M. T. Hughes, R. Brown, M. Massa, N. Ratanawongsa, and M. C. Beach. 2011. A video-intervention to improve clinician attitudes toward patients with sickle cell disease: The results of a randomized experiment. *Journal of General Internal Medicine* 26(5):518–523.

Haywood, Jr., C., P. Tanabe, R. Naik, M. C. Beach, and S. Lanzkron. 2013. The impact of race and disease on sickle cell patient wait times in the emergency department. *American Journal of Emergency Medicine* 31(4):651–656.

HHS (U.S. Department of Health and Human Services). 2019. *National Health Service Corps loan repayment program.* https://nhsc.hrsa.gov/sites/default/files/NHSC/loan-repayment/nhsc-lrp-fact-sheet.pdf (accessed February 3, 2020).

HHS. 2020a. *National Health Service Corps scholarship program: School year 2020–2021 application & program guidance.* https://nhsc.hrsa.gov/sites/default/files/NHSC/scholarships/nhsc-scholarship-application-program-guidance.pdf (accessed March 6, 2020).

HHS. 2020b. *National Health Service Corps substance use disorder loan repayment program.* https://nhsc.hrsa.gov/sites/default/files/NHSC/loan-repayment/sud-lrp-application-guidance.pdf (accessed March 6, 2020).

HHS. n.d. *STAMP: Sickle Cell Disease Training and Mentoring Program.* https://www.minorityhealth.hhs.gov/sicklecell/#stamp (accessed February 3, 2020).

Hill, S., G. Maslow, L. Walker, S. Johnson, and N. Shah. 2014. Growing pains—Determination of transfer and transition from pediatrics to adult outpatient clinics for patients with sickle cell disease (SCD). *Blood* 124(21):3518.

Hood, A. M., A. A. King, M. E. Fields, A. L. Ford, K. P. Guilliams, M. L. Hulbert, J. M. Lee, and D. A. White. 2019. Higher executive abilities following a blood transfusion in children and young adults with sickle cell disease. *Pediatric Blood & Cancer* 66(10):e27899.

Hoots, W. K., J. L. Abkowitz, B. S. Coller, and D. M. DiMichele. 2015. Planning for the future workforce in hematology research. *Blood* 125(18):2745–2752.

Horn, L., E. Koehler, J. Gilbert, and D. H. Johnson. 2011. Factors associated with the career choices of hematology and medical oncology fellows trained at academic institutions in the United States. *Journal of Clinical Oncology* 29(29):3932–3938.

Hunt, S. E., and N. Sharma. 2010. Transition from pediatric to adult care for patients with sickle cell disease. *JAMA* 304(4):408–409; author reply 409.

Hunt, V., D. Layton, and S. Prince. 2015. *Why diversity matters.* https://www.mckinsey.com/business-functions/organization/our-insights/why-diversity-matters (accessed October 28, 2019).

Hussain, S., F. Nichols, L. Bowman, H. Xu, and C. Neunert. 2015. Implementation of transcranial Doppler ultrasonography screening and primary stroke prevention in urban and rural sickle cell disease populations. *Pediatric Blood & Cancer* 62(2):219–223.

Improving Sickle Cell Care in North Carolina and Community Care of North Carolina. n.d. *SCD toolbox: A sickle cell disease toolbox to improve care.* https://www.acep.org/globalassets/uploads/uploaded-files/acep/by-medical-focus/hematology---edsc3/scd-toolbox-flier_v2-final.pdf (accessed January 9, 2020).

IOM (Institute of Medicine). 2001. *Crossing the quality chasm: A new health system for the 21st century.* Washington, DC: National Academy Press.

IOM. 2003. *Unequal treatment: Confronting racial and ethnic disparities in health care.* Washington, DC: The National Academies Press.

IOM. 2008. *Retooling for an aging America: Building the health care workforce.* Washington, DC: The National Academies Press.

IOM. 2011a. *Clinical practice guidelines we can trust.* Washington, DC: The National Academies Press.

IOM. 2011b. *Relieving pain in America: A blueprint for transforming prevention, care, education, and research.* Washington, DC: The National Academies Press.

Jabour, S. M., S. Beachy, S. Coburn, S. Lanzkron, and M. N. Eakin. 2019. The role of patient–physician communication on the use of hydroxyurea in adult patients with sickle cell disease. *Journal of Racial and Ethnic Health Disparities* 6(6):1233–1243.

Jacob, E., C. Childress, and J. D. Nathanson. 2016. Barriers to care and quality of primary care services in children with sickle cell disease. *Journal of Advanced Nursing* 72(6):1417–1429.

JHM (Johns Hopkins Medicine). n.d. *Johns Hopkins sickle cell disease ECHO.* https://www.hopkinsmedicine.org/Medicine/sickle/providers/index.html?_ga=2.65953070.1018478254.1561329500-1735271705.1561329500 (accessed January 9, October 28, 2020).

Jordan, L., P. Swerdlow, and T. D. Coates. 2013. Systematic review of transition from adolescent to adult care in patients with sickle cell disease. *Journal of Pediatric Hematology and Oncology* 35(3):165–169.

JUH (Jefferson University Hospitals). n.d. *Comprehensive sickle cell program.* https://hospitals.jefferson.edu/departments-and-services/comprehensive-sickle-cell-program.html (accessed 2019).

Kanter, J., C. Dampier, I. Agodoa, R. Howard, S. Wade, V. Noxon, and S. K. Ballas. 2017. Quality of care in United States children with sickle cell anemia. *Blood* 130(Suppl 1):2098.

Keller, S., M. Yang, C. Evensen, T. Cowans, and the American Institutes for Research. 2017. *Adult sickle cell quality of life measurement information system: ASCQ-Me user's manual.* http://www.healthmeasures.net/images/ASQMe/ASCQ-Me_Scoring_Manual.pdf (accessed February 27, 2020).

Kelly, A. M., B. Kratz, M. Bielski, and P. M. Rinehart. 2002. Implementing transitions for youth with complex chronic conditions using the medical home model. *Pediatrics* 110(Suppl 3):1322–1327.

Lebensburger, J. D., C. J. Bemrich-Stolz, and T. H. Howard. 2012. Barriers in transition from pediatrics to adult medicine in sickle cell anemia. *Journal of Blood Medicine* 3:105–112.

Lee, J., W. Callon, J. C. Haywood, S. M. Lanzkron, P. Gulbrandsen, and M. C. Beach. 2018. What does shared decision making look like in natural settings? A mixed methods study of patient–provider conversations. *Communication & Medicine* 14(3):217–228.

Liem, R. I., S. Lanzkron, T. D. Coates, L. DeCastro, A. A. Desai, K. I. Ataga, R. T. Cohen, J. Haynes, Jr., I. Osunkwo, J. D. Lebensburger, J. P. Lash, T. Wun, M. Verhovsek, E. Ontala, R. Blaylark, F. Alahdab, A. Katabi, and R. A. Mustafa. 2019. American Society of Hematology 2019 guidelines for sickle cell disease: Cardiopulmonary and kidney disease. *Blood Advances* 3(23):3867–3897.

Loren, A. 2009. Hematology and Goliath: Ensuring the future of benign hematology in a world of combined hematology–oncology fellowships. *Hematologist* 16(4):2.

Mainous, A. G., R. J. Tanner, C. A. Harle, R. Baker, N. K. Shokar, and M. M. Hulihan. 2015. Attitudes toward management of sickle cell disease and its complications: A national survey of academic family physicians. *Anemia* 2015:853835.

Mandan, J., H. S. Sidhu, and A. Mahmood. 2016. Should a clinical rotation in hematology be mandatory for undergraduate medical students? *Advances in Medical Education and Practice* 7:519–521.

Marshall, A. L., S. Jenkins, J. Mikhael, and S. D. Gitlin. 2018. Determinants of hematology–oncology trainees' postfellowship career pathways with a focus on nonmalignant hematology. *Blood Advances* 2(4):361–369.

Matthias, M. S., A. L. Parpart, K. A. Nyland, M. A. Huffman, D. L. Stubbs, C. Sargent, and M. J. Bair. 2010. The patient–provider relationship in chronic pain care: Providers' perspectives. *Pain Medicine* 11(11):1688–1697.

Matthie, N., C. Jenerette, and S. McMillan. 2015. Role of self-care in sickle cell disease. *Pain Management Nursing* 16(3):257–266.

McIntosh, I. D. 2016. Health human resources guidelines: Minimum staffing standards and role descriptions for Canadian cystic fibrosis healthcare teams. *Canadian Respiratory Journal* 2016:PMC4904508.

Molter, B. L., and K. Abrahamson. 2015. Self-efficacy, transition, and patient outcomes in the sickle cell disease population. *Pain Management Nursing* 16(3):418–424.

Mulimani, P., S. K. Ballas, A. B. L. Abas, and L. Karanth. 2016. Treatment of dental complications in sickle cell disease. *Cochrane Database of Systematic Reviews* 2016(12):CD011633.

Naik, R. P., and C. Haywood, Jr. 2015. Sickle cell trait diagnosis: Clinical and social implications. *Hematology: American Society of Hematology—Education Program* 2015:160–167.

Naik, R. P., K. Marrone, S. Merrill, R. Donehower, and R. Brodsky. 2018a. Single-board hematology fellowship track: A 10-year institutional experience. *Blood* 131(4):462–464.

Naik, R. P., K. Smith-Whitley, K. L. Hassell, N. I. Umeh, M. de Montalembert, P. Sahota, C. Haywood, Jr., J. Jenkins, M. A. Lloyd-Puryear, C. H. Joiner, V. L. Bonham, and G. J. Kato. 2018b. Clinical outcomes associated with sickle cell trait: A systematic review. *Annals of Internal Medicine* 169(9):619–627.

NASEM (National Academies of Sciences, Engineering, and Medicine). 2018. *Crossing the global quality chasm: Improving health care worldwide.* Washington, DC: The National Academies Press.

NASEM. 2019. *The role of nonpharmacological approaches to pain management: Proceedings of a workshop.* Washington, DC: The National Academies Press.

Neunert, C. E., R. W. Gibson, P. A. Lane, P. Verma-Bhatnagar, V. Barry, M. Zhou, and A. Snyder. 2016. Determining adherence to quality indicators in sickle cell anemia using multiple data sources. *American Journal of Preventive Medicine* 51(1 Suppl 1):S24–S30.

NHLBI (National Heart, Lung, and Blood Institute). 2002. *The management of sickle cell disease.* https://www.nhlbi.nih.gov/files/docs/guidelines/sc_mngt.pdf (accessed September 22, 2019).

NIH (National Institutes of Health). 2008. *Research portfolio online reporting tools (RePORT).* https://report.nih.gov/crs/View.aspx?Id=713 (accessed September 22, 2019).

NIH Division of Loan Repayment. n.d. *Eligibility and programs.* https://www.lrp.nih.gov/eligibility-programs (accessed February 3, 2020).

NLM (National Library of Medicine). 2018. *About the newborn screening coding and terminology guide.* https://newbornscreeningcodes.nlm.nih.gov/nb/sc/about (accessed March 5, 2020).

NQF (National Quality Forum). 2018. *Strengthening the core set of healthcare quality measures for children enrolled in Medicaid and CHIP, 2018: Final report.* Washington, DC: U.S. Department of Health and Human Services.

NQF. n.d.a. *What NQF endorsement means.* https://www.qualityforum.org/Measuring_Performance/ABCs/What_NQF_Endorsement_Means.aspx (accessed February 27, 2020).

NQF. n.d.b. *National Quality Partners™ shared decision making action team.* http://www.qualityforum.org/National_Quality_Partners_Shared_Decision_Making_Action_Team_.aspx (accessed February 28, 2020).

NQF. n.d.c. *NQF's history.* http://www.qualityforum.org/about_nqf/history (accessed March 12, 2020).

Okpala, I., V. Thomas, N. Westerdale, T. Jegede, K. Raj, S. Daley, H. Costello-Binger, J. Mullen, C. Rochester-Peart, S. Helps, E. Tulloch, M. Akpala, M. Dick, S. Bewley, M. Davies, and I. Abbs. 2002. The comprehensiveness care of sickle cell disease. *European Journal of Haematology* 68(3):157–162.

Okumura, M. J., M. Heisler, M. M. Davis, M. D. Cabana, S. Demonner, and E. A. Kerr. 2008. Comfort of general internists and general pediatricians in providing care for young adults with chronic illnesses of childhood. *Journal of General Internal Medicine* 23(10):1621–1627.

Okwerekwu, I., and J. A. Skirvin. 2018. Sickle cell disease pain management. *U.S. Pharmacists* 43(3):12–18.

Oyeku, S. O., and E. Z. Faro. 2017. Rigorous and practical quality indicators in sickle cell disease care. *Hematology* 2017(1):418–422.

Panepinto, J. A., S. Torres, C. B. Bendo, T. L. McCavit, B. Dinu, S. Sherman-Bien, C. Bemrich-Stolz, and J. W. Varni. 2013. PedsQL™ sickle cell disease module: Feasibility, reliability, and validity. *Pediatric Blood & Cancer* 60(8):1338–1344.

Panepinto, J. A., S. Torres, C. B. Bendo, T. L. McCavit, B. Dinu, S. Sherman-Bien, C. Bemrich-Stolz, and J. W. Varni. 2014. PedsQL™ multidimensional fatigue scale in sickle cell disease: Feasibility, reliability, and validity. *Pediatric Blood & Cancer* 61(1):171–177.

Prabhakar, H., C. Haywood, Jr., and R. Molokie. 2010. Sickle cell disease in the United States: Looking back and forward at 100 years of progress in management and survival. *American Journal of Hematology* 85(5):346–353.

Public Health England. 2019. *Sickle cell and thalassaemia screening programme: Standards.* https://www.gov.uk/government/publications/sickle-cell-and-thalassaemia-screening-programme-standards (accessed March 5, 2020).

Raphael, J. L., P. B. Shetty, H. Liu, D. H. Mahoney, and B. U. Mueller. 2008. A critical assessment of transcranial Doppler screening rates in a large pediatric sickle cell center: Opportunities to improve healthcare quality. *Pediatric Blood & Cancer* 51(5):647–651.

Raphael, J. L., T. L. Rattler, M. A. Kowalkowski, B. U. Mueller, T. P. Giordano, and D. C. Brousseau. 2013. Associations of care in a medical home and health care utilization among children with sickle cell disease. *Journal of the National Medical Association* 105(2):157–165.

Reeves, S. L., H. J. Fullerton, K. J. Dombkowski, M. L. Boulton, T. M. Braun, and L. D. Lisabeth. 2015. Physician attitude, awareness, and knowledge regarding guidelines for transcranial Doppler screening in sickle cell disease. *Clinical Pediatrics* 54(4):336–345.

Reeves, S. L., B. Madden, G. L. Freed, and K. J. Dombkowski. 2016. Transcranial Doppler screening among children and adolescents with sickle cell anemia. *JAMA Pediatrics* 170(6):550–556.

Reeves, S. L., A. C. Tribble, B. Madden, G. L. Freed, and K. J. Dombkowski. 2018. Antibiotic prophylaxis for children with sickle cell anemia. *Pediatrics* 141(3):e20172182.

Rohlfing, J., R. Navarro, O. Z. Maniya, B. D. Hughes, and D. K. Rogalsky. 2014. Medical student debt and major life choices other than specialty. *Medical Education Online* 19(1):25603.

Salm, N., E. Yetter, and A. Tluczek. 2012. Informing parents about positive newborn screen results: Parents' recommendations. *Journal of Child Health Care* 16(4):367–381.

Sambunjak, D., S. E. Straus, and A. Marusic. 2010. A systematic review of qualitative research on the meaning and characteristics of mentoring in academic medicine. *Journal of General Internal Medicine* 25(1):72–78.

Santhosh, L., and J. M. Babik. 2020. Trends in racial and ethnic diversity in internal medicine subspecialty fellowships from 2006 to 2018. *JAMA Network Open* 3(2):e1920482.

Sarri, G., M. Bhor, S. Abogunrin, C. Farmer, S. Nandal, R. Halloway, and D. A. Revicki. 2018. Systematic literature review and assessment of patient-reported outcome instruments in sickle cell disease. *Health and Quality of Life Outcomes* 16(1):99.

Scott, A. W. 2016. Ophthalmic manifestations of sickle cell disease. *Southern Medical Journal* 109(9):542–548.

Shapiro, B. S., L. J. Benjamin, R. Payne, and G. Heidrich. 1997. Sickle cell-related pain: Perceptions of medical practitioners. *Journal of Pain and Symptom Management* 14(3):168–174.

Sharma, D., N. Wallace, E. A. Levinsohn, A. L. Marshall, K. Kayoumi, J. Madero, M. Homer, R. Reynolds, J. Hafler, N. A. Podoltsev, and A. I. Lee. 2019. Trends and factors affecting the U.S. adult hematology workforce: A mixed methods study. *Blood Advances* 3(22):3550–3561.

Shook, L. M., C. B. Farrell, K. A. Kalinyak, S. C. Nelson, B. M. Hardesty, A. G. Rampersad, K. L. Saving, W. J. Whitten-Shurney, J. A. Panepinto, R. E. Ware, and L. Crosby. 2016. Translating sickle cell guidelines into practice for primary care providers with Project ECHO. *Medical Education Online* 21(1):33616.

Sickle Cell Society. 2018. *Standards for the clinical care of adults with sickle cell disease in the UK.* https://www.sicklecellsociety.org/wp-content/uploads/2018/05/Standards-for-the-Clinical-Care-of-Adults-with-Sickle-Cell-in-the-UK-2018.pdf (accessed March 5, 2020).

Simon, E., B. Long, and A. Koyfman. 2016. Emergency medicine management of sickle cell disease complications: An evidence-based update. *Journal of Emergency Medicine* 51(4):370–381.

Singh, A. P., C. Haywood, Jr., M. C. Beach, M. Guidera, S. Lanzkron, D. Valenzuela-Araujo, R. E. Rothman, and A. F. Dugas. 2016. Improving emergency providers' attitudes toward sickle cell patients in pain. *Journal of Pain and Symptom Management* 51(3):628–632.

Sinha, C. B., N. Bakshi, D. Ross, and L. Krishnamurti. 2019. Management of chronic pain in adults living with sickle cell disease in the era of the opioid epidemic: A qualitative study. *JAMA Network Open* 2(5):e194410.

Sivaguru, H., S. M. Kemp, R. Crowley, G. Hann, D. A. Yardumian, M. Roberts-Harewood, and O. Wilkey. 2015. An evaluation of the transition to adult care for young patients with sickle cell disease. *Archives of Disease in Childhood* 100(Suppl 3):A168–A169.

Smith, L. A., S. O. Oyeku, C. Homer, and B. Zuckerman. 2006. Sickle cell disease: A question of equity and quality. *Pediatrics* 117(5):1763–1770.

Sobota, A., E. J. Neufeld, P. Sprinz, and M. M. Heeney. 2011. Transition from pediatric to adult care for sickle cell disease: Results of a survey of pediatric providers. *American Journal of Hematology and Oncology* 86(6):512–515.

Sobota, A. E., N. Shah, and J. W. Mack. 2017. Development of quality indicators for transition from pediatric to adult care in sickle cell disease: A modified Delphi survey of adult providers. *Pediatric Blood Cancer* 64(6).

Soffer, E., and W. K. Hoots. 2018. Challenges facing the benign hematology physician–scientist workforce: Identifying issues of recruitment and retention. *Blood Advances* 2(3):308.

Stacey, D., F. Légaré, K. Lewis, M. J. Barry, C. L. Bennett, K. B. Eden, M. Holmes-Rovner, H. Llewellyn-Thomas, A. Lyddiatt, R. Thomson, and L. Trevena. 2017. Decision aids for people facing health treatment or screening decisions. *Cochrane Database of Systematic Reviews* 2017(4):CD001431.

Straus, S. E., M. O. Johnson, C. Marquez, and M. D. Feldman. 2013. Characteristics of successful and failed mentoring relationships: A qualitative study across two academic health centers. *Academic Medicine* 88(1):82–89.

Sullivan, K. M., M. Horwitz, I. Osunkwo, N. Shah, and J. J. Strouse. 2018. Shared decision-making in hematopoietic stem cell transplantation for sickle cell disease. *Biology of Blood and Marrow Transplantation* 24(5):883–884.

Sweet, D. n.d. *Value of credentialing.* https://aahivm.org/value-of-credentialing (accessed March 6, 2020).

Tanabe, P., A. Stevenson, L. DeCastro, L. Drawhorn, S. Lanzkron, R. E. Molokie, and N. Artz. 2013. Evaluation of a train-the-trainer workshop on sickle cell disease for ED providers. *Journal of Emergency Nursing* 39(6):539–546.

Tejaswini, D. 2015. Post-fellowship career decision-making in a changing hematology practice landscape. *Hematologist* 12(3):14–15.

Telfair, J., L. R. Alexander, P. S. Loosier, P. L. Alleman-Velez, and J. Simmons. 2004a. Providers' perspectives and beliefs regarding transition to adult care for adolescents with sickle cell disease. *Journal of Health Care for the Poor and Underserved* 15(3):443–461.

Telfair, J., J. E. Ehiri, P. S. Loosier, and M. L. Baskin. 2004b. Transition to adult care for adolescents with sickle cell disease: Results of a national survey. *International Journal of Adolescent Medicine and Health* 16(1):47–64.

Telfer, P., and B. Kaya. 2017. Optimizing the care model for an uncomplicated acute pain episode in sickle cell disease. *Hematology: American Society of Hematology—Education Program* 2017(1):525–533.

Ter-Minassian, M., S. Lanzkron, A. Derus, E. Brown, and M. A. Horberg. 2019. Quality metrics and health care utilization for adult patients with sickle cell disease. *Journal of the National Medical Association* 111(1):54–61.

Therrell, Jr., B. L., M. A. Lloyd-Puryear, J. R. Eckman, and M. Y. Mann. 2015. Newborn screening for sickle cell diseases in the United States: A review of data spanning 2 decades. *Seminars in Perinatology* 39(3):238–251.

Thompson, A. 2014. Is the NIH expert report on sickle cell disease a "clinical practice guideline we can trust?" *The Hematologist* 11(6):14.

Todd, R. F., S. D. Gitlin, and L. J. Burns. 2004. Subspeciality training in hematology and oncology, 2003: Results of a survey of training program directors conducted by the American Society of Hematology. *Blood* 103(12):4383–4388.

Treadwell, M., J. Telfair, R. W. Gibson, S. Johnson, and I. Osunkwo. 2011. Transition from pediatric to adult care in sickle cell disease: Establishing evidence-based practice and directions for research. *American Journal of Hematology* 86(1):116–120.

Treadwell, M. J., K. Hassell, R. Levine, and S. Keller. 2014. Adult Sickle Cell Quality-of-Life Measurement Information System (ASCQ-ME): Conceptual model based on review of the literature and formative research. *Clinical Journal of Pain* 30(10):902–914.

Treadwell, M., S. Johnson, I. Sisler, M. Bitsko, G. Gildengorin, R. Medina, F. Barreda, K. Major, J. Telfair, and W. R. Smith. 2016. Self-efficacy and readiness for transition from pediatric to adult care in sickle cell disease. *International Journal of Adolescent Medicine and Health* 28(4):381–388.

Treadwell, M., M. DeBaun, and J. Tirnauer. 2018. *Transition from pediatric to adult care: Sickle cell disease.* https://www.uptodate.com/contents/transition-from-pediatric-to-adult-care-sickle-cell-disease (accessed April 12, 2020).

Tubman, V. N., and J. J. Field. 2015. Sickle solubility test to screen for sickle cell trait: What's the harm? *Hematology: American Society of Hematology—Education Program* 2015:433–435.

Utuama, O., K. Carter-Wicker, J. Herbert, R. Gibson, A. Kutlar, A. Logan, M. M. Kabongo, and T. Adamkiewicz. 2015. Sickle cell disease: Challenges and comfort in providing care by family physicians: *Blood* 126(23):5570.

Varni, J. W., M. Seid, and P. S. Kurtin. 2001. PedsQL™ 4.0: Reliability and validity of the Pediatric Quality of Life Inventory™ version 4.0 generic core scales in healthy and patient populations. *Medical Care* 39(8):800–812.

Vichinsky, E. P. 1991. Comprehensive care in sickle cell disease: Its impact on morbidity and mortality. *Seminars in Hematology* 28(3):220–226.

Wallace, P. J., N. T. Connell, and J. L. Abkowitz. 2015. The role of hematologists in a changing United States health care system. *Blood* 125(16):2467–2470.

Wallace, N. H., J. P. Hafler, M. E. Hurwitz, N. A. Podoltsev, J. Lacy, and A. I. Lee. 2016. Factors influencing hematology career choice in hematology and oncology fellows at a major academic institution. *Blood* 128(22):3538.

Wang, C. J., P. L. Kavanagh, A. A. Little, J. B. Holliman, and P. G. Sprinz. 2011. Quality-of-care indicators for children with sickle cell disease. *Pediatrics* 128(3):484–493.

Wilkie, D. J., B. Johnson, A. K. Mack, R. Labotka, and R. E. Molokie. 2010. Sickle cell disease: An opportunity for palliative care across the life span. *Nursing Clinics* 45(3):375–397.

Williams, C. P., C. H. Smith, K. Osborn, C. J. Bemrich-Stolz, L. M. Hilliard, T. H. Howard, and J. D. Lebensburger. 2015. Patient-centered approach to designing sickle cell transition education. *Journal of Pediatric Hematology and Oncology* 37(1):43–47.

Wilson, I. B., and P. D. Cleary. 1995. Linking clinical variables with health-related quality of life: A conceptual model of patient outcomes. *JAMA* 273(1):59–65.

Yang, W., J. H. Williams, P. F. Hogan, S. S. Bruinooge, G. I. Rodriguez, M. P. Kosty, D. F. Bajorin, A. Hanley, A. Muchow, N. McMillan, and M. Goldstein. 2014. Projected supply of and demand for oncologists and radiation oncologists through 2025: An aging, better-insured population will result in shortage. *Journal of Oncology Practice* 10(1):39–45.

Yawn, B. P., and J. John-Sowah. 2015. Management of sickle cell disease: Recommendations from the 2014 expert panel report. *American Family Physician* 92(12):1069–1076.

Yawn, B. P., G. R. Buchanan, A. N. Afenyi-Annan, S. K. Ballas, K. L. Hassell, A. H. James, L. Jordan, S. M. Lanzkron, R. Lottenberg, W. J. Savage, P. J. Tanabe, R. E. Ware, M. H. Murad, J. C. Goldsmith, E. Ortiz, R. Fulwood, A. Horton, and J. John-Sowah. 2014. Management of sickle cell disease: Summary of the 2014 evidence-based report by expert panel members. *JAMA* 312(10):1033–1048.

Yusuf, H. R., H. K. Atrash, S. D. Grosse, C. S. Parker, and A. M. Grant. 2010. Emergency department visits made by patients with sickle cell disease: A descriptive study, 1999–2007. *American Journal of Preventive Medicine* 38(4 Suppl):S536–S541.

Zempsky, W. T., E. A. O'Hara, J. P. Santanelli, T. M. Palermo, T. New, K. Smith-Whitley, and J. F. Casella. 2013. Validation of the Sickle Cell Disease Pain Burden Interview–Youth. *Journal of Pain* 14(9):975–982.

7

Developing and Delivering the Next Generation of Therapies

We should be aggressive about pursuing the research and learning more and pushing ahead, because while the road may be murky, it's there, and there's reason for optimism and so we should just keep plugging until we get there....

—Celia W. (Open Session Panelist)

Chapter Summary

- After decades of relatively little progress being made in therapeutic innovations for sickle cell disease (SCD), an influx of pipeline products has been introduced in recent years.
- New therapies for SCD, including curative therapies, target a number of different mechanisms, thus offering a wide variety of options for SCD patients. There is still a need for targeted SCD therapies that address the underlying cause of the disease.
- Scientific and medical research advances need to be coupled with health care delivery and payment policies to ensure universal access to pipeline products.
- Patient-centric research approaches, which seek to engage and educate patients about clinical trials and therapeutic innovations, are needed to dispel decades of patient mistrust and misconceptions about new therapies.

Over the past two decades a great deal of scientific and medical research effort has resulted in progress toward developing new treatments—including potential cures—of sickle cell disease (SCD), but research is just one aspect of making novel therapies a reality. Developing the most effective therapies will require input and support from the sickle cell community, including from individuals living with the disease. This input can help guide researchers to develop new, effective treatments that are accepted by the sickle cell community. Testing new treatments in clinical trials will require a different set of considerations, including strategies for encouraging participation in trials and determining which endpoints to use as measures of success. Once novel therapies are approved by the U.S. Food and Drug Administration (FDA), considerations such as health care delivery policies and reimbursement for treatment costs will be important considerations. In each of these steps, the SCD patients' concerns, preferences, and well-being should be given first priority.

PATIENT PERSPECTIVES

Any effort to develop a treatment or cure for SCD must start with the patient. Understanding the experiences and beliefs of individuals living with SCD, their families, and the associated community will be integral to developing effective treatments that target the most important outcomes to those stakeholders. Similarly, it is vital to understand patient perspectives concerning curative therapies to completely realize their benefits.

Although the literature in this area is lacking, researchers have identified some pervasive perspectives and attitudes within the sickle cell community and reported on the impacts of these beliefs on health outcomes. Recurring themes from this research include a distrust of the medical profession, fear of the adverse effects of therapies, inadequate SCD education and awareness, a minimization of the role of patients in shared decision making (SDM), and perceived barriers to experimental clinical studies (Bakshi et al., 2017; Haywood et al., 2011; Long et al., 2011; Scharff et al., 2010). SCD is also widely perceived to be an orphan disease that lacks sufficient resources or attention—and many believe that social factors (e.g., a majority of SCD patients are African American) explain much of this marginalized status (Bulgin et al., 2018).

Bonham et al. (2007) examined the interconnectedness of race and disease using "SCD as a prism for understanding the historical connections between genetic diseases and racial diseases, and the consequences of these connections" and viewing SCD as a foundation for "comprehending the attitudes of African Americans toward genetic research" (p. 311). Social, political, and cultural factors combined to shape the conceptualization of SCD (which has been widely seen as a "black disease") and influence the care given to individuals living with the disease. A study by Treadwell et al. (2006) documented general misconceptions about SCD among the African American community and also described the existence of SCD stigma and a lack of compassion and cultural sensitivity among those in the medical profession. The stigma attached to SCD, which has its roots in racism and racist attitudes, has detrimental consequences for patient health and negatively affects patient–provider relationships and care-seeking behaviors (Bulgin et al., 2018; Wailoo, 2017).

In a study examining the attitudes and beliefs of African Americans toward genetics and genetic testing, Long et al. (2011) found a lower-than-desired uptake of SCD education but reported that collaborations involving trusted sources of information, such as family members, community physicians and leaders, the church, and those with personal experiences, could help mitigate this gap. When investigating SCD patients' perspectives on gene therapy, Strong et al. (2017) found a lack of awareness, fear and uncertainty about side effects, and concerns about the HIV-derived viral vector, infertility risks, and the potential risk for cancer. Persaud et al. (2019) investigated the perspectives of patients, parents, and clinicians toward somatic genome editing and found that patients expressed being both hopeful and fearful about the topic and also feeling insufficiently informed. The findings revealed that patients were more likely to have a positive attitude toward gene therapy when there was better education, prior participation in clinical trials, and perceived benefit. Persaud and Bonham (2018) also found that when patients have a trustful relationship with health providers, they are more likely to seek advice from providers and expect better outcomes from medical care.

Trust is a core element shaping the patient–health provider relationship, and a patient's level of trust or distrust can affect his or her attitudes toward therapies and health outcomes. African Americans in general report higher levels of distrust of the medical community than white Americans, and sickle cell patients report concerns about biased treatment, being seen as drug seeking, and experiencing other forms of marginalization (Bonham et al., 2007; Strong et al., 2017; Wailoo, 2017). SCD patients' trust in health teams is increased when team members are better able to relate to and communicate with them (Haywood et al., 2014; Strong et al., 2017).

A key—but often ignored—factor influencing SCD patient perspectives is how they receive information about the disease. Studies of information-seeking behaviors among African Americans have found that they rely on familial sources and other trusted sources, such as their church or peers (i.e., others living with the disease) (Acharya et al., 2009; Long et al., 2011). SCD patients report that their preferred way of receiving information about SCD is through direct interactions with medical providers, although they are also open to other sources, such as the Internet, books and pamphlets, and DVDs, as long as the information is clear, truthful, and preferably accompanied by illustrations (Omondi et al., 2013; Strong et al., 2017). The community also recognizes the complexities of the decision-making process associated with options for disease-modifying strategies and expects to be included in that process. When deciding whether to pursue allogenic hematopoietic stem cell transplantation (HSCT), for example, patients were primarily influenced by the disease burden (particularly when it reached a critical point), consultation with HSCT clinicians, and familial support (Khemani et al., 2018). In a qualitative study of clinicians who were experts in SCD and their attitudes toward sharing decision making with patients and families regarding whether to pursue disease-modifying therapies, the clinicians were found to take a collaborative (discussing all plans) or proponent (advocating a predetermined plan) approach, depending on the disease severity and treatment urgency (Bakshi et al., 2017).

In summary, the sickle cell community has made it clear that certain factors will be key in aiding individuals with SCD to make informed decisions about curative and disease-modifying therapies, as well as effective management strategies to ensure high-quality health care. Those factors include access to trusted sources of information and resources; clear and transparent dissemination of information from the medical community, including results from clinical trials; an active and meaningful role in decision making for patients; a prioritization of patient needs; the establishment of partnerships between advocacy organizations and trusted providers; and the creation of mechanisms for building trust among providers, researchers, and the community (Lebensburger et al., 2013, 2015; Liem et al., 2010; Persaud et al., 2019). Individuals living with SCD should be empowered to advocate for themselves, must be better enabled to interact effectively with health care providers, and need an enhanced ability to navigate the health care system. Better education is needed not only for the SCD community but also for health care providers, particularly regarding patient needs, effective management, and innovative programs to ease the transition to adult care. Providers also need the training and means to address any implicit and institutional biases and other forms of systemic racism and inequities in health care.

In 2017 the American Society of Hematology (ASH) initiated an aggressive advocacy campaign related to SCD and sickle cell trait, and it set research priorities that included developing novel therapies and strengthening curative therapies. In September 2018 the National Heart, Lung, and Blood Institute of the National Institutes of Health (NIH) launched the Cure Sickle Cell Initiative to accelerate genetic therapies (NIH, 2018). These efforts bode well for the sickle cell community, as each initiative is patient-focused and committed to engaging patients, families, advocates, and organizations in the cause. While these new developments give increased attention to curing SCD, overcoming the complicated history of race and health will be challenging.

THERAPIES UNDER DEVELOPMENT

The goal of research into new treatments is to find more effective ways to prevent or ameliorate the various manifestations of SCD—and, ultimately, to cure it altogether. The specific goals of the therapies include preventing and treating its complications, decreasing its morbidity, minimizing the numbers of crises and hospitalizations, lowering its symptom burden, prolonging life, improving quality of life (QOL), and, with a cure, eliminating SCD's root cause. Even with an effective cure, though, ameliorative therapies will still be needed because those who have lived with the disease for years will have to address any lingering SCD-related health concerns.

As of December 2019, hydroxyurea (HU), L-glutamine, voxelotor, and crizanlizumab are disease-modifying drugs available for those with SCD, and HSCT is the only established non-experimental curative therapy (Bernaudin et al., 2007; FDA, 2019; Hsieh et al., 2009; Kutlar et al., 2019; Strouse et al., 2008). In 2017 L-glutamine became the second drug approved by FDA to prevent crises in individuals 5 years of age or older living with SCD (FDA, 2017; Riley et al., 2018), and voxelotor and crizanlizumab have been approved only recently (November 2019). None of the available therapies represent a completely satisfactory option for people affected by SCD. In particular, none of the drugs reduce the number of vaso-occlusive episodes (VOEs) by more than 50 percent. However, building on decades of research, efforts are under way to develop novel pathophysiology-related agents and novel genetic approaches to a cure. This section reviews the SCD therapies, both therapeutic and curative, that are now under development.

New Drugs for SCD

In 1998, when FDA approved HU to treat acute VOEs, it was the first drug specifically for SCD—and it would remain the only such drug for nearly two decades. This was not for lack of trying, however. In the early part of the 21st century, the sickle cell community was keenly aware of the need for additional or alternate disease-modifying therapies. The adoption of HU by providers and patients alike had been associated with a number of problems, including concerns about numerous potential side effects, the need for close monitoring, the required daily long-term dosing, and concerns about long-term toxicity (Halsey and Roberts, 2003; McGann and Ware, 2015; Steinberg, 2002). Furthermore, some patients experienced

incomplete responses—or even no response—underlining the need for additional therapies (Steinberg, 1999; Stuart and Nagel, 2004). Nevertheless,
drug development in SCD proceeded slowly.

Over the past two decades, however, mounting evidence from the mouse
models of SCD, particularly the Berkley and Townes transgenic humanized
sickle mice, has led to a more nuanced and in-depth understanding of the
complex pathophysiology of SCD. The primacy of hemoglobin polymerization and red blood cell (RBC) sickling in the phenotype has not been
challenged, but multiple complex and interlinked downstream mechanisms
have been identified, in large part—and in some cases exclusively—based
on preclinical evidence. Thus, compounding hemoglobin polymerization,
cellular hyperadhesion, endothelial activation, hemolysis, hemostatic activation, oxidant stress, sterile inflammation, and hyperviscosity are now
all recognized as critical determinants of the phenotype (Du et al., 2018;
Kalpatthi and Novelli, 2018). This has led to a number of drugs that target
specific aspects of the pathogenic cascade (see Figure 7-1).

These drugs, along with their novel therapeutic strategies, are
typically classified into six categories, as summarized in the table in

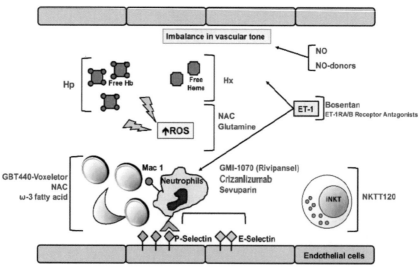

FIGURE 7-1 Schematic diagram of the mechanisms of action of pathophysiology-
based new therapeutic options for treatment of SCD and sickle cell vasculopathy.
NOTE: Ab = antibody; ET-1 = endothelin-1; ET-R = endothelin-1 receptor; Hb =
hemoglobin; Hp = haptoglobin; Hx = hemopexin; iNKT = invariant natural killer
T cells; NAC = N-Acetyl-cysteine; NKTT120 = humanized monoclonal antibody
specifically depleting iNKT; NO = nitric oxide; ROS = reactive oxygen species.
SOURCE: Matte et al., 2019.

Appendix I: anti-sickling agents, anti-adhesion agents, antioxidant agents, anti-inflammatory agents, anticoagulant and antiplatelet agents, and nitric-oxide (NO)-related agents. All of these treatments share certain limitations: they do not address the genetic cause (the hemoglobin S [HbS] mutation), they each address only certain manifestations of the disease, they do not specifically target chronic pain, and they cannot reverse end-organ damage. Nonetheless, they hold promise for interrupting the pathophysiologic mechanisms in SCD and thus decreasing organ-specific complications, reducing morbidity and mortality, and improving QOL. More details can be found in Ballas et al. (2012), which provides an extensive review of SCD management based on the complications and notes the variation among patients and in the same patient over time. Other reviews discuss advances in treatment strategies targeting inflammation, oxidative injury, vascular tone, hemoglobin polymerization, and adhesion (Ataga and Desai, 2018; Kapoor et al., 2018; Steinberg and Brugnara, 2003; Telen et al., 2019).

Agents That Block HbS Polymerization

HbS polymerizes in RBCs to create fibers that reduce the flexibility of RBCs leading to hemolysis and other downstream complications, so one approach to treating SCD is to block HbS polymerization. There are various approaches to doing this. One is to increase fetal hemoglobin (HbF) production. High intracellular HbF levels prevent or reduce HbS polymerization, as evidenced by individuals with congenital hereditary persistence of HbF co-inherited with SCD, although the protection from sickling is usually not complete. In addition to HU, whose role in therapy is well established and has been confirmed by strong evidence obtained in the United States (Charache et al., 1995; Steinberg et al., 2010) and throughout the world (Tshilolo et al., 2019; Voskaridou et al., 2010), other drugs, such as decitabine (Molokie et al., 2017), histone deacetylase inhibitors (Shearstone et al., 2016), sodium 2,2-dimethylbutyrate (Kutlar et al., 2013), and metformin (Han et al., 2019), have been found to boost HbF levels and are under investigation for SCD.

Another strategy to reduce HbS polymerization involves modulating the oxygen affinity of hemoglobin. Voxelotor (GBT440), which was approved by FDA for SCD in November 2019, increases the oxygen affinity of hemoglobin (Vichinsky et al., 2019). By increasing the oxygen affinity of hemoglobin, voxelotor maintains hemoglobin in the oxygenated state and reduces polymerization and sickling (Vichinsky et al., 2019). Clinical trials in adults and children have shown reduced hemolysis and improved hemoglobin, although these changes were not accompanied by a statistically significant reduction in VOEs (Vichinsky et al., 2019). While voxelotor does not appear to adversely affect oxygen delivery, according to measurements of erythropoietin levels in study patients, more research may be needed in children at a high risk of stroke, in whom cerebral oxygenation partly relies on increased oxygen extraction. There are also lingering concerns that increasing the total hemoglobin without reducing the intracellular concentration of HbS may lead to hyperviscosity and its attendant complications (Estepp, 2018).

Anti-Adhesion Agents

Cellular hyperadhesion is a critical component of vaso-occlusion. In the proinflammatory milieu of SCD, the endothelium and the blood cells overexpress activated adhesion molecules (integrins), which promote the binding of sickle RBCs, reticulocytes, leukocytes, and platelets to the endothelium and to one another. The complex network of interactions between cellular elements and the endothelium is amply documented in animal models (Sundd et al., 2019). The translational relevance of paradigms developed from mouse research has now been validated in humans. Among the most promising approaches are those that target selectins. P-selectin, E-selectin, and several integrins mediate cellular adhesions in mice (reviewed in Telen, 2007). FDA approved crizanlizumab for SCD in November 2019 (FDA, 2019). Crizanlizumab, a monoclonal antibody that targets P-selectins, has been tested in humans and found to prevent VOEs, as predicted by the evidence in mouse models. High-dose crizanlizumab reduced the rate of VOEs to a median of 1.63/year compared with 2.98/year with placebo (a 45.3 percent lower rate, $p = 0.01$) (Ataga et al., 2017; Kutlar et al., 2019). In addition, "the median time to the first crisis was significantly longer with high-dose crizanlizumab than with placebo (4.07 versus 1.38 months, $p = 0.001$), as was the median time to the second crisis (10.32 versus 5.09 months, $p = 0.02$)" (Ataga et al., 2017, p. 429). Rivipansel, unlike crizanlizumab, is a pan-selectin inhibitor with particular activity against E-selectin (Chang et al., 2010). Rivipansel has shown clinical benefit in a Phase II trial, where it reduced cumulative intravenous opiate requirements by 83 percent in patients hospitalized with VOEs (Telen et al., 2015); however, in a major setback for the field, Pfizer recently announced that the Phase III trial (RESET) did not meet the primary endpoint of time to readiness for discharge and the key secondary efficacy endpoints of time-to-discharge, cumulative IV opioid consumption, and time to discontinuation of IV opioids (Pfizer, 2019). The reason for the negative trial results may lie in either the inferiority of E-selectin blockade (as compared to P-selectin blockade) as a strategy to block VOEs or in the difficulty of aborting a VOE once it has started. If the latter hypothesis is correct, preventive approaches will remain more successful. A third selectin inhibitor, sevuparin, which has predominant activity against L-selectin, is also under investigation (White et al.,

2019). While side effects in the anti-selectin trials were relatively modest, heightened surveillance for hemorrhagic and infectious complications will be warranted in clinical use, given the role of selectins in hemostasis and immunity. Finally, intravenous immunoglobulins are under investigation for their capacity to block neutrophil adhesion to RBCs and the endothelium.

Antioxidant Agents

Oxidant stress is the by-product of multiple disturbed pathways in SCD. Both reactive oxygen and nitrogen species are elevated and natural antioxidant mechanisms are depleted in the plasma and tissues. Enzymatic sources of reactive oxygen species (ROS), including xanthine oxidase (Aslan et al., 2001), nicotinamide adenine dinucleotide phosphate oxidase (George et al., 2013), and NO synthase (Kaul et al., 2000), are upregulated in SCD and promote oxidant damage in response to ischemia-reperfusion injury. Autoxidation of RBCs and platelet mitochondrial ROS production (Cardenes et al., 2014) are also sources of oxidant stress. Finally, hemolysis leads to free hemoglobin quenching NO in the vasculature by the Fenton reaction (Minneci et al., 2005). Restoring the balance of oxidants and antioxidants is a viable therapeutic strategy in SCD that is finally bearing fruit. L-glutamine is an antioxidant and precursor of NO that was approved as the second disease-modifying drug (Niihara et al., 2018). While its benefit is more modest than that obtained with HU (25 percent versus 50 percent reduction in VOEs), L-glutamine has a much more favorable side-effect profile (Charache et al., 1995; Niihara et al., 2018). Omega-3 fatty acids also have antioxidant and anti-inflammatory properties and have been shown to reduce VOE frequency by approximately 50 percent (Tomer et al., 2001); they are currently being investigated in larger, randomized studies.

Anti-Inflammatory Agents

A chronic state of sterile inflammation is a cardinal feature of SCD. Its role is most evident in acute chest syndrome (ACS), where inflammation triggers capillary leak and acute lung injury (Sundd et al., 2019), but the hallmarks of inflammation are present at steady state, where levels of inflammatory cytokines, leukocytes, and other pro-inflammatory molecules are elevated as compared with individuals without SCD (Schimmel et al., 2013). By-products of hemolysis (i.e., hemin) and ischemia-reperfusion injury are responsible for activating vascular cells and producing damage-associated molecular products and proinflammatory cytokines (Chen et al., 2014; Dutra et al., 2014). Intensive research in mice has identified multiple pathways of inflammation, including hemin-TLR4, multiple mediators of the inflammasome complex, and the nuclear factor kappa-light-chain-enhancer of activated B cells (NF-κB)[1] family of transcriptional factors, leukotrienes, and mast cells (Belcher et al., 2014; Kaul and Hebbel, 2000). There are many compounds under development that target specific aspects of inflammation. Corticosteroids could potentially target multiple pathways, but their role in SCD remains controversial after clinical evidence of rebound pain and VOE emerged following their use in severe ACS (Griffin et al., 1994). Clinical trials are ongoing with efforts to modulate specific mediators of inflammation, which could potentially lead to drugs with more limited and predictable side-effect profiles. The drugs under investigation include leukotriene inhibitors (e.g., zileuton and montelukast), inhibitors of mast cell activation (e.g., imatinib and cromolyn sodium), inhibitors of natural killer cells (e.g., rogadenoson and adenosine A_{2A} receptor activators), inhibitors of NF-κB (e.g., sulfasalazine), and components of the inflammasome complex (e.g., canakinumab and NLRP3 inhibitors) (Field et al., 2017; Telen, 2016; Vincent et al., 2013).

Anticoagulant and Antiplatelet Agents

Hemostatic activation is present at baseline in SCD and worsens during VOEs. Virtually all components of the coagulation cascade are affected in SCD (Ataga and Key, 2007; Ataga et al., 2008; De Franceschi et al., 2011; Peters et al., 1994; Setty et al., 2008; Singer and Ataga, 2008; Stuart and Setty, 2001; Whelihan et al., 2016). Externalization of RBC prothrombotic phospholipids (Franck et al., 1985), RBC and platelet microparticle shedding (Allan et al., 1982; Wun et al., 1998), hemolysis-mediated platelet activation (Cardenes et al., 2014; Villagra et al., 2007), and the reduced clearance of prothrombotic cells post-splenectomy (Crary and Buchanan, 2009) are all documented mechanisms of hemostatic activation in SCD. Clinical studies in large administrative databases, smaller case series, and single-institution reports have shown a higher prevalence and incidence of pulmonary thrombosis and intravascular catheter-related thrombosis in SCD, particularly in hospitalized patients (Brunson et al., 2017, 2019; Naik et al., 2013, 2014; Novelli et al., 2012; Stein et al., 2006). Yet, the association between hemostatic activation and SCD complications is less clear. Theoretically, antiplatelets and anticoagulants should reduce vaso-occlusion by dampening hyperadhesion and platelet recruitment. However, clinical studies of anticoagulants and antiplatelet agents have largely been disappointing (Noubouossie et al., 2016). There is ongoing research on recently approved drugs, including the newer direct oral anticoagulants,

---

[1] NF-κB (nuclear factor kappa-light-chain-enhancer of activated B cells) is a protein complex that controls transcription of DNA, cytokine production, and cell survival.

which are currently being investigated in clinical trials for their potential to mitigate the SCD phenotype. It remains to be determined whether antiplatelet agents may be beneficial in subsets of patients with a more pronounced hemostatic activation profile and as a part of multidrug interventions. For instance, in the Determining Effects of Platelet Inhibition on Vaso-occlusive Events clinical trial of prasugrel, an agent that inhibits platelet activation, a subset analysis of the pediatric study population showed a possible benefit in the adolescent group (12–17 years old) (Heeney et al., 2016).

Nitric Oxide

NO metabolism and metabolites are profoundly altered in SCD and central to its pathophysiology. NO therapeutics, including inhaled NO, L-arginine, and sildenafil (a phosphodiesterase inhibitor), have been tested in clinical trials. The results have been mixed, with the DeNOVO trial being unquestionably negative (Gladwin et al., 2011) and others inconclusive or terminated early due to toxicity (Walk-PHaSST) (Machado et al., 2011) or low enrollment (Children's Hospital Los Angeles and Hope Pharmaceuticals, 2009). Yet, NO modulation remains an attractive therapeutic strategy, particularly for specific complications or in the subset of patients with particularly brisk hemolysis. Two potential treatments under investigation are a topical nitrite preparation for leg ulcers, and the oral soluble guanylate cyclase stimulator riociguat for patients with a hyperhemolysis phenotype (STERIO-SCD trial) (Kato, 2015). There is also preliminary evidence that L-arginine, a NO precursor, may reverse platelet mitochondrial ROS production and thereby reduce platelet activation and other downstream effects (e.g., hyperadhesion). L-arginine reduced the frequency of VOEs in children (Morris et al., 2013) and is under investigation in a larger study.

Defining a Cure

As noted above, neither the drugs already approved by FDA for use in SCD nor any of the drugs under development address the root cause. They focus instead on addressing the manifestations of the disease. Thus, much attention has been paid to developing a "cure" that would eliminate the underlying mutation and shut down the pathways that lead to the various manifestations. Ideally, a cure would permanently correct the mutation and thus eliminate VOEs, arrest progressive organ damage, and possibly even reverse some pre-existing organ damage. However, even such a therapy would not completely "cure" those whose bodies have been damaged by SCD; they would likely still have organ damage, experience chronic pain, and continue to require treatments.

There are currently two basic approaches to curing SCD, one available now and another, seen as more promising, that is still under development. The first is HSCT. It is the only curative therapy available, but it has short-comings that limit its value, including difficulties finding suitable donors, the possibility of the transplant being rejected, and short-term morbidity and mortality risks (Gluckman et al., 2017; Hsieh et al., 2014; Thompson, 2013; Walters, 2015). The second is the "holy grail" of gene therapy, or gene editing, which does not rely on donors and circumvents the challenges of graft-versus-host-disease (GVHD) and the need for immunosuppression past transplantation (Walters, 2005). It is still in the experimental stages, however, and is not widely available; it has its own set of challenges; and it has been met with a somewhat less than enthusiastic response from the SCD community because of insufficient education and a fear of known and unknown risks (Persaud et al., 2019; Strong et al., 2017).

Stem Cell Transplant

Since the 1990s, stem cell transplant has offered the potential for an SCD cure. More than 1,000 patients, predominantly in the United States and Europe, have now been treated with allogeneic transplantation with excellent results (Gluckman et al., 2017; Hsieh et al., 2014; Walters et al., 1996, 2001). The finding that even modest levels of donor chimerism (i.e., 20 percent myeloid engraftment) result in significant levels of donor hemoglobin that prevent HbS polymerization has led to the development of non-myeloablative or reduced-intensity conditioning regimens; the cumulative outcomes of both remain encouraging. The outcome of transplants from matched siblings has been particularly impressive. The European Blood and Marrow Transplant, Eurocord, and the Center for International Blood and Marrow Trans-plant Research reported the results on 1,000 recipients of human leukocyte antigen (HLA)-identical sibling transplants performed between 1986 and 2013 and found a 5-year event-free and overall survival of 91.4 percent (95% confidence interval [CI] 89.6–93.3) and 92.9 percent (95% CI 91.1–94.6), respectively (Gluckman et al., 2017). Event-free survival was lower with increasing age at transplantation (hazard ratio [HR] = 1.09; $p < 0.001$) and higher for transplantations performed after 2006 (HR = 0.95, $p = 0.013$) (Gluckman et al., 2017). Increasing age was associated with higher rates of acute and chronic GVHD (4 percent and 2 percent higher HR for every 1 year of age increment) and graft failure or death (10 percent higher HR for each year) (Gluckman et al., 2017). The higher risk of chronic GVHD and need for fertility preservation may be indications for non-myeloablative conditioning in older patients (Bernaudin et al., 2019).

Patients who have stable donor engraftment are cured and no longer experience VOEs and other acute complications. However, chronic pain lingers in those who were significantly affected by it before the transplant, and it is unclear whether and to what extent the organ damage can be reversed by transplantation. Stem cell transplantation has largely remained limited to patients with matched siblings, performed outside of clinical trials, and out of reach for most adults with organ dysfunction. Long-term toxicity and reproductive risks also remain a concern. Newer research avenues aim to develop safer conditioning regimens, effective GVHD prevention strategies, more widely available means of fertility preservation, and to expand access to those without matched siblings.

Unrelated-donor stem cell sources are actively sought to expand access to transplantation in SCD and other benign and malignant hematological conditions. While the probability of identifying fully matched donors in the bone marrow registry is low for African Americans (19 percent), allowing for a partial mismatch at one of eight HLA loci increases the likelihood of finding a donor to more than 70 percent (Gragert et al., 2014). Immunologic mismatch leads, however, to a higher incidence of GVHD. While this may be a tolerable side effect in transplant recipients with hematologic malignancies due to the concurrent graft-versus-leukemia effect, it is highly undesirable in patients with benign hematologic conditions, who do not derive any appreciable benefit from GVHD. A recent report shows that when a sibling donor is not available, the outcome of transplantation from different sources is similar. Event-free survival between recipients of transplants from haplo-identical related donors (HR = 1.43, 95% CI 0.81–2.50; p = 0.21) or mismatched unrelated donors (HR = 1.17, 95% CI 0.67–2.05; p = 0.58) versus HLA-matched unrelated donors, or mismatched unrelated donors versus haplo-identical related donors (HR = 1.22, 95% CI 0.65–2.27; p = 0.98), was not statistically significantly different (Eapen et al., 2019). Umbilical cord blood has been explored as a stem cell source due to its lower risk of inducing GVHD (Bernaudin et al., 2007), but its longer time to engraftment and the resulting delayed hematological and immune recovery and low graft cell volume have yielded high graft rejection rates (Kamani et al., 2012; Saraf et al., 2016). Techniques to expand the umbilical cord graft volume ex vivo are under development (Horwitz et al., 2014).

Side Effects and Risks

The side effects and risks of allogeneic stem cell transplant are similar to those observed in other diseases, but they are compounded by SCD-specific factors. For instance, the toxicity of conditioning regimens and immuno-suppressive agents after transplantation may be poorly tolerated by organs (e.g., kidneys or organs in the cardiovascular system) whose physiologic functional reserve is depleted by SCD. The immune reactivity of the transplant recipient is also affected by chronic transfusion regimens, which may result in HLA and RBC alloimmunization and alterations in the bone marrow microenvironment from marrow infarction and stress erythropoiesis. There are recent guidelines for the screening and early recognition of complications after transplantation for hemoglobinopathies (Shenoy et al., 2018).

Stem cell transplant in SCD also poses unusual ethical concerns. Unlike hematologic malignancies, which are often rapidly lethal without curative transplantation, SCD is a chronic disease, and certain subgroups discussed in Chapter 1, such as those with HbSC, HbS/beta thalassemia, or HbSS with hereditary persistence of fetal hemoglobin, have life expectancies that may be comparable to those of unaffected African Americans (Platt et al., 1994). In other patients, existing and developing disease-modifying strategies offer the promise of long-term survival with tolerable morbidity and acceptable QOL. Thus, the side effects of stem cell transplantation need to be assessed in the context of the patient's individual experience with SCD and projected disease course. With matched sibling transplantation, the side effects are relatively modest, and long-term, disease-free survival is the norm. However, as the immunological mismatch becomes more pronounced, the risks of severe toxicity, such as GVHD, rise dramatically, particularly in adults. Opportunistic infections caused by the immunosuppressive regimens also remain a concern although they have been mitigated by non-myeloablative and reduced intensity conditioning regimens.

Stem cell transplant has profound psychosocial repercussions from pre-transplant through the post-transplant phase that must be prevented or managed. An assessment of the psychological well-being of the transplant recipient should be conducted early on, and pre-/post-transplant assessments should include evaluations by social workers and other mental health professions. It is critical to carefully address the family and socioeconomic support available to the transplant candidate. Caregivers' perspectives may weigh significantly in decisions and should be solicited (Khemani et al., 2018). Thus, an SDM model that includes that patient's support system should be adopted throughout the process of informed consent and the treatment and follow-up period. Potential barriers to adherence to anti-rejection regimens should be addressed. It is unrealistic to expect that most patients on long-term opiates will be able to transition to non-opiate analgesia in the immediate post-transplant period. First, certain painful complications, such as avascular necrosis, are not reversible, nor is neuropathic pain. Second, central sensitization and the interplay among decreased executive function, mood disorders, and pain are also expected to have long-term repercussions. Thus, opiate therapy before transplant should be streamlined, and an effort should be made to ease transition by exploring non-pharmacological analgesic strategies, optimizing mental health, and addressing spiritual and existential concerns in advance. Even when stem cell transplant is relatively uneventful and a cure is attained, there should be ongoing attention to the psychological needs of the recipients. As a chronic, lifelong, life-threatening illness, SCD shapes self-identity and psychological ownership. In other words, it may become part of the patient's "identity" (Karnilowicz, 2011), which can then be questioned or threatened by a cure.

Implications for Fertility and Other Reproductive Issues

Gonadotoxic conditioning regimens with busulfan, other myeloablative drugs (e.g., cyclophosphamide), and radiation affect fertility and carry a risk of ovarian failure (prevalence of 65–84 percent) (Joshi et al., 2014; Loren et al., 2011), particularly in post-pubertal individuals. Furthermore, transfusional hemosiderosis arising from repeated transfusions in the pre-transplantation period also predisposes to endocrinopathy and reduced fertility. Thus, fertility preservation should be discussed up front and offered by means of ovarian and testicular tissue cryopreservation whenever possible and as recommended by the Practice Committee of the American Society for Reproductive Medicine 2013 guidelines (ASRM, 2013), with the caveat that it may not be covered by health insurers outside of a clinical trial. In European countries where the procedure is at no cost to the patient, such preservation is performed systematically in all SCD transplant patients (Bernaudin et al., 2019). However, both laparoscopic unilateral oophorectomy and testicular tissue explant are invasive and require general anesthesia, which predisposes patients to vaso-occlusive complications in the post-operative period. Thus, adequate precautions to minimize post-procedure complications should be enacted. For settings where pre-transplantation sperm and ovarian cryopreservation are unavailable or unaffordable, fertility-preserving conditioning regimens are being developed, and gonadal shielding during irradiation is an option.

Another reproductive concern related to stem cell transplant is the need for subsequent hormonal therapy to develop secondary sexual characteristics in prepubertal children, particularly girls (Dallas et al., 2013; Walters et al., 2000). It is important to frame the discussion of the reproductive risks of stem cell transplantation (Xue et al., 2019) within the broader context of the risks deriving from untreated SCD, which is known to affect sexual maturation and fertility, and alternative treatments that may also affect fertility, such as HU (Joseph et al., 2019; Pecker et al., 2019).

Expanding Access to Non-Matched Donors and Others

Access to stem cell transplant continues to be very limited. Only 14 percent of individuals with SCD will have an HLA-matched sibling donor (Walters, 2015). Similarly, only 19 percent will have a well-matched unrelated donor, far lower than the 75 percent likelihood for Caucasian patients

(Walters, 2015). In contrast, it is estimated that more than 50 percent of patients will have a haplo-identical donor. Haplo-identical transplant for nonmalignant diseases has expanded exponentially over the past few years thanks to new conditioning strategies, such as the addition of thyotepa to the preparative regimen (de la Fuente et al., 2019), graft preparation by T-cell depletion and CD34+ selection to reduce GVHD, and post-transplant cyclophosphamide to modulated alloreactivity (Brodsky et al., 2008). While relatively few patients with SCD have received a haplo-identical graft, the results have been encouraging. The rates of GVHD and graft rejection are lower than initially predicted (although long-term follow-up data are not yet available), and the majority of patients have experienced resolution of their anemia and other SCD-related complications (Cairo et al., 2019). Several clinical trials of haplo-identical transplantation with improved conditioning regimens or posttransplant immunosuppression are under way (Limerick and Fitzhugh, 2019; Tanhehco and Bhatia, 2019).

Long-Term Outcomes

Studies of the long-term outcomes after transplantation have explored the potential to stop disease progression or reverse the most severe complications. There is emerging evidence that both neurological and cardiovascular complications may either remain stable or improve. Secondary strokes have not occurred after transplantation (Bernaudin et al., 2007; Walters et al., 2010), and overall cerebral vasculopathy, including silent cerebral infarcts and lacunar infarcts, has remained stable, as recorded by magnetic resonance imaging (MRI) (Green et al., 2017), except in those patients with the highest cerebrovascular disease burden (Dallas et al., 2013). Transplant-related neurological toxicity, such as posterior reversible leukoencephalopathy syndrome, may sometimes complicate the assessment of neurological outcomes after transplantation.

Pulmonary hypertension is a major risk factor for early mortality, with a tricuspid regurgitant jet velocity > 2.5 m/s conferring a relative risk (RR) of 10 for mortality (Gladwin et al., 2004). After transplantation, tricuspid regurgitant jet velocity improved from 2.84 m/s (95% CI 2.71–2.99) before HSCT to 2.33 (95% CI 2.14–2.51) over 3 years in adults (Hsieh et al., 2014). Pulmonary function tests also showed stable deficits or improved biomarkers (Gilman et al., 2017; Walters et al., 2010).

A major caveat concerning studies of long-term transplant outcomes is that a control group receiving best supportive care, transfusions, or HU has not generally been available for comparison.

Research Gap: Outcomes for Pediatric Patients Versus Adults

The optimal timing of transplantation in children with an identical HLA-matched sibling remains unknown, but mounting research evidence suggests that outcomes are superior in patients younger than 10 years old. There is also a strong rationale to carry out transplants in patients before complications and irreversible organ damage have occurred. In both children and adults, common indications for transplantation have included a severe phenotype despite HU or transfusion therapy or any severe complication, such as pulmonary hypertension or progressive cerebral vasculopathy (Kassim and Sharma, 2017; Walters et al., 1996). Yet criteria to recommend transplantation mostly rest on expert opinion, without any validated tools to determine optimal timing or suitability. Biomarkers to predict disease course, major outcomes, and mortality are still needed (Kalpatthi and Novelli, 2018).

Research is needed on patients' QOL after transplant, particularly in adults; extensive studies documenting QOL pre- and post-transplant are not yet available. Algorithms and decision trees based on biomarkers of disease severity are also not available and are urgently needed for use in selecting candidates for transplantation. Ideally, transplantation should be prioritized in those patients with a severe phenotype despite disease-modifying therapies but whose organ function remains adequate to withstand the physiologic demands of the procedure. Decisions concerning transplantation opportunity and timing will become even more complex once the new biological therapies under development become available. A future is foreseeable where multiple medications used sequentially or in combination may significantly mitigate the phenotype to the point that stem cell transplantation offers no added value. Funding for biomarker development is imperative for generating the information needed to navigate these complex scenarios.

Another important area of research concerns whether transplantation can reverse specific complications. In particular, it will be important to ascertain whether the progressive deterioration in neurocognitive function in SCD can be slowed or reversed.

Research on chronic pain and its effects on mood in SCD is urgently needed and will be important in dissecting the multifaceted pain that patients often continue to experience after transplantation. In general, research on the psychological impact of transplantation will be needed, particularly in the arena of self-identity and perceptions of the self in relation to others.

Finally, more studies are needed to analyze the patients' and caregivers' perspectives on important factors that affect decision making in transplantation (Khemani et al., 2018).

Gene Therapy

Gene therapy was an unattainable goal for SCD until the past decade. However, successes with primary immunodeficiency syndromes and hemophilia have spurred interest in gene therapy approaches for hemoglobinopathies. Since the 1990s, the use of viral vectors has allowed ex vivo gene therapy (via the insertion of genes into autologous hematopoietic stem cells). Most recently, the development of clustered regularly interspaced short palindromic repeats (CRISPR)/CRISPR-associated protein 9 (Cas9) technology has offered the promise of a cure (Jinek et al., 2012). Both approaches are preferable to stem cell transplant because they overcome the problem of a lack of suitable donors and also the risk of transplant-related complications, such as GVHD and opportunistic infections from prolonged immunosuppression. The principal methods of gene therapy under development are (1) the addition of β-globin or βT87Q-globin to produce hemoglobin (HbA) or γ-globin to enhance HbF levels, (2) HbF induction by editing of globin regulatory elements or knockdown of HbF repressors, and (3) direct gene correction of the SCD mutation with programmable nucleases (Demirci et al., 2019).

Gene Replacement

The introduction of replication-defective, HIV-1-based lentiviral vectors (LVs) has overcome many of the limitations of older gammaretroviral vectors, including the inability to transduce quiescent hematopoietic stem cells and to carry large gene constructs, such as β-globin and its regulatory elements. Genetic transfer of an anti-sickling β-globin LV into hematopoietic stem cells followed by myeloablative transplant cured one child (Ribeil et al., 2017), but it was not successful in seven subsequent adults with sickle cell anemia, which led to modifying the intensity of the conditioning regimen and improving the stem cell dose and gene transfer protocol (Kanter, 2017). Promising preliminary reports have been presented at the ASH annual meeting in 2018, in 2019 at the American Society of Gene and Cell Therapy meeting, and at European Hematology Association meetings. One study is a Phase I/II trial of modified gamma globin LV-based gene therapy in two adults with SCD after a reduced-intensity conditioning regimen. In this trial, the expression of a modified HbF (HbF^G16D) was shown to be 20 percent for the first patient 1 year post-transplant, with a similar trajectory for the second patient, who was still in the early phase of post-transplant at the time of publication of the results; these findings were associated with a reduction in acute pain episodes (Malik et al., 2018). Another study, a Phase I trial of lentiviral-based gene transduction of a β-globin with an anti-sickling substitution

(T87Q) into bone marrow harvested or plerixafor-mobilized stem cells in 15 patients (Tisdale et al., 2018) showed more robust production of HbA^{T87Q} (Kanter et al., 2019; Mpara et al., 2019). In four patients with more than 6 months follow-up, HbA^{T87Q} was 47–60 percent of total hemoglobin, almost equaling or exceeding HbS levels (Kanter et al., 2019), and it was accompanied by an improvement in the SCD phenotype. Based on up to 3 years of follow-up, insertional mutagenesis and oncogenesis, also major concerns with gammaretroviral vectors, have not materialized in patients with thalassemia or SCD treated with lentiviral-based gene therapy, but longer follow-up is required.

Given the variability of results with the ongoing gene therapy approaches, stopping points for trials need to be defined and criteria developed to prevent the possibility that noncurative studies (where the gene product is not likely to be expressed to a level necessary to achieve a cure) are misclassified as curative.

Gene Editing

CRISPR/Cas9 has revolutionized gene editing by providing an efficient, easy-to-design approach that is less costly than those that rely on nucleases. Gene-editing strategies aim at suppressing HbS polymerization via the following major mechanisms: (1) inducing HbF by inhibiting the binding of transcriptional repressors BAF chromatin remodeling complex subunit BCL11A (BCL11A) and leukemia/lymphoma-related factor, or targeting transcriptional regulators of HbF, (2) correcting the HbS mutation, or (3) inserting an anti-sickling beta-globin cDNA (betaAS3). Approaches are being developed to target hematopoietic stem cells and inducible pluripotent stem cells. Concerns exist about the potential immunogenicity of guide RNAs or Cas9 and the efficiency and specificity of editing. The most advanced gene editing approach involves deleting BCL11A; it is part of an ongoing Phase I/II clinical trial by CRISPR Therapeutics and Vertex Pharmaceuticals. In October 2019, CRISPR appeared to be successful in restoring the functional bone marrow cells in the first patient with SCD to undergo this gene editing technique (Stein, 2019).

Ethical Issues and Other Considerations

Gene therapy shares some of the concerns surrounding stem cell transplantation because it requires a conditioning regimen, with the attendant risks of infertility and secondary malignancies, particularly when myeloablative regimens are employed, as in ongoing gene therapy approaches. In gene therapy, as in allogeneic transplantation, there are also uncertainties as to the optimal source of stem cells. Mobilizing autologous peripheral blood stem cells in patients with SCD is now feasible thanks to plerixafor, a molecule that releases stem cells from their marrow niches into the circulation and, unlike filgrastim, does not appear to cause side effects (Boulad et al., 2018; Esrick et al., 2018; Hsieh and Tisdale, 2018; Lagresle-Peyrou et al., 2018). It remains to be determined whether peripheral blood or bone marrow is the optimal source of autologous stem cells for gene transfer or editing. Maximizing the stem cell yield is critical, because many gene transfer approaches require culturing stem cells ex vivo, which may lead to a loss of repopulating potential and ultimately an inadequate number of cells harboring the transgene for reinfusion.

A well-publicized ethical concern surrounding all gene therapy approaches is their potential to be adapted to germ line editing (in human embryos). NIH and many regulatory agencies throughout the world do not support this application of the technologies (Evitt et al., 2015). There are additional ethical considerations about safety, particularly surrounding immunogenicity in CRISPR/Cas9 and the lingering concerns about mutagenesis, given the relatively short duration of the follow-up of the treated patients to date. When devising therapies for a disease that is disproportionally common in low- to middle-income areas of the world, it also behooves investigators and policy makers to promote widely applicable approaches that do not rely on highly specialized infrastructure and expertise. Thus, approaches should also be developed that target stem cells in vivo, a less technically challenging procedure.

Finally, similar to the situation with stem cell transplantation, the SCD community has lower risk tolerance for gene therapy due to the availability of effective alternative therapies and the absence of long-term outcomes data for most patients. Thus, it is paramount that gene therapy trials receive the appropriate oversight by both an FDA-appointed and a non-FDA panel of experts. There also needs to be greater assurance for postmarket evaluation and controlled use because in rare diseases, such as SCD, widespread use of novel disease modifiers by providers not familiar with the disease can lead to dangerous and devastating outcomes. The analysis of long-term data and expert guided therapy will be crucial.

The technical limitations of current gene therapy approaches need to be underscored. First, all current strategies involve ex vivo gene transduction or editing, which involve the ex vivo manipulation of stem cells, with their potential loss of repopulating potential, and myeloablative chemotherapy to accommodate the auto transplant. Ideally, both problems will be overcome by in vivo gene therapy approaches, where the viral vector will be directly injected into the patient, as it is the case in techniques that are under investigation for hemophilia (Nienhuis et al., 2017). Second, it is important to note that gene therapy does not necessarily equate to a cure (i.e., the permanent and complete suppression of HbS polymerization and its attendant complications) and should never be labeled and presented as such to the patients and other stakeholders. Based on the preliminary results of the ongoing gene therapy trials, it is unlikely that any of the current gene therapy approaches will result in a cure, although it is hoped that progressive technical advances will eventually achieve a cure in the next decades.

Family Privacy Concerns

Any procedure that accesses DNA poses ethical concerns—related to privacy, confidentiality, subsequent use, and disclosure to significant others—that have legal and societal repercussions (NASEM, 2017a).

CLINICAL TRIALS AND THE DRUG APPROVAL PROCESS

The final step in the drug development process is the clinical trials necessary to receive approval from FDA to make the drug widely available, and the drugs in development can face some special challenges arising from SCD characteristics and affected individuals' circumstances. One set of challenges is related to the African American community's experiences with the U.S. health care system and the resulting lack of trust that many members have for doctors and the entire health care system. A second set of challenges stems from the multiplicity and complexity of SCD symptoms, which makes it difficult to determine the best way to measure a treatment's efficacy.

Patient Mistrust and Lack of Awareness

Clinical trials require an awareness of the existence of the trials and the willing participation of individuals with the disease, which in turn requires a certain level of trust among those individuals. Addressing these issues will help smooth the way for successful clinical trials of the SCD treatments now in development. Because individuals of African descent are significantly more likely to have the SCD mutation than people whose ancestors come from other parts of the world, U.S. clinical trials of SCD drugs will inevitably require large percentages of African Americans among the trial participants, but African Americans have many reasons to distrust the health care system.

First, the history of human experimentation in the United States has been marked by racism and inequality, as epitomized by the infamous U.S. Public Health Service Syphilis Study (CDC, 2015). Furthermore, many African Americans have experienced institutionalized racism in health care and the research community. Patients with SCD, specifically, have suffered from the stigma of an inherited disease that causes intractable pain (Blake et al., 2018; Bulgin et al., 2018); because that pain is almost never "objectively" documented, legitimate requests for opiates have often been misconstrued as "drug seeking" behavior, particularly in emergency departments (EDs) (Shapiro et al., 1997). These misperceptions among health care providers of addiction and abuse are now being compounded by a regulatory and institutional environment that curtails opiate prescribing to control the U.S. opiate crisis (NASEM, 2017b), with SCD patients at risk of experiencing unintended effects in this climate. Regular misunderstandings between SCD patients and health care providers over pain control have often generated mutual mistrust (Puri et al., 2016). None of this is conducive to a successful partnership between patients and providers to test novel SCD treatments.

Compounding the issue of mistrust, decreased access to care among African Americans and a lack of clinicians specializing in caring for patients with SCD have resulted in a lack of awareness of new therapies and clinical trials among SCD patients. In response, ASH has recently developed several initiatives to increase access to care, educate providers across the nation, and bolster research infrastructure, including developing a clinical trial network (Michaelis, 2019).

Social media is emerging as a powerful tool with which to disseminate health care information and help shape opinions. For instance, two Facebook groups, the Sickle Cell Warriors and Sickle Cell Unite, boast thousands of users and have become important resources for the community through the information and support they provide to members and users. The discussions in these groups can also provide insight into perceptions among stakeholders, such as their opinions on the efficacy of HU. One published analysis of common themes among Facebook group members reported that some patients and caregivers perceived HU as masking symptoms (e.g., by artificially improving blood counts), thereby making it more difficult for patients to receive necessary acute care for pain, while others thought of HU as a "cancer drug" (its original approved use); both perceptions likely make patients less willing to take the drug (Walker et al., 2019). One implication of this research is that social media could be leveraged by health care providers to advance sickle cell research agendas and dispel misconceptions about clinical trials.

Clinical Evidence for Approval

Clinical trials require an objective way to measure the outcomes achieved with the tested therapy and compare those outcomes with those that were achieved with other therapies or no therapy. However, this is not always a straightforward process for SCD.

Determining Which Endpoints to Use

A key question that must be answered before running a clinical trial is which endpoints will be used to judge the outcome. With SCD, however, developing biomarkers to use as endpoints in research or in the clinic has been hampered by the complexity of the phenotype, which is determined by a myriad of genetic and epigenetic factors and a complex pathogenetic mechanism (Kalpatthi and Novelli, 2018). For example, even though VOEs are extremely disabling and the most common cause of hospitalization in SCD, self-reported pain scores remain the only indicator in humans, despite the fact that mouse models of SCD have allowed intravital imaging and characterization of the molecular events that lead to SCD (Sundd et al., 2019). This is a major limitation because self-reported pain is highly subjective and a notoriously poor biomarker. Indeed, both drug development and clinical care are hampered by the absence of objective, quantifiable biomarkers of SCD (Kalpatthi and Novelli, 2018).

Thus, it would be extremely valuable to develop new markers of acute pain for both clinical research and clinical care. Objective biomarkers would help validate self-reports and reduce mutual mistrust between patients and health care providers. In addition, there is a need for patient-centered, technology-based approaches that can capture distinctive changes in pain intensity and quality, such as the use of abstract animations, which have been shown to be less affected by age, literacy level, or language than visual analog score scales (Jonassaint et al., 2018a,b).

Patients are also afflicted by chronic pain. In the Pain in Sickle Cell Epidemiology Study (PiSCES), pain occurred daily in approximately half of study participants (McClish et al., 2017). Chronic pain is not typically included as an outcome in clinical research, yet it profoundly affects QOL. Thus, the development of a biomarker for chronic pain would be useful. Novel biomarkers under investigation include those based on brain imaging with functional MRI (Karafin et al., 2019).

SCD severity scores (Burke et al., 2016) and composite biomarker signatures (Du et al., 2018) are now being developed to address the limitations of existing VOE-based biomarkers.

To develop other endpoints for clinical research, investigators should focus on identifying biomarkers of specific pathogenic processes. The experience gained in the senicapoc trial indicates that hemolysis alone is not an adequate biomarker of efficacy for investigational drugs (Ataga et al., 2011). However, biomarkers that measure hyperadhesion, oxidant stress, or hemostatic activation could be employed to predict and measure response to drugs that specifically target those pathways (Kalpatthi and Novelli, 2018). In an effort to inform the field, ASH partnered with FDA to conduct work to identify clinical trial endpoints. The work, which was informed by seven panels of clinicians, researchers, and patients, resulted in the publication of two consensus recommendations on (1) endpoints for patient-reported outcomes (PROs), pain, and the brain; and (2) endpoints for renal and cardiopulmonary, cure, and low-resource settings (Farrell et al., 2019).

Outcome Measures in SCD

There is an ongoing debate on clinically relevant endpoints for SCD research. The consensus is that the endpoints traditionally used in SCD clinical trials are limited and poorly represent the heterogeneity of the disease. Well-characterized biomarkers and relevant surrogate endpoints are scarce. While the validity of transcranial Doppler velocity to assess stroke risk and cerebral vasculopathy (Adams, 2007) and of tricuspid regurgitant jet velocity to assess mortality risk are undisputed, most other complications lack adequate biomarkers (Gladwin et al., 2004). VOE represents the most blatant example of a complication that has posed significant challenges for clinical trial design. Most studies have employed the duration and severity of VOE as clinical endpoints, yet both are difficult to operationalize.

One strategy to develop more valuable outcome measures has been to invest in developing tools for PROs. In particular, QOL measures and PROs that capture certain complications have not been adequately incorporated in clinical research. For instance, PRO instruments that include cognition, depressive symptoms, sexual dysfunction, and sleep disturbances have been lacking and are sorely needed. Other areas of development include measures that can be applied to younger and older populations and measures that capture the totality of acute and chronic pain. Examples of recommended PROs include the Brief Pain Inventory, the ASCQ-Me, and the Adult Sickle Cell Quality of Life Measurement Information System (ASCQ-Me) Quality of Care.[2]

HEALTH CARE DELIVERY POLICY

Once a new therapy has been developed, it must be provided to patients, which raises the next question: the most effective approaches for delivery. This is particularly important for new curative therapies, as these will typically involve different treatment regimens—a one-time treatment, for example, rather than daily dosing—and will likely be significantly more expensive than therapeutic drugs.

---

[2] For more information on the tools, see http://www.ascq-me.org (accessed July 6, 2020) and https://www.mdanderson.org/documents/Departments-and-Divisions/Symptom-Research/BPI_UserGuide.pdf (accessed July 6, 2020).

Implications of Curative Therapy for Delivery System Innovation

Because traditional fee-for-service models of reimbursement provide little direct incentive for physicians to maximize quality or avoid wasteful spending, several recent reforms have attempted to strengthen physician incentives for quality and efficiency. Such reforms remain nascent in the SCD context, however. High-cost curative therapy may also pose unique challenges that could further stifle such delivery system reform innovations in SCD. This section considers these issues and potential solutions.

Patient-centered medical homes (PCMHs) are provider-centered care delivery models that encourage care coordination (AHRQ, n.d.), and they show promise for SCD care. Under this model, care is accessible, continuous, comprehensive, family-centered, coordinated, compassionate, and culturally effective (AAP, 2002; Raphael et al., 2013). Typically, care is coordinated by a personal physician or a provider in the community. Some evidence suggests that PCMHs improve outcomes for SCD patients. A study of 150 children in a large children's hospital found that SCD children receiving PCMH had half the rate of ED visits (incident rate ratio [IRR] = 0.51, 95% CI 0.33–0.78) and just more than half the rate of hospitalizations (IRR = 0.56, 95% CI 0.33–0.93) compared with children not receiving such care (Raphael et al., 2013). The study found that the comprehensive care component of the PCMH was the one that significantly reduced ED visits and hospitalizations. This suggests that PCMH may hold promise as a delivery system reform. Caution is nonetheless warranted. While the PCMH may prove beneficial in the pediatric context, it may not be a viable method for improving the delivery of medical care for adults (Ballas and Vichinsky, 2015). The PCMH is centered around having a personal provider who will coordinate care as the primary criterion. Given the well-known problems that arise in transitioning from pediatrics to adult care, the PCMH model may be harder to establish in the adult care setting.

Another prominent delivery system reform is the use of the accountable care organization (ACO), which is a partnership between a third-party payer and a set of providers, typically including a primary care provider, specialists, hospitals, rehabilitation centers, and long-term care facilities, that seeks to provide coordinated care (CMS, 2019). ACOs receive a fixed base payment from the insurer plus a share in the savings if they achieve cost and quality targets for their patients. The goal is to encourage high-quality care and avoid unnecessary costs. One example is New York City's Kings County ACO, which identified advanced SCD as a priority subpopulation due to the high number of readmissions (Stine et al., 2017). In response, the primary care and hematology departments partnered to create a multidisciplinary high-risk clinic to deal with advanced SCD patients. Systematic data on the performance of such ACOs in SCD care could better inform an overall delivery reform strategy.

Bundled payments are a third prominent reform type, designed to achieve lower costs, higher quality, and better health (Oyeku and Faro, 2017). Also known as "episode-based payments," bundled payments are designed to encourage high-value care by encouraging providers to improve coordination, efficiency, and care quality and outcomes (*NEJM Catalyst*, 2018). Under bundled payments, the total health care costs for an episode are prospectively determined, and providers receive no marginal compensation for any services within the bundle. Thus, providers take a loss when the cost exceeds the prospective bundled payment level, but they can share in the savings if they achieve costs below the target (conditional on meeting quality standards). While there are examples of SCD bundles (e.g., the Cleveland Clinic Children's SCD discharge bundle), they are relatively scarce. The Center for Medicare & Medicaid Innovation has developed more than 50 different payment and delivery models since its establishment via the Patient Protection and Affordable Care Act of 2010, but individuals with rare conditions such as SCD have been left behind.[3]

Delivery system innovation in SCD has not been rapid, and recent curative therapies pose additional challenges. If gene therapies or other curative therapies involve high up-front costs for health care providers (e.g., as in chimeric antigen receptor T-cell therapy for cancer treatment), in which hospitals must pay in advance to acquire the drug and then wait for reimbursement, it may discourage health systems and other provider organizations from delivery system innovation that might benefit (and thus attract) more SCD patients. A solution might be helping providers finance the up-front costs of high-cost therapies and care. Public and private payers might be tapped as a source of financing, especially since delays in reimbursement create the need for financing.

Curative therapies also pose a challenge for bundled payments. Incorporating these in a bundled payment would likely discourage their use because the fixed payment may be insufficient. On the other hand, excluding them might encourage overuse because the bundled payment itself penalizes overuse. Criteria for use of these new therapies would help address this problem, for example, reducing the number of "marginal" cases where patients may or may not benefit would help mitigate overuse, even if the curative therapies are not bundled.

It may be tempting to believe that curative therapy would eliminate the need for intensive, coordinated care, but this may not be the case. "Cured" individuals may still experience pain throughout their lives and may also require genetic counseling because they could pass the mutation to future generations. Experience with HSCT patients suggests that a fraction of

---

[3] For a list of innovation models for payment and service delivery, see https://innovation.cms.gov/innovation-models#views=models (accessed July 8, 2020).

them continue to have chronic pain (Darbari et al., 2019). SCD patients may also continue to suffer the consequences of earlier organ damage.

Treatment innovation could even increase the need for specialized care. Curative therapies might be administered primarily or even solely by SCD specialists. If so, then access to specialists will limit therapy availability. Among commercially insured SCD patients, less than half see a specialist in a given year; that rate is less than one-sixth for Medicaid patients (Dampier et al., 2017). Unless access to specialists is particularly well correlated with eligibility for a therapy, barriers to specialist care will slow the diffusion of novel curative therapies. The solution must lie in either expanding specialist access or establishing protocols for nonspecialists—perhaps with some additional training, specialist support, or other resources.

Shared Decision Making

There are various reasons for believing that the best approach to making decisions about SCD care will be one in which patients and clinicians work together. For example, Ross et al. (2016) present qualitative research indicating that patients prefer collaborative decision-making processes over decisions made solely by clinicians. Patients also believe that clinicians should consider their personal preferences for care, listen to their perspective, and provide information about complications, long-term outcomes, side effects, and other relevant factors. The desire for SDM is likely to be even more acute in the context of curative therapy. "Cures" offer the chance of a substantial and durable clinical benefit, but they generally come with considerable uncertainty surrounding the degree of benefit and long-term side effects, and both the adverse effects and benefits are hard to gauge. The optimal clinical decision will depend at least in part on the patient's tolerance for uncertainty and ambiguity. All of these factors suggest that an SDM approach is best.

Existing studies on SDM in the SCD context provide a basis for specific research relative to curative SCD therapy. Khemani et al. (2018) conducted qualitative research designed to elicit the factors influencing the choice of HSCT. Identifying the key decision factors helps facilitate more productive conversations between providers and patients about treatment choice. Crosby et al. (2015) set forth a set of six strategies designed to facilitate SDM in the context of weighing the benefits and side effects of HU treatment. Finally, an ongoing Patient-Centered Outcomes Research Institute study is comparing alternative approaches to facilitating SDM concerning treatment options for pediatric SCD patients (PCORI, 2019). The launch of an innovative curative therapy should be accompanied by careful research and guidance on strategies for SDM.

REIMBURSEMENT POLICY

Decisions about new SCD therapies will also depend strongly on various economic factors, such as the price of treatment, cost–benefit considerations, and, in particular, reimbursement policies. While it is impossible to offer any specifics about the economic future for novel SCD therapies, other areas of medicine offer a sense of the general economic considerations that will shape the uptake of these new SCD treatments and cures.

It is difficult to predict how curative therapies for SCD will be priced, but the relevant factors will include the size of the eligible patient population and the expected take-up, the expected rate of treatment response, and the extent of irreversible sequelae (e.g., organ damage). If the expected take-up is low, the budget impact of even an expensive therapy might be relatively limited for an individual payer; this would mitigate pushback on price. In addition, the expected clinical value will play a role in the price negotiations between pharmaceutical manufacturers and third-party payers. There remains considerable uncertainty around all of these factors.

This caveat notwithstanding, there is some insight from studying the lifetime cost of caring for SCD patients using chronic therapy. A "perfect" cure would be worth at least this much to third-party payers. For example, the average lifetime cost of treating a person with hepatitis C virus (HCV) is estimated to be $64,490, with higher costs for individuals with longer-than-average life expectancies (Razavi et al., 2013). Sofosbuvir (Sovaldi), which cured HCV in more than 90 percent of patients (Cholongitas and Papatheodoridis, 2014), launched with a list price of about $84,000, although payers likely paid somewhat less after rebates (particularly after competitors arrived) (ICER, 2015; Pollack, 2015; U.S. Senate Committee on Finance, 2015). Partially effective cures could be valued similarly, on a pro-rata basis. Note that these are minimum values because they disregard the value of health gains to patients, caregivers, employers, and other stakeholders. Nonetheless, they provide a fixed point for thinking about the potential cost and budget impact of cures at a time when details about their clinical benefits remain scarce.

Kauf et al. (2009) estimated the total lifetime cost of care for an SCD Medicaid patient to be more than $450,000. This is a conservative estimate because commercially insured patients cost more than Medicaid patients. Thus, in the current pricing environment, a perfect cure might cost upward of $450,000 per patient; $1 billion would treat just more than 2,000 patients, a fraction of those with SCD. Given these numbers, it is difficult to imagine that a large subset of patients would receive curative therapy without significant changes to the structure of pricing contracts or price levels. It is similarly unlikely that third-party payers will make investments of this size and scope without an evidence base assessing the value of therapy—especially in light of growing willingness by U.S. payers to price according to measured effectiveness (CVSHealth, 2018). For curative therapies to be widely adopted, strategies will be required to stimulate the development of evidence on value and new approaches to payment.

Aligning Endpoints for Approval and Reimbursement

It is well understood that regulatory agencies and third-party payers differ in their incentives and demands for evidence on efficacy, safety, and value (Bognar et al., 2017). For example, FDA does not consider cost or value for money in its approval decisions. U.S. third-party payers, on the other hand, are increasingly considering value in their reimbursement decisions. Within the past year, the pharmacy benefit manager CVS Caremark proposed allowing clients to exclude pharmaceuticals that have a launch price that is higher than $100,000 per quality-adjusted life-year (QALY) gained due to the therapy (CVSHealth, 2018). Other payers are routinely using cost-per-QALY evidence in their price negotiations. A survey of 422 formulary decision makers from U.S. payers found that 45 percent were likely or extremely likely to request a rebate to align a drug's net price with the recommended value-based price calculated by the Institute for Clinical and Economic Review (ICER) and that around 59 percent of payers have used an ICER report as a basis for clinical and economic outcomes thresholds when creating an outcomes-based contract (ICON, 2018).

Clinical trials will always feature endpoints likely to satisfy regulators. However, patients may lose out on access to new therapies if those endpoints do not also permit third-party payers to assess value. The dominant method for value assessment today is measuring cost per QALYs gained or some variant of that, such as cost per life-year saved or healthy life-year gained. This is not to suggest that the cost per QALY is or should be the only criterion for reimbursement. Rather, payers are more likely to cover a new therapy generously if there is evidence of value for the money.

The extant cost-effectiveness literature on SCD therapies is somewhat sparse; a search of PubMed generated only 62 results, and very few of them used QALYs to measure benefit. Spackman et al. (2014) did so, reporting the cost per QALY gained by preoperative transfusion. Other studies have used alternatives to the QALY as a measure of benefit. For example, Panepinto et al. (2000) estimated the cost per additional life-year saved by universal SCD screening compared with targeted screening. Other studies have reported cost per healthy life-year gained (Cunningham-Myrie et al., 2015; McGann et al., 2015).

Controversy persists around whether QALYs are the best way to measure health benefits (Lakdawalla et al., 2018). However, the increasing adoption of cost-per-QALY criteria by U.S. payers suggests that evidence on QALYs can ease the path toward access for patients. A critical step will be to map clinical endpoints to "health utility levels." Very briefly, each health state (e.g., the number of pain crises per month) is enumerated and then valued relative to a perfectly healthy life-year. Spending 1 year in a state that is 80 percent as valuable as a perfectly healthy life-year is worth 0.8 QALYs, and so on. Innovators should anticipate the demand for studies on value by generating studies that map their clinical trial endpoints of interest to QALYs. Producing evidence on value more quickly will facilitate a more rapid uptake of new therapies (Lakdawalla et al., 2018).

There is a limited body of evidence estimating QALYs in the sickle cell context. A few studies have estimated health utility levels for SCD patients (Anie et al., 2002; McClish et al., 2017; Woods et al., 1997). The United Kingdom's National Institute for Health and Care Excellence (NICE) reviewed this literature and calculated that the weighted average QALY for SCD was 0.732 (i.e., 1 year spent with SCD is estimated to be worth 0.732 perfectly healthy life-years) (NICE, 2012). This study also extrapolated utility levels associated with two complications, ACS and stroke; because of the absence of SCD-specific data, these were based on estimates obtained in non-SCD patient populations.

The growing importance of QALYs, along with the relatively limited literature on QALY measurement in SCD, suggests the importance of generating data that can readily assess the value of new SCD therapies. In addition, clinical trial endpoints must align with the published methods for estimating QALYs. For example, an innovator may conduct a clinical trial showing that a new drug reduces the number of monthly pain crises. This permits an assessment of value only if studies exist that compute health utility levels and QALYs against monthly pain crises.

Value assessments include both estimated QALYs gained and the incremental costs of a new therapy. Cost estimates include the direct cost of a new intervention and of supportive care as well as the cost offsets associated with, for example, reduced health care use due to health benefits. The International Society for Pharmacoeconomics and Outcomes Research published guidelines in 2015 recommending that collecting cost data should be fully integrated into clinical trials (Ramsey et al., 2015). Including costs as a secondary endpoint in pivotal randomized clinical trials would expedite the collection of these data and the associated assessment of value.

Novel Payment Mechanisms for Curative Therapies

Lessons from Other Disease Areas

Curative therapies may provide substantial long-term benefits but with high up-front costs. Several noteworthy examples in other disease areas provide insights into the kinds of access constraints that SCD cures may face and the potential for solutions.

Sovaldi, as noted earlier, cured HCV in more than 90 percent of patients (Cholongitas and Papatheodoridis, 2014). The treatment was initially priced at about $84,000 for a 12-week course in the United States. While the price fell in the months following launch, it remained relatively high (ICER, 2015; Pollack, 2015). Significantly, Sovaldi provided value for money (NICE, 2014). NICE deemed the United Kingdom price of about GBP 35,000 to be cost-effective (Hirschler, 2014; NICE, 2014). Despite the evidence on value, Sovaldi's price multiplied by the number of HCV patients resulted in a substantial potential budget impact (Henry, 2018; Touchot and Flume, 2015). During the first 9 months of 2014, the total U.S. health care expenditures were $6.6 billion, making Sovaldi the highest-revenue drug in the country during that period (Schumock et al., 2015).

At the same time, reports emerged of payers denying coverage of Sovaldi or approving access only after fibrotic changes had been documented in the liver (Do et al., 2015). Several private insurers implemented stringent prior authorization systems to limit their spending on Sovaldi, to the point that 25 percent of patients prescribed it were initially denied access (Schumock et al., 2015), even though many did receive it later (Do et al., 2015).

Sovaldi presents a case of a likely cost-effective drug whose uptake was limited by its substantial budget impact. This raises the question of whether novel financing arrangements can blunt the problem of high up-front costs. One direct approach is an annuity pricing model, sometimes referred to as a "drug mortgage" (Sachs et al., 2018). For example, Bluebird Bio has developed a gene-replacement therapy for thalassemia that may feature a seven-figure up-front cost. Perhaps as a result, it has announced plans for an annuity payment model, in which third-party payers would pay on a 5-year installment plan, with the installments also partially tied to the continuing durable effectiveness of the drug (Walker, 2019). Other firms have also tied the price of cures to their effectiveness. Spark Therapeutics prices its gene therapy for childhood retinal dystrophy at $850,000. Given the uncertainty about its long-term effectiveness and its high price tag, the company has proposed an outcomes-based pricing contract that offers a partial refund if the patient's eyesight deteriorates (Richards, 2019). Spark Therapeutics also proposed a payment option that, in addition to the outcomes-based rebates, spreads out payments over time. Because current government price-reporting requirements do not explicitly account for the possibility of these amortized payments, Spark Therapeutics has proposed this novel payment mechanism as a Centers for Medicare & Medicaid Services (CMS) demonstration project (Spark Therapeutics, 2018). The obstacles created by federal price-reporting requirements for novel payments are considered in more detail below. Another pricing approach is to negotiate a fixed total cost that can help payers reduce the risk of unexpectedly large budget impacts. For example, Louisiana's Medicaid program is experimenting with a "Netflix-style" pricing model: for a fixed monthly subscription fee, it receives a license for unrestricted use of AbbVie's, Gilead's, or Merck's HCV treatments (Louisiana Department of Health, 2019). Medicaid programs are in a better position than private payers to avoid regulatory pitfalls, so they may present a potential test bed for novel payment mechanisms.

Finally, while this issue is not unique to curative therapies, prior authorization rules for new therapies might become a barrier to patient access, particularly if there is no published evidence of value. Prior authorization rules require physicians or hospitals to submit formal requests to payers before providing certain treatments (AMCP, 2012). This tool is implemented as a cost-cutting strategy; in principle, it limits an expensive treatment to patients deemed genuinely in need. However, in a recent survey of physicians by the American Medical Association, 47 percent of respondents reported that prior authorization, when required, often or always delayed access to necessary treatments; 91 percent reported that it significantly or somewhat negatively affected patient clinical outcomes, and 28 percent reported that it led to a serious adverse event (e.g., death, hospitalization, disability/permanent bodily damage, or other life-threatening event) (AMA, 2018). Prior authorization becomes more likely when the case for value is weaker; it is a tool for limiting use rather than allocating treatment to patients likely to receive demonstrable higher value from it.

Innovative Payment Models for Curative or High-Cost Therapies

The examples above touch on a few of the numerous possible alternative payment mechanisms for curative therapies.

Annuity-style payment models allow health plans to spread out payments for treatments over time through installments up to a contractual ceiling (Carr and Bradshaw, 2016). Annuity-style payments suit treatments that provide value for money but have exceptionally high budget impacts because of large patient populations or high up-front costs. Annuity models can also be tied to outcomes, as in the thalassemia example above. Performance-based risk-sharing (PBRS) agreements have been around since the early 2000s (Carlson et al., 2017). PBRS agreements tie payments to the real-world performance of the annuity model. Because payers and manufacturers share the risk, PBRS agreements provide a means for addressing uncertainty about long-term therapeutic benefits or side effects. A study by Carlson et al. (2017) identified around 62 PBRS agreements in the United States between 1993 and 2016, of which 68 percent were active or presumed active in 2016: 47 percent were for pharmaceutical products, 34 percent for devices, and 19 percent for diagnostics. PBRS agreements do require a clinical endpoint that can be measured in real-world data; pain crises might be one example, although a wider range of options would help facilitate outcomes-based pricing in different treatment contexts.

Another example, which has been used in solid organ and stem cell transplantation, is reinsurance (Slocomb and Werner, 2017). The health plan can enter into a financial arrangement—with either a manufacturer or third-party reinsurer—to cap total spending at some agreed-upon maximum. Reinsurance from a manufacturer simply caps spending at an agreed-upon level. Third-party reinsurance offloads spending above the threshold to the third party.

A related alternative is risk pooling. Under this scheme, payers would pay a certain share of their beneficiaries' premiums into a fund devoted to high-cost therapies (Slocomb and Werner, 2017). If therapy costs exceed a prespecified threshold, the payer would receive compensatory funds from the pool. The pool could be administered by a nonprofit third party, the government, or the reinsurer, and it could be supported partially by the government to ensure patient access to high-cost treatments.

Enabling Innovative Contracting Arrangements

While there are a handful of innovative payment models, the idea remains nascent in the U.S. marketplace. New data—and policy and regulatory reforms—could help accelerate adoption.

As noted above, real-world data on effectiveness can insure payers against nonresponse or declining effectiveness over time. This requires identifying measurable endpoints that reflect patient well-being as comprehensively as possible.

Manufacturers have also shown some hesitation to enter into novel payment mechanisms due to Medicaid's "best-price rule" (Sachs et al., 2018), under which Medicaid is legally entitled to pay the lowest price observed in the entire national marketplace for a drug. The implications for outcomes-based pricing remain slightly hazy. For example, with a contract that offers a full refund to a payer for a therapy that fails to work, if that refund is triggered for one patient in the plan, would that immediately entitle Medicaid to a price of zero? CMS could clarify the issue without congressional action. The Medicaid best-price statute does not specify the unit of analysis for a best-price calculation, that is, it does not stipulate whether the price paid for an individual patient or dose serves as a possible "best price." Thus, for an outcomes-based contract, CMS could specify that the best price should be calculated as the weighted average of the prices the manufacturer receives (Sachs et al., 2018).

Clarity concerning the Anti-Kickback Statute, which bars manufacturers from offering federal health care programs anything of value in an attempt to induce the purchase of a therapy (HEAT, n.d.), would also help in the case of Medicaid and Medicare payments. In principle, an outcomes-based rebate to Medicaid or Medicare might be construed as a kickback. Survey evidence shows that 57 percent of payers and 83 percent of manu-facturers viewed clarifying the Anti-Kickback Statute as a high-impact, urgent need (Duhig et al., 2018).

Finally, annuity-style payment models might be hampered by the short duration of insurance contracts. SCD cures may have benefits that last for, say, 30 years. A natural response would be to spread payments out over this entire timeframe to mitigate the budget impact as much as possible. However, 17 percent of insurance beneficiaries switch their plan each year (Cunningham and Kohn, 2000). It is not entirely clear how to deal with an annuity payment obligation after a patient switches insurers. One solu-tion would be to facilitate longer-term insurance contracts, but that would require far-reaching changes to the U.S. health insurance system (Bhattacha-rya et al., 2013). Another sweeping reform would be to create a system in which obligations can be transferred from one payer to another. Basu (2015) has proposed that payers receive a valuable tradable asset when they pay for a curative therapy. The value of this asset would reflect the total value of the cure to Medicare and Medicaid. This effectively rewards the payer for some or all of the benefits of the cure that accrue after the beneficiary enters public health insurance. It also enables the government to compensate commercial payers for some of the benefits that commercial payers are providing to public insurers.

Creating incentives for long-term health investments ought to be viewed as an important, long-term goal of health policy, but it must be supplemented with practical short-term steps as well. Existing examples suggest that shortening the annuity payout period may be a simpler, albeit less comprehensive, solution in the short term.

CONCLUSIONS AND RECOMMENDATIONS

Conclusion 7-1: For many African Americans (the predominant population group affected by SCD), efforts to advance medical science are still marred by historical exploitation. Yet, many are also willing to participate in clinical trials, and, somewhat paradoxically, there is evidence that recruitment efforts lag for this population. Researchers must be especially vigilant in their adherence to standards and practices in the consent and participation of those with SCD in research. Recruitment efforts for trials need to be equitable, including the use of community-based organizations to recruit and support participants. Communication with potential participants should be geared toward clarity and education, and, over the long term, research results should be conveyed to participants whether the trial has been successful or not. This is especially warranted as new therapies (e.g., genetic modification, stem cell transplant) become widely available to treat and potentially cure those with SCD.

Conclusion 7-2: Many new disease-modifying drugs for SCD will become available in the next decades. Biomarkers are needed to predict response, prioritize certain treatments over others, and guide combination therapy. Comparative effectiveness research is needed to guide health care/insurance coverage policies, particularly for very expensive biological agents.

Conclusion 7-3: Allogeneic transplant from a sibling-matched donor carries limited toxicity and a high success rate. When HLA-matched siblings are available, stem cell transplant should be discussed and offered in early childhood, before complications have arisen. As new drugs that may obviate the need for curative treatment become available, biomarker-based decision trees are urgently needed to determine the appropriate timing and suitability of stem cell transplant. Additionally, there is a need for research on the impact of stem cell transplantation on organ dysfunction in adults.

Conclusion 7-4: Stem cell transplant carries a high psychosocial impact. Holistic care that addresses the psychological, economic, social, and spiritual impact of transplantation is critical and should become the standard of care from the pre-transplantation period to the post-transplant long-term follow-up stage.

Conclusion 7-5: Gene therapy advances and clinical trials are proceeding at a fast pace. Education and patient-facing materials on the risks and benefits of gene therapy are urgently needed, as is research to elucidate the long-term implications of gene therapy.

Conclusion 7-6: The current delivery and payment system could serve as an impediment to diffusion of and access to therapeutic innovations. There is a need for delivery system and payment reforms, including training of SCD specialists to facilitate the diffusion of new, curative, and other SCD therapies.

Recommendation 7-1: The Centers for Medicare & Medicaid Services in collaboration with private payers should identify approaches to financing the up-front costs of curative therapies.

Recommendation 7-2: The U.S. Department of Health and Human Services should encourage and reimburse the practice of shared decision making and the development of decision aids for novel, high-risk, potentially highly effective therapies for individuals living with sickle cell disease.

Recommendation 7-3: The National Institutes of Health, U.S. Food and Drug Administration, pharmaceutical industry, and research community should establish an organized, systematic approach to encourage participation in clinical trials by including affected individuals in the design of trials, working with community-based organizations to disseminate information and recruit participants, and conducting other targeted activities.

REFERENCES

AAP (American Academy of Pediatrics). 2002. The medical home. *Pediatrics* 110(1 Pt 1):184–186.

Acharya, K., C. W. Lang, and L. F. Ross. 2009. A pilot study to explore knowledge, attitudes, and beliefs about sickle cell trait and disease. *Journal of the National Medical Association* 101(11):1163–1172.

Adams, R. J. 2007. Hydroxyurea lowers TCD—and also stroke? *Blood* 110 (3):789–790.

AHRQ (Agency for Healthcare Research and Quality). n.d. *Defining the PCMH.* https://pcmh.ahrq.gov/page/defining-pcmh (accessed January 10, 2020).

Allan, D., A. R. Limbrick, P. Thomas, and M. P. Westerman. 1982. Release of spectrin-free spicules on reoxygenation of sickled erythrocytes. *Nature* 295(5850):612–613.

AMA (American Medical Association). 2018. *2018 AMA prior authorization (PA) physician survey.* https://www.ama-assn.org/system/files/2019-02/prior-auth-2018.pdf (accessed January 9, 2020).

AMCP (Academy of Managed Care Pharmacy). 2012. *Prior authorization.* http://www.amcp.org/prior_authorization (accessed April 13, 2020).

Anie, K. A., A. Steptoe, and D. H. Bevan. 2002. Sickle cell disease: Pain, coping and quality of life in a study of adults in the UK. *British Journal of Health Psychology* 7(Part 3):331–344.

Aslan, M., T. M. Ryan, B. Adler, T. M. Townes, D. A. Parks, J. A. Thompson, A. Tousson, M. T. Gladwin, R. P. Patel, M. M. Tarpey, I. Batinic-Haberle, C. R. White, and B. A. Freeman. 2001. Oxygen radical inhibition of nitric oxide-dependent vascular function in sickle cell disease. *Proceedings of the National Academy of Sciences* 98(26):15215–15220.

ASRM (American Society for Reproductive Medicine). 2013. Fertility preservation in patients undergoing gonadotoxic therapy or gonadectomy: A committee opinion. *Fertility and Sterility* 100(5):1214–1223.

Ataga, K. I., and P. C. Desai. 2018. Advances in new drug therapies for the management of sickle cell disease. *Expert Opinion on Orphan Drugs* 6(5):329–343.

Ataga, K. I., and N. S. Key. 2007. Hypercoagulability in sickle cell disease: New approaches to an old problem. *Hematology: American Society of Hematology—Education Program* 91–96.

Ataga, K. I., C. G. Moore, C. A. Hillery, S. Jones, H. C. Whinna, D. Strayhorn, C. Sohier, A. Hinderliter, L. V. Parise, and E. P. Orringer. 2008. Coagulation activation and inflammation in sickle cell disease-associated pulmonary hypertension. *Haematologica* 93(1):20–26.

Ataga, K. I., M. Reid, S. K Ballas, Z. Yasin, C. Bigelow, L. S. James, W. R. Smith, F. Galacteros, A. Kutlar, J. H. Hull, J. W. Stocker, and the ICA-17043-10 study investigators. 2011. Improvements in haemolysis and indicators of erythrocyte survival do not correlate with acute vaso-occlusive crises in patients with sickle cell disease: A Phase III randomized, placebo-controlled, double-blind study of the Gardos channel blocker senicapoc (ICA-17043). *British Journal of Haematology* 153(1):92–104.

Ataga, K. I., A. Kutlar, J. Kanter, D. Liles, R. Cancado, J. Friedrisch, T. H. Guthrie, J. Knight-Madden, O. A. Alvarez, V. R. Gordeuk, S. Gualandro, M. P. Colella, W. R. Smith, S. A. Rollins, J. W. Stocker, and R. P. Rother. 2017. Crizanlizumab for the prevention of pain crises in sickle cell disease. *New England Journal of Medicine* 376(5):429–439.

Bakshi, N., C. B. Sinha, D. Ross, K. Khemani, G. Loewenstein, and L. Krishnamurti. 2017. Proponent or collaborative: Physician perspectives and approaches to disease modifying therapies in sickle cell disease. *PLOS ONE* 12(7):e0178413.

Ballas, S. K., and E. P. Vichinsky. 2015. Is the medical home for adult patients with sickle cell disease a reality or an illusion? *Hemoglobin* 39(2):130–133.

Ballas, S. K., M. R. Kesen, M. F. Goldberg, G. A. Lutty, C. Dampier, I. Osunkwo, W. C. Wang, C. Hoppe, W. Hagar, D. S. Darbari, and P. Malik. 2012. Beyond the definitions of the phenotypic complications of sickle cell disease: An update on management. *Scientific World Journal* 2012:949535.

Basu, A. 2015. Financing cures in the United States. *Expert Review of Pharmacoeconomics and Outcomes Research* 15(1):1–4.

Belcher, J. D., C. Chen, J. Nguyen, L. Milbauer, F. Abdulla, A. I. Alayash, A. Smith, K. A. Nath, R. P. Hebbel, and G. M. Vercellotti. 2014. Heme triggers TLR4 signaling leading to endothelial cell activation and vaso-occlusion in murine sickle cell disease. *Blood* 123(3):377–390.

Bernaudin, F., G. Socie, M. Kuentz, S. Chevret, M. Duval, Y. Bertrand, J. P. Vannier, K. Yakouben, I. Thuret, P. Bordigoni, A. Fischer, P. Lutz, J. L. Stephan, N. Dhedin, E. Plouvier, G. Margueritte, D. Bories, S. Verlhac, H. Esperou, L. Coic, J. P. Vernant, E. Gluckman, and SFGM-TC. 2007. Long-term results of related myeloablative stem-cell transplantation to cure sickle cell disease. *Blood* 110(7):2749–2756.

Bernaudin, F., J. H. Dalle, D. Bories, R. Peffault de Latour, M. Robin, Y. Bertrand, C. Pondarre, J. P. Vannier, B. Neven, M. Kuentz, S. Maury, P. Lutz, C. Paillard, K. Yakouben, I. Thuret, C. Galambrun, N. Dhedin, C. Jubert, P. Rohrlich, J. O. Bay, F. Suarez, N. Raus, J. P. Vernant, E. Gluckman, C. Poirot, G. Socié, and Société Francaise de Greffe de Moelle et de Thérapie Cellulaire. 2019. Long-term event-free survival, chimerism and fertility outcomes in 234 patients with sickle-cell anemia younger than 30 years after myeloablative conditioning and matched-sibling transplantation in France. *Haematologica* 105(1):91–101.

Bhattacharya, J., A. Chandra, M. Chernew, D. Goldman, A. Jena, D. Lakdawalla, A. Malani, and T. Philipson. 2013. *Best of both worlds: Uniting universal coverage and personal choice in health care.* https://www.aei.org/wp-content/uploads/2014/09/-best-of-both-worlds-uniting-universal-coverage-and-personal-choice-in-health-care_105214167938.pdf (accessed January 9, 2020).

Blake, A., V. Asnani, R. R. Leger, J. Harris, V. Odesina, D. L. Hemmings, D. A. Morris, J. Knight-Madden, L. Wagner, and M. R. Asnani. 2018. Stigma and illness uncertainty: Adding to the burden of sickle cell disease. *Hematology* 23(2):122–130.

Bognar, K., J. A. Romley, J. P. Bae, J. Murray, J. W. Chou, and D. N. Lakdawalla. 2017. The role of imperfect surrogate endpoint information in drug approval and reimbursement decisions. *Journal of Health Economics* 51:1–12.

Bonham, V. L., C. Haywood, and V. N. Gamble. 2007. Sickle cell disease: The past, present and future social and ethical dilemmas. In B. Pace (ed.), *Renaissance of sickle cell disease research in the genome era.* London: Imperial College Press. Pp. 311–323.

Boulad, F., T. Shore, K. van Besien, C. Minniti, M. Barbu-Stevanovic, S. W. Fedus, F. Perna, J. Greenberg, D. Guarneri, V. Nandi, A. Mauguen, K. Yazdanbakhsh, M. Sadelain, and P. A. Shi. 2018. Safety and efficacy of plerixafor dose escalation for the mobilization of CD34+ hematopoietic progenitor cells in patients with sickle cell disease: Interim results. *Haematologica* 103(5):770–777.

Brodsky, R. A., L. Luznik, J. Bolanos-Meade, M. S. Leffell, R. J. Jones, and E. J. Fuchs. 2008. Reduced intensity HLA-haploidentical BMT with post transplantation cyclophosphamide in nonmalignant hematologic diseases. *Bone Marrow Transplantation* 42(8):523–527.

Brunson, A., A. Lei, A. S. Rosenberg, R. H. White, T. Keegan, and T. Wun. 2017. Increased incidence of VTE in sickle cell disease patients: Risk factors, recurrence and impact on mortality. *British Journal Haematology* 178(2):319–326.

Brunson, A., T. Keegan, A. Mahajan, R. White, and T. Wun. 2019. High incidence of venous thromboembolism recurrence in patients with sickle cell disease. *American Journal of Hematology* 94(8):862–870.

Bulgin, D., P. Tanabe, and C. Jenerette. 2018. Stigma of sickle cell disease: A systematic review. *Issues in Mental Health Nursing* 39(8):675–686.

Burke, L., J. C. Hobart, K. Fox, J. Lehrer-Graiwer, K. Bridges, M. Kraus, and E. Ramos. 2016. The 10-item sickle cell disease severity measure (SCDSM-10): A novel measure of daily SCD symptom severity developed to assess benefit of GBT440, an experimental HbS polymerization inhibitor. *Blood* 128(22):4760.

Cairo, M. S., J. A. Talano, T. B. Moore, Q. Shi, R. S. Weinberg, B. Grossman, and S. Shenoy. 2019. Familial haploidentical stem cell transplant in children and adolescents with high-risk sickle cell disease: A Phase 2 clinical trial. *JAMA Pediatrics*, December 9 [Epub ahead of print].

Cardenes, N., C. Corey, L. Geary, S. Jain, S. Zharikov, S. Barge, E. M. Novelli, and S. Shiva. 2014. Platelet bioenergetic screen in sickle cell patients reveals mitochondrial complex V inhibition, which contributes to platelet activation. *Blood* 123(18):2864–2872.

Carlson, J. J., S. Chen, and L. P. Garrison, Jr. 2017. Performance-based risk-sharing arrangements: An updated international review. *Pharmacoeconomics* 35(10):1063–1072.

Carr, D. R., and S. E. Bradshaw. 2016. Gene therapies: The challenge of super-high-cost treatments and how to pay for them. *Regenerative Medicine* 11(4):381–393.

CDC (Centers for Disease Control and Prevention). 2015. *U.S. Public Health Service syphilis study at Tuskegee: The Tuskegee timeline*. https://www.cdc.gov/tuskegee/timeline.htm (accessed August 1, 2019).

Chang, J., J. T. Patton, A. Sarkar, B. Ernst, J. L. Magnani, and P. S. Frenette. 2010. GMI-1070, a novel pan-selectin antagonist, reverses acute vascular occlusions in sickle cell mice. *Blood* 116(10):1779–1786.

Charache, S., M. L. Terrin, R. D. Moore, G. J. Dover, F. B. Barton, S. V. Eckert, R. P. McMahon, D. R. Bonds, and Investigators of the Multicenter Study of Hydroxyurea in Sickle Cell Anemia. 1995. Effect of hydroxyurea on the frequency of painful crises in sickle cell anemia. *New England Journal of Medicine* 332(20):1317–1322.

Chen, G., D. Zhang, T. A. Fuchs, D. Manwani, D. D. Wagner, and P. S. Frenette. 2014. Heme-induced neutrophil extracellular traps contribute to the pathogenesis of sickle cell disease. *Blood* 123(24):3818–3827.

Children's Hospital Los Angeles and Hope Pharmaceuticals. 2009. *Safety and efficacy of sodium nitrite in sickle cell disease*. https://clinicaltrials.gov/ct2/show/NCT01033227 (accessed January 9, 2020).

Cholongitas, E., and G. V. Papatheodoridis. 2014. Sofosbuvir: A novel oral agent for chronic hepatitis C. *Annals of Gastroenterology* 27(4):331–337.

CMS (Centers for Medicare & Medicaid Services). 2019. *Accountable care organizations (ACOs): General information*. https://innovation.cms.gov/initiatives/aco (accessed January 9, 2020).

Crary, S. E., and G. R. Buchanan. 2009. Vascular complications after splenectomy for hematologic disorders. *Blood* 114(14):2861–2868.

Crosby, L. E., L. M. Shook, R. E. Ware, and W. B. Brinkman. 2015. Shared decision making for hydroxyurea treatment initiation in children with sickle cell anemia. *Pediatric Blood & Cancer* 62(2):184–185.

Cunningham, P. J., and L. Kohn. 2000. Health plan switching: Choice or circumstance? *Health Affairs* 19(3):158–164.

Cunningham-Myrie, C., A. Abdulkadri, A. Waugh, S. Bortolusso Ali, L. G. King, J. Knight-Madden, and M. Reid. 2015. Hydroxyurea use in prevention of stroke recurrence in children with sickle cell disease in a developing country: A cost effectiveness analysis. *Pediatric Blood & Cancer* 62(10):1862–1864.

CVSHealth. 2018. *Current and new approaches to making drugs more affordable.* https://cvshealth.com/sites/default/files/cvs-health-current-and-new-approaches-to-making-drugs-more-affordable.pdf (accessed January 9, 2020).

Dallas, M. H., B. Triplett, D. R. Shook, C. Hartford, A. Srinivasan, J. Laver, R. Ware, and W. Leung. 2013. Long-term outcome and evaluation of organ function in pediatric patients undergoing haploidentical and matched related hematopoietic cell transplantation for sickle cell disease. *Biology of Blood and Marrow Transplantation* 19(5):820–830.

Dampier, C., J. Kanter, R. Howard, I. Agoda, S. Wade, V. Noxon, and S. K. Ballas. 2017. Access to care for Medicaid and commercially-insured United States patients with sickle cell disease. *Blood* 130(Suppl 1):4660.

Darbari, D. S., J. Liljencrantz, A. Ikechi, S. Martin, M. C. Roderick, C. D. Fitzhugh, J. F. Tisdale, S. L. Thein, and M. Hsieh. 2019. Pain and opioid use after reversal of sickle cell disease following HLA-matched sibling haematopoietic stem cell transplant. *British Journal of Haematology* 184(4):690–693.

De Franceschi, L., M. D. Cappellini, and O. Olivieri. 2011. Thrombosis and sickle cell disease. *Seminars in Thrombosis and Hemostasis* 37(3):226–236.

de la Fuente, J., N. Dhedin, T. Koyama, F. Bernaudin, L. Kuentz, L. Karnik, G. Socie, K. A. Culos, R. A. Brodsky, M. R. DeBaun, and A. A. Kassim. 2019. Haploidentical bone marrow transplantation with post-transplantation cyclophosphamide plus thiotepa improves donor engraftment in patients with sickle cell anemia: Results of an international learning collaborative. *Biology of Blood and Marrow Transplantation* 25(6):1197–1209.

Demirci S., A. Leonard, J. J. Haro-Mora, N. Uchida, and J. F. Tisdale. 2019. CRISPR/Cas9 for sickle cell disease: Applications, future possibilities, and challenges. *Advances in Experimental Medicine and Biology* 1144:37–52.

Do, A., Y. Mittal, A. Liapakis, E. Cohen, H. Chau, C. Bertuccio, D. Sapir, J. Wright, C. Eggers, K. Drozd, M. Ciarleglio, Y. Deng, and J. K. Lim. 2015. Drug authorization for sofosbuvir/ledipasvir (Harvoni) for chronic HCV infection in a real-world cohort: A new barrier in the HCV care cascade. *PLOS ONE* 10(8):e0135645.

Du, M., S. Van Ness, V. Gordeuk, S. M. Nouraie, S. Nekhai, M. Gladwin, M. H. Steinberg, and P. Sebastiani. 2018. Biomarker signatures of sickle cell disease severity. *Blood Cells, Molecules, and Diseases* 72(Suppl 1):1–9.

Duhig, A. M., S. Saha, S. Smith, S. Kaufman, and J. Hughes. 2018. The current status of outcomes-based contracting for manufacturers and payers: An AMCP membership survey. *Journal of Managed Care and Specialty Pharmacy* 24(5):410–415.

Dutra, F. F., L. S. Alves, D. Rodrigues, P. L. Fernandez, R. B. de Oliveira, D. T. Golenbock, D. S. Zamboni, and M. T. Bozza. 2014. Hemolysis-induced lethality involves inflammasome activation by heme. *Proceedings of the National Academy of Sciences* 111(39):E4110–E4118.

Eapen, M., R. Brazauskas, M. C. Walters, F. Bernaudin, K. Bo-Subait, C. D. Fitzhugh, J. S. Hankins, J. Kanter, J. J. Meerpohl, J. Bolanos-Meade, J. A. Panepinto, D. Rondelli, S. Shenoy, J. Williamson, T. L. Woolford, E. Gluckman, J. E. Wagner, and J. F. Tisdale. 2019. Effect of donor type and conditioning regimen intensity on allogeneic transplantation outcomes in patients with sickle cell disease: A retrospective multicentre, cohort study. *Lancet Haematology* 6(11):e585–e596.

Esrick, E. B., J. P. Manis, H. Daley, C. Baricordi, H. Trebeden-Negre, F. J. Pierciey, M. Armant, S. Nikiforow, M. M. Heeney, W. B. London, L. Biasco, M. Asmal, D. A. Williams, and A. Biffi. 2018. Successful hematopoietic stem cell mobilization and apheresis collection using plerixafor alone in sickle cell patients. *Blood Advances* 2(19):2505–2512.

Estepp, J. H. 2018. Voxelotor (GBT440), a first-in-class hemoglobin oxygen-affinity modulator, has promising and reassuring preclinical and clinical data. *American Journal of Hematology* 93(3):326–329.

Evitt, N. H., S. Mascharak, and R. B. Altman. 2015. Human germline CRISPR-Cas modification: Toward a regulatory framework. *American Journal of Bioethics* 15(12):25–29.

Farrell, A. T., J. Panepinto, C. P. Carroll, D. S. Darbari, A. A. Desai, A. A. King, R. J. Adams, T. D. Barber, A. M. Brandow, M. R. DeBaun, M. J. Donahue, K. Gupta, J. S. Hankins, M. Kameka, F. J. Kirkham, H. Luksenburg, S. Miller, P. A. Oneal, D. C. Rees, R. Setse, V. A. Sheehan, J. Strouse, C. L. Stucky, E. M. Werner, J. C. Wood, and W. T. Zempsky. 2019. End points for sickle cell disease clinical trials: Patient-reported outcomes, pain, and the brain. *Blood Advances* 3(23):3982–4001.

FDA (U.S. Food and Drug Administration). 2017. *FDA approved L-glutamine powder for the treatment of sickle cell disease.* https://www.fda.gov/drugs/resources-information-approved-drugs/fda-approved-l-glutamine-powder-treatment-sickle-cell-disease (accessed January 9, 2020).

FDA. 2019. *FDA approves crizanlizumab-tmca for sickle cell disease.* https://www.fda.gov/drugs/resources-information-approved-drugs/fda-approves-crizanlizumab-tmca-sickle-cell-disease (accessed January 9, 2020).

Field, J. J., E. Majerus, V. R. Gordeuk, M. Gowhari, C. Hoppe, M. M. Heeney, M. Achebe, A. George, H. Chu, B. Sheehan, M. Puligandla, D. Neuberg, G. Lin, J. Linden, and D. G. Nathan. 2017. Randomized Phase 2 trial of regadenoson for treatment of acute vaso-occlusive crises in sickle cell disease. *Blood Advances* 1(20):1645–1649.

Franck, P. F., E. M. Bevers, B. H. Lubin, P. Comfurius, D. T. Chiu, J. A. Op den Kamp, R. F. Zwaal, L. L. van Deenen, and B. Roelofsen. 1985. Uncoupling of the membrane skeleton from the lipid bilayer. The cause of accelerated phospholipid flip-flop leading to an enhanced procoagulant activity of sickled cells. *Journal of Clinical Investigation* 75(1):183–190.

George, A., S. Pushkaran, D. G. Konstantinidis, S. Koochaki, P. Malik, N. Mohandas, Y. Zheng, C. H. Joiner, and T. A. Kalfa. 2013. Erythrocyte NADPH oxidase activity modulated by Rac GTPases, PKC, and plasma cytokines contributes to oxidative stress in sickle cell disease. *Blood* 121(11):2099–2107.

Gilman, A. L., M. J. Eckrich, S. Epstein, C. Barnhart, M. Cannon, T. Fukes, M. Hyland, K. Shah, D. Grochowski, E. Champion, and A. Ivanova. 2017. Alternative donor hematopoietic stem cell transplantation for sickle cell disease. *Blood Advances* 1(16):1215–1223.

Gladwin, M. T., V. Sachdev, M. L. Jison, Y. Shizukuda, J. F. Plehn, K. Minter, B. Brown, W. A. Coles, J. S. Nichols, I. Ernst, L. A. Hunter, W. C. Blackwelder, A. N. Schechter, G. P. Rodgers, O. Castro, and F. P. Ognibene. 2004. Pulmonary hypertension as a risk factor for death in patients with sickle cell disease. *New England Journal of Medicine* 350(9):886–895.

Gladwin, M. T., G. J. Kato, D. Weiner, O. C. Onyekwere, C. Dampier, L. Hsu, R. W. Hagar, T. Howard, R. Nuss, M. M. Okam, C. K. Tremonti, B. Berman, A. Villella, L. Krishnamurti, S. Lanzkron, O. Castro, V. R. Gordeuk, W. A. Coles, M. Peters-Lawrence, J. Nichols, M. K. Hall, M. Hildesheim, W. C. Blackwelder, J. Baldassarre, J. F. Casella, and N. I. De. 2011. Nitric oxide for inhalation in the acute treatment of sickle cell pain crisis: A randomized controlled trial. *JAMA* 305(9):893–902.

Gluckman, E., B. Cappelli, F. Bernaudin, M. Labopin, F. Volt, J. Carreras, B. Pinto Simoes, A. Ferster, S. Dupont, J. de la Fuente, J. H. Dalle, M. Zecca, M. C. Walters, L. Krishnamurti, M. Bhatia, K. Leung, G. Yanik, J. Kurtzberg, N. Dhedin, M. Kuentz, G. Michel, J. Apperley, P. Lutz, B. Neven, Y. Bertrand, J. P. Vannier, M. Ayas, M. Cavazzana, S. Matthes-Martin, V. Rocha, H. Elayoubi, C. Kenzey, P. Bader, F. Locatelli, A. Ruggeri, and M. Eapen. 2017. Sickle cell disease: An international survey of results of HLA-identical sibling hematopoietic stem cell transplantation. *Blood* 129(11):1548–1556.

Gragert, L., M. Eapen, E. Williams, J. Freeman, S. Spellman, R. Baitty, R. Hartzman, J. D. Rizzo, M. Horowitz, D. Confer, and M. Maiers. 2014. HLA match likelihoods for hematopoietic stem-cell grafts in the U.S. registry. *New England Journal of Medicine* 371(4):339–348.

Green, N. S., M. Bhatia, E. Y. Griffith, M. Qureshi, C. Briamonte, M. Savone, S. Sands, M. T. Lee, A. Lignelli, and A. M. Brickman. 2017. Enhanced long-term brain magnetic resonance imaging evaluation of children with sickle cell disease after hematopoietic cell transplantation. *Biology of Blood and Marrow Transplantation* 23(4):670–676.

Griffin, T. C., D. McIntire, and G. R. Buchanan. 1994. High-dose intravenous methylprednisolone therapy for pain in children and adolescents with sickle cell disease. *New England Journal of Medicine* 330(11):733–737.

Halsey, C., and I. A. Roberts. 2003. The role of hydroxyurea in sickle cell disease. *British Journal of Haematology* 120(2):177–186.

Han, J., S. L. Saraf, R. E. Molokie, and V. R. Gordeuk. 2019. Use of metformin in patients with sickle cell disease. *American Journal of Hematology* 94(1):E13–E15.

Haywood, C., Jr., M. C. Beach, S. Bediako, C. P. Carroll, L. Lattimer, D. Jarrett, and S. Lanzkron. 2011. Examining the characteristics and beliefs of hydroxyurea users and nonusers among adults with sickle cell disease. *American Journal of Hematology* 86(1):85–87.

Haywood, C., Jr., S. Lanzkron, S. Bediako, J. J. Strouse, J. Haythornthwaite, C. P. Carroll, M. Diener-West, G. Onojobi, M. C. Beach, and the IMPORT Investigators. 2014. Perceived discrimination, patient trust, and adherence to medical recommendations among persons with sickle cell disease. *Journal of General Internal Medicine* 29(12):1657–1662.

HEAT (Health Care Fraud Prevention and Enforcement Action Team). n.d. *Comparison of the Anti-Kickback Statute and Stark Law.* https://oig.hhs.gov/compliance/provider-compliance-training/files/starkandakscharthandout508.pdf (accessed Januay 9, 2020).

Heeney, M. M., C. C. Hoppe, M. R. Abboud, B. Inusa, J. Kanter, B. Ogutu, P. B. Brown, L. E. Heath, J. A. Jakubowski, C. Zhou, D. Zamoryakhin, T. Agbenyega, R. Colombatti, H. M. Hassab, V. N. Nduba, J. N. Oyieko, N. Robitaille, C. I. Segbefia, and D. C. Rees. 2016. A multinational trial of prasugrel for sickle cell vaso-occlusive events. *New England Journal of Medicine* 374(7):625–635.

Henry, B. 2018. Drug pricing & challenges to hepatitis C treatment access. *Journal of Health and Biomed Law* 14:265–283.

Hirschler, B. 2014. UK cost body backs pricey Gilead hepatitis pill for some patients. *Reuters*, August 14. https://www.reuters.com/article/uk-health-hepatitis-gilead-sciences/uk-cost-body-backs-pricey-gilead-hepatitis-pill-for-some-patients-idUKKBN0GF05P20140815 (accessed April 15, 2020).

Horwitz, M. E., N. J. Chao, D. A. Rizzieri, G. D. Long, K. M. Sullivan, C. Gasparetto, J. P. Chute, A. Morris, C. McDonald, B. Waters-Pick, P. Stiff, S. Wease, A. Peled, D. Snyder, E. G. Cohen, H. Shoham, E. Landau, E. Friend, I. Peleg, D. Aschengrau, D. Yackoubov, J. Kurtzberg, and T. Peled. 2014. Umbilical cord blood expansion with nicotinamide provides long-term multilineage engraftment. *Journal of Clinical Investigation* 124(7):3121–3128.

Hsieh, M. M., and J. F. Tisdale. 2018. Hematopoietic stem cell mobilization with plerixafor in sickle cell disease. *Haematologica* 103(5):749–750.

Hsieh, M. M., E. M. Kang, C. D. Fitzhugh, M. B. Link, C. D. Bolan, R. Kurlander, R. W. Childs, G. P. Rodgers, J. D. Powell, and J. F. Tisdale. 2009. Allogeneic hematopoietic stem-cell transplantation for sickle cell disease. *New England Journal of Medicine* 361(24):2309–2317.

Hsieh, M. M., C. D. Fitzhugh, R. P. Weitzel, M. E. Link, W. A. Coles, X. Zhao, G. P. Rodgers, J. D. Powell, and J. F. Tisdale. 2014. Nonmyeloablative HLA-matched sibling allogeneic hematopoietic stem cell transplantation for severe sickle cell phenotype. *JAMA* 312(1):48–56.

ICER (Institute for Clinical and Economic Review). 2015. *New lower prices for Gilead hepatitis C drugs reach CTAF threshold for high health system value.* https://icer-review.org/announcements/new-lower-prices-for-gilead-hepatitis-c-drugs-reach-ctaf-threshold-for-high-health-system-value (accessed January 10, 2020).

ICON. 2018. *Industry perceptions and expectations: The role of ICER as an independent HTA organisation.* https://www.iconplc.com/insights/value-based-healthcare/the-role-of-icer-as-an-independent-hta-organisation (accessed January 10, 2020).

Jinek, M., K. Chylinski, I. Fonfara, M. Hauer, J. A. Doudna, and E. Charpentier. 2012. A programmable dual-RNA-guided DNA endonuclease in adaptive bacterial immunity. *Science* 337(6096):816–821.

Jonassaint, C. R., C. Kang, D. M. Abrams, J. J. Li, J. Mao, Y. Jia, Q. Long, M. Sanger, J. C. Jonassaint, L. De Castro, and N. Shah. 2018a. Understanding patterns and correlates of daily pain using the Sickle Cell Disease Mobile Application to Record Symptoms via Technology (SMART). *British Journal of Haematology* 183(2):306–308.

Jonassaint, C. R., N. Rao, A. Sciuto, G. E. Switzer, L. De Castro, G. J. Kato, J. C. Jonassaint, Z. Hammal, N. Shah, and A. Wasan. 2018b. Abstract animations for the communication and assessment of pain in adults: Cross-sectional feasibility study. *Journal of Medical Internet Research* 20(8):e10056.

Joseph, L., S. Manceau, C. Pondarré, A. Habibi, F. Bernaudin, S. Allali, M. De Montalembert, C. Chalas, J. B. Arlet, C. Jean, and V. Brousse. 2019. Effect of hydroxyurea exposure before puberty on sperm parameters in males with sickle cell disease. *Blood* 134(Suppl 1):889.

Joshi, S., B. N. Savani, E. J. Chow, M. H. Gilleece, J. Halter, D. A. Jacobsohn, J. Pidala, G. P. Quinn, J. Y. Cahn, A. A. Jakubowski, N. R. Kamani, H. M. Lazarus, J. D. Rizzo, H. C. Schouten, G. Socie, P. Stratton, M. L. Sorror, A. B. Warwick, J. R. Wingard, A. W. Loren, and N. S. Majhail. 2014. Clinical guide to fertility preservation in hematopoietic cell transplant recipients. *Bone Marrow Transplant* 49(4):477–484.

Kalpatthi, R., and E. M. Novelli. 2018. Measuring success: Utility of biomarkers in sickle cell disease clinical trials and care. *Hematology: American Society of Hematology—Education Program* 2018(1):482–492.

Kamani, N. R., M. C. Walters, S. Carter, V. Aquino, J. A. Brochstein, S. Chaudhury, M. Eapen, B. M. Freed, M. Grimley, J. E. Levine, B. Logan, T. Moore, J. Panepinto, S. Parikh, M. A. Pulsipher, J. Sande, K. R. Schultz, S. Spellman, and S. Shenoy. 2012. Unrelated donor cord blood transplantation for children with severe sickle cell disease: Results of one cohort from the Phase II study from the blood and marrow transplant clinical trials network (BMT CTN). *Biology of Blood Marrow Transplantation* 18(8):1265–1272.

Kanter, J., M. C. Walters, M. Hsieh, L. Krishnamurti, J. L. Kwiatkowski, R. Kamble, C. von Kalle, M. Joseney-Antoine, F. J. Pierciey, W. Shi, M. Asmal, A. A. Thompson, and J. F. Tisdale. 2017. Interim results from a Phase 1/2 clinical study of lentiglobin gene therapy for severe sickle cell disease. *Blood* 130(Suppl 1):527.

Kanter, J., A. Thompson, M. Mapara, J. Kwiatkowski, L. Krishnamurti, M. Schmidt, A. Miller, F. Pierciey, W. Huang, J. Ribeil, M. Walters, and J. Tisdale. 2019. Updated results from the HGB-206 study in patients with severe sickle cell disease treated under a revised protocol with lentiglobin gene therapy using plerixafor-mobilised haematopoietic stem cells. *HemaSphere* 3(S1):754–755.

Kapoor, S., J. A. Little, and L. H. Pecker. 2018. Advances in the treatment of sickle cell disease. *Mayo Clinic Proceedings* 93(12):1810–1824.

Karafin, M. S., G. Chen, N. J. Wandersee, A. M. Brandow, R. W. Hurley, P. Simpson, D. Ward, S. J. Li, and J. J. Field. 2019. Chronic pain in adults with sickle cell disease is associated with alterations in functional connectivity of the brain. *PLOS ONE* 14(5):e0216994.

Karnilowicz, W. 2011. Identity and psychological ownership in chronic illness and disease state. *European Journal of Cancer Care (Engl)* 20(2):276–282.

Kassim, A. A., and D. Sharma. 2017. Hematopoietic stem cell transplantation for sickle cell disease: The changing landscape. *Hematology/Oncology Stem Cell Therapy* 10(4):259–266.

Kato, G. 2015. *A multi-center study of riociguat in patients with sickle cell diseases.* https://clinicaltrials.gov/ct2/show/NCT02633397 (accessed January 10, 2020).

Kauf, T. L., T. D. Coates, L. Huazhi, N. Mody-Patel, and A. G. Hartzema. 2009. The cost of health care for children and adults with sickle cell disease. *American Journal of Hematology* 84(6):323–327.

Kaul, D. K., and R. P. Hebbel. 2000. Hypoxia/reoxygenation causes inflammatory response in transgenic sickle mice but not in normal mice. *Journal of Clinical Investigation* 106(3):411–420.

Kaul, D. K., X. D. Liu, M. E. Fabry, and R. L. Nagel. 2000. Impaired nitric oxide-mediated vasodilation in transgenic sickle mouse. *American Journal of Physiology Heart and Circulatory Physiology* 278(6):H1799–H1806.

Khemani, K., D. Ross, C. Sinha, A. Haight, N. Bakshi, and L. Krishnamurti. 2018. Experiences and decision making in hematopoietic stem cell transplant in sickle cell disease: Patients' and caregivers' perspectives. *Biology of Blood and Marrow Transplantation* 24(5):1041–1048.

Kutlar, A., M. E. Reid, A. Inati, A. T. Taher, M. R. Abboud, A. El-Beshlawy, G. R. Buchanan, H. Smith, K. I. Ataga, S. P. Perrine, and R. G. Ghalie. 2013. A dose-escalation Phase IIa study of 2,2-dimethylbutyrate (HQK-1001), an oral fetal globin inducer, in sickle cell disease. *American Journal of Hematology* 88(11):E255–E260.

Kutlar, A., J. Kanter, D. K. Liles, O. A. Alvarez, R. D. Cancado, J. R. Friedrisch, J. M. Knight-Madden, A. Bruederle, M. Shi, Z. Zhu, and K. I. Ataga. 2019. Effect of crizanlizumab on pain crises in subgroups of patients with sickle cell disease: A SUSTAIN study analysis. *American Journal of Hematolgy* 94(1):55–61.

Lagresle-Peyrou, C., F. Lefrere, E. Magrin, J. A. Ribeil, O. Romano, L. Weber, A. Magnani, H. Sadek, C. Plantier, A. Gabrion, B. Ternaux, T. Felix, C. Couzin, A. Stanislas, J. M. Treluyer, L. Lamhaut, L. Joseph, M. Delville, A. Miccio, I. Andre-Schmutz, and M. Cavazzana. 2018. Plerixafor enables safe, rapid, efficient mobilization of hematopoietic stem cells in sickle cell disease patients after exchange transfusion. *Haematologica* 103(5):778–786.

Lakdawalla, D. N., J. A. Doshi, L. P. Garrison, C. E. Phelps, A. Basu, and P. M. Danzon. 2018. Defining elements of value in health care—A health economics approach: An ISPOR special task force report. *Value in Health* 21(2):131–139.

Lebensburger, J. D., R. F. Sidonio, M. R. Debaun, M. M. Safford, T. H. Howard, and I. C. Scarinci. 2013. Exploring barriers and facilitators to clinical trial enrollment in the context of sickle cell anemia and hydroxyurea. *Pediatric Blood & Cancer* 60(8):1333–1337.

Lebensburger, J. D., L. M. Hilliard, L. E. Pair, R. Oster, T. H. Howard, and G. R. Cutter. 2015. Systematic review of interventional sickle cell trials registered in clinicaltrials.Gov. *Clinical Trials (London, England)* 12(6):575–583.

Liem, R. I., A. H. Cole, S. A. Pelligra, M. Mason, and A. A. Thompson. 2010. Parental attitudes toward research participation in pediatric sickle cell disease. *Pediatric Blood & Cancer* 55(1):129–133.

Limerick, E., and C. Fitzhugh. 2019. Choice of donor source and conditioning regimen for hematopoietic stem cell transplantation in sickle cell disease. *Journal of Clinical Medicine* 8(11):1997.

Long, K. A., S. B. Thomas, R. E. Grubs, E. A. Gettig, and L. Krishnamurti. 2011. Attitudes and beliefs of African-Americans toward genetics, genetic testing, and sickle cell disease education and awareness. *Journal of Genetic Counseling* 20(6):572–592.

Loren, A. W., E. Chow, D. A. Jacobsohn, M. Gilleece, J. Halter, S. Joshi, Z. Wang, K. A. Sobocinski, V. Gupta, G. A. Hale, D. I. Marks, E. A. Stadtmauer, J. Apperley, J. Y. Cahn, H. C. Schouten, H. M. Lazarus, B. N. Savani, P. L. McCarthy, A. A. Jakubowski, N. R. Kamani, B. Hayes-Lattin, R. T. Maziarz, A. B. Warwick, M. L. Sorror, B. J. Bolwell, G. Socie, J. R. Wingard, J. D. Rizzo, and N. S. Majhail. 2011. Pregnancy after hematopoietic cell transplantation: A report from the Late Effects Working Committee of the Center for International Blood and Marrow Transplant Research (CIBMTR). *Biology of Blood and Marrow Transplantation* 17(2):157–166.

Louisiana Department of Health. 2019. *Department of Health receives three proposals for hepatitis C payment model.* http://ldh.la.gov/index.cfm/newsroom/detail/5072 (accessed January 13, 2020).

Machado, R. F., R. J. Barst, N. A. Yovetich, K. L. Hassell, G. J. Kato, V. R. Gordeuk, J. S. R. Gibbs, J. A. Little, D. E. Schraufnagel, L. Krishnamurti, R. E. Girgis, C. R. Morris, E. B. Rosenzweig, D. B. Badesch, S. Lanzkron, O. Onyekwere, O. L. Castro, V. Sachdev, M. A. Waclawiw, R. Woolson, J. C. Goldsmith, M. T. Gladwin, and walk-PHaSST Investigators and Patients. 2011. Hospitalization for pain in patients with sickle cell disease treated with sildenafil for elevated TRV and low exercise capacity. *Blood* 118(4):855–864.

Malik, P., M. Grimley, C. T. Quinn, A. Shova, L. Courtney, C. Lutzko, T. A. Kalfa, O. Niss, P. A. Mehta, S. Chandra, E. Grassman, J. C. M. Van der Loo, S. Witting, D. Nordling, A. Shreshta, S. Felker, C. Terrell, L. Reeves, D. Pillis, L. Anastacia, F. D. Bushman, J. Knight-Madden, K. Kalinyak, S. M. Davies, and M. Asnani. 2018. Gene therapy for sickle cell anemia using a modified gamma globin lentivirus vector and reduced intensity conditioning transplant shows promising correction of the disease phenotype. *Blood* 132(Suppl 1):1021.

Matte, A., F. Zorzi, F. Mazzi, E. Federti, O. Olivieri, and L. De Franceschi. 2019. New therapeutic options for the treatment of sickle cell disease. *Mediterranean Journal of Hematology and Infectious Diseases* 11(1):e2019002.

McClish, D. K., W. R. Smith, J. L. Levenson, I. P. Aisiku, J. D. Roberts, S. D. Roseff, and V. E. Bovbjerg. 2017. Comorbidity, pain, utilization, and psychosocial outcomes in older versus younger sickle cell adults: The PiSCES project. *Biomed Research International* 2017:4070547.

McGann, P. T., and R. E. Ware. 2015. Hydroxyurea therapy for sickle cell anemia. *Expert Opinion on Drug Safety* 14(11):1749–1758.

McGann, P. T., S. D. Grosse, B. Santos, V. de Oliveira, L. Bernardino, N. J. Kassebaum, R. E. Ware, and G. E. Airewele. 2015. A cost-effectiveness analysis of a pilot neonatal screening program for sickle cell anemia in the Republic of Angola. *Journal of Pediatrics* 167(6):1314–1319.

Michaelis, M. C. 2019. The Sickle Cell Clinical Trials Network: One year in. *The Hematologist* 16(4):1.

Minneci, P. C., K. J. Deans, H. Zhi, P. S. Yuen, R. A. Star, S. M. Banks, A. N. Schechter, C. Natanson, M. T. Gladwin, and S. B. Solomon. 2005. Hemolysis-associated endothelial dysfunction mediated by accelerated NO inactivation by decompartmentalized oxyhemoglobin. *Journal of Clinical Investigation* 115(12):3409–3417.

Molokie, R., D. Lavelle, M. Gowhari, M. Pacini, L. Krauz, J. Hassan, V. Ibanez, M. A. Ruiz, K. P. Ng, P. Woost, T. Radivoyevitch, D. Pacelli, S. Fada, M. Rump, M. Hsieh, J. F. Tisdale, J. Jacobberger, M. Phelps, J. D. Engel, S. Saraf, L. L. Hsu, V. Gordeuk, J. DeSimone, and Y. Saunthararajah. 2017. Oral tetrahydrouridine and decitabine for noncytotoxic epigenetic gene regulation in sickle cell disease: A randomized Phase 1 study. *PLOS Medicine* 14(9):e1002382.

Morris, C. R., F. A. Kuypers, L. Lavrisha, M. Ansari, N. Sweeters, M. Stewart, G. Gildengorin, L. Neumayr, and E. P. Vichinsky. 2013. A randomized, placebo-controlled trial of arginine therapy for the treatment of children with sickle cell disease hospitalized with vaso-occlusive pain episodes. *Haematologica* 98(9):1375–1382.

Mpara, M., J. Tisdale, J. Kanter, J. Kwiatkowski, L. Krishnamurti, M. Schmidt, A. Miller, F. Pierciey, W. Shi, J. Ribeil, M. Asmal, A. Thompson, and M. C. Walters. 2019. Lentiglobin gene therapy in patients with sickle cell disease: Updated interim results from HGB-206. *Biology of Blood and Marrow Transplantation* 25(3):S64–S65.

Naik, R. P., M. B. Streiff, C. Haywood, Jr., J. A. Nelson, and S. Lanzkron. 2013. Venous thromboembolism in adults with sickle cell disease: A serious and under-recognized complication. *American Journal of Medicine* 126(5):443–449.

Naik, R. P., M. B. Streiff, C. Haywood, Jr., J. B. Segal, and S. Lanzkron. 2014. Venous thromboembolism incidence in the cooperative study of sickle cell disease. *Journal of Thrombosis and Haemostasis* 12(12):2010–2016.

NASEM (National Academies of Sciences, Engineering, and Medicine). 2017a. *Human genome editing: Science, ethics, and governance.* Washington, DC: The National Academies Press.

NASEM. 2017b. *Pain management and the opioid epidemic: Balancing societal and individual benefits and risks of prescription opioid use.* Washington, DC: The National Academies Press.

NEJM Catalyst. 2018. *What are bundled payments?* https://catalyst.nejm.org/what-are-bundled-payments (accessed January 13, 2020).

NICE (National Institute for Health and Care Excellence). 2012. *Sickle cell acute painful episode: Management of an acute painful sickle cell episode in hospital.* https://www.ncbi.nlm.nih.gov/books/NBK126761/pdf/Bookshelf_NBK126761.pdf (accessed March 6, 2020).

NICE. 2014. *NICE consults on further draft guidance on the drug sofosbuvir (Sovaldi) for treating hepatitis C.* https://www.nice.org.uk/news/press-and-media/NICE-consults-on-draft-guidance-on-the-drug-sofosbuvir-for-treating-hepatitis-C (accessed January 13, 2020).

Nienhuis, A. W., A. C. Nathwani, and A. M. Davidoff. 2017. Gene therapy for hemophilia. *Molecular Therapies* 25(5):1163–1167.

NIH (National Institutes of Health). 2018. *NIH launches initiative to accelerate genetic therapies to cure sickle cell disease.* https://www.nih.gov/news-events/news-releases/nih-launches-initiative-accelerate-genetic-therapies-cure-sickle-cell-disease (accessed March 6, 2020).

Niihara, Y., S. T. Miller, J. Kanter, S. Lanzkron, W. R. Smith, L. L. Hsu, V. R. Gordeuk, K. Viswanathan, S. Sarnaik, I. Osunkwo, E. Guillaume, S. Sadanandan, L. Sieger, J. L. Lasky, E. H. Panosyan, O. A. Blake, T. N. New, R. Bellevue, L. T. Tran, R. L. Razon, C. W. Stark, L. D. Neumayr, E. P. Vichinsky, and investigators of the Phase 3 Trial of L-glutamine in Sickle Cell Disease. 2018. A Phase 3 trial of L-glutamine in sickle cell disease. *New England Journal of Medicine* 379(3):226–235.

Noubouossie, D., N. S. Key, and K. I. Ataga. 2016. Coagulation abnormalities of sickle cell disease: Relationship with clinical outcomes and the effect of disease modifying therapies. *Blood Reviews* 30(4):245–256.

Novelli, E. M., C. Huynh, M. T. Gladwin, C. G. Moore, and M. V. Ragni. 2012. Pulmonary embolism in sickle cell disease: A case–control study. *Journal of Thrombosis Haemostasis* 10(5):760–766.

Omondi, N. A., S. E. Ferguson, N. S. Majhail, E. M. Denzen, G. R. Buchanan, A. E. Haight, R. J. Labotka, J. D. Rizzo, and E. A. Murphy. 2013. Barriers to hematopoietic cell transplantation clinical trial participation of African American and black youth with sickle cell disease and their parents. *Journal of Pediatric Hematology/Oncology* 35(4):289–298.

Oyeku, S. O., and E. Z. Faro. 2017. Rigorous and practical quality indicators in sickle cell disease care. *Hematology: American Society of Hematology—Education Program* 2017(1):418–422.

Panepinto, J. A., D. Magid, M. J. Rewers, and P. A. Lane. 2000. Universal versus targeted screening of infants for sickle cell disease: A cost-effectiveness analysis. *Journal of Pediatrics* 136(2):201–208.

PCORI (Patient-Centered Outcomes Research Institute). 2019. *Comparing two ways to help parents of children with sickle cell disease decide on treatment with their doctors.* https:// www.pcori.org/research-results/2017/comparing-two-ways-help-parents-children-sickle-cell-disease-decide-treatment (accessed January 10, 2020).

Pecker, L. H., E. Salzberg, S. Chaturvedi, N. Zhao, M. S. Christianson, and S. M. Lanzkron. 2019. Anti-Mullerian hormone, a measure of ovarian reserve, is low in female subjects in the multi-center study of hydroxyurea. *Blood* 134(Suppl 1):890.

Persaud, A., and V. L. Bonham. 2018. The role of the health care provider in building trust between patients and precision medicine research programs. *American Journal of Bioethics* 18(4):26–28.

Persaud, A., S. Desine, K. Blizinsky, and V. L. Bonham. 2019. A CRISPR focus on attitudes and beliefs toward somatic genome editing from stakeholders within the sickle cell disease community. *Genetics in Medicine* 21(8):1726–1734.

Peters, M., B. E. Plaat, H. ten Cate, H. J. Wolters, R. S. Weening, and D. P. Brandjes. 1994. Enhanced thrombin generation in children with sickle cell disease. *Thrombosis and Haemostasis* 71(2):169–172.

Pfizer. 2019. *Pfizer announces Phase 3 top-line results for rivipansel in patients with sickle cell disease experiencing a vaso-occlusive crisis.* https://www.pfizer.com/news/press-release/press-release-detail/pfizer_announces_phase_3_top_line_results_for_rivipansel_in_patients_with_sickle_cell_disease_experiencing_a_vaso_occlusive_crisis (accessed March 6, 2020).

Platt, O. S., D. J. Brambilla, W. F. Rosse, P. F. Milner, O. Castro, M. H. Steinberg, and P. P. Klug. 1994. Mortality in sickle cell disease. Life expectancy and risk factors for early death. *New England Journal of Medicine* 330(23):1639–1644.

Pollack, A. 2015. *Sales of Sovaldi, new Gilead hepatitis C drug, soar to $10.3 billion.* https:// www.nytimes.com/2015/02/04/business/sales-of-sovaldi-new-gilead-hepatitis-c-drug-soar-to-10-3-billion.html (accessed January 10, 2020).

Puri, A., C. Haywood, M. C. Beach, M. Guidera, S. Lanzkron, D. Valenzuela-Araujo, R. E. Rothman, and A. F. Dugas. 2016. Improving emergency providers' attitudes toward sickle cell patients in pain. *Journal of Pain and Symptom Management* 51(3):628–632.

Ramsey, S. D., R. J. Willke, H. Glick, S. D. Reed, F. Augustovski, B. Jonsson, A. Briggs, and S. D. Sullivan. 2015. Cost-effectiveness analysis alongside clinical trials II—An ISPOR Good Research Practices Task Force report. *Value in Health* 18(2):161–172.

Raphael, J. L., T. L. Rattler, M. A. Kowalkowski, B. U. Mueller, T. P. Giordano, and D. C. Brousseau. 2013. Association of care in a medical home and health care utilization among children with sickle cell disease. *Journal of the National Medical Association* 105(2):157–165.

Razavi, H., A. C. Elkhoury, E. Elbasha, C. Estes, K. Pasini, T. Poynard, and R. Kumar. 2013. Chronic hepatitis C virus (HCV) disease burden and cost in the United States. *Hepatology* 57(6):2164–2170.

Ribeil, J. A., S. Hacein-Bey-Abina, E. Payen, A. Magnani, M. Semeraro, E. Magrin, L. Caccavelli, B. Neven, P. Bourget, W. El Nemer, P. Bartolucci, L. Weber, H. Puy, J. F. Meritet, D. Grevent, Y. Beuzard, S. Chretien, T. Lefebvre, R. W. Ross, O. Negre, G. Veres, L. Sandler, S. Soni, M. de Montalembert, S. Blanche, P. Leboulch, and M. Cavazzana. 2017. Gene therapy in a patient with sickle cell disease. *New England Journal of Medicine* 376(9):848–855.

Richards, S. E. 2019. When a treatment costs $450,000 or more, it had better work. *The Atlantic*, April 22.

Riley, T. R., A. Boss, D. McClain, and T. T. Riley. 2018. Review of medication therapy for the prevention of sickle cell crisis. *Pharmacy and Therapeutics* 43(7):417–437.

Ross, D., N. Bakshi, K. Khemani, C. Sinha, G. Loewenstein, and L. Krishnamurti. 2016. What are the expectations of patients in decision making process for disease modifying therapies for sickle cell disease: Do they care about shared decision making? *Blood* 128(22):5968.

Sachs, R., N. Bagley, and D. N. Lakdawalla. 2018. Innovative contracting for pharmaceuticals and Medicaid's best-price rule. *Journal of Health Politics, Policy and Law* 43(1):5–18.

Saraf, S. L., A. L. Oh, P. R. Patel, Y. Jalundhwala, K. Sweiss, M. Koshy, S. Campbell-Lee, M. Gowhari, J. Hassan, D. Peace, J. G. Quigley, I. Khan, R. E. Molokie, L. L. Hsu, N. Mahmud, D. J. Levinson, A. S. Pickard, J. G. Garcia, V. R. Gordeuk, and D. Rondelli. 2016. Nonmyeloablative stem cell transplantation with alemtuzumab/low-dose irradiation to cure and improve the quality of life of adults with sickle cell disease. *Biology of Blood and Marrow Transplantation* 22(3):441–448.

Scharff, D. P., K. J. Mathews, P. Jackson, J. Hoffsuemmer, E. Martin, and D. Edwards. 2010. More than Tuskegee: Understanding mistrust about research participation. *Journal of Health Care for the Poor and Underserved* 21(3):879–897.

Schimmel, M., E. Nur, B. J. Biemond, G. J. van Mierlo, S. Solati, D. P. Brandjes, H. M. Otten, J. J. Schnog, S. Zeerleder, on behalf of the Curama Study Group. 2013. Nucleosomes and neutrophil activation in sickle cell disease painful crisis. *Haematologica* 98(11):1797–1803.

Schumock, G. T., E. C. Li, K. J. Suda, M. D. Wiest, J. Stubbings, L. M. Matusiak, R. J. Hunkler, and L. C. Vermeulen. 2015. National trends in prescription drug expenditures and projections for 2015. *American Journal of Health-System Pharmacy* 72(9):717–736.

Setty, B. N., S. G. Betal, J. Zhang, and M. J. Stuart. 2008. Heme induces endothelial tissue factor expression: Potential role in hemostatic activation in patients with hemolytic anemia. *Journal of Thrombosis and Haemostasis* 6(12):2202–2209.

Shapiro, B. S., L. J. Benjamin, R. Payne, and G. Heidrich. 1997. Sickle cell-related pain: Perceptions of medical practitioners. *Journal of Pain Symptom Management* 14(3):168–174.

Shearstone, J. R., O. Golonzhka, A. Chonkar, D. Tamang, J. H. van Duzer, S. S. Jones, and M. B. Jarpe. 2016. Chemical inhibition of histone deacetylases 1 and 2 induces fetal hemoglobin through activation of GATA2. *PLOS ONE* 11(4):e0153767.

Shenoy, S., J. Gaziev, E. Angelucci, A. King, M. Bhatia, A. Smith, D. Bresters, A. E. Haight, C. N. Duncan, J. de la Fuente, A. C. Dietz, K. S. Baker, M. A. Pulsipher, and M. C. Walters. 2018. Late effects screening guidelines after hematopoietic cell transplantation (HCT) for hemoglobinopathy: Consensus statement from the Second Pediatric Blood and Marrow Transplant Consortium International Conference on Late Effects after Pediatric HCT. *Biology of Blood and Marrow Transplantation* 24(7):1313–1321.

Singer, S. T., and K. I. Ataga. 2008. Hypercoagulability in sickle cell disease and beta-thalassemia. *Current Molecular Medicine* 8(7):639–645.

Slocomb, T., and M. Werner. 2017. *New payment and financing models for curative regenerative medicines.* https://invivo.pharmaintelligence.informa.com/IV005132/New-Payment-And-Financing-Models-For-Curative-Regenerative-Medicines (accessed January 10, 2020).

Spackman, E., M. Sculpher, J. Howard, M. Malfroy, C. Llewelyn, L. Choo, R. Hodge, T. Johnson, D. C. Rees, K. Fijnvandraat, M. Kirby-Allen, S. Davies, and L. Williamson. 2014. Cost-effectiveness analysis of preoperative transfusion in patients with sickle cell disease using evidence from the taps trial. *European Journal of Haematology* 92(3):249–255.

Spark Therapeutics. 2018. *Spark Therapeutics announces first-of-their-kind programs to improve patient access to Luxturna™ (voretigene neparvovecrzyl), a one-time gene therapy treatment.* http://ir.sparktx.com/news-releases/news-release-details/spark-therapeutics-announces-first-their-kind-programs-improve (accessed January 10, 2020).

Stein, P. D., A. Beemath, F. A. Meyers, E. Skaf, and R. E. Olson. 2006. Deep venous thrombosis and pulmonary embolism in hospitalized patients with sickle cell disease. *American Journal of Medicine* 119(10).

Stein, R. 2019. The CRISPR revolution: A patient hopes gene-editing can help with pain of sickle cell disease. *National Public Radio (WAMU 88.5)*. https://www.npr.org/sections/health-shots/2019/11/19/780510277/gene-edited-supercells-make-progress-in-fight-against-sickle-cell-disease (accessed January 30, 2020).

Steinberg, M. H. 1999. Management of sickle cell disease. *New England Journal of Medicine* 340(13):1021–1030.

Steinberg, M. H. 2002. Hydroxyurea treatment for sickle cell disease. *Scientific World Journal* 2:1706–1728.

Steinberg, M. H., and C. Brugnara. 2003. Pathophysiological-based approaches to treatment of sickle cell disease. *Annual Review of Medicine* 54:89–112.

Steinberg, M. H., W. F. McCarthy, O. Castro, S. K. Ballas, F. D. Armstrong, W. Smith, K. Ataga, P. Swerdlow, A. Kutlar, L. DeCastro, M. A. Waclawiw, Investigators of the Multi-center Study of Hydroxyurea in Sickle Cell Anemia, and MSH Patients Follow-Up. 2010. The risks and benefits of long-term use of hydroxyurea in sickle cell anemia: A 17.5 year follow-up. *American Journal of Hematology* 85(6):403–408.

Stine, N., D. A. Chokshi, J. Knudsen, M. Cunningham, and R. Wilson. 2017. How America's largest safety-net health system built a high performance Medicare ACO. *Health Affairs*, November 7. https://www.healthaffairs.org/do/10.1377/hblog20171106.437941/full (accessed April 13, 2020).

Strong, H., M. J. Mitchell, A. Goldstein-Leever, L. Shook, P. Malik, and L. E. Crosby. 2017. Patient perspectives on gene transfer therapy for sickle cell disease. *Advances in Therapy* 34(8):2007–2021.

Strouse, J. J., S. Lanzkron, M. C. Beach, C. Haywood, H. Park, C. Witkop, R. F. Wilson, E. B. Bass, and J. B. Segal. 2008. Hydroxyurea for sickle cell disease: A systematic review for efficacy and toxicity in children. *Pediatrics* 122(6):1332–1342.

Stuart, M. J., and R. L. Nagel. 2004. Sickle-cell disease. *Lancet* 364(9442):1343–1360.

Stuart, M. J., and B. N. Setty. 2001. Hemostatic alterations in sickle cell disease: Relationships to disease pathophysiology. *Pediatric Pathology and Molecular Medicine* 20(1):27–46.

Sundd, P., M. T. Gladwin, and E. M. Novelli. 2019. Pathophysiology of sickle cell disease. *Annual Review of Pathology* 14(1):263–292.

Tanhehco, Y. C., and M. Bhatia. 2019. Hematopoietic stem cell transplantation and cellular therapy in sickle cell disease: Where are we now? *Current Opinion on Hematology* 26(6):448–452.

Telen, M. J. 2007. Role of adhesion molecules and vascular endothelium in the pathogenesis of sickle cell disease. *Hematology: American Society of Hematology—Education Program* 2007:84–90.

Telen, M. J. 2016. Beyond hydroxyurea: New and old drugs in the pipeline for sickle cell disease. *Blood* 127(7):810–819.

Telen, M. J., T. Wun, T. L. McCavit, L. M. De Castro, L. Krishnamurti, S. Lanzkron, L. L. Hsu, W. R. Smith, S. Rhee, J. L. Magnani, and H. Thackray. 2015. Randomized Phase 2 study of GMI-1070 in SCD: Reduction in time to resolution of vaso-occlusive events and decreased opioid use. *Blood* 125(17):2656–2664.

Telen, M. J., P. Malik, and G. M. Vercellotti. 2019. Therapeutic strategies for sickle cell disease: Towards a multi-agent approach. *Nature Reviews Drug Discovery* 18(2):139–158.

Thompson, A. A. 2013. Ideal donors, imperfect results in sickle cell disease. *Blood* 122(6):858–859.

Tisdale, J. F., J. Kanter, M. Y. Mapara, J. L. Kwiatkowski, L. Krishnamurti, M. Schmidt, A. L. Miller, F. J. Pierciey, Jr., W. Shi, J.-A. Ribeil, M. Asmal, A. A. Thompson, and M. C. Walters. 2018. Current results of lentiglobin gene therapy in patients with severe sickle cell disease treated under a refined protocol in the Phase 1 HGB-206 study. *Blood* 132(Suppl 1):1026.

Tomer, A., S. Kasey, W. E. Connor, S. Clark, L. A. Harker, and J. R. Eckman. 2001. Reduction of pain episodes and prothrombotic activity in sickle cell disease by dietary n-3 fatty acids. *Thrombosis and Haemostasis* 85(6):966–974.

Touchot, N., and M. Flume. 2015. The payers' perspective on gene therapies. *Nature Biotechnology* 33(9):902–904.

Treadwell, M. J., L. McClough, and E. Vichinsky. 2006. Using qualitative and quantitative strategies to evaluate knowledge and perceptions about sickle cell disease and sickle cell trait. *Journal of the National Medical Association* 98(5):704–710.

Tshilolo, L., G. Tomlinson, T. N. Williams, B. Santos, P. Olupot-Olupot, A. Lane, B. Aygun, S. E. Stuber, T. S. Latham, P. T. McGann, and R. E. Ware, for the REACH investigators. 2019. Hydroxyurea for children with sickle cell anemia in sub-Saharan Africa. *New England Journal of Medicine* 380(2):121–131.

U.S. Senate Committee on Finance. 2015. *The price of Sovaldi and its impact on the U.S. health care system.* https://www.finance.senate.gov/imo/media/doc/1%20The%20Price%20of%20Sovaldi%20and%20Its%20Impact%20on%20the%20U.S.%20Health%20Care%20System%20(Full%20Report).pdf (accessed March 6, 2020).

Vichinsky, E., C. C. Hoppe, K. I. Ataga, R. E. Ware, V. Nduba, A. El-Beshlawy, H. Hassab, M. M. Achebe, S. Alkindi, R. C. Brown, D. L. Diuguid, P. Telfer, D. A. Tsitsikas, A. Elghandour, V. R. Gordeuk, J. Kanter, M. R. Abboud, J. Lehrer-Graiwer, M. Tonda, A. Intondi, B. Tong, J. Howard, and Hope Trial investigators. 2019. A Phase 3 randomized trial of voxelotor in sickle cell disease. *New England Journal of Medicine* 381(6):509–519.

Villagra, J., S. Shiva, L. A. Hunter, R. F. Machado, M. T. Gladwin, and G. J. Kato. 2007. Platelet activation in patients with sickle disease, hemolysis-associated pulmonary hypertension, and nitric oxide scavenging by cell-free hemoglobin. *Blood* 110(6):2166–2172.

Vincent, L., D. Vang, J. Nguyen, M. Gupta, K. Luk, M. E. Ericson, D. A Simone, and K. Gupta. 2013. Mast cell activation contributes to sickle cell pathobiology and pain in mice. *Blood* 122(11):1853–1862.

Voskaridou, E., D. Christoulas, A. Bilalis, E. Plata, K. Varvagiannis, G. Stamatopoulos, K. Sinopoulou, A. Balassopoulou, D. Loukopoulos, and E. Terpos. 2010. The effect of prolonged administration of hydroxyurea on morbidity and mortality in adult patients with sickle cell syndromes: Results of a 17-year, single-center trial (LASHS). *Blood* 115(12):2354–2363.

Wailoo, K. 2017. Sickle cell disease—A history of progress and peril. *New England Journal of Medicine* 376(9):805–807.

Walker, A. L., L. M. Gaydos, R. Farzan, L. De Castro, and C. Jonassaint. 2019. Social media discussions provide new insight about perceptions of hydroxyurea in the sickle cell community. *American Journal of Hematology* 94(5):E134–E136.

Walker, J. 2019. *Biotech proposes paying for pricey drugs by installment.* https://www.wsj.com/articles/biotech-proposes-paying-for-pricey-drugs-by-installment-11546952520 (accessed January 13, 2020).

Walters, M. C. 2005. Stem cell therapy for sickle cell disease: Transplantation and gene therapy. *Hematology: American Society of Hematology—Education Program* 2005:66–73.

Walters, M. C. 2015. Update of hematopoietic cell transplantation for sickle cell disease. *Current Opinion in Hematology* 22(3):227–233.

Walters, M. C., M. Patience, W. Leisenring, J. R. Eckman, J. P. Scott, W. C. Mentzer, S. C. Davies, K. Ohene-Frempong, F. Bernaudin, D. C. Matthews, R. Storb, and K. M. Sullivan. 1996. Bone marrow transplantation for sickle cell disease. *New England Journal of Medicine* 335(6):369–376.

Walters, M. C., R. Storb, M. Patience, W. Leisenring, T. Taylor, J. E. Sanders, G. E. Buchanan,
Z. R. Rogers, P. Dinndorf, S. C. Davies, I. A. Roberts, R. Dickerhoff, A. M. Yeager, L.
Hsu, J. Kurtzberg, K. Ohene-Frempong, N. Bunin, F. Bernaudin, W. Y. Wong, J. P. Scott,
D. Margolis, E. Vichinsky, D. A. Wall, A. S. Wayne, C. Pegelow, R. Redding-Lallinger,
J. Wiley, M. Klemperer, W. C. Mentzer, F. O. Smith, and K. M. Sullivan. 2000. Impact
of bone marrow transplantation for symptomatic sickle cell disease: An interim report.
Multicenter investigation of bone marrow transplantation for sickle cell disease. *Blood*
95(6):1918–1924.

Walters, M. C., M. Patience, W. Leisenring, Z. R. Rogers, V. M. Aquino, G. R. Buchanan, I. A.
Roberts, A. M. Yeager, L. Hsu, T. Adamkiewicz, J. Kurtzberg, E. Vichinsky, B. Storer, R.
Storb, K. M. Sullivan, and the Multicenter Investigation of Bone Marrow Transplantation
for Sickle Cell Disease. 2001. Stable mixed hematopoietic chimerism after bone marrow
transplantation for sickle cell anemia. *Biology of Blood and Marrow Transplantation*
7(12):665–673.

Walters, M. C., K. Hardy, S. Edwards, T. Adamkiewicz, J. Barkovich, F. Bernaudin, G. R.
Buchanan, N. Bunin, R. Dickerhoff, R. Giller, P. R. Haut, J. Horan, L. L. Hsu, N.
Kamani, J. E. Levine, D. Margolis, K. Ohene-Frempong, M. Patience, R. Redding-
Lallinger, I. A. Roberts, Z. R. Rogers, J. E. Sanders, J. P. Scott, K. M. Sullivan, for the
Multicenter Study of Bone Marrow Transplantation for Sickle Cell Disease. 2010. Pul-
monary, gonadal, and central nervous system status after bone marrow transplantation
for sickle cell disease. *Biology of Blood and Marrow Transplantation* 16(2):263–272.

Whelihan, M. F., M. Y. Lim, M. J. Mooberry, M. G. Piegore, A. Ilich, A. Wogu, J. Cai,
D. M. Monroe, K. I. Ataga, K. G. Mann, and N. S. Key. 2016. Thrombin generation
and cell-dependent hypercoagulability in sickle cell disease. *Journal of Thrombosis and
Haemostasis* 14(10):1941–1952.

White, J., M. Lindgren, K. Liu, X. Gao, L. Jendeberg, and P. Hines. 2019. Sevuparin blocks
sickle blood cell adhesion and sickle-leucocyte rolling on immobilized L-selectin in a dose
dependent manner. *British Journal of Haematology* 184(5):873–876.

Woods, K., M. Miller, M. Johnson, A. Tracy, A. Kutlar, and C. Cassel. 1997. Functional status
and well-being in adults with sickle cell disease. *Journal of Clinical Outcomes Management* 4(5):15–21.

Wun, T., T. Paglieroni, A. Rangaswami, P. H. Franklin, J. Welborn, A. Cheung, and
F. Tablin. 1998. Platelet activation in patients with sickle cell disease. *British Journal of
Haematology* 100(4):741–749.

Xue, C., X. Wang, Q. Qu, H. Qu, X. Fang, X. Sui, X. Liu, Y. Li, and Y. Jiang. 2019. Sexual
dysfunction and abnormal androgen level after hematopoietic stem cell transplantation.
Blood 134(Suppl 1):5691.

8

Community Engagement and Patient Advocacy

The community-based organizations are valued. I would consider them like the gatekeepers to the sickle cell disease community. They definitely have their finger on the pulse of the community.

—Shauna W. (Open Session Panelist)

Chapter Summary

- There is a long history of community-based organizations (CBOs) and patient organizations advocating for and serving the needs of the sickle cell disease (SCD) population and generating awareness about SCD and sickle cell trait (SCT).
- The current landscape of SCD patient groups includes several organizations at the national, state, and local levels, with very different structures, that improve the lives of individuals with SCD within a defined sphere but lack the needed unified voice to effect large-scale change for individuals with SCD and SCT.
- SCD CBOs perform a crucial function in the SCD care delivery ecosystem, but their efforts are hampered by a lack of financial resources and infrastructural challenges.
- Models of patient advocacy from other rare diseases offer key takeaways for improving the organization and effectiveness of SCD patient advocacy groups and CBOs.

continued

- To truly move from local-level impact to system-level change, the organization of SCD CBOs and patient advocacy groups needs to be restructured, their capabilities defined, and their role embedded within the care delivery system.
- Funding sources for these groups also need to be diversified, and more funds must be made available for CBOs' work from both federal and private sources.

HISTORICAL PERSPECTIVE

Individuals living with sickle cell disease (SCD) and sickle cell trait (SCT) often experience racism, stigma, and implicit bias within and outside the health care system. SCD-specific community-based organizations (CBOs) have been and continue to be important in mitigating these experiences and therefore have a critical role in any strategic initiative to improve care and services for this population.

As discussed in earlier chapters of this report, individuals living with SCD and SCT were and continue to be socially stigmatized and neglected in the health care system because of the lack of general understanding of the disease and its consequences. This current state is best understood in the context of the historical experiences that have shaped advocacy and community engagement. In response to social activism in the 1960s regarding the poor health of African Americans, an activism that was catalyzed by the Black Panther Party, President Nixon told Congress in a 1971 speech that "a second targeted disease for concentrated research should be sickle cell anemia.... It is a sad and shameful fact that the causes of this disease have been largely neglected throughout our history. We cannot rewrite this record of neglect, but we can reverse it" (Gold, 2017).

In conjunction with this increased attention to SCD, 12 states and the District of Columbia enacted mandatory sickle cell screening laws for African Americans. Most of these laws equated SCT with SCD. These laws led to stigmatizing people with carrier status, resulting in such things as denial of health and life insurance, poorer employment opportunities, and rejection from the U.S. Air Force Academy (Markel, 1992). In 1972, the call for a special effort to address SCD led to the passage of the National Sickle Cell Anemia Control Act (Public Law 92-294) (Manley, 1984). One important aspect of the act is that it ended mandatory genetic testing for SCD. The act made testing voluntary; provided $6 million dollars toward research into and treatment of SCD; and authorized education, information, screening, testing, genetic counseling, research, and treatment programs to improve understanding (Manley, 1984).

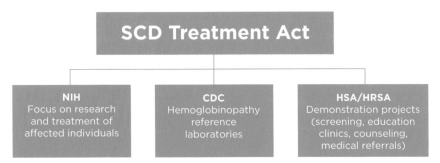

FIGURE 8-1 Federal agencies involved in SCD and SCT activities stemming from the Sickle Cell Treatment Act.
NOTE: CDC = Centers for Disease Control and Prevention; HRSA = Health Resources and Services Administration; HSA = Health Services Administration; NIH = National Institutes of Health; SCD = sickle cell disease.

The decade after the National Sickle Cell Control Act was passed featured increased awareness of and efforts to educate the public about SCD and SCT and to develop and evaluate new therapies. In the early 1970s the federal efforts focused on SCD and SCT involved three major agencies (see Figure 8-1): the National Institutes of Health (NIH); the Health Services Administration (HSA), later renamed the Health Resources and Services Administration (HRSA), and the Centers for Disease Control and Prevention (CDC).

NIH focused on research and treatment. HSA and HRSA translated this work and established demonstration projects for screening, education clinics for counseling, and medical referral for those diagnosed with SCD, specifically through the Maternal and Child Health Bureau (MCHB). CDC focused on developing hemoglobinopathy laboratories and training programs to provide proficiency testing and also to serve as reference laboratories. Under the administration of NIH, the comprehensive SCD treatment centers were established, with the goal of reducing morbidity and mortality (Manley, 1984).

The HSA sickle cell clinics were the nexus of connectivity with the community and offered genetic counseling and awareness education, referring those identified as having SCD to the NIH comprehensive centers. The centers were supported by an interagency transfer of funds from NIH that began in 1972 with $1.9 million, increasing to $3.4 million in 1974. The number of centers rapidly expanded from 19 in 1972 to 26 in 1975, with the majority located in the southeast United States, where there was a dense population of African Americans. This initiative established a protocol for education and counseling for SCD through the sickle cell clinics. In 1976 the Genetic Disease Act was passed, with a mandate to provide genetic services for all genetic conditions, including SCD, affording MCHB a platform to establish structures for serving individuals with SCD. By 1982 a reported 1.6 million clients had been educated and 860,000 clients screened. The concept of the SCD CBO was an integral part of the original design of SCD services introduced by the National Sickle Cell Control Act.

Unfortunately, federal funding appropriation was far less than what was needed to provide services for all genetic diseases. In addition, it was delegated to states to incorporate sickle cell into their genetics service delivery networks and MCHB programs. Further restructuring of the funding mechanisms for genetic diseases inherently modified the clinic structure and functions and the overall delivery of SCD services; this dismantled the robust infrastructure established by the federal mandate, giving rise to a fragmented SCD care delivery system in which individual states controlled screening and follow-up with other services, such as data collection, research, and clinical services, split among various federal agencies.

Despite the National Sickle Cell Control Act, discrimination borne out of misinformation and a lack of knowledge about persons with SCD and SCT did not end. National funding for SCD was tied to congressional appropriations, which resulted in a "push–pull" on research funding between SCD and other disease groups. Failure to distinguish SCT, the carrier state affecting millions of Americans, from SCD led to an incorrect labeling of SCT as SCD and resulted in needless fears and discrimination for many individuals. The general public and some physicians reinforced this medical mismanagement and bias, resulting in individuals with SCT being denied education, insurance, and employment opportunities (Scott, 1981). Moreover, the poorly conceived design and inadequate resources of the clinics may have contributed to improper and inadequate testing procedures, incorrect interpretation of test results, and misinformed genetic counseling. There was little supervision of the interpretation of genetic testing results by trained medical professionals, and counseling services were inconsistent, causing undue harm from miscommunication and misinterpretation of results (Scott, 1981).

To avoid a repeat of the negative consequences associated with the National Sickle Cell Control Act, any national strategy that addresses identified priorities for SCD and SCT requires critical information and feedback from the SCD community. However, the work of the advocates/advocacy groups and CBOs (formerly housed within the clinics) is hampered by important obstacles discussed in this chapter, which will need to be addressed if the full potential of the community is to be harnessed and the relevant stakeholders to be engaged in advancing care, outcomes, and resources for the SCD population. Most importantly, there is a need to develop a structured and scalable value framework for the contribution that CBOs provide toward improving care outcomes that will allow adequate infrastructure and financial support for their continued existence.

SICKLE CELL COMMUNITY-BASED ORGANIZATIONS AND PATIENT ADVOCACY GROUPS

SCD is the largest of the rare genetic diseases, yet it lacks the coordinated efforts and unified patient voice needed to make a difference. The current landscape of SCD patient organizations is complex. There are multiple stakeholders operating at various levels (federal, state, and local), and they may conduct brick-and-mortar or virtual (not bound by geography) activities or a combination of both. There are community- and health system–based support groups for individuals living with SCD and their families, and there are smaller groups established by individuals affected by SCD and their families. Patient advocates or groups may influence policy, programs, resource allocation, and messaging to relevant stakeholders and the general public about the interests, needs, and well-being of the SCD population.

SCD CBOs encompass a wide variety of entities, from independent individual advocates to small local groups focused on sickle cell awareness and education to large national groups, including organizations delivering enabling services. These organizations are also involved in community engagement, which is the "inclusion of local health system users and community resources in all aspects of design, planning, governance, and delivery of health care services" (PHCPI, 2018). Patient advocates, advocacy groups, and CBOs may liaise between the SCD population and the care delivery system; as discussed later in this chapter, most diseases, especially rare and inheritable diseases, have benefited from the work of strong patient organizations. CBOs and advocacy groups carry out sets of activities based on their organizational structures, but the lack of coordination among these groups results in a duplication of activities, primarily because the various organizations typically operate independently. This has limited their overall effectiveness and served as an impediment to having a far-reaching impact.

National efforts that encompass the interests of all CBOs and advocacy groups regardless of size, infrastructure, mission, and capacity are challenging, particularly in SCD, where all entities are under-resourced. The CDC National Resource Directory (CDC, 2019b) identifies two SCD resources working at the national level to advance awareness, care, and outcomes: the Sickle Cell Disease Association of America (SCDAA) and the Sickle Cell Community Consortium (SCCC). These two groups are vastly different in focus, structure, and scope.

There are several CBOs and advocacy groups operating at the state and local levels to advocate for and support the SCD community. Some of these organizations may be members and affiliates of SCDAA or other national organizations discussed later in this chapter, but they still operate independently. Appendix K lists CBOs and advocacy resource groups related to SCD, identified using publicly available information and online sources, including all state-level chapters of SCDAA. However, this list is not fully inclusive; it is only meant to provide an overview of SCD patient organizations by state. There is no available comprehensive listing or registry of SCD CBOs or advocacy groups, nor is there a standardized classification of precisely which services each offers. Thus, there is an opportunity to create a comprehensive cataloguing of CBOs and community resources available for the SCD population and to develop a formal characterization and classification of the various services that each offers.

Services Offered by SCD Community-Based Organizations

SCD CBOs provide a myriad of services beyond awareness about SCD and SCT and advocacy that support and complement health care for children and adults; these include education, counseling, care coordination, and enabling services (see Table 8-1). The influence and overall impact of the SCD CBOs remains invisible in the scientific literature because community participation, engagement, and support are not typically measured with the current scientific publications. CBOs, by dint of their defined scope and sphere, are embedded in their communities, understand the dynamics and needs of these communities, and can tailor their offerings accordingly.

The activities in Table 8-1 can be categorized into three key categories of functions discussed in the next sections: providing public education and awareness, providing enabling services to the SCD population, and bridging the SCD population and the scientific and clinical community.

Providing Public Education and Awareness

Public awareness and information serve to demystify a health condition. This is especially needed for SCD/SCT, as alluded to in preceding chapters. Public awareness and understanding of the disease are limited, which places the burden on individuals to educate those in their milieu (e.g., health care, schools, places of employment, clinics). It is also important to ensure that public information about SCT is factually accurate and that misinformation is promptly debunked so as to avoid a repeat of the 1970s situation when SCT was confounded with SCD, resulting in stigmatizing people with carrier status. CBOs and other patient advocacy groups assume the collective voice of individuals with SCD and SCT and play a pivotal role in educating the public and key stakeholders, especially legislators. These groups require access to appropriate and accurate information and education and the necessary counseling and health education skills to ensure that

TABLE 8-1 Community-Based Organization Services Supporting the Needs of Children and Adults with SCD and SCT, Not Including Advocacy

Service	Description of Activities
SCD and SCT education	• SCD/SCT education individually or at the community level
Genetic counseling services	• Counseling services for SCT and other hemoglobinopathy traits, such as C, E, and beta-thalassemia o Consumers are referred to hospital-based genetic counselors for full reproductive counseling
Psychosocial support	• Support groups • Peer support networks • Social networks • Information-sharing networks, such as SCDAA's Get Connected • Hospital visitation • Recreational and social activities, such as picnics and other social outings
Camps	• Support for children and young adults to participate in external camps • Annual SCD-specific camps
Care coordination	• Care coordination at the individual or population level for adolescents and young adults or older adults • Case management o A few CBOs can provide in-home nurse case management services to support the hospital-to-home transition and reduce avoidable admissions
Case finding and referral to care	• Assisting state health departments and health systems/hospitals with finding newborns with positive newborn screening results for SCD • Finding individuals lost to care/follow-up and referring back to health care • Assisting sickle cell programs with finding patients lost to care • Assisting individuals with SCD in finding a medical home, particularly a primary care provider and/or a sickle cell expert
Enabling services	• Transportation to and from medical and dental appointments • Assistance with the maintenance of basic needs, such as housing, utilities, and food • Caregiver support • Bereavement support • Linkage to community resources • Child care • Tutoring
Clinical trial education and recruitment	• Partnering with private industry and hospitals to educate consumers on clinical trial participation • Recruitment for open clinical trials
Transition assistance	• Education on transition • Assessment of transition readiness • Accompanying young adults to first adult-focused care visit

NOTE: CBO = community-based organization; SCD = sickle cell disease; SCDAA = Sickle Cell Disease Association of America; SCT = sickle cell trait.

they communicate accurate and up-to-date information about SCD and SCT to broad audiences. The optimal purpose of such public awareness campaigns is to share accurate information with all.

In a recent campaign about self-management education awareness, CDC demonstrated that the important components of public awareness efforts include having a clear, concise, and simple message; engaging all relevant partners and stakeholders; and providing access to additional (vetted) readily available informational resources in various accessible formats for individuals and stakeholders. A similar structured process to communicate awareness messages for use by all SCD CBOs and advocacy groups would result in less misinformation and fewer potentially conflicting messages. One way to ensure consistency and accuracy in messaging would be to develop a centralized toolkit that all advocacy and CBO groups could use to provide evidence-based, culturally appropriate information at the appropriate literacy level in their awareness campaigns. The federal government, in collaboration with relevant organizations, could develop such a toolkit.

Providing Enabling Services to the SCD Population

CBOs and patient advocacy groups are best positioned to provide certain enabling services, including social and peer support, hospital visitation, and recreational and social activities, to address the isolation and need for community that individuals with SCD have expressed. CBOs may also provide services tailored to mitigating various nonmedical social needs, such as transportation to and from medical appointments; assistance with basic needs, such as housing, utilities, food, child care, and tutoring; and linkage to other community resources, such as vocational training and legal clinics to help with disability insurance. Many of these services are provided by community health workers (CHWs) who work within CBOs or medical centers.

Many CBOs provide an annual SCD camp, which is an important enabling service. For children with chronic disease, the summer camp experience can support education and quality-of-life (QOL) benefits through opportunities for peer modeling, disease education, and reduced isolation. The committee heard from young adult panelists in the open session of the fourth meeting that an SCD camp is a valuable service that not only addresses the significant isolation that individuals experience but also serves as a pipeline for SCD advocates who attended camp as children, returned as camp counselors, and continue on to find their niche as advocates in the SCD community.

There are several categories of camp experiences for children and young adults with SCD. Many involve 1- to 2-week experiences for children, with or without their siblings. The camps are staffed by the sponsoring CBO and volunteers. There are also national camps that provide experiences for children with chronic illnesses in general. Many of these camps offer "sickle cell only" weeks on their properties supported by their regular camp staff and have medical teams on site that are familiar with the care of children and adults with SCD. Local health care systems work alongside CBOs locally to ensure that when campers have pain or fever, physicians and nurses are on site to provide care and to aid in transport to nearby health centers (Narcisse et al., 2018). Some providers use camp as an opportunity to strengthen the provider–patient relationship (DiDomizio and Gillard, 2018). Parents and caregivers are reassured and comforted when their local medical teams or others familiar with SCD are on staff. This provides opportunities for these children whose families might have limited their camp experiences otherwise. Expenses and charges for camp participation are supplemented or fully covered by philanthropy or grant funding. Finally, providing counselor-in-training and counselor positions for, respectively, teens and adults with SCD offers informal peer-mentoring and patient support systems.

Although sickle cell camps have been in existence for more than four decades, very little has been published on their key elements or on how the experience affects the lives of individuals living with SCD. The benefit of camps for children with chronic disease has been well demonstrated for inflammatory bowel disease (Salazar and Heyman, 2014; Shepanski et al., 2005), cancer (Wu et al., 2016), burns (Bakker et al., 2011), and pediatric diabetes (Bultas et al., 2016). Generally, camp experiences increase self-esteem, as participants learn that there are other children with SCD who may share similar problems. Campers enjoy the opportunity to play, participate in sports, swim, and live with other children with SCD without being forced to think about their illness. Some camps offer only recreational activities, while others provide opportunities to learn disease self-management, increase sickle cell knowledge, prepare for transition from pediatric to adult care, or learn life skills needed to get ready for college and vocations.

Narcisse et al. (2018) published on summer camps for SCD, highlighting the importance of appropriate staff training in adapting the camp schedule, activities, and environment to minimize the potential for exacerbating a vaso-occlusive episode (VOE). For example, camps can arrange for temperature control, access to water for liberal hydration, and schedules that allow for frequent breaks in order to prevent overexertion, which can trigger a VOE. The authors also recommend developing and disseminating standardized manuals to guide the operational structure and functions of an SCD-specific camp, including staff training, recruiting young adults with SCD as counselors, the appropriate medical team infrastructure based on camper census, and standardization of suitable educational material and resources. It is imperative that research on the care needs of the SCD population, adolescent transition, and various QOL metrics, such as self-management, coping, and isolation, be conducted to guide resources offered at SCD camps.

Client engagement across the life span is difficult for any CBO serving a community with a chronic inherited condition. Camp may be the first time that a child with SCD has an experience involving the local CBO. This experience helps the CBO develop a relationship with the child before the transition to young adulthood. Relationships formed at camp can often be a source of support when a youth with SCD is hospitalized or struggling to keep up in school. These positive camp experiences cultivate participation in tutoring, reunions, seasonal parties, and other events.

Serving as a Bridge Between the SCD Population and the Scientific and Clinical Community

The final and key role of CBOs and patient advocacy groups is to connect individuals with SCD and SCT to the health care system. This function begins with newborn screening (NBS), for which some states partner with CBOs and patient advocacy groups to follow up with families of newborns with positive SCD results and link them with needed care. Although the committee was unable to find existing models for joint training, having CBO staff and medical practitioners participate together in training on how to work collaboratively would only enhance the relationship between the two.

CBOs also provide education about SCD and SCT to individuals and to the community to help with clinical and reproductive decision making. CBOs may partner with researchers at academic medical centers or private pharmaceutical manufacturers to disseminate information about clinical trials and recruit participants. This a crucial role for CBOs, especially in light of the historical injustices that African Americans have suffered in participating in investigational clinical research, which has fostered deep mistrust between the community and the health care system and has historically contributed to an unwillingness to participate in clinical trials.

Some CBOs offer services to aid young adults transitioning from pediatric to adult care by assessing transition readiness and providing education. Some organizations may even accompany young adults to their first adult clinical visit. CBOs also provide care coordination and case referral services. As discussed in Chapters 4, 5, and 6, the complexities of SCD and its associated complications necessitate care from a multidisciplinary team, resulting in a situation that may be overwhelming for individuals and their families to navigate on their own. CBOs can assist people in finding a medical home that supports their whole-person needs (see Chapter 5) and with scheduling and coordinating services among multiple medical providers. When liaising between the SCD population and the health care system, CBOs often rely on CHWs, as other staff members may not be as facile at navigating the health care system. The CHW's role is discussed in the next section.

The liaison role of the CBO and SCD advocacy groups should never be considered unilateral. While the focus is on supporting access to care for the individuals affected, historically CBOs have always been in a position of "supporter," with no quid pro quo benefit. CBOs are often not included in scientific publications, even though they provide researchers with invaluable help in both developing strong grant applications and securing access to affected individuals. Their role as a liaison to the health care system and to research efforts is generally invisible. Without equal visibility as part of the research team in scientific publications, CBOs are relegated to the acknowledgment section of manuscripts and remain undervalued. While CBOs may lack the infrastructure to produce scientific literature, they are strong cultural brokers within the SCD community and are necessary for most scientific research advances. True partnership with the medical community will require redefining roles and their ascribed values, with clear guidelines for infrastructure and capacity building within CBOs to support their key function as a bridge between the SCD community and the health care system.

Community Health Workers

CHWs are also known as "outreach workers," *promotores/as de salud,* "community health representatives," and "patient navigators" (Rosenthal et al., 2010). Clinician scientists and several SCD CBOs across the country recently coproduced a publication that described the role of nonclinical CHWs in SCD care (Hsu et al., 2016). The authors cited the high socioeconomic and health burden of SCD as a public health concern and suggested that public health approaches might be able to mitigate the socio-ecological barriers that result in poor outcomes (which CHWs can address). Because care delivery for SCD, as with most chronic conditions, is complicated by disparities in health care access, delivery, services, and cultural provider–patient mismatches, the authors propose using CHWs to support case management, social support, and health system navigation (Hsu et al., 2016). CHWs would address multiple barriers faced in accessing the health care system and serve seven core roles in improving patients' health, as detailed in Figure 8-2 (Hsu et al., 2016).

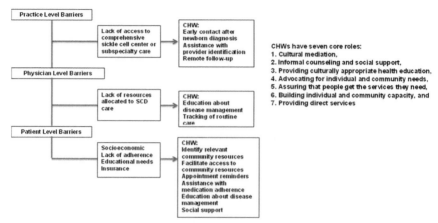

FIGURE 8-2 Multiple barriers can be addressed by community health workers for SCD.
NOTE: CHW = community health worker; SCD = sickle cell disease.
SOURCE: Hsu et al., 2016.

There is evidence from the literature indicating that it may be effective to use CHWs to support and manage care for individuals with other chronic conditions, but there is very limited evidence for the SCD population (Otero-Sabogal et al., 2010; Rhodes et al., 2007; Rosenthal et al., 2010).

Examples of Community-Based Organizations and Patient Advocacy Groups and Services Provided

The capabilities and activities at CBOs and patient advocacy groups vary greatly. This section provides an overview of select CBOs and groups that are recognized for their active programming and patient advocacy efforts in the SCD population. Because there is little research and few publications on the contributions of such CBOs, the groups described here were identified through open session speaker remarks, information provided to the committee and National Academies team, and discussions with relevant stakeholders. Information on the groups' activities was drawn from the public information on their websites.

Sickle Cell Disease Association of America

SCDAA was founded in 1971 as the National Association for Sickle Cell Disease (it updated its name in 1994). The association's mission is "to advocate for people affected by sickle cell conditions and empower CBOs to maximize QOL and raise public consciousness while advancing the search for a universal cure" (SCDAA, 2019). SCDAA has a network of state and local affiliated member organizations that are independent CBOs, which it works with to advance its mission (see Appendix K).

SCDAA supports a number of programs, including the CHW training program, a leadership academy that provides leadership skills, organizational effectiveness, and technical support for member CBOs, and also the National Sickle Cell Advocacy Network, which educates and empowers patients, families, caregivers, clinicians, stakeholders, and experts who are themselves affected by the disease or who want to advocate, educate, and help people living with SCD. The organization hosts an annual convention, which has been running for more than four decades and offers a platform for collaboration for more than 300 attendees (CBO member organizations, individuals living with SCD and SCT, health care professionals, and researchers) to share and learn from each other. SCDAA also developed Get Connected, the first patient-powered registry.

SCDAA is funded by a variety of sources, including federal grants, such as HRSA's Sickle Cell Disease Newborn Screening Follow-Up Program, which provides the resources for the organization to work with CBOs across the country in order to improve access to quality care for the SCD population, and it has strategic partnerships with various other philanthropic organizations. A major SCDAA initiative is the organization's national advocacy day, where the community works strategically on legislation that will foster improved research and access to care.

Sickle Cell Disease Foundation of California

The Sickle Cell Disease Foundation of California (SCDFC), founded in 1957, was the first social service nonprofit founded to focus on the needs of the SCD population (Sickle Cell Disease Foundation, n.d.). Perhaps because of its longevity, the SCDFC offers a strong model of successful patient advocacy at the state level. SCDFC works collaboratively with the Center for Inherited Blood Disorders (CIBD), a safety net clinic in southern California that provides health care services for individuals with blood disorders. SCDFC and CIBD successfully advocated for adding $15 million to the state budget specifically to establish comprehensive sickle cell centers. Using data from their involvement in the CDC Sickle Cell Disease Data Project (CDC, 2019a), SCDFC spearheaded the advocacy efforts. It also led efforts by participating in the Pacific Regional Sickle Cell Collaborative, one of five regional grantees funded by HRSA as part of the U.S. Sickle Cell Disease Treatment Demonstration Program (SCDTDP), to expand access to health care through the establishment of the MLK Jr. Outpatient Center for Adults with SCD (Sickle Cell Disease Foundation, n.d.). SCDFC provides support services, patient education, and public awareness and fundraising activities;

it works according to an established, highly effective model that can offer insights for other patient advocacy groups.

Sickle Cell Foundation of Georgia

> *Camp New Hope really keeps a lot of kids together;*
> *it keeps them feeling as though there is family, a community for us,*
> *that we all have something.*

—Gregory G. (Open Session Panelist)

Since 1971 the Sickle Cell Foundation of Georgia (SCFGA) has served individuals with SCD and SCT in a variety of ways. In 2018, SCFGA provided services to 2,067 individuals in 64 counties across the state (SCFGA, 2018), including care coordination through the use of CHWs, assistance with applying to federal programs, testing and counseling to individuals with SCT, support groups, health fairs, and awareness events targeting the broader community. The Sickle Cell Road Race/Walk at Welcome All Park in Atlanta has been an annual awareness and fundraising event since 1979. SCFGA has a mobile trait testing unit, first donated by baseball legend Hank Aaron in 1973, which serves the entire state, providing access to trait testing and genetic counseling to rural areas.

Part of SCFGA's mission is to provide education, awareness, and support to health care providers of all categories (physicians, advanced practice providers, nurses, residents, and medical students) through its partnerships with Emory University, Children's Healthcare of Atlanta, and the Morehouse School of Medicine. It has developed a robust pediatric-to-adult transition support services program, working collaboratively with the Children's Healthcare of Atlanta hospital and Grady Hospital SCD program to facilitate the education and engagement of young adults who are transitioning into adult care.

This initiative has been expanded to include support for youth beyond the transition age, whom it has mentored and trained to support its mission and objectives, including its role as a co-investigator on the Patient-Centered Outcomes Research Institute–funded transition study. It recently launched an initiative to build capacity among non-specialty providers to treat individuals with SCD in Georgia using a structured continuing medical education webinar and in-person curriculum and by broadly disseminating the American Society of Hematology (ASH) pocket guides for SCD clinical practice and various informational sheets about SCD therapies, such as hydroxyurea (HU) and Endari. In 2015 it established a CHW program funded through the HRSA/SCDAA NBS program to provide care coordination support to help link individuals with primary care medical homes.

It built partnerships with federally qualified health centers located in communities with the largest access to care gaps across 75 counties in Georgia.

For more than 40 years SCFGA has hosted a camp for children with SCD. The first day camp was sponsored in 1973, and the day camps later became retreats and (beginning in 1990) a week-long away camp. Camp New Hope, which patient speakers referenced as a source of support at the committee's open session meeting, is staffed by volunteers, most of whom are living with SCD and attended the camp in the past. In 2018 the 1-week camp hosted 114 participating youth. In addition to relying on volunteers as camp counselors, the camp also ran a 24-hour infirmary staffed by 25 volunteers—12 physicians, 12 nurses, and 1 social worker (SCFGA, 2018). SCFGA also organizes charity events to promote public awareness and education and to advocate for legislation.

The Children's Sickle Cell Foundation of Pittsburgh

The Children's Sickle Cell Foundation launched a legislative agenda with an Advocacy Luncheon in 2009. Through the Pennsylvania Sickle Cell Provider's Network (PASCPN), five CBOs work with four hospitals on issues directly affecting the sickle cell population across the state. PASCPN coordinates efforts to educate lawmakers during the Pennsylvania Supports Sickle Cell Disease Advocacy Day. Each year approximately 350 attendees wearing bright red shirts that read "PA Supports SCD" flock to the Pennsylvania State Capitol. Planning the advocacy day takes several months, and a core team consisting of a few representatives of the network works to reach consensus on the legislative priorities, talking points, program agenda, and logistics.

The Pennsylvania Legislative Black Caucus is an engaged partner and secures the venue for the morning press conference, lunch, and afternoon roundtable discussion with its key members. Each CBO arranges visits to important legislators and those representing its home district around the program schedule. Physicians, CBO leaders, individuals living with SCD, and parents and other family members meet with legislators or their staffers to speak directly from the talking points on their unique perspectives. Each meeting lasts about 15 minutes and usually ends with a photograph of the group and legislator.

One critical aspect of this legislative advocacy effort is to be intentional about including a follow-up plan. The legislative office provides a card with a follow-up contact, and it is important to reach out within a week or two to clarify any points or to simply offer thanks for their time and support.

In 2011 PASCPN responded to the proposed budget collapse of the sickle cell line item into a broader category line item, which would have resulted in removing dedicated funds for SCD. This issue was added to the legislative priorities that year, and as a result of educating both Democrat and Republican leaders the line item (and dedicated funding) was preserved.

This galvanized PASCPN, which continues to be successful in reaching and educating lawmakers and receiving support on issues of HU education and, most currently, addressing the effects of the opioid crisis on those in the state with SCD. Models like this help develop best practices that should be shared throughout the nation to help other states address these issues.

Sickle Cell Disease Association of Illinois

The Sickle Cell Disease Association of Illinois (SCDAI) was founded in 1971. SCDAI details a list of milestones that the organization has accomplished, including a grant awarded by HRSA to conduct NBS and a memorandum of understanding with the Illinois Department of Public Health NBS program to provide follow-up services to parents of newborns with positive SCD or SCT results. SCDAI also partners with the University of Illinois at Chicago sickle cell centers to provide free hemoglobinopathy screenings to more than 500 families, disease self-management training for individuals with SCD, and care coordination training for parents of children with SCD. The organization undertakes philanthropic and charity events, such as bowling and golfing tournaments, to raise awareness and runs an annual toy drive and holiday event to provide gifts to more than 5,000 children living with SCD (SCDAI, n.d.).

Sickle Cell Disease Association of America, Michigan Chapter, Inc.

The Sickle Cell Disease Association of America, Michigan Chapter, Inc. (SCDAAMI) provides education, social work, and care coordination services. The organization works with a psychologist and social worker at the Children's Hospital to help patients access appropriate services, including career planning, and to navigate relevant Social Security Administration programs. SCDAAMI also has camps for children aimed at fostering independence, and it receives funding from HRSA to run the NBS program in the state. The organization has several support and wellness programs for adolescents living with SCD, including Project Enrich (which provides tutors for students twice per week and offers nutritional education, yoga, and other wellness activities), and the organization also offers homework aid for hospitalized children. SCDAAMI has prepared information to educate legislators. In addition to receiving federal funding for specific programs, SCDAAMI organizes annual fundraising activities, such as walks for SCD (SCDAAMI, n.d.).

Sickle Cell Association of Texas Marc Thomas Foundation

The Sickle Cell Association of Texas Marc Thomas Foundation offers care coordination and case management services, including health screening, transportation, basic needs assistance, emergency financial assistance, and counseling (Sickle Cell Association of Texas Marc Thomas Foundation, n.d.). The organization also runs a variety of free camps targeted at different age groups, including Camp Next Level, described as a 4-day intense transitional program for 15- to 19-year-olds. The foundation also provides medical case management, screening and education for trait and disease status, and education to professionals (e.g., social workers, clinicians, and teachers) on stigma, prejudice, mental health, and ethics.

Sickle Cell Community Consortium

SCCC is a relatively young organization that originated in the 2014 Patient-Focused Drug Development Initiative from the U.S. Food and Drug Administration (FDA). The consortium was formed to "harness and amplify the power of the patient voice" (SCCC, n.d.). The consortium, in partnership with its sister organization, Sickle Cell Warriors, acts as an organizing entity for SCD CBOs, patient and caregiver advocates, community partners, and medical and research advisers, with the goal of having them work together to identify needs and gaps in the SCD community, strategies to address those needs, and the partners best positioned to implement those strategies (SCCC, n.d.). SCCC's activities are educational, and its constituents are primarily individuals and CBOs that liaise directly with the SCD population. The consortium's annual leadership summit convenes patients, caregivers, and CBOs to engage in training opportunities and lectures that are designed to equip and empower them in their advocacy work. The consortium also organizes the annual Sickle Cell Warriors Convention, with input from the patient community, which is designed to educate and empower patients, and also Warrior University, an online repository of educational resources that the SCD population and caregivers curate for the general public. It is unclear from publicly available information how the consortium funds its activities, but its annual meetings are sponsored and supported by industry partners and federal agencies.

Summary

The organizations detailed above have made enormous strides in their states in advancing the policy priorities for the SCD population, and they are making an impact in local SCD communities. Local awareness activities, such as charity walks, runs, and golf outings (especially during September, which is National Sickle Cell Disease Awareness Month, and June, which includes June 19 as World Sickle Cell Day), have still not managed to garner as much national momentum for SCD awareness as has happened for other diseases. This could be attributed to the fact that there is little to no coordination among national, state, or local organizations. In addition to the state and local SCD agencies listed on the SCDAA and CDC National Resource Directory and in Appendix K, there are many more advocacy groups online, leveraging the power of social media to spread awareness and provide patient support and education to thousands of individuals with SCD and their families.

Individuals with SCD and Their Families Advocating for Themselves

As far as empowerment, first it starts with you.

—Unknown (Open Session Participant)

Self-advocacy is the act of communicating one's needs within the scope of the issue at hand in order to have them met in a timely and appropriate manner (Ramos Salazar, 2018; Wiltshire et al., 2006). This can be applied in every aspect of life: educational, social, medical, and employment. Successful self-advocacy is based on building effective relationships with the various stakeholders who can influence or meet these needs. In the SCD community, individuals with SCD are often not viewed as "advocates" unless they speak at a conference or participate in a steering committee or professional or governmental working group. However, this belief is misguided; individuals and sometimes their caregivers may be best positioned to represent their own needs and preferences. Self-advocacy is effective because individuals understand their disease, know their body, and can articulate their symptoms, which sometimes may lead to the right diagnosis, pain relief, treatment of the underlying medical condition, and appropriate enabling services to improve QOL (Ramos Salazar, 2018; Wiltshire et al., 2006). For a caregiver's perspective, see Box 8-1.

Developing self-advocacy skills should begin early in childhood and continue throughout the life course. As discussed in Chapter 2, health literacy limitations, socioeconomic status, race, ethnicity, stigma, and discrimination are all potential impediments to effective self-advocacy for persons living with SCD. These obstacles are further reinforced by the general power imbalance within the health care system, where the power lies with the physician or other health care provider. Even in the realm of "patient-centered care," where the patient is the key member of the care team, the existing culture means that patients and their families do not have an equal voice in the decision-making process. The medical team is perceived and purported to be in charge, and it ultimately makes the key decisions, thus minimizing the emphasis on patient engagement and shared decision making in care delivery.

Another barrier to self-advocacy may be that at the point of care, in either the emergency department or the hospital, the individual with SCD

BOX 8-1
A Caregiver's Story
Andrea M.

As a mother of a child with sickle cell disease (SCD), I had a lot of questions about how services were provided to me and my family, stemming from my experience the moment that I received a phone call with the diagnosis of SCD for my youngest son. Something just didn't seem right with receiving a phone call with this incredibly disturbing news. I thought many times that there had to be a more sensitive way to deliver that message. As I tucked those feelings away, they never left me. As I look back, I realize the desire to change that one, very important moment. Later, as I sat in a class at the University of Pittsburgh as a member of the Parents' Consortium for Advocacy and Change, I learned that what I was feeling wasn't new, but it was exciting. This class was for parents of children with special needs who saw a systems-level need but lacked the experience needed to make significant change. There were about 15 parents who participated in the class. What I didn't realize right away was [that] the feeling that I had about SCD was common among other families of children who were facing a number of challenges, from autism to learning disabilities, and what we all had in common was finding our Voices, both individual and collective. I was searching for my Voice. The first book on my reading list was *Stick Your Neck Out: A Street-Smart Guide to Change in Your Community and Beyond*. I will never forget the call to action and the feeling of empowerment that rushed over my entire body as I turned each page of the self-guided manual. I became determined to learn as much as I could about SCD, from the health care providers who cared for my child to the other parents that I met in the waiting area of the sickle cell clinic. I learned that true advocacy begins with knowledge and awareness of the issues facing individuals living with SCD, their families (not just my own), [and] understanding the systems of care and the challenges that the medical teams were facing in order to care for persons with SCD. I gained knowledge, tools, and confidence to impact the sickle cell world.

---

may be too incapacitated to be effective. Even when individuals with SCD attempt to effectively self-advocate, they may be disbelieved or referred to as difficult or non-compliant, particularly with respect to pain management. It is not unusual for well-informed and activated individuals to share their individualized pain management plans with providers and, rather than be applauded for being actively engaged and invested in their chronic disease care, be accused of drug-seeking for requesting a specific pain medication, dose, and interval of administration.

The committee was unable to find any studies on self-advocacy in the SCD population. However, the patient and panelists meetings at the committee's open sessions underscored the resilience of individuals with SCD, as many of them have been able to leverage their diagnosis to become advocates for themselves and others with the disease. Research from the general patient population shows that patient self-advocacy is a predictor of patient satisfaction and is an essential skill in chronic disease management (Ramos Salazar, 2018; Wiltshire et al., 2006). One study, however, found that the African American women in the study sample were less likely to advocate for themselves than white or Hispanic women by discussing health information that they have obtained with their providers, highlighting an opportunity to equip patients to be better self-advocates (Wiltshire et al., 2006).

Other Organizations Addressing the Needs of the SCD Population

There are myriad other stakeholders that may not be formally recognized as SCD patient advocates but whose functions may confer the same benefits of patient advocacy. For example, health care professional associations may also seek to promote the well-being and interests of the patient. One example of this in SCD is the ASH Sickle Cell Disease Coalition (SCDC)—a disease-focused initiative to address the burden of SCD, both in the United States and globally. ASH established SCDC in 2016 to "help amplify the voice of the SCD stakeholder community, promote awareness, and improve outcomes for individuals with SCD" (ASH, 2017). SCDC is made up of multiple stakeholders in the SCD sphere, including patient advocacy groups. ASH's activities are multifaceted and include SCD community engagement workshops and focus groups (individuals with SCD in eight cities around the United States) to inform a handbook on the appropriate design and conduct of patient-centered clinical trials (from communications with ASH staff).

Patient advocacy groups that are not specific to SCD but that advocate for individuals with rare and inheritable diseases also contribute to the advocacy efforts for SCD. According to its website, the National Organization for Rare Diseases (NORD) works with its approximately 280 patient member organizations to offer education, advocacy, research, and patient services, with the goal of identifying, treating, and curing rare diseases, including SCD. In addition to advocating for legislation for rare diseases and provider education, NORD offers patient-specific programs, with education for patients and families, and patient services, such as financial assistance for drug access and travel and lodging assistance for clinical trials (NORD, 2020).

The Genetic Alliance is another national organization that supports individuals, families, and communities affected by rare genetic diseases. It advocates for these rare disease populations and connects individuals to advocacy outlets that help make their voices heard. The Genetic Alliance has a research arm that ensures that patient groups and activated communities are truly leading and driving the research effort. It supports its own bio-bank, institutional review board, patient registry, and engagement platform and provides education and advocacy support for organizations to foster participants becoming research drivers.

CHALLENGES FACED BY SICKLE CELL ADVOCATES AND GROUPS

Individuals and organizations advocating for the population of individuals living with SCD face several obstacles that may limit their effectiveness in accomplishing their goals. The first obstacle, which was alluded to earlier in this chapter, is that many of these organizations operate at the local level and in silos and are thus unable to effect change at the broader level. Currently, none of the SCD CBOs or patient advocacy groups are empowered to influence change for all aspects of the population's needs, in contrast with groups focused on hemophilia and cystic fibrosis (CF), as discussed later in this chapter. The other barriers pertain to a lack of human and financial resources.

Financial Sustainability

To diversify funding sources for CBOs and SCD advocacy groups, outreach has to be deliberate and focused.

—Derek R. (Open Session Panelist)

The sources of funding for SCD CBOs and patient advocacy groups are few and fail to provide sustainability. These organizations may be funded by federal grants, state entities, the pharmaceutical industry, or charitable events (see Figure 8-3).

Some CBOs and patient advocacy groups receive funding from the federal government in the form of grants for specific projects. In 2017, SCDAA was awarded a $11.6 million, 4-year grant through HRSA (HRSA, 2016); SCDAA also works as the National Coordinating Center to provide technical assistance to 15 CBOs that are sub-awardees to the HRSA grant. The CBOs, including SCFGA, SCDAA–Mobile Chapter in Alabama, Sickle Cell Disease Association of America/Ohio Sickle Cell and Health Association, and the Children's Sickle Cell Foundation, collaborate with other organizations in their states to conduct NBS follow-up to ensure that individuals diagnosed with SCD are appropriately referred to and are receiving necessary services, such as counseling, education, and other enabling services (SCDAA, n.d.). Grants such as HRSA's NBS follow-up program are time-bound, so there is no continuity, and funding for the programming

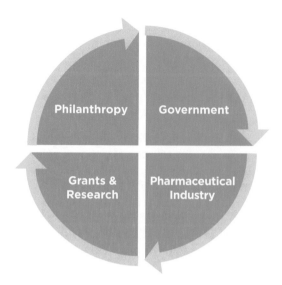

FIGURE 8-3 Funding sources for SCD patient organizations.
NOTE: Funding from the sources is not proportional.

ends when the grant period does, fostering discontinuity if grants are not renewed. HRSA also funds the five regional collaboratives through the SCDTDRCP. Each collaborative is composed of a range of partners, including CBOs working on the grant goals of improving access to high-quality comprehensive SCD care, provider training, and data collection on SCD quality metrics (PSCRC, 2019).

Collaborative efforts between the two groups are difficult to discern. The role of CBOs within SCDTDRCP varies across the five regional collaboratives. Grant support is usually allocated for specific programs and does not pay for hiring staff or capacity building. The funding available to CBOs through these grants is limited, which promotes competition. The federal grant process also excludes many CBOs because they do not have the appropriate fiduciary infrastructure or staff with the grant writing skills to develop a competitive application in response to a call for proposals.

Some CBOs and patient advocacy groups receive state funding, including SCFGA (Georgia), Piedmont Health Services and Sickle Cell Agency (North Carolina), and SCDAAMI. Most state funds are also for specific programs and do not facilitate capacity building to support the myriad of other services needed by the local SCD population.

The pharmaceutical industry is also a funding source for several SCD CBOs and advocacy groups. Most often, these organizations provide support for specific programs, such as conferences or workshops. For instance,

SCDAAMI lists Sanofi, Genzyme, Emmaus, Pfizer, and other pharmaceutical companies as sponsors on its website (SCDAAMI, n.d.). Certain pharmaceutical companies also have set aside funds that they make available to CBOs through competitive grants. The Access to Excellent Care for Sickle Cell Patients Pilot Program through Global Blood Therapeutics (GBT) is one such example; it provides up to $50,000 during a 12-month period to CBOs and patient advocacy groups serving individuals with SCD and their families with the aim of piloting a variety of models to deliver high-quality health care (GBT, n.d.). Pilots may be focused on expanding CBO capacity by partnering with federally qualified health centers, improving transition from pediatric to adult care, and innovative training programs for clinicians. Novartis also announced the Solutions to Empower Patients (STEP) program in 2018, which provided up to $50,000 to encourage CBOs, patient advocacy groups, and other entities to innovate. The preceding year's STEP grants were targeted at organizations for metastatic breast cancer (Novartis, 2018), indicating that the funding source is not specific to SCD and likely not a long-term source of funding. Some have highlighted the inherent conflict that CBOs and SCD patient advocacy groups face in relying on pharmaceutical companies because the funds may not support their programmatic needs. Finally, CBOs and patient advocacy organizations may also fundraise through charity events, such as annual galas, sports events, and conferences.

In summary, there are a variety of ways that these CBOs and other nonprofits support their activities. These funding mechanisms are not robust, available funds are limited for a defined range of activities, and they are possibly unable to support much needed organizational development to help CBOs scale their services to reach more individuals. As a result, these funding opportunities may inadvertently lead to mission creep, fragmentation, and inefficiency. It is important that SCD advocacy groups remain mission-focused, but this is a current challenge. Thus, there is a need to diversify funding sources at all levels—federal, state, and private— and to identify dedicated sources of funding that will support sustained programming.

Infrastructure

Most CBOs and patient advocacy groups operate with very few staff and rely on volunteers for their daily operations and activities. The challenge with this model is that programming is contingent on volunteer availability. In 2018 SCFGA reported using 3,990 (750 non-camp) hours of donated time (3–100 hours per volunteer) (SCFGA, 2018). The limited staffing levels also mean that the organization may not have the necessary expertise for its programming, including not having enough adequately

trained staff to provide patient and community education, sufficient CHWs
to conduct outreach in the community, the necessary expertise for grant
writing and fundraising, or other core capabilities necessary for success.
CBOs should have access to technical support that broadens staff skills
and services. Programs are needed to support grant writing, budgeting and
finances, legal counseling, client engagement, care coordination, and support for research participation.

Individual Challenges

Patient advocates may face a number of challenges as well. Some advocates may be worried that their activities will disrupt their relationship with
their health care providers. In a focus group with ovarian cancer patients,
for example, those who wanted to self-advocate identified locating relevant
health information as one of their major challenges and also expressed hesitation at taking any action that might upset their relationships with their
health care providers (Hagan and Medberry, 2016). Yet, data suggest that
patient self-advocacy is a predictor of patient satisfaction. A 2018 study of
522 patients found that patients' education about their disease and their
ability to assert their needs positively influenced their satisfaction with their
physicians (Ramos Salazar, 2018). This finding has important implications
for the SCD population, considering the issues with the patient–provider
relationship that were discussed in Chapter 2. Second, advocates often carry
out their activities in addition to their current work and life responsibilities.
This may lead to their involvement waxing and waning over time, as they
may have limited time or energy for advocacy activities at times. Third,
advocates living with SCD may find that their health affects their ability to
participate in advocacy activities.

MODELS OF PATIENT ADVOCACY FROM
OTHER RARE DISEASES

Two diseases referred to throughout this report, hemophilia and CF,
offer valuable models for patient advocacy and community engagement
for the SCD population. However, the trajectory of these diseases has been
different from that of SCD, so these models may not be entirely applicable.
Some of what distinguishes these diseases from SCD is the minimal role the
pharmaceutical industry has played in SCD, in part because the mainstay
drugs for the disease (penicillin and HU) were generic when adopted for
SCD. Both hemophilia and CF provide important examples about patient
advocacy for rare diseases.

Chelation therapies are the primary agents developed in the past
two decades in which the SCD community has interacted directly with

the pharmaceutical industry. It is worth considering how patient advocacy has contributed to the awareness, funding levels for research and patient services, and improvements for individuals living with the conditions and addressing components that could pertain to SCD.

Hemophilia

Hemophilia is an inheritable blood disorder that prevents the blood from clotting, ultimately causing severe bleeding from any minor injury. Because hemophilia has no cure, it requires constant, high-quality care from providers at hemophilia treatment centers (HTCs), which are partially funded by CDC, HRSA, MCHB of HRSA, and other federal agencies. The pharmaceutical industry has partnered with the hemophilia organizations for more than four decades in developing agents to ameliorate hemophilia complications. CDC funding supports programs for research, surveillance, and prevention for bleeding and clotting disorders (NHF, 2020d). HTCs are unique in that they provide comprehensive specialty care for hemophilia and related disorders and also function as an additional resource for a primary care provider (PCP), dentist, or other specialist to ensure best care practices. HTCs provide genetic counseling, medical and psychosocial care, and other services to patients and their families.

The Hemophilia Patient Advocacy Model

The hemophilia patient support landscape is dominated by four well-known organizations: the National Hemophilia Foundation (NHF), the Coalition for Hemophilia B, the Hemophilia Federation of America (HFA), and the World Federation of Hemophilia (WFH) (Azevedo, 2017). As its name suggests, the Coalition for Hemophilia B focuses on treatment and improving the QOL for individuals with hemophilia B. The discussion in this section focuses on the other three organizations whose efforts are targeted at individuals with all forms of hemophilia.

Global efforts WFH, which leads global advocacy efforts for hemophilia, was established in 1963 to improve care and treatment globally. The founding patient associations for WFH included groups from Argentina, Australia, Belgium, Canada, Denmark, France, Germany, Japan, the Netherlands, Sweden, the United Kingdom, and the United States (WFH, 2020b). WFH established its global presence when it became a member of the World Health Organization in 1969. In 2019 WFH had programs in 22 countries (excluding the United States) in 6 regions of the world, with objectives organized around the six key areas in its comprehensive development model: government support, care delivery, medical expertise and laboratory diagnosis, treatment products, patient organization, and data collection and outcomes research (WFH, 2020a). WFH's work in the United States is conducted through WFH USA, its U.S. affiliate. The two entities collaborate on the other WFH programs: humanitarian aid, research and data collection, and training and education. As part of the humanitarian aid program, WFH distributes donated pharmaceutical products to individuals with hemophilia in developing nations. The World Bleeding Disorders Registry (WBDR), a longitudinal, prospective patient registry that provides patient-level clinical and outcome data, was established in 2018 as part of WFH's research and data collection efforts. WBDR issued its first report in May 2019 (WFH, 2020c). WFH uses WBDR data collected to strengthen its efforts to educate key stakeholders and generate awareness about the needs of the hemophilia population (WFH USA, 2020). Finally, WFH training and education efforts focus on training health care professionals and community leaders through workshops delivered primarily through its eLearning platform.

WFH and WFH USA's work is bolstered by in-kind medication and financial donations by partners such as Sanofi Genzyme, Sobi, CSL Behring, GC Pharma, and Grifols (WFH USA, 2018). Products donated to WFH and WFH USA in 2018 totaled approximately $378 million. Financial donations from corporate and community partners in 2018 totaled approximately $1.57 million (WFH USA, 2018). WFH USA partners with members of NHF through the NHF Chapter Challenge, which asks NHF chapters to provide support for the WFH humanitarian aid program. Since its launch in 2016, the NHF Chapter Challenge has raised $482,462 (WFH USA, 2018).

Efforts in the United States The other two main organizations working to support individuals with hemophilia in the United States are NHF and HFA. Established in 1948, NHF is the oldest organization advancing awareness and promoting better treatment and cures. It is believed to have made substantial contributions to improving awareness for hemophilia, including advocating for more resources for research, encouraging access to high-quality care, and providing patient and family support.

When the organization was established, the life expectancy for hemophilia was approximately 30 years; with access to appropriate therapy, life expectancy is now normal. NHF has a national, state, and local presence through its 51 nationwide chapter affiliates, 7 of which are owned by the foundation (NHF, 2017).

At a broader level, NHF and chapter organizations' activities focus on ensuring better treatments and a cure for inheritable bleeding disorders through education, research, and advocacy. NHF has initiatives in state and federal legislation on access to health care, payer education, educating workers and the public, and other advocacy issues. The foundation also promotes shared decision making between physicians and patients, family support networks that pair patients with mentors for peer support, community groups that provide support and education, and self-infusion. At the state level, NHF monitors issues of priority to the hemophilia population, such as Medicaid-managed care to ensure that costs remain affordable (NHF, 2020a). It also provides training and strategic planning courses to state hemophilia chapters and coalitions.

NHF has been instrumental in advancing the organization and delivery of high-quality care nationwide. In 1973 NHF spearheaded a 2-year campaign that led to creating the network of comprehensive HTCs (NHF, 2020b). Currently, there are 141 HTCs that are part of the U.S. Hemophilia Treatment Center Network providing comprehensive care to individuals with hemophilia throughout the United States and its territories (CDC, 2018a) (see Chapter 5 for the hemophilia care model). Since 1974, Congress has supported the HTCs through HRSA to provide "comprehensive multidisciplinary services not typically covered by insurance, such as physical therapy assessments, social work, and case management services," and through CDC to "support research, surveillance, and prevention for bleeding and clotting disorders, including hemophilia" (NHF, 2020d). The NHF Medical and Scientific Advisory Council (MASAC), a group of expert scientists, physicians, allied health professionals, patients, and government liaisons from the relevant federal agencies within the U.S. Department of Health and Human Services, advances the standard of clinical care and issues treatment recommendations for all bleeding disorders (NHF, 2020c). "MASAC guidelines [issued as recommendations] set the standard of care and are frequently referred to by an international array of physicians, medical schools, pharmacists, emergency room personnel, insurance companies, patients, and others" (Skinner et al., 2014, p. e545).

NHF also promotes the interests of individuals with hemophilia and their families by partnering with affiliated chapters to develop policy agendas at the federal and state levels on issues pertaining to "improved access to high-quality medical care, a safe blood supply, access to the full range of safe and effective treatments, adequate reimbursement at the public and private levels, and expanded federal funding for hemophilia treatment centers" (NHF, 2020c). These agendas are used to guide the organization's educational, policy making, and public awareness campaigns and other activities. NHF supports chapters in serving their local communities, including liaising to build relationships between chapters and HTCs, providing grants for educational programs and staffing, and assisting with grant writing. NHF also offers national, regional, and local training to chapters (NHF, 2020c).

According to its 2017 financial statements, NHF's activities are funded primarily by pharmaceutical companies (82 percent of revenues) (NHF, 2018), and the organization has reported net assets of $23,210,450.

HFA was established in 1994 to "address the evolving needs of the bleeding disorders community" (HFA, n.d.), triggered by the contamination of blood products in the late 1970s through mid-1980s with HIV and the hepatitis C virus (HCV), which posed a particular burden for individuals with bleeding disorders. In the 1980s approximately 90 percent of people with severe hemophilia were infected with HIV, and almost all people living with hemophilia who used factor products before 1988 were infected with HCV, complicating their care (HFA, n.d.). HFA's goal was to create a voice for the patient in light of this devastation to the hemophilia population. Many of HFA's programming and educational activities mirror those undertaken by NHF. In fact, the majority, if not all, of the 40 state and local CBOs that are HFA members are also part of NHF. NHF and HFA release joint statements on key policy issues pertaining to the hemophilia population and in accordance with their missions. The reported net assets for HFA in 2017 were $5,422,183 (HFA, 2017). In 2010 the HFA board of directors reversed the association's stance of refusing funding from pharmaceutical companies producing therapeutic products for hemophilia; it currently lists Takeda, Genentech, Bayer Healthcare, CSL Behring, Novo Nordisk, Sanofi Genzyme, HEMA Biologics, Kedrion Biopharma, and Pfizer Rare Disease among its top supporters.

Key Takeaways from Hemophilia Patient Organizations for SCD

There are factors that have contributed to the effectiveness of CBOs and national organizations serving the hemophilia population. Some of these may not immediately be applicable to SCD organizations, but hemophilia organizations had to overcome challenges with public awareness, patient and provider education, lack of funding, and accessing high-quality, comprehensive care similar to those that now confront the SCD population, so there are some worthy takeaways that could inform the patient advocacy landscape for SCD.

Defined leadership and concerted efforts There are several organizations working independently to promote research, education, and care and to meet the overall needs of individuals with hemophilia, but the three organizations discussed in this section emerge as leading these efforts in the United States and globally. CBOs that support the needs of children and adults with hemophilia and their families at the state and local levels also work closely with these organizations to ensure a unified voice in messaging and education to policy makers, providers, and other relevant stakeholders. NHF is also influential in informing high-quality care through MASAC, which sets clinical guidelines. The coordinated efforts of hemophilia organizations are evident even at the state level, as demonstrated by the Hemophilia Council of California (Hemophilia Council of California, n.d.). SCD CBOs and their patient advocacy efforts are currently siloed, with no organizational model of how the national, state, local, and virtual organizations are working together to address the shared goal of advancing important issues. The result is duplicated efforts, diversification of the limited resources that exist, and a lack of a unified voice and message in support of the SCD population.

Funding In 2018 there were an estimated 28 different hemophilia drugs available in the United States, with another 21 in development (Terry, 2018). The number of pharmaceutical companies engaged in therapeutic development for hemophilia is a source of support for the relevant CBOs and patient advocacy groups. The public awareness that hemophilia has gained over the decades has also translated into additional financial support for research and other activities.

In contrast, most funding for SCD patient advocacy is from federal sources in the form of grants for specific projects rather than organizational development, capacity building, and programming. Some pharmaceutical companies, such as GBT and Novartis, are funding SCD CBOs' work, but these funds are still limited, competitive, and available to only a few organizations. There is the potential for diversified sources of financial support—both private and federal—for SCD patient organizations. Public awareness, education, and understanding of SCD and the burden on the community could generate more private-sector support for SCD organizations. As mentioned, the lack of a defined model of organization and centralized leadership for SCD CBO efforts is a potential impediment.

Role within the care delivery system for hemophilia Creating HTCs and the definition of standards of care delivered by HTCs established hemophilia CBOs as part of the hemophilia ecosystem. *Standards and Criteria for the Care of Persons with Congenital Bleeding Disorders*, published by NHF's MASAC, identifies opportunities to engage CBOs in health care (NHF, 2002). For example, the standards call for enhanced communication among the health care team and patients, consultants, PCPs, and other community-based health care workers to support the patient's needs; for the establishment of a community network to link CBOs with HTCs to maximize resources and minimize duplication of services; and for referrals from HTCs, with the consent of the patient, to social services and CBOs that are positioned to address basic human needs, such as food, clothing, and transportation (NHF, 2002). Currently, SCD CBOs operate in parallel with the health care system. Health system–based social workers and CHWs provide supportive functions to individuals living with SCD, but most are also mired in administrative activities, care for a full panel of patients, and are unable to dedicate sufficient attention to SCD individuals' needs. CBOs and their staff are best positioned to support their patients as they transition out of the health care system into the community. However, there is a void between the health system and the community-based resources that partially results from the lack of a unified effort among organizations serving the SCD population, thereby making it difficult to identify the appropriate CBOs for handoff. A well-defined model of organization for CBOs and other organizations will streamline efforts and offer guidance for how to leverage their capabilities in the comprehensive care model proposed by the committee in this report.

Policy and historical impetus for action Finally, it is worth noting that several policy and historical events have contributed to the effectiveness of hemophilia patient advocacy and community groups. Congress authorized funding in 1975 to establish comprehensive hemophilia clinics, which was later expanded; that was influenced by—but also spurred on—the efforts to improve care and outcomes. The AIDS and hepatitis C crises in the later 1970s and the 1980s also galvanized efforts by creating urgency for improved testing for clotting agents and empowering individuals living with hemophilia and communities to advocate for themselves (Baker et al., 2005). These events cannot be replicated for SCD, but SCD may be at a tipping point. CBOs and patient groups are best positioned to engage with the efforts related to several therapeutic products in the pipeline, the move for universal curative therapies (which will necessitate patient and provider education about scientific developments to inform treatment decision making), and the need to ensure access to beneficial therapeutic products that will soon arrive on the market.

Cystic Fibrosis

The CF community is small but highly active, thanks in part to the national patient advocacy group. The Cystic Fibrosis Foundation (CFF) was established in 1955, when affected individuals were not expected to survive childhood. As of 2012, life expectancy was approximately 41 years because of CFF's activities to find a cure and prolong healthy lives (CFF, n.d.f; Mogayzel et al., 2014). CFF leads efforts to improve care, to increase access to beneficial therapies, to increase public education and awareness, and to improve the delivery of support services. CFF differs from other patient advocacy groups in that it directly oversees aspects of the care organization and of the delivery, data collection, therapeutic product development, and services for health-related social needs.

The CF Care Center Network was established in 1961 when CFF accredited two CF centers based on criteria established by its center committee, which developed the standards for care, research, and teaching that each center must implement and sustain for accreditation. These requirements included convening a team of experts to treat inpatient and outpatient clinical needs, implementing care guidelines developed by CF clinical experts, and treating people with CF to improve the knowledge of the center's medical team (Mogayzel et al., 2014). In 2019 there were more than 130 care centers (CFF, n.d.b), which are reviewed each year and undergo periodic visits from the center committee to maintain accreditation. CFF also funds care centers to enable them to participate in clinical research and in training multidisciplinary care teams about clinical best practices.

In 1966 CFF created a patient registry to collect data with which to track the impact of the CF care standards on individuals' health. Providers at the care centers enter health data on consenting patients. Today the patient registry provides key information to the care centers and the CF community about the natural history of the disease, its complications, the impact of care delivery, and important clinical outcomes. This information feeds into the creation of a learning health system, where real-time data are used to refine and improve clinical care. Factors identified as important for survival, such as CF-related diabetes, nutrition, and lung function, then inform the quality improvement efforts at the care centers (Mogayzel et al., 2014).

CFF launched into drug development in 2000 when it provided investments to the first pharmaceutical manufacturer to conduct research to identify compounds that might alter genetic errors in people with CF (CFF, n.d.c). This investment began CFF's venture philanthropy model for drug development. The impetus for this model was the lack of progress made by the late 1990s in developing therapeutic products that addressed the underlying cause of the disease (CFF, n.d.c). As is the case with most rare diseases, most pharmaceutical companies were reluctant to invest time and resources into clinical research to identify therapies that would benefit only a small population. The venture philanthropy model was CFF's response to that obstacle: funding drug development with for-profit companies. Since the initial investment, CFF has funded several biopharmaceutical companies, including Pfizer, Genzyme, Editas, and Corbus, and invested $425 million to accelerate drug development for CF (CFF, n.d.c). CFF's investment has led to the approval of several drugs, with many more in the pipeline (CFF, n.d.e). The venture philanthropy model has also funded CFF for further research, the care centers, and services to the CF population. CFF enters into agreements with drug companies in which it invests to receive royalties related to drugs developed as a result of its funding (CFF, n.d.e). This model, with CFF taking the lead in funding drug development and using the payoff from its investments to underwrite its activities, is unique because the drug development function has traditionally been kept separate from other functions in health care in order to protect the patient's interests.

The drug development process is the main source of funding for CFF. In 2014 CFF "sold royalty rights for CF treatments developed by Vertex for $3.3 billion" (CFF, n.d.c), making it the nation's largest disease-focused charity by net assets (Tozzi, 2015). In 2018 CFF also raised more than $80 million from the CF community in the form of charity events, such as walks and golf outings (Tozzi, 2015).

CFF is actively involved in funding health-related services for individuals with CF and their families through its Compass program, which helps individuals with CF navigate insurance requirements; identify financial resources to defray copays, deductibles, and other financial obstacles to accessing care; apply for benefits, including Social Security and disability; acquire legal information for employment, education, and other government benefits; and identify resources to address a variety of social determinants of health, including transportation to and from care, and housing, living, and food expenses (CFF, n.d.d).

CFF works with its 70 chapters and branch offices across the country to raise funds and support the CF community. However, it is unclear from the publicly available information how the chapters are organized and operate in conjunction with CFF.

CFF, care centers, and chapters are actively involved in generating awareness and working at all levels of government to shape public policy and increase awareness resources. At the federal level CFF has pushed for expanded funding for NIH and FDA to support basic and translational research and requested greater resources for the drug approval process, which increases the chances of finding a cure. At the state level, CFF joined forces with CF care centers and patient advocates around the United States to rally for programs like Medicaid to express the need for constructive insurance coverage policies for care and therapies. The organization spoke to lawmakers about the complications of CF and the need for access to the appropriate treatments. In addition, it also turned its focus to legislation that influenced health programs essential to high-quality CF care (CFF, n.d.a).

Public awareness of CF has been bolstered by the influence of high-profile personalities. Canadian singer Celine Dion has been an advocate, dedicating her time and money to the CF community in Canada for more than 30 years (Global Genes, 2015). The tragic loss of her niece at the age of 16 to CF sparked her to become an advocate for the CF community. She has appeared in multiple CF campaigns and is a known advocate for CF NBS. Dion has pressed lawmakers to support efforts for NBS through service announcements and public appearances, hosted benefit concerts and galas, and donated much of her personal funds toward research and awareness (Global Genes, 2015). During his 2015 State of the Union address,

President Obama "cited the story of CF as an example of how nonprofits, the pharmaceutical industry, researchers, patients, and their families can work together to produce more targeted and effective treatments for diseases" (CFF, n.d.c).

Key Takeaways from Cystic Fibrosis Patient Organizations for SCD

The CFF model of patient advocacy is unique in its scope of activities and also reflects a model for how patient advocacy groups can drive efforts in response to the perceived needs, as opposed to change being driven by external factors. This model is not entirely replicable because of the level of risk that the organization assumes. The CFF venture philanthropy model is now emulated by organizations for other rare diseases, and NIH has adopted CFF's strategies to advance drug development for rare diseases.

The influx of pharmaceutical companies into therapeutic development for CF means that this approach is probably not warranted for SCD. However, there is an opportunity for CBOs and other organizations working to create awareness for and address the needs of the SCD population to actively define and shape the provision of high-quality care for the SCD population. Some organizations, such as ASH, have taken steps by developing clinical practice guidelines for SCD care, but there is currently no mechanism to translate these guidelines into practice (see Chapter 6). The disparate efforts under way with multiple organizations are also a potential barrier to meaningfully influencing care, outcomes, and change for the SCD population.

OPPORTUNITIES TO MOVE FROM LOCAL
TO SYSTEM-LEVEL CHANGE

*If you're going to advocate for something, I would advocate for
more than minimal.*

—Amy S. (Open Session Panelist)

Patient advocacy groups and CBOs clearly play an integral role in SCD, providing the necessary health-related services; educating individuals and their families, providers, legislators, and other key stakeholders; and helping to generate awareness in the process. There is an opportunity to leverage these organizations as key stakeholders in any action to improve care and outcomes, especially in delivering the comprehensive, person-centric care that the committee recommends. There are four opportunities to establish CBOs and patient advocacy groups as key stakeholders in SCD action.

Integrate Community-Based Organizations and Advocacy Groups as an Integral Part of the Care Delivery Process

You have to have support; even if you don't have family that understands, having a community of support is integral.

—Tosin O. (Open Session Panelist)

CBOs and patient advocacy groups are already actively contributing to the care delivery process, from the initial stages (identifying individuals who screened positive for SCD or SCT for clinical follow-up), to CHWs entering the community to assist individuals who are unable to reach care, to providing education to help individuals manage their care. This role can be strengthened through formalized handoffs from the health care system to the community and vice versa. Health system–based CHWs and social workers primarily assist individuals with navigating insurance and scheduling appointments. However, their role does not extend into the community because they cannot follow individuals after they leave the health care system. CBOs could take over once a person is back in the community. Formal handoffs will ensure that no one is lost after departing the health care system. By having a community partner assist, individuals with SCD may also be able to effectively manage their care and minimize disease complications.

Leverage Community-Based Organizations and Advocacy Groups to Address the Social Needs of Individuals Living with SCD

There is also an opportunity to leverage the strength of CBOs and advocacy groups in addressing the social and health-related needs of individuals with SCD and their families. Most CBOs are already addressing these needs but are limited in their ability to do so due to the aforementioned challenges.

Integrate Community-Based Organizations and Advocacy Groups into Clinical Trials and Research Processes

It is necessary to create opportunities for advocacy groups to be an important part of the care delivery and research process—from helping to inform clinical trial design and recruitment to facilitating patient access to health care services.

TABLE 8-2 Proposed Classification System for Stratification of Services Provided by an SCD Community-Based Organization

	Advocacy and Awareness	Genetic Counseling and Screening Education	Direct Enabling Services
Tier A	Engage a professional in lobbying efforts as a consultant or staff	Health professional for oversight of certified genetic counselors' onsite screening; organized education and oversight for genetic counseling	Care coordination, referral to medical home, transportation, and other resources
Tier B	Organize state-level advocacy efforts	Trait testing on site, state newborn screening follow-up, and certified genetic counselors	Transportation services, case finding, and referral to medical home
Tier C	Hold periodic local awareness events	Referral to state department for testing and education about sickle cell disease/sickle cell trait	Referrals to community resources

Standardize Structure for SCD Community-Based Organizations and Patient Organizations

There is a need for a system that classifies SCD CBOs according to the type and breadth of services provided. Table 8-2 categorizes the range of services that CBOs may provide, including advocacy and awareness (e.g., health fairs, SCD/SCT awareness events, national lobbying), education and counseling (e.g., trait testing on site, NBS tracking and follow-up referrals, health professional on site to provide complex genetic counseling), direct enabling (e.g., direct care coordination, transportation, funeral support, utilities), and a combination of any of the above. These services are arranged in tiers, with Tier A representing the highest level and breadth of service delivery. (A CBO in Tier A could also incorporate components from Tiers B and C.)

Classifying CBOs by their capabilities and activities also streamlines outreach by patients, funders, and health care systems, which are able to identify the patient organizations best positioned for different functions. Finally, a classification system could eliminate the siloing of CBOs and SCD patient organizations by helping those performing different functions to learn from each other and share best practices. The absence of a unified voice is one reason for a lack of meaningful impact at a broader level for SCD advocacy groups.

SUMMARY

This chapter summarizes the historical context surrounding the establishment of the SCD CBO and patient advocacy groups for SCD and describes the evolving landscape of SCD CBOs, with a combination of the traditional CBO model, hybrid models that include individual advocates and support groups, and a primarily virtual model. The chapter also details the various services and initiatives currently in the scope of work of SCD CBOs and patient groups, underlining the fact that there is currently no formal classification system or standardization process of protocols that is universally used among these organizations. Because SCD is by its nature influenced by stigma, racism, and discrimination, this report is not complete without a uniquely defined role for the cultural brokers within the SCD community, the CBOs, or patient advocates.

The committee acknowledges that SCD CBOs provide enabling services that support the physical, mental, and social health of individuals affected by SCD; however, despite their critical importance in the cultural broker- age ecosystem, SCD CBOs are primarily under-resourced in the African American community, underfunded, and dependent on fundraising for their existence, as the business model is focused more on finding funds than on planning activities and then seeking funding sources consistent with those activities. There is a need to identify a sustainable funding mechanism to support the continued existence of SCD CBOs in order to reverse the cur- rent fragmentation resulting from a lack of sustainable funding and a stan- dard classification system. CBOs will need a concerted initiative to build consistent and measurable infrastructure, to develop a clear definition of their scope of services based on infrastructure capacity, and build the neces- sary skills to foster the sustainability of the newly acquired infrastructure.

Finally, an SCD CBO will best thrive in an environment of trust, respect, and equal partnership with other stakeholders in the SCD com- munity. Currently, SCD CBOs struggle to gain recognition from health care systems, state health departments, and local hospitals, largely due to variations in services, an under-resourced infrastructure, and a lack of transparency regarding governance, mission, and fiduciary responsibility. This creates challenges for partnerships at every level, leading to a vicious cycle of continued lack of funding and resources. There is criticism over what SCD CBOs do not provide for their communities when very few have access to the skills and resources needed to brand their organizations, publicize their work, and publish data on their programs. When hospitals do not trust CBOs to provide enabling services and social support, the hospitals work to create them internally. This further stresses the partner- ships between stakeholders and CBOs because hospital-based entities are competing for funding through grants and philanthropy.

These challenges are not unique to the SCD community. Therefore, solutions from other chronic diseases should be considered when trying to plan future efforts. One of the initial steps to improving the ability of SCD CBOs to develop long-lasting, proactive partnerships will be to rely on a national organization that can validate their capabilities and services. This organization could be similar to NHF in structure, provide funding and technical assistance to local member CBOs according to a classification system, and meet certain criteria, including those based on the skill sets of CBO staff. The certification of genetic counselors and CHWs, already existing for SCD, could be expanded and incorporated into criteria for accreditation, with the appropriate required recertification to remain up to date in the knowledge base and the appropriate oversight to ensure counseling competency.

Ideally, this national organization would work to build relationships with other community members, such as health care systems, thereby facilitating partnerships at the local level that would be strategically positioned in communities that contain large numbers of individuals living with SCD. If an organization develops infrastructure, outlines mission-driven programs and services with transparent measurable objectives, trains and certifies staff, and receives accreditation from the national organization, that will bolster the foundation for building a healthy respectful partnership. Maintaining certification and accreditation will require a bidirectional flow of funds between the local and the national organizations. However, federal, private industry, third-party payers, and health system funding, primarily driven from the national level down, will alleviate some of the burden for fundraising at the local level. Quality metrics developed for accreditation will encourage SCD CBOs to collect and store programmatic and service data for reporting. This will help in making CBO-specific data public so that individuals living with SCD can identify the CBOs that provide the services they need. This information will be useful for not only consumer use but also organizational strategic planning, policy development, branding, and marketing. This would further "legitimize" the SCD CBOs among SCD stakeholders broadly and help establish CBO participation in SCD learning networks as valid team members in service provision, patient engagement, and information dissemination.

Community expectations for SCD CBOs are daunting (see this chapter's introduction). Developing the capacity of the national organization for technical assistance in all areas will require tremendous commitment, dedication, resources, and funding. In the past, funding at the national and local levels for SCD programming and initiatives has come through grants and direct gifts, which are difficult to sustain due to competition. The SCD community will realize that collaboration and partnership must culminate in supporting one or two national or "umbrella" CBOs. The CF and hemophilia communities have handled this well, and available funding is robust. However, in the SCD community funding is sparse, largely due to the minimal development of drugs and technologies. When adopted for use in SCD, penicillin and HU were generic, and procedures (e.g., apheresis) and laboratory tests (e.g., high-performance liquid chromatography) were fully developed. Recently, SCD drug development has soared. This provides an opportunity for new resources and funding mechanisms for CBOs. All stakeholders might benefit if a well-positioned national organization were to establish a transparent mechanism to fund virtual and local CBOs and measure, monitor, and track how they help children and adults with SCD.

Role of the SCD Community-Based Organization in a National Awareness Campaign

Education and awareness gaps remain in the SCD community, and there is a dire need for robust educational campaigns to address this limited understanding about the origins, impact, and consequences of SCD and the difference between SCD and SCT to avoid a recurrence of the damage done in the 1970s by the poor planning and execution of the SC clinics. An awareness campaign is clearly necessary, in part to dispel the myth in the African American community and beyond that SCD has "gone away" because they do not hear about it anymore. CBOs could play a key role, particularly if a unified message adopted by all stakeholders could be used as the primary campaign message.

The attention that new drugs and curative therapies will bring could be harnessed into messaging, thus procuring funding and resources from private industry. A well-designed campaign would be broad, dispel myths and stigma, attract positive attention, and work to unite the community. Recent media attention has not resulted in positive feedback from adults with SCD and caregivers of children. Awareness "messaging" will require full participation from those affected by SCD, those working toward improving their QOL, and media and news production professionals who understand the African American and Latinx American communities to determine how messaging may be best received by the public. In the interim, targeting inclusion in other public awareness campaigns will improve exposure. For example, CDC sponsors a campaign, Self-Management Education: Learn More, Feel Better, to increase public awareness of disease self-management education that could easily incorporate SCD (CDC, 2018b).

Targeting dissemination in the SCD community would increase awareness of self-management education in the community and also the visibility of SCD in the broader CDC and U.S. chronic illness community. Another example is the #MAKEITVISIBLE movement of the U.S. Pain Society (U.S. Pain Foundation, 2017). Improving the ability to partner with others in chronic illness awareness may benefit the SCD community and foster partnerships at the national and local levels.

National and local projects to raise awareness should identify and address barriers at each level: individuals with SCD and their families, systems of care, and urban and rural communities. Literacy skills and unequal access to resources must be considered. Campaigns should be within the framework of health promotion but tempered with compassion when discussing prevention, so as not to further stigmatize those living with SCD. National mass media campaigns should be synergistic and consistent with longer-term local CBO action and patient engagement initiatives.

Finally, it is important to recognize the role of the virtual SCD CBO and advocacy groups in supporting awareness, advocacy, and education to help eliminate the isolation that individuals with SCD experience around not just their disease but being involved with and invited to participate in interventions to improve and support SCD. The mantra "Nothing for us without us" should be taken literally when addressing a strategic plan and action blueprint for SCD. There are a vast number of "invisible warriors," individuals living with SCD and SCT who are not in formal advocacy or community groups but find their sense of community via Facebook, Instagram, Snapchat, and other virtual platforms. They are the informal grassroots network of SCD advocates who should intentionally be sought out, albeit via nontraditional means, and their voice should be included in defining the way forward.

CONCLUSIONS AND RECOMMENDATIONS

Conclusion 8-1: SCD CBOs provide enabling services that support the physical, mental, and social health of individuals affected by SCD; however, despite their critical importance in the cultural brokerage ecosystem, SCD CBOs are primarily under-resourced in the African American community, under-funded, and dependent on fundraising for their existence, as the business model is focused more on finding funds than planning activities and finding funding sources consistent with those activities.

Conclusion 8-2: Funding mechanisms for SCD CBOs and patient organizations are not sustainable and competitive.

Conclusion 8-3: The current organization and structure of SCD CBOs is fractured and fragmented, thereby resulting in inefficiencies and duplication of activities. There is a need for a clear definition of scope of services based on infrastructure capacity and skill building to foster the sustainability of the newly acquired infrastructure.

Conclusion 8-4: Despite the role they play in serving as a liaison between the health system and community resources for individuals with SCD, currently SCD CBOs struggle to gain recognition from health care systems, state health departments, and local hospitals, largely due to variation in services, under-resourced infrastructure, and transparency regarding governance, mission, and fiduciary responsibility.

Recommendation 8-1: The U.S. Department of Health and Human Services, in collaboration with health professional associations, health care providers, and other key stakeholders, should partner with community-based organizations and patient advocates to translate and disseminate emerging clinical research information to people living with sickle cell disease and their families in order to improve health literacy and empower them to engage in the care and treatment decision-making process.

Recommendation 8-2: The U.S. Department of Health and Human Services, in collaboration with state health departments and health care providers, should partner with community-based organizations and community health workers to engage the sickle cell disease (SCD) population in designing educational and advocacy programs and policies and in disseminating information on health and community services to individuals living with SCD and their caregivers.

REFERENCES

ASH (American Society of Hematology). 2017. *About the sickle cell disease coalition.* http://www.scdcoalition.org/about.html (accessed July 20, 2020).

Azevedo, M. 2017. 4 hemophilia support organizations you should know about. *Hemophilia News Today,* August 3. https://hemophilianewstoday.com/2017/08/03/8566 (accessed April 20, 2020).

Baker, J. R., S. O. Crudder, B. Riske, V. Bias, and A. Forsberg. 2005. A model for a regional system of care to promote the health and well-being of people with rare chronic genetic disorders. *American Journal of Public Health* 95(11):1910–1916.

Bakker, A., P. G. Van der Heijden, M. J. Van Son, R. Van de Schoot, and N. E. Van Loey. 2011. Impact of pediatric burn camps on participants' self esteem and body image: An empirical study. *Burns* 37(8):1317–1325.

Bultas, M. W., A. D. Schmuke, V. Moran, and J. Taylor. 2016. Psychosocial outcomes of participating in pediatric diabetes camp. *Public Health Nursing* 33(4):295–302.

CDC (Centers for Disease Control and Prevention). 2018a. *HTC population profile.* Atlanta, GA: Centers for Disease Control and Prevention.

CDC. 2018b. *Self-management education (SME) programs for chronic health conditions.* https://www.cdc.gov/learnmorefeelbetter/programs/index.htm (accessed May 16, 2019).

CDC. 2019a. *California SCDC program data.* https://www.cdc.gov/ncbddd/hemoglobinopathies/scdc-state-data/california.html (accessed May 16, 2019).

CDC. 2019b. *Sickle cell disease national resource directory.* https://www.cdc.gov/ncbddd/sicklecell/map/map-nationalresourcedirectory.html (accessed May 16, 2019).

CFF (Cystic Fibrosis Foundation). n.d.a. *Advocacy achievements.* https://www.cff.org/About-Us/Our-Approach-to-Federal-State-and-Local-Policy/Our-Advocacy-Work/Advocacy-Achievements (accessed January 13, 2020).

CFF. n.d.b. *Care centers.* https://www.cff.org/Care/Care-Centers (accessed January 13, 2020).

CFF. n.d.c. *CF foundation venture philanthropy model.* https://www.cff.org/About-Us/About-the-Cystic-Fibrosis-Foundation/CF-Foundation-Venture-Philanthropy-Model (accessed January 13, 2020).

CFF. n.d.d. *What is compass?* https://www.cff.org/Assistance-Services/About-Compass/What-Is-Compass (accessed July 20, 2020).

CFF. n.d.e. *Drug development pipeline.* https://www.cff.org/Trials/pipeline (accessed January 13, 2020).

CFF. n.d.f. *Our history.* https://www.cff.org/About-Us/About-the-Cystic-Fibrosis-Foundation/Our-History (accessed January 13, 2020).

DiDomizio, P. G., and A. Gillard. 2018. Perceptions of health care professionals on the effects of residential summer camp in their patients. *Journal of Pediatric Nursing* 40:37–46.

GBT (Global Blood Therapeutics). n.d. *Access to Excellent Care for Sickle Cell Patients pilot program (ACCEL).* https://www.gbt.com/patients/funding-and-support (accessed April 20, 2020).

Global Genes. 2015. RARE on the red carpet: Celine Dion pitches in for cystic fibrosis. *RARE Daily*, January 25. https://globalgenes.org/2015/01/25/rare-red-carpet-celine-dion-pitches-cystic-fibrosis (accessed April 20, 2020).

Gold, J. 2017. *Sickle cell patients suffer discrimination, poor care—and shorter lives.* https://mlk50.com/sickle-cell-patients-suffer-discrimination-poor-care-and-shorter-lives-f85abe11bb67 (accessed January 13, 2020).

Hagan, T. L., and E. Medberry. 2016. Patient education vs. patient experiences of self-advocacy: Changing the discourse to support cancer survivors. *Journal of Cancer Education* 31(2):375–381.

Hemophilia Foundation of California. n.d. *About.* https://www.hemophiliaca.org/about (accessed January 13, 2020).

HFA (Hemophilia Foundation of America). 2017. *2017 annual report.* Washington, DC: Hemophilia Federation of America.

HFA. n.d. *What is HFA?* https://www.hemophiliafed.org/our-role-and-programs/what-is-hfa (accessed January 15, 2020).

HRSA (Health Resources and Services Administration) Maternal and Child Health Bureau. 2016. *Sickle cell disease newborn screening follow-up program.* https://www.hrsa.gov/library/sickle-cell-disease-newborn-screening-follow-program (accessed April 20, 2020).

Hsu, L. L., N. S. Green, E. Donnell Ivy, C. E. Neunert, A. Smaldone, S. Johnson, S. Castillo, A. Castillo, T. Thompson, K. Hampton, J. J. Strouse, R. Stewart, T. Hughes, S. Banks, K. Smith-Whitley, A. King, M. Brown, K. Ohene-Frempong, W. R. Smith, and M. Martin. 2016. Community health workers as support for sickle cell care. *American Journal of Preventive Medicine* 51(1 Suppl 1):S87–S98.

Manley, A. F. 1984. Legislation and funding for sickle cell services, 1972–1982. *American Journal of Pediatric Hematology/Oncology* 6(1):67–71.

Markel, H. 1992. The stigma of disease: Implications of genetic screening. *American Journal of Medicine* 93(2):209–215.

Mogayzel, P. J., J. Dunitz, L. C. Marrow, and L. A. Hazle. 2014. Improving chronic care delivery and outcomes: The impact of the cystic fibrosis care center network. *BMJ Quality & Safety* 23(Suppl 1):i3.

Narcisse, L., E. A. Walton, and L. L. Hsu. 2018. Summer camps for children with sickle cell disease. *Ochsner Journal* 18(4):358–363.

NHF (National Hemophilia Foundation). 2002. *Standards and criteria for the care of persons with congenital bleeding disorders.* https://www.hemophilia.org/Researchers-Healthcare-Providers/Medical-and-Scientific-Advisory-Council-MASAC/MASAC-Recommendations/Standards-and-Criteria-for-the-Care-of-Persons-with-Congenital-Bleeding-Disorders (accessed January 15, 2020).

NHF. 2017. *2017 annual report.* New York: National Hemophilia Foundation.

NHF. 2018. *2017 annual report.* https://www.hemophilia.org/sites/default/files/document/files/Accomplishments_2017.pdf (accessed July 20, 2020).

NHF. 2020a. *Advocacy & healthcare coverage.* https://www.hemophilia.org/Advocacy-Healthcare-Coverage/Advocacy-Priorities (accessed January 15, 2020).

NHF. 2020b. *Comprehensive medical care: Htcs.* https://www.hemophilia.org/Researchers-Healthcare-Providers/Comprehensive-Medical-Care-Hemophilia-Treatment-Centers (accessed January 15, 2020).

NHF. 2020c. *Fast facts.* https://www.hemophilia.org/About-Us/Fast-Facts (accessed January 15, 2020).

NHF. 2020d. *Federal hemophilia programs.* https://www.hemophilia.org/Advocacy-Healthcare-Coverage/Advocacy-Priorities/Federal-Priorities/Federal-Hemophilia-Programs (accessed January 15, 2020).

NORD (National Organization for Rare Diseases). 2020. *Programs and services.* https://rarediseases.org/about/what-we-do/programs-services (accessed January 15, 2020).

Novartis. 2018. *Novartis to fund five innovative ideas to support patients and the sickle cell community.* https://www.pharma.us.novartis.com/news/media-releases/novartis-fund-five-innovative-ideas-support-patients-and-sickle-cell-community (accessed January 15, 2020).

Otero-Sabogal, R., D. Arretz, S. Siebold, E. Hallen, R. Lee, A. Ketchel, J. Li, and J. Newman. 2010. Physician–community health worker partnering to support diabetes self-management in primary care. *Quality in Primary Care* 18(6):363–372.

PHCPI (Primary Health Care Performance Initiative). 2018. *Community engagement.* https://improvingphc.org/community-engagement (accessed March 11, 2020).

PSCRC (Pacific Sickle Cell Regional Collaborative). 2019. *About.* https://pacificscd.org/about (accessed January 15, 2020).

Ramos Salazar, L. 2018. The effect of patient self-advocacy on patient satisfaction: Exploring self-compassion as a mediator. *Communication Studies* 69(5):567–582.

Rhodes, S. D., K. L. Foley, C. S. Zometa, and F. R. Bloom. 2007. Lay health advisor interventions among Hispanics/Latinos: A qualitative systematic review. *American Journal of Preventive Medicine* 33(5):418–427.

Rosenthal, E. L., J. N. Brownstein, C. H. Rush, G. R. Hirsch, A. M. Willaert, J. R. Scott, L. R. Holderby, and D. J. Fox. 2010. Community health workers: Part of the solution. *Health Affairs* 29(7):1338–1342.

Salazar, G., and M. B. Heyman. 2014. Benefits of attending a summer camp for children with inflammatory bowel disease. *Journal of Pediatric Gastroenterology and Nutrition* 59(1):33–38.

SCCC (Sickle Cell Community Consortium). n.d. *Who we are.* https://sicklecellconsortium.org/who-we-are (accessed January 15, 2020).

SCDAA (Sickle Cell Disease Association of America). 2019. *Mission & vision.* https://www.sicklecelldisease.org/mission (accessed January 15, 2020).

SCDAA. n.d. *Grant project.* http://sicklecelldisease.net/grant-project (accessed January 15, 2020).

SCDAAMI (Sickle Cell Disease Association of America, Michigan Chapter, Inc.). n.d. *Home page.* https://www.scdaami.org (accessed January 15, 2020).

SCDAI (Sickle Cell Disease Association of Illinois). n.d. *About us.* https://www.sicklecelldisease-illinois.org/about_us (accessed January 15, 2020).

SCFGA (Sickle Cell Foundation of Georgia). 2018. *Operations report 2018.* Atlanta, GA: Sickle Cell Foundation of Georgia.

Scott, R. B. 1981. Whither sickle cell disease in the 1980s. *Journal of the National Medical Association* 73(4):307–308.

Shepanski, M. A., L. B. Hurd, K. Culton, J. E. Markowitz, P. Mamula, and R. N. Baldassano. 2005. Health-related quality of life improves in children and adolescents with inflammatory bowel disease after attending a camp sponsored by the Crohn's and Colitis Foundation of America. *Inflammatory Bowel Diseases* 11(2):164–170.

Sickle Cell Association of Texas Marc Thomas Foundation. n.d. *Home page.* https://www.sicklecelltx.org (accessed January 15, 2020).

Sickle Cell Disease Foundation. n.d. *MLK Jr. Outpatient Center for Adults with SCD.* http://www.scdfc.org/scd-clinic-at-mlk.html (accessed January 15, 2020).

Skinner, M. W., J. M. Soucie, and K. McLaughlin. 2014. The National Haemophilia Program standards, evaluation and oversight systems in the United States of America. *Blood Transfusion* 12(Suppl 3):e542–e548.

Terry, M. 2018. A look at hemophilia drug prices and the market. *BioSpace*, July 3. https://www.biospace.com/article/a-look-at-hemophilia-drug-prices-and-the-market (accessed April 20, 2020).

Tozzi, J. 2015. This medical charity made $3.3 billion from a single pill. *Bloomberg*, July 7. https://www.Bloomberg.Com/news/features/2015-07-07/this-medical-charity-made-3-3-billion-from-a-single-pill (accessed April 20, 2020).

U.S. Pain Foundation. 2017. *#makeitvisible movement raises awareness, funding for invisible illness.* http://uspainfoundation.org/press-release/makeitvisible-movement-raises-awareness-funding-invisible-illness/#makeitvisible (accessed January 15, 2020).

WFH (World Federation of Hemophilia). 2020a. *Country programs.* https://www.wfh.org/en/our-work-reg-national/country-programs (accessed January 15, 2020).

WFH. 2020b. *Over 50 years of advancing treatment for all.* https://www.wfh.org/en/about/history (accessed January 15, 2020).

WFH. 2020c. *Research and data collection.* https://www.wfh.org/usa/programs/research-and-data-collection (accessed January 15, 2020).

WFH USA. 2018. *WFH USA year-end report.* Albany, NY: World Federation of Hemophilia.

WFH USA. 2020. *Evidence-based advocacy.* https://www.wfh.org/usa/programs/research-data-collection-evidence-based-advocacy (accessed January 15, 2020).

Wiltshire, J., K. Cronin, G. E. Sarto, and R. Brown. 2006. Self-advocacy during the medical encounter: Use of health information and racial/ethnic differences. *Medical Care* 44(2):100–109.

Wu, Y. P., J. McPhail, R. Mooney, A. Martiniuk, and M. D. Amylon. 2016. A multisite evaluation of summer camps for children with cancer and their siblings. *Journal of Psychosocial Oncology* 34(6):449–459.

9

Strategic Plan and Blueprint for Sickle Cell Disease Action

We need a roadmap, we need a system, we need something that is going to give us what many people already have, and what this country is going to need more of, as there are more people that are going to be living longer and living better with this new science.

—Adrienne S. (Open Session Panelist)

The strategic plan and blueprint for sickle cell disease (SCD) action identifies the strategic vision, strategies, and action steps for improving health care and health outcomes for individuals living with SCD. The fundamental vision of the framework is to advance and extend healthy, productive lives for individuals living with SCD and to advance understanding of sickle cell trait (SCT).

In developing the strategic plan, the committee found that most of the key messages from the Institute of Medicine (IOM) report *Crossing the Quality Chasm: A New Health System for the 21st Century* (IOM, 2001) still hold true today for the SCD population. Furthermore, SCD has not benefited in significant ways from medical advances compared with the general population or even other populations living with rare and heritable diseases, such as cystic fibrosis (CF) and hemophilia. Despite advances that have helped children living with SCD live longer, mortality and morbidity increase sharply in young adulthood (Treadwell et al., 2018) (see Chapter 1). Pregnant women with SCD are more likely to die or suffer adverse outcomes than the general population (ASH, 2015).

There is insufficient research and information about the needs of the SCD population, which makes it difficult to appropriately inform programming and policies to address their needs. However, there are evidence-based interventions (preventive, acute, and post-acute services) that every individual living with SCD should receive, although many do not. Clinical practice guidelines developed for SCD management are not applied consistently; even where there is strong evidence for certain services, not everyone with SCD receives them. People with SCD are dying at a much higher rate than the rest of the population, as discussed in Chapter 1 (IHME, 2020). One reason for these poor health outcomes is that the health care delivery system is not organized to address the health needs of individuals with SCD as they transition from pediatric to adult care. As the longevity of people living with SCD increases, so do the number and types of complications requiring comprehensive and coordinated care from a multidisciplinary team of experts and an array of health and non-health services. Only a limited number of health care professionals is willing and able to provide the necessary SCD care, and the health care delivery system is poorly organized to facilitate the needs of this population. As a result, people living with SCD often resort to episodic acute care to manage pain, the hallmark of the disease, as well as other acute complications. Lacking for this population is a system of care that can provide comprehensive coordinated care management aimed at preventing SCD complications and reducing the disease burden.

The sociopolitical and historical contexts underpinning the disease compound these problems. As discussed earlier, the roots of SCD in the United States can be traced back to the slave trade, where some African slaves transported involuntarily may have carried the gene. Because of persistent racism and discrimination, the disease was not addressed for years after it was discovered in the United States. This racism persists, and individuals with SCD and SCT have had to contend with discrimination in the health care system. Those living with SCD are also stigmatized in both health care and non–health care settings, in social circles, in places of employment, and schools. The far-reaching health and health-related social implications of SCD and SCT for those who live with these conditions and their families necessitate expansive action that takes into account the inherent complexities of the disease.

Taking these factors into consideration, the committee determined that, at a minimum, the strategic plan should ensure that the SCD population receives the same high-quality health care to which every American is entitled. The strategic plan (see Figure 9-1) is composed of a strategic vision, eight strategies in support of the vision, and foundational principles, which undergird the strategic plan.

The committee based the foundational principles on the six aims for the health care system identified in the IOM report *Crossing the Quality*

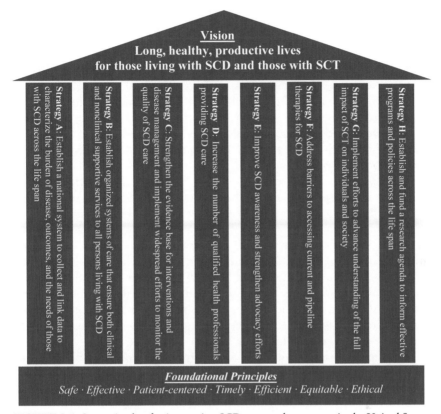

FIGURE 9-1 Strategic plan for improving SCD care and outcomes in the United States.
NOTE: SCD = sickle cell disease; SCT = sickle cell trait.

Chasm: safe, effective, patient-centered, timely, efficient, and equitable
(IOM, 2001). According to the IOM report, "a health care system that
achieves major gains in these six areas would be far better at meeting
patient needs" (IOM, 2001, p. 6). The committee, however, believed that
due to the history of marginalization and racism that has affected the
majority of the population impacted by SCD, it was important to add a
seventh principle: ethical. The seven foundational principles for action for
SCD in the United States are described below.

1. *Safe*: avoiding injuries to patients from the care that is intended to
   help them;
2. *Effective*: providing services based on scientific knowledge to all
   who could benefit and refraining from providing services to those
   not likely to benefit;

3. *Patient-centered*: providing care that is respectful of and responsive to individual patient preferences, needs, and values and ensuring that patient values guide all clinical decisions;
4. *Timely*: reducing waits and sometimes harmful delays for both those who receive and those who give care;
5. *Efficient*: avoiding waste, including waste of equipment, supplies, ideas, and energy;
6. *Equitable*: providing care that does not vary in quality because of personal characteristics, such as gender, ethnicity, geographic location, and socioeconomic status; and
7. *Ethical*: providing care that is free of provider prejudice or bias, avoiding unfair treatment because of SCD diagnosis and trait status, and addressing patient mistrust in the health care system.

The vision for the strategic plan is to assure "long, healthy, productive lives for those living with SCD and those with SCT." The committee identified eight overarching strategies or "pillars" to support the attainment of this vision. These strategies take into account the multifaceted needs of the SCD and SCT population and the equally multidimensional interventions required to meet these needs. The strategies are equally important and need to all be approached with the same level of urgency.

The committee also proposes a blueprint for implementing the strategic plan. The blueprint offers action steps for each of the strategies in the strategic plan. The actions reflect the committee's recommendations identified in the report's preceding chapters after a thorough review of the available evidence. The action steps or recommendations are enumerated with the chapter that contains the supporting evidence. The committee recognizes that it will not be feasible to tackle all of the actions simultaneously and as such, offers timeframes for accomplishing each of the recommendations. The timeframes take into account the complexity of the activity, the level of resources needed to accomplish the task, and the existence of current programs that can serve as a vehicle for advancing action. Activities are also prioritized by actions that need to occur sequentially.

Each of the recommendations will require multistakeholder engagement, and the committee identifies some of the partners who need to be involved to achieve each action step. The committee, however, believes that in order to make meaningful and sustained progress on the strategic plan, it is critical that there be central oversight from the Office of the Assistant Secretary for Health (OASH) at the U.S. Department of Health and Human Services (HHS). OASH should appoint an oversight body with members from across HHS agencies to oversee the implementation of the strategic plan and action blueprint. The appointment of the oversight body should be immediate, and the current HHS Sickle Cell Disease Workgroup, which has representation from 11 HHS agencies, is one option for such an interagency group (Azar and Giroir, 2019). The oversight group should be charged with advancing the strategic plan and blueprint by engaging and convening other stakeholders, developing interim milestones and monitoring progress, identifying funding sources, and overseeing other necessary activities.

To ensure continued progress, the oversight body should conduct regular assessments of the implementation of the strategic plan, with the first evaluation occurring no more than 5 years after the release of this report.

Strategy A: Establish a national system to collect and link data to characterize the burden of disease, outcomes, and the needs of those with SCD across the life span. This strategy will be achieved by establishing robust and well-supported longitudinal data collection systems that include the majority of those living with the disease. A comprehensive data collection system will help inform the burden of the disease, care needs, and outcomes. The recommended action steps to achieve this strategy are listed below.

Recommendation 3-1: The Centers for Disease Control and Prevention should work with all states to develop state public health surveillance systems to support a national longitudinal registry of all persons with sickle cell disease.
In addition to expanding the Centers for Disease Control and Prevention (CDC) Sickle Cell Data Collection (SCDC) program currently under way, additional efforts to collect data on all persons living with SCD in all states should be undertaken. CDC should collaborate with professional associations, such as the American Society of Hematology (ASH), which just launched a clinical trials network; other federal entities, such as the Health Resources and Services Administration (HRSA) and the National Institutes of Health (NIH); and other stakeholders, such as researchers and providers. Data can be gathered about SCD patients and their care and health outcomes tracked over their lifetimes. CDC's previous data collection efforts, such as the California Registry and Surveillance System for Hemoglobinopathies and the current SCDC, can serve as models. Similarly, state-led surveillance and registry efforts as well as other disease registries, such as the Surveillance, Epidemiology, and End Results Program for cancer and the CF and hemophilia treatment centers' registries, offer valuable insights that can be scaled through appropriate resourcing and standardization.

The Cystic Fibrosis Foundation (CFF) supports its registry with private donations, pharmaceutical company donations, and investments. This can serve as a model for the SCD community. Additionally, given that

California and Georgia already have experience with linking health records for individuals living with SCD, they could serve as initial longitudinal registries which can then be expanded to all other states.
Timeframe: 1–2 years

Recommendation 3-2: The Health Resources and Services Administration, the National Institutes of Health, and the Agency for Healthcare Research and Quality should develop a clinical data registry for sickle cell disease. The registry would allow for identifying best practices for care delivery and outcomes.

NIH, in partnership with federal agencies such as HRSA and the Agency for Healthcare Research and Quality, and entities such as the Patient-Centered Outcomes Research Institute (PCORI), which is currently funding demonstration projects to improve the care and treatment of SCD, should define and implement systems to validate and implement standards of health care and measures of desired clinical outcomes and patient-reported outcomes (PROs). Efforts to improve measures of access, use, and health-related disease burden should also be included. Emphasis should be placed on fostering research and clinical learning networks to identify and disseminate common protocols and best practices for health care delivery. Existing comprehensive SCD care centers and HRSA's SCD treatment demonstration regional collaboratives are existing mechanisms that can be standardized into formal learning networks, in collaboration with health care systems, providers, and health care professional associations.
Timeframe: 1–2 years

Recommendation 3-3: The Office of the Assistant Secretary for Health should establish a working group to identify existing and disparate sources of data that can be immediately linked and mined. These data can be used to provide needed information on sickle cell disease health care services usage and costs in the short term.

Administrative datasets, such as hospital datasets, state-specific datasets, national datasets, and health insurance claims databases, can also be mined to inform the data gaps in SCD health services use. Individual hospitals and state hospital associations collect administrative data on emergency department (ED) use, ambulatory clinical data, and inpatient records, which can be linked with other datasets to provide insights on the SCD population in specific geographic areas. Similarly, data available at the national level such as the National Hospital Discharge Survey and the Health Care Utilization Project and state-level data can enable researchers to obtain valuable information about the SCD population.
Timeframe: 1–2 years

Strategy B: Establish organized systems of care assuring both clinical and nonclinical supportive services to all persons living with SCD. Such systems would ensure access to high-quality, evidence-based, comprehensive primary and specialty (acute and chronic) care delivered by multidisciplinary teams; to supplemental enabling services; and to behavioral health and social services. The following action steps will be necessary to achieve this strategy.

Recommendation 2-1: The Social Security Administration should review disability insurance qualifications to ensure that the qualification criteria reflect the burden of the disease borne by individuals with sickle cell disease.
In 2015 the Social Security Administration (SSA) altered its listings of impairments for both children and adults, making them more difficult to meet. Changes in these listings are crucial, as they control the standards for automatic eligibility for disability benefits health insurance, which is much needed by the SCD population. Existing disability insurance qualifications for SCD do not reflect the full impact of SCD on functional status. The current Supplemental Security Income (SSI) criteria penalize patients for obtaining high-quality care that reduces disability but do not recognize the burden placed on patients who consequently lose insurance coverage and can no longer access needed services. These standards need to be revised in the next review period in 2020. SSA should engage health professional associations and SCD providers to assess the full functional impact of SCD on the patient in order to inform amendments to the SSI eligibility criteria. SSA should consider stakeholder feedback received during the proposed rulemaking period. In the short term, SSA should consider other approaches, such as soliciting needed information for adjudicating cases directly from providers to ascertain level of disease severity.
Timeframe: 1–2 years

Recommendation 2-2: States should expand and enhance vocational rehabilitation programs for individuals with sickle cell disease who need additional training in order to actively participate in the workforce.
Some individuals may experience silent cerebral infarcts into adulthood, which can have long-lasting impact on cognitive function. Frequent pain crises and hospitalizations could also make it difficult for individuals to succeed professionally. Accommodations may require vocational rehabilitation services to support effective participation in the job market.
Timeframe: 2–3 years

Recommendation 5-1: The Office of the Assistant Secretary for Health, through the Office of Minority Health, should convene a panel of relevant stakeholders to delineate the elements of a comprehensive system of sickle cell disease (SCD) care, including community supports to improve health outcomes, quality of life, and health inequalities. Relevant stakeholders may include the National Minority Quality Forum, National Medical Association, American Society of Pediatric Hematology/Oncology, American Academy of Pediatrics, American Board of Pediatrics, American College of Physicians, American Society of Hematology, Sickle Cell Disease Association of America Inc., Sickle Cell Adult Provider Network, and other key clinical disciplines and stakeholders engaged in SCD care; health systems; and individuals living with SCD and their families.

ImproveCareNow, a collaborative community to transform health care for children and young adults with Crohn's disease and inflammatory bowel disease, offers a model. Crucial elements to be delineated by the panel include the following:

- Responsibility for geographically defined populations of individuals living with SCD (e.g., regionally, statewide);
- Guidance for using newborn screening (NBS) data to facilitate linkage to care for all positive screens in geographic area; and
- The types of services that should be delivered at comprehensive centers and at the community level.

HRSA should use the product of this activity to develop a process for certifying comprehensive SCD centers with linkages to community, nonurban, and stand-alone providers. These centers should develop strategies to enhance SCD care in geographically defined regions. Such strategies may include shared protocols for managing crises in community EDs, explicit guidelines for primary care providers, community health workers (CHWs) to assist individuals living with SCD, telemedicine access, and continuing education activities.

An essential component of certifying SCD comprehensive care centers is creating consensus workforce requirements similar to those used by CFF. To achieve high-quality care as defined by the National Heart, Lung, and Blood Institute (NHLBI) consensus guidelines and ASH clinical guidelines, individuals with SCD should receive treatment from a multidisciplinary team. Using this type of model would support wellness and long-term preventive strategies, including health screenings, education on pain management and disease management, individual counseling, coordination with community resources, the development of a healthy lifestyle and eating habits, and resources for advocacy and support.

The committee recommends that SCD center certification include a requirement that the center's team include, at minimum, the first-level core team members listed in Table 6-1 in Chapter 6. However, the team may need to expand based on individual patient needs; thus, Table 6-1 also describes other recommended team members.
Timeframe: 2–3 years

Recommendation 5-2: The Centers for Medicare & Medicaid Services should work with state Medicaid programs to develop and pilot reimbursement models for the delivery of coordinated sickle cell disease health care and support services.
The payment system in the United States is often an impediment to the delivery of coordinated, multidisciplinary care for individuals living with lifelong diseases. The Centers for Medicare & Medicaid Services (CMS) and private payers have implemented disease-specific models, and the Center for Medicare & Medicaid Innovation (CMMI) continues to pilot several payment models. Payers need to work with SCD providers to facilitate the implementation of a comprehensive model for SCD care, as outlined in Chapter 5. Specifically, the committee recommends that CMS, as the leading insurer through the Medicaid program for most of the SCD population, should take the lead in exploring novel payment models that support comprehensive care for individuals with SCD in the following ways:

- CMMI should pilot novel payment models to encourage and pay for coordinated comprehensive health care delivered by certified SCD centers.
- CMS should develop novel payment approaches that facilitate the delivery of coordinated care for conditions, such as SCD, that are rare, require coordinate comprehensive long-term care, and have high-budget impact therapeutic options.

Timeframe: 3–4 years

Recommendation 5-3: The U.S. Department of Education should collaborate with state departments of health and education and local school boards to develop educational materials to provide guidance for teachers, school nurses, school administrators, and primary care providers to support the medical and academic needs of students with sickle cell disease.
The increased risk for learning difficulties and poor performance from the impact of the disease and from absenteeism caused by vaso-occlusive crises and frequent hospitalizations may make children with

SCD eligible for special educational assistance to help them succeed academically. The Individuals with Disabilities Education Act provides for services for children with special educational needs under Part B and Part C. For those in higher education, the Americans with Disabilities Act prohibits discrimination due to disabilities and requires reasonable accommodations for the individual. Individuals who are eligible for special educational services and their families may not be familiar with the services available to them or how to initiate access to these services. State departments of education and local school boards should provide guidance to help simplify the process for parents of children with SCD who wish to obtain the needed educational supports for their children.
Timeframe: 1–2 years

Strategy C: Strengthen the evidence base for interventions and disease management and implement widespread efforts to monitor the quality of SCD care. Existing evidence to support care and management of SCD needs to be updated to reflect the current demographics and needs of the population living with SCD, where patients are living into adulthood and contending with complications that arise later in life. Excess mortality in adulthood can be attributed to not receiving appropriate or quality care. A concerted effort is needed to track and improve the quality of care that accredited comprehensive SCD centers provide (as described in Strategy B). The following action steps support this strategy.

Recommendation 4-1: Private and public funders and health professional associations should fund and conduct research to close the gaps in the existing evidence base for sickle cell disease care in order to inform the development of clinical practice guidelines and indicators of high-quality care.
Specific areas for research include understanding the health and psychosocial needs of SCD patients and the impact of the disease over time. NIH should collaborate with stakeholders, such as ASH, that have developed SCD guidelines to identify and fund studies to fill the gaps in the existing evidence base. Guidelines for SCD preventive, acute/subacute, and chronic care have been developed and provide the field with benchmarks for SCD care. The evidence base for some of these guidelines, such as screening for pulmonary hypertension, screening for retinopathy, and the use of exchange transfusions for acute chest syndrome, is weak. There is a need to generate evidence to address the gaps to help standardize and promote the delivery of high-quality care.
Timeframe: 3–5 years

Recommendation 5-4: The National Heart, Lung, and Blood Institute; Health Resources and Services Administration; Centers for Disease Control and Prevention; and U.S. Food and Drug Administration should collaborate with the American Society for Hematology, Pediatric Emergency Care Applied Research Network, Patient-Centered Outcomes Research Institute, and private funders of quality improvement initiatives to foster the development of quality improvement collaboratives.

These quality improvement collaboratives could stem from the clinical research network being developed by ASH and other groups that have a record of running strong and active quality improvement programs. At a minimum, standards of care for the list of indicators known to be effective and consensus-driven must be included: (1) transcranial Doppler (TCD) screening, (2) prophylactic antibiotics for children with SCD between the ages of 3 months and 5 years old, (3) pain management, (4) vaccinations, (5) hydroxyurea (HU) use, and (6) successful transitioning from pediatric to adult care. An adapted learning network that builds on existing efforts (e.g., a registry developed by CDC, treatment demonstration programs funded by HRSA, and the implementation consortium funded by NHLBI) is recommended.
Timeframe: 3–5 years

Recommendation 6-1: Federal agencies including the Agency for Healthcare Research and Quality; National Heart, Lung, and Blood Institute; Health Resources and Services Administration; Centers for Disease Control and Prevention; and U.S. Food and Drug Administration should work together with and fund researchers and professional associations to develop and track a series of indicators to assess the quality of sickle cell disease care including patient experience, the prevention of disease complications, and health outcomes.

Specific indicators for chronic health care maintenance, acute/subacute care, and chronic care are needed. PROs, including experience of care (the Consumer Assessment of Healthcare Providers and Systems), should be incorporated into quality indicators and routinely monitored. Efforts should begin with a list of indicators known to be effective and consensus driven: (1) TCD screening, (2) prophylactic antibiotics for children with SCD between the ages of 3 months and 5 years old, (3) pain management, (4) vaccinations, (5) HU use, and (6) successful transitioning from pediatric to adult care. To promote patient-centered and equitable care, a core set of patient self-management indicators, identified via literature review, expert consensus, clinicians in practice, and SCD patients and their families, should be developed and implemented. Federal and private funders should support the development of patient self-management support tools (e.g., decision aids, educational materials, apps, e-health interventions) to achieve optimal quality of life and treatment benefits. *Timeframe: 1–2 years (to identify and develop list of quality indicators); 3–5 years (to implement monitoring program to track performance of those indicators)*

Recommendation 6-2: The Centers for Medicare & Medicaid Services and private payers should require the reporting of expert consensus-driven sickle cell disease (SCD) quality measures and other metrics of health care quality for persons with SCD.
Efforts must be undertaken to standardize the quality of care at a high level and to reduce variations that are driven by problems with the interpersonal nature of health care. This has been well studied in the context of acute pain management. Other quality measures should be defined, measured, and reported.
Timeframe: 3–5 years

Recommendation 6-3: The U.S. Department of Health and Human Services should fund efforts to identify and mitigate potentially modifiable disparities in mortality and health outcomes. Specific subgroups to consider include young adults in transition from pediatric to adult care, pregnant women, and older adults.
CDC should lead efforts to examine high mortality in these subpopulations via a surveillance or registry system. HHS (specifically, NIH, HRSA, and CDC) should fund health care services research and quality improvement initiatives aimed at decreasing disparities in outcomes for these subpopulations.
Timeframe: 1–2 years

Strategy D: Increase the number of qualified health professionals providing SCD care by enhancing existing health professional training and accreditation programs and incentivizing providers to provide compassionate and high-quality care. This objective can be achieved through the following action steps.

Recommendation 6-4: The National Institutes of Health should disseminate information on loan repayment opportunities to incentivize health care professionals interested in conducting research on sickle cell disease (SCD). The Health Resources and Services Administration should add populations with SCD as a designated population health professional shortage area under the National Health Service Corps program and create a loan repayment program for health care professionals working with SCD populations.

Given the shortage of highly qualified providers to treat individuals living with SCD, HHS should designate SCD as a health disparity population and set aside specific funds to support fellows and young professionals who commit to working clinically or conducting research in this area. Other programs supporting young investigators and clinicians, such as those run by ASH and the American Society of Pediatric Hematology/Oncology, are also encouraged to expand.

Timeframe: 1-2 years (to disseminate information about existing programs); 3–5 years (to develop criteria for loan repayment and similar programs for health professionals working specifically with the SCD population)

Recommendation 6-5: Health professional associations (American Society of Hematology, American College of Obstetricians and Gynecologists, American College of Emergency Physicians, American Academy of Family Physicians, American Academy of Pediatrics, National Medical Association, American College of Physicians) and organizations for other relevant health professionals such as advanced practice providers, nurses, and community health workers should convene an Academy of Sickle Cell Disease (SCD) Medicine to support SCD providers through education, credentialing, networking, and advocacy.

The SCD academy, through its multifaceted activities, will play a key role in increasing the available workforce to care for SCD patients. Primarily it should be instrumental in augmenting education for SCD providers, including those outside of the hematology and emergency medicine specialty areas, by educating new providers and offering continuing medical education to existing providers. This training may be TeleECHO participation (telementoring with hematologists), modules developed collaboratively by participating organizations (e.g., ASH, NHLBI, American Association of Medical Colleges, Academy of Managed Care Pharmacy, American Academy of Nursing, American Academy of Physician Assistants), web-based/didactic training, or social media (e.g., hematologist-led blogs/discussion boards, dissemination of clinical research findings via Twitter).

Minimally, training should include information on sociocultural factors that affect the provider–patient relationship (e.g., implicit bias, structural determinants of health, systemic racism), current treatment guidelines, issues with transitions from pediatric to adult care, and advances in SCD research. Training should be designed to address provider educational gaps and biases that erode the provider–patient relationship. Providers who participate in ongoing educational programs should be incentivized to become SCD experts, as has been done with

other chronic diseases. The HIV academy run by the Association of HIV Medicine provides a model for such an academy.
Timeframe: 2–3 years

Recommendation 6-6: Health professional associations and graduate and professional schools should develop early and effective mentoring programs to link early career health professionals with seasoned providers to generate interest in sickle cell disease care.
ASH has an effective mentoring program (ASH Ambassador) that could be replicated by other associations or medical and graduate schools. Special emphasis should be placed on identifying and recruiting underrepresented minority trainees. The goal is to stimulate and support interest in working with patients who are living with SCD by fostering mentoring relationships and networking opportunities.
Timeframe: 3–5 years

Strategy E: Improve SCD awareness and strengthen advocacy efforts through targeted education and strategic partnerships among HHS, health care providers, advocacy groups and community-based organizations, professional associations, and other key stakeholders (e.g., media and state health departments). The goal is to demystify the disease, alleviate bias and stigma faced by those living with SCD, and increase empathy through education. Strategic partnerships with advocacy groups and community-based organizations (CBOs) will enhance their capacity to provide supportive services and acknowledge their value as partners in promoting patient-centered policies and programs. The following action steps will be necessary to achieve this objective.

Recommendation 2-3: The U.S. Department of Health and Human Services should engage with media to improve awareness about the disease and address misconceptions about the disease and those affected.
Studies indicate that, globally, significant gaps in the public's knowledge about SCD continue to perpetuate stigma that confronts individuals living with it. The mainstream media is an important vehicle for disseminating factually correct information about SCD and SCT to the general public to dispel misconceptions about SCD and is an important partner for sharing information about scientific advances in treating SCD to inform those affected and also the general public.
Timeframe: 1–2 years

Recommendation 8-1: The U.S. Department of Health and Human Services, in collaboration with health professional associations, health care providers, and other key stakeholders, should partner with

community-based organizations and patient advocates to translate and disseminate emerging clinical research information to people living with sickle cell disease and their families in order to improve health literacy and empower them to engage in the care and treatment decision-making process.

All educational interventions for individuals living with SCD should be culturally and linguistically relevant. This includes eHealth (including mHealth), whose promise for increasing health literacy, addressing cognitive impairments, and promoting the self-management of SCD should be explored on a larger scale. Funding should be provided to develop multimedia (e.g., print, text, video, games, mHealth, web-based) educational materials for individuals with SCD and their caregivers.
Timeframe: 2–3 years

Recommendation 8-2: The U.S. Department of Health and Human Services, in collaboration with state health departments and health care providers, should partner with community-based organizations and community health workers to engage the sickle cell disease (SCD) population in designing educational and advocacy programs and policies and in disseminating information on health and community services to individuals living with SCD and their caregivers.

Engaging patients in developing and implementing educational programs and materials increases their feasibility and acceptability. Research supports the benefits of peer-based programs (e.g., peer mentoring, camps, transition programs) and CHWs in increasing disease knowledge and self-management for youth and adults with chronic diseases, including SCD. Successful local and state advocacy programs should be replicated in other communities with funding and support from strategic partners. Several CBOs have programs that reach out to individuals with SCD; however, there is a need for additional funding and capacity building to enhance CBOs' infrastructure to enable them to reach out to individuals who can benefit from the resources that they offer. Federal and private funders, particularly SCD pharmaceutical manufacturers, should complement each other's efforts to fund and develop programs for individuals living with SCD and promote advocacy for individuals living with SCD.
Timeframe: 1–2 years

Strategy F: Address barriers to accessing current and pipeline therapies for SCD, with the goal of ensuring widespread patient access to beneficial therapies. The following action steps will be necessary to achieve this objective.

Recommendation 7-1: The Centers for Medicare & Medicaid Services in collaboration with private payers should identify approaches to financing the up-front costs of curative therapies.
Financial barriers to accessing therapies, including costly palliative care, can be addressed through the following approaches:

- Develop clear criteria for use of novel curative therapies to minimize the potential for economic incentives to push the use or non-use of curative therapy.
- Enable providers to finance the up-front costs of curative therapies, potentially via establishing a pool of payer-contributed funds earmarked for this purpose.
- CMS should issue guidance clarifying how Medicaid best-price rules would apply to outcomes-based pricing, annuity pricing, and other salient novel pricing arrangements.
- Encourage and reimburse the practice of shared decision making for novel, high-risk, potentially highly effective therapies, including
  o informed consent for clinical trial participation; and
  o patient counseling on the uptake of high-risk, curative therapies.

CMS and state Medicaid agencies could also consider the 340B program for SCD therapies in the pipeline, which are expected to carry high up-front costs. Current covered entities eligible to participate in the 340B program, including children's hospitals, community hospitals, and federally qualified health centers, are all sources of care frequented by SCD patients.
Timeframe: 2–3 years

Recommendation 7-2: The U.S. Department of Health and Human Services should encourage and reimburse the practice of shared decision making and the development of decision aids for novel, high-risk, potentially highly effective therapies for individuals living with sickle cell disease.
In addition to active support for informed consent for clinical trial participation, emphasis should be placed on counseling patients on the uptake of therapies that are high risk and curative, that have high clinical uncertainty, or that are preference sensitive, such as discussions about fertility preservation. Reimbursement should take into consideration tools and knowledge that foster provider–patient shared decision making about comprehensive care that addresses the psychological, economic, social and spiritual, and short- and long-term impacts for individuals living with SCD.

In the short term (1–2 years), there is an urgent need to identify and synthesize the criteria for the use of recently approved medication, with the goal of providing guidance for providers and patients and improving uptake of these drugs. OASH should engage health professionals, payers, patients, and other relevant stakeholders in developing guidance for the use of new medication. Current efforts by HRSA and the NIH implementation science group can also inform this work. Within 3–5 years, this work should evolve to include the development and funding of shared decision-making tools with input from pharmaceutical companies, payers, and other relevant stakeholders.
Timeframe: 1–2 years (to identify and synthesize criteria for the use of new medications); 3–5 years (to develop guidance for shared decision making and tools for implementation)

Recommendation 7-3: The National Institutes of Health, U.S. Food and Drug Administration, pharmaceutical industry, and research community should establish an organized, systematic approach to encourage participation in clinical trials by including affected individuals in the design of trials, working with community-based organizations to disseminate information and recruit participants, and conducting other targeted activities.
PCORI, ASH, the U.S. Food and Drug Administration, and NIH all have existing activities to foster patient-centric clinical trials design. The lessons and best practices from these disparate efforts need to be standardized, scaled, and adopted for inclusion in every clinical trial involving individuals living with SCD.
Timeframe: 2–3 years

Strategy G: Implement efforts to advance understanding of the full impact of SCT on individuals and society. Unlike SCD, which is associated with debilitating pain and life-shortening complications, individuals with SCT inherit only one gene for abnormal hemoglobin and one normal gene. Individuals with SCT typically live normal, pain-free, productive lives. However, in recent years concerns about complications have prompted the mandatory screening of subgroups, such as athletes. Additionally, while SCT status information is collected as part of the NBS process, there is no indication that it is communicated to the parents and, eventually, to the individual to inform future decision making. The committee identified the following action steps but cautions that all activities pertaining to collecting and using data to raise awareness and improve interventions should be performed so as not to stigmatize those living with SCT in any way.

Recommendation 3-4: The Health Resources and Services Administration should work with states to standardize the communication of and use of newborn screening positive results in genetic counseling and should create a mechanism for communicating this information across the life span and ensuring access to needed support and services.

SCT status information is collected as part of NBS in all 50 states and the District of Columbia. Communication of SCT status is not standardized in the United States, and there is no indication that the information is passed along to individuals or families across the life span and used for further action, such as genetic counseling. There is an opportunity to systematize the communication and appropriate use of SCT information.

Timeframe: 2–3 years

Recommendation 4-2: The National Institutes of Health should fund research to elucidate the pathophysiology of sickle cell trait.

There have been indications that SCT may be a risk factor for health complications and sudden death in certain rare, extreme instances, such as severe dehydration and high-intensity physical activity. These adverse outcomes include exertional rhabdomyolysis and sudden death, chronic renal dysfunction, and venous thromboembolism. With 1–3 million Americans and 8–10 percent of African Americans living with SCT, there is a need for further studies to understand the extent of these complications and to determine what actions need to be taken to completely eliminate the risks for them.

Timeframe: 2–3 years

Recommendation 4-3: The Office of the Assistant Secretary for Health should partner with community-based organizations, the media, and other relevant stakeholders to disseminate information to promote awareness and education about the potential risks associated with sickle cell trait.

As discussed in Chapter 4, SCT is not a disease, and individuals with it can live long, healthy lives. However, there are indications that individuals with carrier status may be predisposed to certain health complications. This has resulted in subpopulation screening for pregnant women, National Collegiate Athletic Association student-athletes, and military personnel. Currently, there is a lack of evidence-based research supporting subpopulation screening and appropriate use of screening results, which means that there is a potential for inefficiencies in the approach for screening and for the use of results to discriminate against individuals.

Timeframe: 1–2 years

Strategy H: Establish and fund a research agenda to inform effective programs and policies across the life span. Federal and private funders should collaborate to provide funding to clinician scientists and scholars with expertise in SCD, race, and stigma to advance research on pressing topics. The oversight body established by OASH should collaborate with health professional associations, researchers, patients, and funders to develop a robust research agenda with priority topics that need to be studied. Organizations such as ASH have developed a comprehensive list of SCD research priorities that can serve as a starting point for this strategy. The committee also identified the following research topics from its assessment of the literature. The list below is not intended to be comprehensive but to provide an example of some of the areas with substantial knowledge gaps:

Societal and Structural Contributors (Chapter 2)
- Research on the nature and impacts of racism and stigma on individuals living with SCD. This work should facilitate or be in conjunction with developing effective tools and approaches for educating providers and patients on identifying, managing, and preventing stigma, racism, and other biases that affect the care and well-being of individuals with SCD.
- Research that supports international "big data" research projects aimed at deciphering and addressing (as needed) the complex genotype–environment interactions (broadly defined) that underlie individual and population differences in the pathophysiology of SCD and responses to treatments and curative therapies.

Current Management Approaches (Chapter 4)
1. Research on the comparative effectiveness of outcomes in existing protocols for SCD clinical research networks and foster the establishment of clinical research networks to evaluate existing treatment approaches and study potential variations.
2. Research on the medical burden and psychosocial impact of SCD as patients age out of pediatric care into adult care and geriatric care.
3. Research to identify strategies to increase uptake of existing evidence-based guidelines.
4. Research on non-pharmacological approaches to managing SCD, including integrative health.
5. Research on the effectiveness of non-opioid based treatments for chronic pain, including cannabis, drugs that act on neuropathic pain, non-steroidal anti-inflammatory drugs, and cognitive behavioral therapy.

Health Care Organization and Use (Chapter 5)
1. Research to identify and understand trends in the use of health care services by children and adults with SCD.

Developing and Delivering the Next Generation of Therapies (Chapter 7)
1. Research that measures health utility for SCD patients and permits the measurement of quality-adjusted life-years for this population.
2. Research by manufacturers that includes clinical endpoints in randomized trials that can be mapped to health utility levels via published studies.
3. Research that includes total health care costs as a secondary endpoint in pivotal clinical trials of new SCD therapy.
4. Research on the development and validation of biomarkers for disease severity and progression that could be contracted upon in outcomes-based pricing arrangements.
5. Research and develop biomarker-based decision trees to determine the appropriate timing and suitability of curative stem cell transplant, particularly as new drugs are becoming available that may obviate the need for it.
    •   Develop biomarkers to predict response, prioritize certain treatments over others, and guide combination therapy.
    •   Develop biomarkers to measure the durability of the treatment effect/persistence of the benefit.
6. Research on the impact of stem cell transplantation on organ dysfunction in adults, particularly for the central nervous system.
7. Research that elucidates chronic pain in SCD, including
    •   incorporating chronic pain as an outcome measure in clinical research;
    •   non-opiate-based treatments for chronic pain;
    •   the interplay of cognition, mood, and pain; and
    •   assessment of benefits of a holistic, palliative care approach to pain in SCD.
8. Research to develop endpoints for clinical trials that capture the complexity of the SCD phenotype.
    •   Quality-of-life endpoints should be incorporated in comparative effectiveness research.
    •   Caution and surveillance are needed when populations not included in the clinical trials are exposed to the new drugs.

9. Research on comparative effectiveness to guide health care/insurance coverage policies, particularly for expensive biological agents.
Timeframe: 1–2 years (to develop research agenda); 3–5 years (to disseminate funding opportunities for researchers)[1]

REFERENCES

ASH (American Society of Hematology). 2015. *Study pinpoints pregnancy complications in women with sickle cell disease.* https://www.hematology.org/Newsroom/Press-Releases/2015/3852.aspx (accessed November 1, 2019).

Azar, A., and B. Giroir. 2019. *Coming together to confront sickle cell disease.* https://www.hhs.gov/blog/2019/06/19/coming-together-to-confront-sickle-cell-disease.html (accessed January 30, 2020).

IHME (Institute for Health Metrics and Evaluation). 2020. *GBD results tool.* http://ghdx.healthdata.org/gbd-results-tool (accessed April 21, 2020).

IOM (Institute of Medicine). 2001. *Crossing the quality chasm: A new health system for the 21st century.* Washington, DC: National Academy Press.

Treadwell, M., M. DeBaun, and J. Tirnauer. 2018. *Transition from pediatric to adult care: Sickle cell disease.* https://www.uptodate.com/contents/transition-from-pediatric-to-adult-care-sickle-cell-disease (accessed November 1, 2019).

---

[1] This text was revised since the prepublication of the report to include the timeline for implementation of this strategy. The prepublication version of the report listed the timeline as "Ongoing."

Appendix A

Public Meeting Agendas and Submissions to the Committee

FIRST PUBLIC MEETING

February 21, 2019
Keck Center of the National Academies
500 Fifth Street, NW
Washington, DC 20001

Open Session

1:15–1:20 p.m.   **Opening Remarks; Conduct of the Open Session**
Marie Clare McCormick, M.D., Sc.D.,
Committee Chair

1:20–2:30   **Charge to the Committee and Discussion**
ADM Brett P. Giroir, M.D., Assistant Secretary for
Health, U.S. Department of Health and Human
Services

CAPT David Wong, M.D., Medical Officer, Office
of Minority Health, U.S. Department of Health and
Human Services

2:30–2:50   **Epidemiology of Sickle Cell Disease in the United States**
Mary Hulihan, Dr.P.H., Health Scientist, Epidemiology
and Surveillance Branch, Division of Blood Disorders,
Centers for Disease Control and Prevention

419

2:50–3:10	Clinical Complications and Care Delivery *Alexis Thompson, M.D., M.P.H., Professor of Pediatrics, Ann & Robert H. Lurie Children's Hospital of Chicago; President, American Society of Hematology*
3:10–3:30	Therapeutic Approaches for Sickle Cell Disease *James G. Taylor VI, M.D., Center for Sickle Cell Disease, Howard University*
3:30–4:00	The Role of Advocacy in Improving the Patient Experience and Outcomes *Shirley Miller, M.A., Patient Advocate, Atrium Health* *Lakiea Bailey, Ph.D., Executive Director, Sickle Cell Community Consortium*
4:00–4:30	Public Comments

SECOND PUBLIC MEETING

April 16, 2019
Keck Center of the National Academies
500 Fifth Street, NW
Washington, DC 20001

Open Session

9:30 a.m.	Welcome and Opening Remarks *Marie Clare McCormick, M.D., Sc.D., Committee Chair*
9:45	Panel 1: The Impact of Sickle Cell Disease on Patients, Families, and Communities *Facilitator: Charmaine Royal, Ph.D., M.S., Committee Member*
9:45–9:50	Panel Introductions
9:50–10:00	*Derek Robertson, M.B.A., J.D., Patient Advocate; Co-Founder, Maryland Sickle Cell Disease Association*
10:00–10:10	*Adrienne Bell-Cors Shapiro, Co-Founder and Science Administrator, Axis Advocacy*

10:10–10:20   *Tosin Ola, RN, BSN, Founder and President, Sickle Cell Warriors*

10:20–10:30   **Beatrice Bowie**, *Patient*

10:30–10:50   Discussion

10:50   Break

11:05   Panel 2: Addressing the Needs of Sickle Cell Patients Across the Life Span
                Facilitator: **Lori Crosby, Psy.D.**, *Committee Member*

11:05–11:10   Panel Introductions

11:10–11:25   *Tracie Bullock Dickson, Ph.D., Education Program Specialist, Office of Special Education and Rehabilitative Services, U.S. Department of Education*

                Carmen Sánchez, *Education Program Specialist, Office of Special Education and Rehabilitative Services, U.S. Department of Education*

11:25–11:35   *Richard P. Weishaupt, J.D., Senior Attorney, Health and Human Services, Community Legal Services of Philadelphia*

11:35–11:45   *Wanda Whitten-Shurney, M.D., Chief Executive Officer and Medical Director, Sickle Cell Disease Association of America, Michigan Chapter, Inc.*

11:45 a.m.–   Discussion
12:05 p.m.

12:05   Lunch

12:45   Panel 3: Health Care for Sickle Cell: Health Professional Awareness and Education
                Facilitator: **Mary Catherine Beach, M.D.**, *Committee Member*

12:45–12:50   Panel Introductions

12:50–1:00   *Barbara Speller-Brown, D.N.P., P.N.P.-B.C., Director,*
               SCD Transition Clinic; Lead Sickle Cell Translational
               Research APN, Children's National Health System

1:00–1:10   *Jeffrey Glassberg, M.D., Associate Professor,*
               Emergency Medicine; Hematology and Medical
               Oncology, Mount Sinai

1:10–1:20   *Charles Jonassaint, Ph.D., Assistant Professor of*
               Medicine, Social Work and Clinical and Translational
               Science, Department of Medicine, University of
               Pittsburgh

1:20–1:40   Discussion

1:40   Break

1:55   **Panel 4: Curative Therapies for Sickle Cell Disease**
               Facilitator: Darius Lakdawalla, Ph.D., Committee
               Member

1:55–2:00   **Panel Introductions**

2:00–2:10   *Betsy Myers, Ph.D., Program Director for Medical*
               Research, Doris Duke Charitable Foundation

2:10–2:20   *Mark Walters, M.D., Program Director, Alpha Stem*
               Cell Clinic; Medical Director, Jordan Family Center
               for Bone Marrow Transplant & Cellular Therapies
               Research, University of California, San Francisco,
               Benioff Children's Hospital of Oakland

2:20–2:30   *Edward Benz, Jr., M.D., Executive Director, National*
               Institutes of Health Cure Sickle Cell Initiative

2:30–2:40   *Celia Witten, Ph.D., M.D., Deputy Director, Center*
               for Biologics Evaluation and Research, U.S. Food and
               Drug Administration

2:40–3:00   Discussion

3:00   **Public Comments**

3:45   Closing Remarks
                Marie Clare McCormick, M.D., Sc.D., Committee Chair

4:00   OPEN SESSION ENDS

THIRD PUBLIC MEETING

June 3, 2019
Keck Center of the National Academies
500 Fifth Street, NW
Washington, DC 20001

Open Session

1:00 p.m.   **Welcome and Opening Remarks**
                Marie Clare McCormick, M.D., Sc.D., Committee Chair

1:15   **Panel 1: Organizing and Managing Care for Sickle Cell
                Disease**
                Facilitator: **Ellen Riker**, *Senior Vice President, CRD
                Associates*
                Panelists:
                    Brynn Bowman, M.P.A., *Vice President of
                    Education, Center to Advance Palliative Care*

                    Kathryn Sabadosa, M.P.H., *Senior Research
                    Director, The Dartmouth Institute; Cystic Fibrosis
                    Foundation's Quality Improvement Initiative*

                    Amy Shapiro, M.D., *Chief Executive Officer and
                    Co-Medical Director, Indiana Hemophilia and
                    Thrombosis Center, Inc.*

                    Emily Riehm Meier, M.D., M.S.H.S., *Pediatric
                    Hematologist and Director, Sickle Cell Research,
                    Indiana Hemophilia and Thrombosis Center, Inc.*

                    Donna McCurry, A.P.R.N., F.N.P.-B.C., *Senior
                    Nurse Practitioner and Program Manager,
                    Comprehensive Sickle Cell Resource Center,
                    Truman Medical Centers, Kansas City, Missouri*

2:25   Break

2:35	**Panel 2: Paying for Sickle Cell Disease Care** *Facilitator:* **Cheryl Damberg, Ph.D.,** *Distinguished Chair in Health Care Payment Policy and Principal Senior Researcher, RAND Corporation* Panelists:

> **Sara van Geertruyden, J.D.,** *Executive Director, Partnership to Improve Patient Care*
>
> **Marc Manley, M.D., M.P.H.,** *Chief Medical Officer, Hennepin Health*
>
> **Stephen Cha, M.D.,** *Chief Medical Officer, UnitedHealthcare Community & State*
>
> **Ruth Krystopolski,** *Senior Vice President, Population Health, Atrium Health*
>
> **Ronald M. Kline, M.D.,** *Medical Officer, Patient Care Models Group, Center for Medicare and Medicaid Innovation, Centers for Medicare & Medicaid Services*

3:55	**Break**
4:05	**Panel 3: Patient Perspectives on Health Care Access, Innovative Therapies, and Other Related Issues** *Facilitator:* **Marie Clare McCormick, M.D., Sc.D.,** *Committee Chair* Panelists:

> **Shauna H. Whisenton**
> **Jennifer Nsenkyire**
> **Teonna Woolford**
> **Jacques (Jackie) Jackson**

5:10	**Public Comments**
5:30	**Closing Remarks** *Marie Clare McCormick, M.D., Sc.D., Committee Chair*
5:45	**OPEN SESSION ENDS**

FOURTH PUBLIC MEETING

July 9, 2019
Parker H. Petit Institute for Bioengineering and Biosciences building
315 Ferst Drive, NW, Atlanta, GA 30332
Suddath Room

Open Session

9:30–10:15 a.m.	Hemophilia of Georgia Center for Bleeding and Clotting Disorders of Emory *Christine L. Kempton, M.D., M.Sc., Director*
10:15–10:45	SCD as a Public Health Issue and CDC Efforts *Mary Hulihan, Dr.P.H., Health Scientist, Epidemiology and Surveillance Branch, Division of Blood Disorders, Centers for Disease Control and Prevention*
10:45–11:00	Break

11:00 a.m.–
12:30 p.m.
	Patient Panel
	Facilitator: **Marie Clare McCormick**, *Committee Chair*
	    Zyekevious (Zye) Barnes
	    Bryan Belcher
	    Marquis Belton
	    Gregory (Greg) Green
	    Jonathan Hamilton
	    Elijah Henry
	    Michael Thomas

12:30–1:30	Lunch
1:30–2:00	Travel to Site Visit Location
2:00–3:15	Site Visit: Grady Memorial Sickle Cell Center

FIFTH PUBLIC MEETING

September 11, 2019
Keck Center of the National Academies
500 Fifth Street, NW
Washington, DC 20001

Open Session

9:00–10:30 a.m.   **Panel: SCD Therapies: Products in Development,
the Regulatory Process, and Considerations for Access**
Facilitator: **Enrico Novelli, M.D.,** *Committee Member*
Panelists:
Bernard Dauvergne, Pharm.D., *Executive Director,
Addmedica*

Brian M. Elliott, M.D., *Clinical Development
Medical Director, Novartis*

Tony Ho, M.D., *Executive Vice President of
Research & Development, CRISPR Therapeutics*

Ted Love, M.D., *President and Chief Executive
Officer, Global Blood Therapeutics*

9:50–10:20 a.m.   **Closing Remarks and Discussion**

Appendix B

Literature Search Terms and Strategy

Search No.	Search Terms	
	Sickle Cell Disease OR Sickle Cell Trait.mp [mp=title, abstract, original title, name of substance word, subject heading word, keyword heading word, protocol supplementary concept word, unique identifier]	
	AND	
	Introduction	# found: 9,588
1	*Legislation OR Law	
2	*Epidemiology	
3	*Prevalence	
4	*Incidence	
5	*Health Outcomes OR Outcome Measures	
6	*Risk Factors	
7	*Complications (stroke, ACS, pain crises, kidney and heart issues, etc.)	
8	*Thalassemia	
9	*Heredity	
10	*Anemia	
11	*Hemoglobinopathy	
12	*Gene	
13	*Pain Crisis/Vaso-Occlusive Crises	
14	*Hemoglobin S	

continued

Search No.	Search Terms	
15	*Homozygosity	
16	*Red Blood Cells	
17	Morbidity	
18	Mortality	
19	Pathophysiology	
20	Global Burden	
	Structural Determinants	# found: 1,373
21	*Economic Burden OR Unmet Need OR Burden of Health OR Burden of Illness	
22	*Health Disparities	
23	*Cost	
24	*Cost of Care	
25	*Financial Impact OR Economic Hardship OR Poverty	
26	*Life Course OR Life Course Perspective OR Life course	
27	*Education	
28	*Employment	
29	Bias (search before 1990)	
30	Health Literacy	
31	Stigma (search before 1990)	
32	Discrimination (search before 1990)	
33	Racism (search before 1990)	
	Screening Surveillance	# found: 1,405
34	*Federal Programs OR State Programs OR Local Programs	
35	*Surveillance	
36	*Registries	
37	*Screening OR Prevention	
38	*Screening (newborn, etc.)	
39	*Limitations	
40	*Bioethics	
41	*Ethics	
42	*Medical Ethics	
43	*Genetic Counseling	
44	*Reproductive Counseling	

Search No.	Search Terms	
	Health Care Organization and Delivery	# found: 2,428
45	*Healthcare Barriers	
46	*Access to Care	
47	*Care Delivery	
48	**Insurance	
49	**Medicaid	
50	**Medicare	
51	**Commercial insurance	
52	**Commercial Payers	
53	**Payers	
54	**Payment policy	
55	*Disease Management	
56	*Care Management	
57	*Pain Management	
58	*Psychosocial Effects	
59	Geographical Barriers	
60	Emergency Care OR Emergency Department	
61	Mental Health	
62	Behavioral Health	
63	Cognitive Deficit OR Cognitive Impairment	
64	Transcranial Doppler	
65	Federally Qualified Healthcare Centers	
	Quality of Care	# found: 715
66	*"Best Practices for Care"	
67	*Pediatric Care	
68	*Adult Care	
69	*Quality of Life	
70	**Patient-centered	
71	**Clinical guidelines	
72	**Primary care providers	
73	**Clinical guidelines	
74	*Patient Engagement OR Family Engagement	

continued

Search No.	Search Terms	
	Workforce Issues	# found: 1,091
75	*Workforce Development OR Workforce Needs	
76	*Community Health Workers	
77	*Employment	
78	**Advanced practice nurse	
79	**Advanced practiced provider	
80	**Nursing OR Nurses OR Nurse Practitioners	
81	**Family physicians	
82	Hospitalists	
83	Benign Hematology	
84	Training (Medical students OR Residents)	
	Internal Medicine	
	Social Workers	
	Psychologists	
	Advocacy and Community Engagement	# found: 569
85	*Patient Advocacy	
86	*Community Engagement	
87	*Funding	
88	*Research	
89	*Patient Education OR Family Education	
90	*Social Support	
91	Policy	
	Current and Innovative Therapeutic Approaches and the Search for a Cure	# found: 5,611
92	*Treatment	
93	*Non-pharmacological Therapies	
94	*Skill-based Therapies	
95	*Educational OR Psychological Therapies	
96	*Gene editing OR Gene Replacement	
97	*Stem Cell Therapy OR Hematopoietic Stem Cells	
98	*Hydroxyurea	
99	*Endari/L-glutamine	
100	*Epigenetics	
101	Clinical Trials	

Search No.	Search Terms	
	NASEM/IOM Studies	# found: 6
102	NIH COPD Action Plan	
103	NASEM: Rare Diseases and Orphan Products: Accelerating Research and Development Report	
104	NASEM: Communities in Action: Pathways to Health Equity Report	
105	NASEM: Epilepsy Across the Spectrum: Promoting Health and Understanding Report	
106	NASEM: A National Strategy for the Elimination of Hepatitis B and C: Phase Two Report	
107	NASEM: Unequal Treatment Report	

Appendix C

Committee and Staff Biographies

COMMITTEE

Marie Clare McCormick, M.D., Sc.D. (*Chair*), is the Sumner and Esther Feldberg Professor of Maternal and Child Health (Emerita), a professor of pediatrics, and a pediatrician with a second doctorate in health services research. Her research has focused on the effectiveness of perinatal and neonatal health services, and the effect they have on the health of women and children. Dr. McCormick's research has also given particular attention to the outcomes of premature infants. She has been a senior investigator on the evaluations of national demonstration programs such as the Robert Wood Johnson Foundation National Perinatal Regionalization Program. She was also an investigator for the federal Healthy Start Program. In addition, she has provided substantial input to the design and conduct of Infant Health and Development Project, which is the largest, multisite randomized trial of early childhood educational intervention. Dr. McCormick received her M.D. and Sc.D. from Johns Hopkins University and her B.A. from Emmanuel College. Dr. McCormick is a member of the National Academy of Medicine and a recipient of the David Rall Medal.

Gilda Barabino, Ph.D., is the president of the Olin College of Engineering. She previously served as the Daniel and Frances Berg Professor and dean of engineering at The City College of New York's (CCNY's) Grove School of Engineering. Prior to joining CCNY, Dr. Barabino served as the associate chair for graduate studies and a professor in the Wallace H. Coulter Department of Biomedical Engineering and the vice provost for academic diversity at Georgia Tech and Emory University. She has also held appointments at Northeastern University. Dr. Barabino is an elected member of the National Academy of Engineering and a member of the National Academies' Committee on Women in Science, Engineering, and Medicine. Dr. Barabino's laboratory focuses on vascular and orthopedic tissue engineering research. She also works to find novel therapeutic strategies that will improve the health of those who suffer from sickle cell disease and related complications. Dr. Barabino received her B.S. in chemistry from Xavier University of Louisiana and her Ph.D. in chemical engineering from Rice University.

Mary Catherine Beach, M.D., M.P.H., is a professor of medicine at the Johns Hopkins University School of Medicine. She holds a joint appointment in health and behavior and society at the Johns Hopkins Bloomberg School of Public Health. Dr. Beach's scholarship about respect and relationships in health care encompasses both empirical and conceptual dimensions. Dr. Beach is currently conducting research on the theoretical foundations of respect and the impact of physician attitudes and patient–physician communication on patients in the primary care setting, in the treatment of HIV and substance abuse, and in the treatment of sickle cell disease. Dr. Beach is on the editorial board for *Patient Education and Counseling* and on the advisory board for Communication in Medicine.

Lori E. Crosby, Psy.D., is a professor of pediatrics and a clinical psychologist. She is the co-director of innovations in community research and co-directs the Cincinnati Clinical Translational Science Award's Community Engagement Core. Dr. Crosby's research focuses on community engagement, self-management, quality improvement, sickle cell disease (SCD), health disparities, and patient-centered outcomes and has been funded by the National Institutes of Health, the Agency for Healthcare Research and Quality, and the Patient-Centered Outcomes Research Institute. She is an elected fellow of the American Psychological Association and a faculty member in the Department of Pediatrics at the University of Cincinnati (UC) College of Medicine, the Division of Behavioral Medicine at Cincinnati Children's Hospital Medical Center, and the Department of Hematology/Oncology at UC Health (adjunct). Dr. Crosby previously served as a member of a National Heart, Lung, and Blood Institute workgroup that developed *2020 Healthy People* objectives for individuals affected by SCD and an American Psychological Association on Advancing Practice. Dr. Crosby received her Psy.D. from Wright State University and completed her pediatric residency/internship at Cincinnati Children's Hospital Medical Center.

Amy Dawson, M.D., M.P.H., FAAFP, is the associate director and the medical director at the Fort Wayne Medical Education Program, a family medicine residency program with dual accreditation by both the Accreditation Council for Graduate Medical Education and the American Osteopathic Association. After earning her M.D. from The Ohio State University, Dr. Dawson trained in family medicine at the Fort Wayne Medical Education Program. Following her training, she spent 3 years in private practice at Brooklyn Medical Associates, followed by 4.5 years as the medical director of the Matthew 25 Health and Dental, and almost 4 years practicing in Quito, Ecuador. In July 2012, she moved back to Indiana and joined the faculty of the Fort Wayne Medical Education Program as the medical director of the Family Medicine Clinic, training new family medicine doctors to provide great health care now and in the future.

Darius Lakdawalla, Ph.D., is the Quintiles Chair in Pharmaceutical Development and Regulatory Innovation at the University of Southern California (USC), where he sits on the faculties of the School of Pharmacy and the Sol Price School of Public Policy. He also serves as the director of research at the Leonard D. Schaffer Center for Health Policy and Economics at USC, one of the nation's premier health policy research centers. Dr. Lakdawalla is currently a research associate at the National Bureau of Economic Research and serves as an associate editor for the *Review of Economics and Statistics*, the *Journal of Health Economics*, and the *American Journal of Health Economics*. He is considered an expert in the field of health policy and economics, with his research focusing primarily on the economics of risks to health, the value and determinants of medical innovation, the economics of health insurance markets, and the industrial organization of health care markets. Dr. Lakdawalla received his Ph.D. in economics from the University of Chicago and his B.A. in mathematics and philosophy from Amherst College.

Bernard (Bernie) Lopez, M.D., M.S., is the executive vice chair in the Department of Emergency Medicine, a team emergency physician for the Philadelphia Flyers, the associate dean of diversity and community engagement at the Sidney Kimmel Medical College, and the associate provost of diversity and inclusion at Thomas Jefferson University. Dr. Lopez's research interests include clinical and basic science aspects of acute vaso-occlusive sickle cell crisis in adult emergency department patients and unconscious bias and its role in health disparities. Dr. Lopez received his M.D. from the Sidney Kimmel (formerly Jefferson) Medical College.

Jonathan D. Moreno, Ph.D., is a David and Lyn Silfen University Professor of Ethics at the University of Pennsylvania in the Department of Medical Ethics and Health Policy. He is the author of several books on ethics. Dr. Moreno received his Ph.D. from Washington University and his B.A.

from Hofstra University. Dr. Moreno is a member of the National Academy of Medicine.

Enrico M. Novelli, M.D., M.S., is an associate professor of medicine at the University of Pittsburgh and an expert in sickle cell disease (SCD). He received his fellowship training in Hematology/Oncology at the University of Pittsburgh Medical Center (UPMC). Dr. Novelli has served as the director of the UPMC Adult Sickle Cell Program since 2007 and as the chief of the section of benign hematology at UPMC since 2018. Dr. Novelli's research focus is on vascular dysfunction and biomarker development in SCD, with a special interest in the area of cognitive dysfunction, for which he has received uninterrupted National Institutes of Health (NIH) funding. He has numerous publications in SCD and has served as a scientific reviewer for many journals, NIH, and the American Heart Association. He is a member of several American Society of Hematology (ASH) committees. Dr. Novelli has been actively interested in advancing hematological care in low-income countries and has led the first two hemophilia symposia in Tanzania under the auspices of a partnership among the World Federation of Hemophilia, the Tanzanian Hemophilia Chapter, and the Hemophilia Center of Western Pennsylvania. In 2015, he was elected as co-chair of the ASH African Newborn Screening and Early Intervention Consortium in SCD. This ambitious initiative aims to bring together institutions in sub-Saharan Africa to introduce standardized practices for screening and early intervention therapies (e.g., penicillin prophylaxis and vaccinations) with the goal of decreasing childhood mortality rates for SCD.

J. Andrew Orr-Skirvin, Pharm.D., BCOP, is an associate clinical professor at Northeastern University in the Department of Pharmacy and the Department of Health Systems Sciences. He specializes in hematology/oncology pharmacy practice. Dr. Orr-Skirvin's research is in supportive care, which includes pain management, nausea and vomiting, neutropenic fever, long-term complication, and growth factor support. He received his Pharm.D. from The University of Texas at Austin and The University of Texas Health Science Center at San Antonio. He received his B.S. in pharmacy from Oregon State University.

Ifeyinwa (Ify) Osunkwo, M.D., M.P.H., is the director for the Sickle Cell Disease Enterprise at Atrium Health's Levine Cancer Institute, serving approximately 1,400 adults and 400 children living with sickle cell disease (SCD). She is a clinical associate professor of medicine at the University of North Carolina at Chapel Hill and a life-span hematologist who specializes in health services outcomes in SCD with a specific focus on transition from pediatrics to adult care chronic pain, health literacy, and patient engagement. She is also an implementation science researcher with a specific focus on SCD. Dr. Osunkwo has more than 25 years of experience in clinical management and population health for SCD as it relates to chronic disease management, quality improvement, and program development. She is a principal investigator on the Education and Mentoring to Bring Access to CarE Network, a regional collaborative focused on increasing access to care for individuals living with SCD in the southeast United States, and leads the Sickle Cell Trevor Thompson Transition Project, a multicenter study to compare the effectiveness of a structured education-based transition program with or without peer mentoring on transition outcomes among emerging adults with SCD. Dr. Osunkwo serves on the board of the Sickle Cell Adult Providers Network and on several committees for the American Society of Hematology (ASH), namely the ASH Communications Committee, the ASH Cardiopulmonary and Renal Guidelines subcommittee, and on the editorial board for *The Hematologist* and *Hematology News*. Dr. Osunkwo received her M.D. from the University of Nigeria and her M.P.H. from the Johns Hopkins Bloomberg School of Public Health. She completed her clinical training at the University of Medicine and Dentistry of New Jersey (pediatric residency) and Columbia University (fellowship in pediatric hematology/oncology and bone marrow transplant).

Susan Paulukonis, M.P.H., M.A., is the program director of the California Rare Disease Surveillance Program at Tracking California, a partnership between the Public Health Institute and the California Department of Public Health. Her expertise is in using population surveillance methodologies to gather information on those affected by rare, non-reportable diseases, determining the incidence and prevalence of such disorders and their outcomes and impact. This work also identifies and highlights those resources that may be needed to improve quality of life for affected populations. The primary focus of her work is sickle cell disease, but the program has also conducted population surveillance in amyotrophic lateral sclerosis, Parkinson's disease, and human health impacts of exposure to cyanotoxins. Dr. Paulukonis was responsible for management of California's Registry and Surveillance System for Hemoglobinopathies and Public Health, Epidemiology, Research and Surveillance in Hemoglobinopathies programs prior to her direction of the state's Sickle Cell Data Collection program. Dr. Paulukonis received her M.P.H. from the University of California, Berkeley, and her M.A. and B.A. from San Francisco State University.

Charmaine Royal, Ph.D., M.S., is an associate professor of African and African American studies, biology, global health, and family medicine and community health at Duke University. She also has appointments in the Duke Initiative for Science & Society, the Kenan Institute for Ethics, and the

Social Science Research Institute, where she directs the Center on Genomics, Race, Identity, Difference and the Center for Truth, Racial Healing & Transformation. Dr. Royal conducts research on scientific, clinical, ethical, social, and policy implications of genetic and genomic research globally, and leads or is involved in a variety of domestic and international projects on sickle cell disease and sickle cell trait. She received her Ph.D. in human genetics and M.S. in genetic counseling from Howard University, and completed postgraduate training at the National Human Genome Research Institute of the National Institutes of Health.

Kim Smith-Whitley, M.D., M.P.H., is the director of the Comprehensive Sickle Cell Center, clinical director of the Division of Hematology, and a professor of pediatrics at the Children's Hospital of Philadelphia. She holds the Elias Schwartz, M.D., Endowed Chair in Hematology. Her research focus is on sickle cell disease (SCD)-related complications, particularly infections and pulmonary issues as well as improving long-term therapies and the transition process from pediatric- to adult-focused care. Through multiple projects and advocacy efforts she hopes to increase access to high-quality care and foster the development of new therapeutics including curative therapies for children and adults with SCD. She is the initiator of two programs at the Children's Hospital of Philadelphia (CHOP): a short-stay at the Hematology Acute Care Unit and The Blue Tie Tag program to recruit blood donors for pediatric transfusions. Dr. Smith-Whitley received her M.D. from The George Washington University School of Medicine then completed residency training at Children's National Hospital and pediatric hematology–oncology fellowship at CHOP.

STAFF

Henrietta Awo Osei-Anto, M.A., M.P.P., is a senior program officer in the Health and Medicine Division at the National Academies of Sciences, Engineering, and Medicine. She previously led the payment and health system transformation Collaborative within the National Academy of Medicine's Leadership Consortium for a Value & Science-Driven Health System. Before joining the National Academies, Ms. Osei-Anto completed a fellowship at Ithaca College where she taught courses on inequalities in the U.S. health care system. She has worked with leaders of multiple sectors of the health care industry on issues of quality improvement, efficiency, and equity in the health care system. She was a senior researcher at the Health Research and Educational Trust of the American Hospital Association, where she managed externally funded projects to implement and evaluate programs to improve quality and reduce cost in the care delivery setting. In this role, she developed tools to help health care leaders effectively prepare their organizations for key health reform provisions pertaining to readmissions, bundled payment, accountable care organizations, and patient-centered medical homes. Ms. Osei-Anto has also served as a consultant to pharmaceutical companies and patient advocacy groups to help them strategically engage in federal health policies. Ms. Osei-Anto earned a bachelor's degree in economics and international studies from Illinois Wesleyan University; a master's degree in public policy and a certificate in health administration and policy from the University of Chicago; and is currently a doctoral candidate in health policy at Brandeis University.

Karen M. Anderson, Ph.D., is a senior program officer in the Health and Medicine Division at the National Academies of Sciences, Engineering, and Medicine. She is the director of the Roundtable on the Promotion of Health Equity and recently directed a consensus study on the potential links among housing, health, and homelessness. She also worked on consensus studies relating to LGBT health and HIV/AIDS. Dr. Anderson earned a Ph.D. in experimental psychology from the University of Pittsburgh. Her professional experiences include positions involving the intersection of social sciences, public health research, and public policy, including time as a staff member in the U.S. House of Representatives for the Committee on Education and Labor, and as a faculty member of the Department of Pediatrics at Howard University. Dr. Anderson has expertise in health disparities, homelessness, adolescent development, reproductive health issues, HIV/AIDS, and LGBT issues.

Cyndi Trang, B.S., is a research associate in the Health and Medicine Division at the National Academies of Sciences, Engineering, and Medicine. She is working on several National Academies studies on sickle cell disease; evidence-based opioid prescribing; and decarbonization, as well as workshops on veterans' health access, biomarkers to establish impairment, and advancing diagnostic excellence. She has also assisted with numerous National Cancer Policy Forum workshops ranging from topics of cancer care in low-resource areas to patient navigation in cancer care. Prior to joining the National Academies, Ms. Trang was a cancer research fellow at the National Cancer Institute, where she worked in the Gene Regulation and Chromosome Biology Laboratory. In addition to her experience in public health policy and laboratory research, Ms. Trang also has experience in the medical field as a former chief scribe at Novant Health. Ms. Trang graduated as an Honors Program Scholar from Marymount University, magna cum laude, with a major in biology, minor in physical science, and a concentration in molecular biology. She is currently pursuing her master's degree in patient safety and health care quality at Johns Hopkins University.

Appendix D

Newborn Screening Results Reporting Protocols for Sickle Cell Disease and Sickle Cell Trait

Background: The Association of Public Health Laboratories (APHL) received a data request from the National Academies of Sciences, Engineering, and Medicine's Addressing Sickle Cell Disease: A Strategic Plan and Blueprint for Action Project—specifically on information on how newborn screening (NBS) programs report screening results for sickle cell disease (SCD) and sickle cell trait (SCT) (i.e., follow-up processes).

Methods: APHL's Newborn Screening and Genetics Program in collaboration with the National Academies SCD committee developed a short survey that would gather information and provide an understanding of what occurs in SCD and SCT NBS results reporting. APHL distributed a PDF version of the survey to six state NBS program representatives (Colorado, Connecticut, Florida, New Jersey, Tennessee, and Washington) of the APHL Hemoglobinopathy Laboratory Workgroup on September 10, 2019. Respondents were asked to review the questions and provide availability for a phone call with APHL staff to answer the survey questions verbally on September 13, 2019.

Results: All six respondents provided answers (five via telephone and one via e-mail). In accordance with APHL's Data Access and Sharing policy, the reports and findings related to the survey will only be released in aggregate without individual identifiers.

Sickle Cell Disease (SCD) NBS Results Reporting

- All six NBS programs have a standardized protocol (written and formal versus informal) for informing parents of their children's SCD status and have a required turnaround time to communicate results.
- The turnaround time for communicating NBS SCD results ranges from 24 hours to a few weeks.
- Communicating SCD results vary in protocol as noted by each NBS program.
- Approximately 98–100 percent of babies who screen positive receive follow-up in 1 year.

Sickle Cell Trait (SCT) NBS Results Reporting

- All six NBS programs have a standardized protocol for informing parents of their children's SCT status and five NBS programs have a required turnaround time to communicate results.
- The turnaround time for communicating NBS SCT results ranges from 1 week to 6 weeks.
- Communicating SCT results vary in protocol as noted by each NBS program.
- The five NBS programs that have a follow-up protocol for SCT are not able to provide the percent of newborns who screen positive for SCT and receive follow-up in 1 year. The five NBS programs distribute letters to parents and/or primary care providers and the NBS program does not get additional information after this.
- One state NBS program provides SCT results to any university or organization that reaches out if properly authorized.

Survey: Newborn Screening Results Reporting Protocols for Sickle Cell Disease and Trait Survey

APHL received a data request from the National Academies SCD committee specifically on information on how NBS programs report screening results for SCD and SCT (i.e., follow-up processes). The purpose of the survey is to gather the requested information. Your participation is vital to providing an understanding of what occurs in results reporting. In accordance with APHL's Data Access and Sharing policy, the reports and findings related to this survey will be released only in aggregate data form without individual identifiers. Thank you for considering this opportunity to make a meaningful contribution.

1. Please tell us who you are:
   - First Name, Last Name
   - Title
   - Phone number, e-mail address

Sickle Cell Disease (SCD):

2. Does your NBS program have a standardized protocol for informing parents of their children's SCD status?
   a. No
   b. Yes
      • If yes, can you share it or point us to it?
3. Is there a required turnaround time for communicating results?
   a. No
   b. Yes
4. What is the average time of returning results?
5. What are the procedures for follow-up once parents have been notified?
6. What percent of babies who screen positive subsequently receive follow-up in 1 year?

Sickle Cell Trait (SCT):

7. Does your NBS program have a standardized protocol for informing parents of their children's SCT status?
   a. No
   b. Yes
      • If yes, can you share it or point us to it?
8. Is there a required turnaround time for communicating results?
   a. No
   b. Yes
9. What is the average time of returning results?
10. What are the procedures for follow-up once parents have been notified?
11. What percent of babies who screen positive subsequently receive follow-up in 1 year?
12. Does your state work with any universities or other organizations to provide SCT screening results for specific groups such as athletes?
    a. No
    b. Yes
       • If yes, please explain.

Appendix E

Sickle Cell Data Collection Program[1]

ABOUT

The Sickle Cell Data Collection (SCDC) program collects information on health status for patients living with sickle cell disease (SCD). The program was developed by the Centers for Disease Control and Prevention (CDC) Foundation in collaboration with the CDC Division of Blood Disorders, the California Rare Disease Surveillance Program, the Georgia Health Policy Center, Pfizer Inc., Global Blood Therapeutics (GBT), Sanofi, and the Doris Duke Charitable Foundation. It is the first program to collect population-based data from multiple sources over an extended number of years. The SCDC program was built on previous surveillance programs from CDC and the National Heart, Lung, and Blood Institute called the Public Health Research, Epidemiology, and Surveillance in Hemoglobinopathies and the Registry and Surveillance System for Hemoglobinopathies.

PROGRAM ORGANIZATION

As of September 2019, only the states of California and Georgia participate in the SCDC program. California's program is called the Public Health Institute's Tracking California program, and Georgia's program is called Georgia State University's Georgia Health Policy Center. Together, they form the SCDC program.

---

[1] CDC (Centers for Disease Control and Prevention). 2020. *Sickle Cell Data Collection (SCDC) program.* https://www.cdc.gov/ncbddd/hemoglobinopathies/scdc.html (accessed March 16, 2020).

FUNDING

Because there are no federal resources able to fund a national surveillance system, the program is funded through a partnership with the CDC Foundation. The CDC Foundation receives its funding support from the following partners: Global Blood Therapeutics, Pfizer Inc., and the Doris Duke Charitable Foundation. Funding supports field staff, partnerships between the states of California and Georgia, and any meetings or project-related travel. The program intends to expand to additional states as resources become available.

PROGRAM PURPOSE AND GOALS

The purpose of the SCDC program is to help understand where people with SCD live in the United States and provide resources for patients to locate the nearest care providers and facilities. The overall goal of the program is to improve the quality of life and life expectancy within the SCD population.

DATA COLLECTION AND USE

Data are collected through newborn screening records, administrative datasets (e.g., hospital discharge, emergency department, and Medicaid), death records, and medical charts. The collected data are used to improve public policy and study long-term trends that may appear in diagnosis, treatment, and health care access within the United States.

PATIENT AND PUBLIC ENGAGEMENT

The SCDC program engages patients and the public by sharing all findings with patients and patient advocates, public health organizations, SCD community organizations, providers, health care administrators, pharmaceutical companies, and policy makers. In addition, the program gives patients the educational resources necessary to make sound decisions about their care. Some educational resources include videos detailing stories of individuals living with SCD, infographics, blog articles, fact sheets, social media content, and quarterly webinars of experts discussing the most recent information regarding SCD. The resources provided by the SCDC program allow patients to properly self-advocate, stay in communication with the larger SCD community, and remain current on recent SCD research findings.

RESULTS

Because of extensive data collection, the SCDC program successfully identifies gaps in the areas of diagnosis, treatment, and health care status for SCD patients and the medical community.

Appendix F

Georgia Comprehensive Sickle Cell Center: A Case Study[1]

July 9, 2019, National Academies SCD Committee Site Visit

ABOUT

The Georgia Comprehensive Sickle Cell Center located at Grady Memorial Hospital in Atlanta, Georgia, was established in 1984. The purpose of the center is to provide the most basic education, clinical research, laboratory diagnosis, counseling, and patient care for sickle cell patients. It was the first comprehensive care clinic in the world to be open 24 hours per day for individuals with sickle cell disease (SCD). To this day, it is still the only comprehensive SCD care center in the state of Georgia.

ORGANIZATION

The Georgia Comprehensive Sickle Cell Center has an outpatient clinic 4 days per week. In addition, it has a 24 hours per day, 7 days per week emergency room with 11 beds specifically for those with SCD. The Center has more than 4,000 visits per year for acute care. Acute care has an admission rate of 16 percent and sends home approximately 84 percent of the individuals seen. The Center is run in collaboration with the Emory University School of Medicine and Grady Memorial Hospital.

---

[1] See https://www.gradyhealth.org/care-treatment/sickle-cell-diseasecenter (accessed December 17, 2019).

FUNDING

The Center is supported by an annual $500,000 grant from the Georgia Department of Public Health.

STAFFING

The Center is staffed by four physicians who provide health care services. Two physicians are full-time and on site while the other two physicians are part-time. The Center also staffs six advanced practice providers, which include nurse practitioners and physician assistants.

PROGRAMS (SERVICES) OFFERED

Services offered include

- acute pain care,
- blood transfusion,
- access to hydrea clinics,
- hydroxyurea treatments, and
- wound care.

DATA COLLECTION AND USE

The Center collects data through the Sickle Cell Data Collection program in Georgia. Data are used to monitor and report the overall health of people in the state with SCD. Orthopedic clinicians at the Georgia Comprehensive Sickle Cell Center are currently involved in research to identify more efficient and effective ways to care for those with SCD.

PATIENT ENGAGEMENT

Patients are engaged through

- sickle cell education,
- monthly group support meetings, and
- pediatric transition classes.

Appendix G

Emory Adult Cystic Fibrosis Program[1]

ABOUT

The Emory+Children's Cystic Fibrosis (CF) Center is the second largest CF Center in the country in terms of patient base according to data from the CF Foundation. The Center includes both pediatric and adult CF programs. The adult clinic has two pulmonary function laboratories and a CF clinical trials office. The Center is in a 14,000 square foot building at Executive Park in Atlanta, Georgia. There are five half-day clinics each week scheduled for Monday, Tuesday, Thursday, and Friday. A comprehensive clinic preview is also held each week on Wednesdays. All adult CF team members are required to attend this preview.

PURPOSE

With having such a large facility, the Center has established a certain protocol to enhance its work. The purpose of the protocol is to ensure the provision of optimal care for CF patients and standardization of care among the different care providers. The protocol includes information specific to responsibilities for the multidisciplinary professionals.

---

[1] See http://medicine.emory.edu/pulmonary-allergy-critical-care/research/adult-cystic-fibrosis. html (accessed December 17, 2019).

STAFFING

Staffing includes two full-time CF nurses; two full-time CF respiratory therapists; one CF nurse practitioner; one CF social worker; one CF mental health counselor; one CF transition coordinator; one CF nutritionist; CF physicians with specific expertise in pulmonary, gastrointestinal, and endocrine medicine; clinical research coordinators; and administrative staff.

PROGRAM ORGANIZATION

The program includes pre-clinic preparation and clinic preview. Pre-clinic preparation calls for the nutritionist to review the patient panel for any annual labs that have yet to be taken and place orders for labs by Tuesday evening of the week before the patient's visit. The registry manager will then compile a list of "short sheets," which detail the patients who are scheduled for the week. If the registry manager is unavailable, these tasks will be completed by the CF director or coordinator. All other care staff will review the patient panels and take the necessary steps specific to their role for clinic preview.

During clinic preview, task folders are distributed to the different care providers (e.g., mental health worker, nurse practitioner). Each care provider will provide a summary of the patient as it relates to their discipline and note whether they need to see the patient. If necessary, the care providers will describe a "clinic goal" for the patient. Task summaries are noted from respiratory therapists, nutritionists, social workers, mental health coordinators, research coordinators, medical doctors, and registered nurses. After clinic preview, the summaries from each care provider are provided to the registry manager. The registry manager will then post the summary from each provider on the day of a patient's clinical visit.

DATA COLLECTION AND USE

The program collects health information from approximately 700 patients with CF. The information is used to inform clinical care and research.

Appendix H

Health Resources and Services Administration Sickle Cell Disease Programs

OVERVIEW OF SICKLE CELL DISEASE PROGRAMS

Sickle Cell Disease Treatment Demonstration Program (SCDTDP): Improve the health outcomes of individuals with sickle cell disease (SCD), reduce morbidity and mortality caused by SCD, reduce the number of individuals with SCD receiving care only in emergency departments, and improve the quality of coordinated and comprehensive services to individuals with SCD and their families.

Sickle Cell Disease Newborn Screening Follow-Up Program: To ensure that individuals diagnosed with SCD through newborn screening receive appropriate follow-up services including counseling, education, access to a medical home, and other support services.

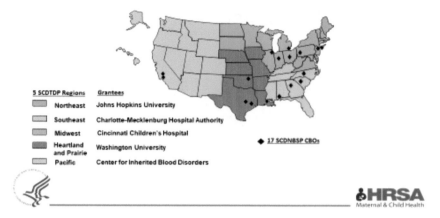

FIGURE H-1 HRSA Sickle Cell Treatment Demonstration Program and Sickle Cell Disease Newborn Screening Follow-Up Program.
NOTE: CBO = community-based organization; SCDNBSP = Sickle Cell Disease Newborn Screening Follow-Up Program; SCDTDP = Sickle Cell Disease Treatment Demonstration Program.
SOURCE: PowerPoint presentation provided via email communication to National Academies staff by Edward Ivy, Medical Officer, Maternal and Child Health Bureau, Health Resources and Services Administration.

TABLE H-1 Programs at a Glance

	Sickle Cell Disease Treatment Demonstration Program	Sickle Cell Disease Newborn Screening Follow-Up Program

Program Objectives	• Support the implementation of five regional networks of care for sickle cell disease (SCD) throughout the United States
	• Use Project Extension for Community Healthcare Outcomes (ECHO), a telementoring program that allows specialists to network and educate other providers, to support strategies to increase the number of providers knowledgeable about evidence-based sickle cell care
	• Increase the number of individuals with SCD receiving hydroxyurea by 10 percent
	• Optional additional activities include efforts to:
	  a. Increase recommended pneumococcal vaccinations
	  b. Increase documented transcranial Doppler ultrasound
	  c. Increase transition plan to an adult provider
		• Provide direct support and financial assistance to a minimum of 15 community-based organizations (CBOs) in 15 states
		• Train 150 community health workers
		• Increase partnerships: Informal and formal, CBOs, hospitals, health systems, state public health departments, primary care providers, federally qualified health centers
		• Serve 15,000 individuals with SCD through:
		  a. Outreach
		  b. Education
		  c. Linkage to medical home
		  d. Referrals to support services
		  e. Care in a patient-centered medical home

Scope	• Progress in State Action Plan Development, Project ECHO, and Data Collection
	• 43 states involved with regions (has yet to reach all 50 states)
	• Building state networks
	• Conducting outreach to providers
	• Five regions have implemented at least one Project ECHO program; eight Project ECHO programs total
	• Data collection through a Provider Survey and Quality Improvement data
		• Technical Assistance:
		  a. Community of Practice—Convene CBOs by region to share successes, challenges, and best practices
		  b. Leadership Academy—Bi-weekly skill-building webinars. Topics include sustainability planning, transition, care coordination, developing patient advocacy, leveraging partnerships, and capacity building
		  c. Partnerships—Identifying national-level strategies that support local CBOs to develop partnerships/memoranda of understanding
		  d. Community Health Workers—Sustainability, recruitment, hiring, retention, ongoing skill building. The Sickle Cell Disease Association of America (SCDAA) will also disseminate best practices and lessons learned

continued

TABLE H-1 Continued

Sickle Cell Disease Treatment Demonstration Program	Sickle Cell Disease Newborn Screening Follow-Up Program

	• Community Health Worker Training
	  a. Virtual Training—SCDAA developed curriculum
	  b. Field Placement—40 hour requirement
	• Peer-to-Peer Mentoring (InquisitHealth)
	  a. Goal is to support individuals and families to access information, resources, and medical care by providing peer-to-peer psychosocial support
	  b. Web-based platform that links peer mentors to individuals and family members
	  c. SCDAA and InquisitHealth developed a sickle cell-specific algorithm that ensures quality coaching and support by utilizing guided conversation guides
	  d. Tracks utilization and contacts
	• Transition Readiness Quality Improvement Project
	  a. Five CBOs will work with more than 200 young adults aged 16–25
	  b. SCDAA will disseminate best practices for improving transition readiness and disseminate to the other 12 CBOs

TABLE H-1 Continued

	Sickle Cell Disease Treatment Demonstration Program	Sickle Cell Disease Newborn Screening Follow-Up Program
Results	Access to care: • Nearly 11,000 patients with SCD received care through the Sickle Cell Disease Treatment Demonstration Regional Collaborative Program (SCDTDRCP) regional networks, reflecting an increase of more than 3,000 patients from baseline • Four states opened clinics in areas of high need. More than 1,000 adults now have access to high-quality care with the newly opened Adult Sickle Cell Clinic at the Martin Luther King, Jr. Outpatient Center in Los Angeles Hydroxyurea use: • Heartland pediatric patients: 12–20 percent; adult patients: 14.3–17.3 percent • Midwest all patients: 48–69 percent • Northeast pediatric patients: 23–34 percent; adult patients: 16–18 percent • Pacific all patients: 29–42 percent Knowledgeable providers: • Telementoring and telehealth initiatives increased provider knowledge across the country • Nearly 100 Project ECHO clinics were held, expanding opportunities for provider education for more than 200 providers	

SOURCES: PowerPoint presentation provided via email communication to National Academies staff by Edward Ivy, Medical Officer, Maternal and Child Health Bureau, Health Resources and Services Administration. Also see https://www.nichq.org/sites/default/files/inline-files/NICHQ-SCDTDP-ImpactStatement_0.pdf (accessed December 17, 2019).

Appendix I

Select Treatments Currently Under Development for Sickle Cell Disease

The table begins on the following page.

Type	Name	Developer/ Sponsor	Research Status (as of December 2019)	Mechanism	Source
Anti-sickling agents	IMR-687	Imara Inc.	• Phase 2a clinical trial—final data collection date for primary outcome measures is estimated for July 2020. • Granted U.S. Orphan Drug Designation, U.S. Rare Pediatric Designation, and Fast Track Designation as of June 2019.	IMR-687 is a selective inhibitor of phosphodiesterase-9 in blood cells. It has the potential to help patients with SCD by reducing red blood cell sickling and red blood cell lysis, reducing white blood cell adhesions, and thus ultimately reducing vaso-occlusive crisis and hospitalizations.	https://clinicaltrials.gov/ct2/show/record/NCT03401112?term=IMR-687&rank=1
	Sanguinate	Prolong Pharmaceuticals	• Phase 2 clinical trial—final data collection date for primary outcome measures was in December 2017. • Granted Orphan Drug Designation.	Sanguinate is a carbon monoxide releasing molecule and oxygen transfer agent under clinical development for the treatment of sickle cell anemia and comorbidities.	https://clinicaltrials.gov/ct2/show/NCT02411708
Anti-adhesion agents	Rivipansel (GMI1070)	Pfizer Inc.	• Phase 3 clinical trial (RESET)—final data collection date for outcome measures was in June 2019. • Granted Orphan Drug status and Fast Track status.	Rivipansel is a glycomimetic drug candidate that acts as a pan-selectin antagonist, meaning it binds to all three members of the selectin family: E-, P- and L-selectin. Rivipansel could reduce cell adhesion, activation, and inflammation that are believed to contribute to reduced blood flow through the microvasculature during vaso-occlusive crisis.	http://glycomimetics.com/pipeline/programs/rivipansel-gmi-1070 https://www.clinicaltrials.gov/ct2/show/record/NCT02187003?term=rivipansel&rank=5

Sevuparin	Modus Therapeutics	• Phase 2 clinical trial—final data collection date for primary outcome measures was in May 2019. It failed to show a meaningful benefit in the total study population. • Modus is considering its options for further development of Sevuparin.	Sevuparin, a novel polysaccharide drug with anti-adhesive, anti-aggregate and anti-inflammatory effects, interacts with multiple targets during a vaso-occlusive crisis. These interactions cause the release of blood components bound to each other and bound to the endothelial wall, preventing further occlusions from occurring.	https://www.clinicaltrials.gov/ct2/show/record/NCT02515838
Gamunex (intravenous gammaglobulin)	Albert Einstein College of Medicine	• Phase I/II clinical trial—estimated final data collection date for primary outcome measures is in September 2022.	Intravenous immunoglobulin reduces neutrophil adhesion to post capillary venular endothelium and adherent neutrophil interactions with circulating red blood cells, thus increasing microcirculatory blood flow and survival.	https://clinicaltrials.gov/ct2/show/NCT01757418
Inclacumab	Global Blood Therapeutics	• Manufacturing under way.	Inclacumab is a novel, fully human monoclonal antibody designed to bind to and selectively inhibit P-selectin, an adhesion molecule found on endothelial cells and platelets that contributes to the cell–cell interactions that are involved in the pathogenesis of vaso-occlusive crisis.	https://www.gbt.com/programs/scd/inclacumab

continued

Type	Name	Developer/ Sponsor	Research Status (as of December 2019)	Mechanism	Source
Antioxidant agents	N-acetylcysteine	Bloodworks Northwest	• Pilot study—final data collection date for primary outcome measures was in December 2018.	N-acetylcysteine can modulate SCD by cleaving hyperactive von Willebrand factor, a vascular adhesion protein.	https://clinicaltrials. gov/ct2/show/NCT018 00526?term=NCT0180 0526&rank=1
Anti-inflammatory agents	Regadenoson	GE Healthcare	• Clinical trial to study the drug's effect on blood flow—estimated final data collection date for primary outcome measures is in January 2022.	Regadenoson is an A2A adenosine receptor agonist that is a coronary vasodilator commonly used in pharmacologic stress testing.	https://clinicaltrials. gov/ct2/show/record/ NCT01566890?term= Regadenoson&cond= sickle&rank=3
Anticoagulant and Antiplatelet agents	Ticagrelor	AstraZeneca	• Phase 3 clinical trial (HESTIA3)—estimated final data collection date for primary outcome measures is in October 2020.	Ticagrelor is an orally administered, direct-acting, reversibly binding P2Y12 receptor antagonist that inhibits adenosine diphosphate-induced platelet aggregation and inhibits cellular uptake of adenosine by inhibiting the equilibrative nucleoside transporter.	https://clinicaltrials. gov/ct2/show/NCT0361 5924?term=Ticagrelor& cond=sickle+cell+anem ia&rank=3
	Rivaroxaban	University of North Carolina at Chapel Hill	• Clinical trial to study the drug's effect on the pathology of SCD—final data collection date for outcome measures was in December 2018.	Inhibition of factor Xa with rivaroxaban will reduce inflammation, coagulation, and endothelial cell activation, and improve microvascular blood flow in patients with SCD during the non-crisis, steady state.	https://clinicaltrials. gov/ct2/show/NCT02 07266?term=Rivarox aban&cond=sickle+cell &rank=1

Nitric oxide	L-Arginine	Emory University	• Phase 2 clinical trials—estimated final data collection date for primary outcome measures is in August 2020.	Low nitric oxide bioavailability contributes to vasculopathy in SCD. L-Arginine is the obligate substrate for nitric oxide production.	https://clinicaltrials.gov/ct2/show/NCT02536170?term=Phase+2+Randomized+Control+Trial+of+Arginine+Therapy+for+Pediatric+Sickle+Cell+Disease+Pain&rank=1
	Riociguat	University of Pittsburgh	• Phase II clinical trials—estimated final data collection date for primary outcome measures is in December 2020.	Riociguat-mediated activation of guanylate cyclase increases the availability of cGMP in the blood vessels within the lungs, which improves blood vessel function and reduces symptoms of SCD.	https://clinicaltrials.gov/ct2/show/NCT02633397
Gene therapy	NCT ID: NCT03282656	Boston Children's Hospital	• Open-label, non-randomized, single center, pilot and feasibility, single arm cohort study of seven patients—estimated final data collection date for primary outcome measures is in February 2020.	The sickle cell gene therapy clinical trial will involve a single infusion of autologous bone marrow-derived CD34+ hematopoietic stem cells transduced with a lentiviral vector containing a short-hairpin RNA targeting BCL11A. This gene therapy technology, developed at Boston Children's Hospital, turns down the expression of the BCL11A protein that normally shuts off production of fetal hemoglobin shortly after birth and represses the expression into childhood and adulthood.	https://clinicaltrials.gov/ct2/show/NCT03282656

continued

Type	Name	Developer/ Sponsor	Research Status (as of December 2019)	Mechanism	Source
	BIVV003	Bioverativ Inc.	• Phase I/IIa clinical trial (PRECIZN-1)—estimated final data collection date for primary outcome measures is September 2022. • The U.S. Food and Drug Administration accepted an investigational new drug application submitted in May 2018.	BIVV003 is a non-viral approach that utilizes zinc finger nuclease gene-editing technology to gene edit a patient's own hematopoietic stem cells. The treatment suppresses sickle hemoglobin production while reactivating the production of fetal hemoglobin to levels that may protect patients against disease progression.	https://clinicaltrials. gov/ct2/show/record/ NCT03653247
	CTX001	CRISPR Therapeutics and Vertex Pharmaceuticals Inc.	• Phase I/II clinical trial— estimated final data collection date for primary outcome measures is February 2021. • Granted Fast Track Designation in January 2019.	An ex vivo gene-edited cell therapy uses a new technology called CRISPR (clustered regularly interspaced short palindromic repeats) to replace stem cells with those engineered to produce high levels of fetal hemoglobin in red blood cells, replacing the damaged hemoglobin.	https://clinicaltrials. gov/ct2/show/ NCT03745287
	LentiGlobin (BB305)	bluebird bio, Inc.	• Phase I/II clinical trial— estimated final data collection date for primary outcome measures is February 2022. • Granted Breakthrough Therapy designation in February 2015.	LentiGlobin BB305 Drug Product aims to treat beta-thalassemia major and severe SCD by inserting a functional human beta-globin gene into the patient's own hematopoietic stem cells ex vivo and then returning those modified cells to the patient through an autologous stem cell transplantation.	https://clinicaltrials. gov/ct2/show/record/ NCT02140554

Transplant	Bone marrow transplant from half-matched related donors	Emory University	• The estimated study completion date is in December 2020.	Participants will receive a bone marrow infusion from a human leukocyte antigen (HLA) half-matched donor through a central venous catheter.	https://clinicaltrials.gov/ct2/show/NCT02757885?term=supplement&cond=sickle+cell&cntry=US&draw=2&rank=17
	Pre-transplant Immunosuppressive Therapy for Haploidentical Transplants	City of Hope Medical Center	• Pilot study—estimated final data collection date for primary outcome measures is February 2023.	Patients will receive a haploidentical hematopoietic stem cell transplant and graft-versus-host-disease prevention with or without pre-transplant immunosuppressive therapy.	https://clinicaltrials.gov/ct2/show/NCT03279094
	Nonmyeloablative Haploidentical Peripheral Blood Mobilized Hematopoietic Precursor Cell Transplantation	National Heart, Lung, and Blood Institute	• The estimated final data collection date for primary outcome measures is September 2025.	Patients will receive a nonmyeloablative allogeneic peripheral blood stem cell transplant with allogeneic peripheral blood stem cells from a haploidentical donor using a novel immunosuppressive regimen.	https://clinicaltrials.gov/ct2/show/NCT03077542
	Mixed Chimerism in Sickle Cell Disease Patients With COH-MC-17	City of Hope Medical Center, California Institute for Regenerative Medicine	• Pilot study—estimated final data collection date for primary outcome measures is December 2022.	Participants will receive COH-MC-17: a 21-day nonmyeloablative conditioning regimen (cyclophosphamide, pentostatin, and rabbit anti-thymocyte globulin), followed by CD4+ T-cell-depleted Haploidentical Hematopoietic Transplant.	https://clinicaltrials.gov/ct2/show/NCT03249831

continued

Type	Name	Developer/Sponsor	Research Status (as of December 2019)	Mechanism	Source
	Reduced Intensity Conditioning for Haploidentical Bone Marrow Transplantation	Medical College of Wisconsin	• Phase II clinical trial—estimated final data collection date for primary outcome measures is December 2023.	A conditioning regimen with Hydroxyurea, rabbit-ATG, Thiotepa, Fludarabine, Cyclophosphamide, Total Body Irradiation, and Mesna will be administered prior to Haploidentical Bone Marrow Transplantation in Eligible patients with a first degree HLA-haploidentical donor.	https://clinicaltrials.gov/ct2/show/NCT03263559
	Familial Haploidentical T-Cell Depleted Transplantation	New York Medical College	• The estimated study completion is in December 2022.	The study investigates host myeloimmunosuppressive conditioning followed by familial haploidentical T-cell depleted allogeneic stem cell transplantation in patients with high risk SCD.	https://clinicaltrials.gov/ct2/show/NCT01461837
	T-Cell Depleted, Alternative Donor Transplantation	Children's Hospital of Pittsburgh	• The estimated final data collection date for primary outcome measures is August 2023.	This study will evaluate the effect of mismatched unrelated volunteer donor and/or haploidentical related donor stem cell transplant on patients with SCD.	https://clinicaltrials.gov/ct2/show/NCT03653338

Supplement				
Vitamin D3	Columbia University	• Phase II clinical trial—the estimated study completion date is December 2019.	Vitamin D helps the immune system to fight infection and to control inflammation and could potentially help prevent respiratory complications in patients with SCD.	https://clinicaltrials.gov/ct2/show/NCT01443728?term=vitamin+d3&cond=sickle+cell&rank=3
Altemia (SC411)	Micelle BioPharma	• Phase IIa clinical trial—the estimated study completion date is January 2022. • Phase III clinical trial (ASCENT)—the estimated study completion date is December 2020. • Granted Orphan Drug designation to the drug back in 2015.	Altemia consists of a complex proprietary mixture of various fatty acids, primarily in the form of Ethyl Cervonate™ (Micelle's proprietary blend of docosahexaenoic acid and other omega-3 fatty acids), and surface active agents formulated using ALT® specifically to address the treatment of SCD. The specific lipids contained in Altemia may restore balance and fluidity to red blood cells and other cells impacted by the disease. Altemia might treat SCD by decreasing blood cell adhesion, chronic inflammation and red blood cell hemolysis, the factors that lead to reduction in pain episodes, vaso-occlusive crises, and organ damage.	https://micellebiopharma.com/sickle-cell-disease-altemia https://clinicaltrials.gov/ct2/show/NCT02973360 https://clinicaltrials.gov/ct2/show/record/NCT02604368

NOTES: There are also psychosocial behavioral interventions and holistic approaches to treat sickle cell disease (see Chapter 4) and additional clinical trials on transplants. This table reflects updates through December 2019. SCD = sickle cell disease.

Appendix J

Other Training Models for Hematologists

Several training models for hematologists currently exist in the field of sickle cell disease (SCD), including

- American Society of Pediatric Hematology/Oncology mentoring program,
- American Society of Hematology Clinical Research Training Institute,
- Program to Increase Diversity Among Individuals Engaged in Health-Related Research,
- American Society of Hematology Committee on Promoting Diversity,
- Johns Hopkins Hematology/Medical Oncology program,
- , Medical College of Wisconsin benign hematology curriculum,
- T32 Training,
- European Hematology Association European Hematology Curriculum, and
- systems-based clinical hematologist.

AMERICAN SOCIETY OF PEDIATRIC HEMATOLOGY/ONCOLOGY MENTORING PROGRAM

New training models have emerged that include "team mentoring" or participation in a "mentoring network." Other models that pair mentors and mentees include the American Society of Pediatric Hematology/Oncology mentoring program that was developed to support early career members. Within this program, mentors and mentees are matched based on mutual agreement with career development and research planning as the most commonly planned goals. Mentorship occurs by phone, e-mail, or in person at annual meetings. Most mentors and mentees are satisfied with the program and perceive a benefit from their participation (Badawy et al., 2017).

AMERICAN SOCIETY OF HEMATOLOGY CLINICAL RESEARCH TRAINING INSTITUTE

Another program with the goal to improve mentorship opportunities is the American Society of Hematology (ASH) Clinical Research Training Institute (CRTI), which is a 1-year experience for senior fellows and junior faculty intent on a career in hematology. The program began in 2003 and begins with a week-long workshop held in August and during the annual ASH meeting. The ASH CRTI is supported by a National Institutes of Health R25 training award (1R25CA168526-01A1) (Sung et al., 2015). Each participant is matched with a faculty member and the summer workshop includes 20 established clinical researchers, 5 or 6 biostatisticians, a library scientist, and representatives from key funding agencies including the National Heart, Lung, and Blood Institute (NHLBI) and the National Cancer Institute. Although the program has had success, with most participants remaining in academic hematology, the diversity of participants is low; only 3 percent identify as black/African American or Hispanic. Steps taken to increase the participation of under-represented minorities to 15 percent include adding participants and collaborating with the ASH Committee on Promoting Diversity on the CRTI Oversight Committee to disseminate information about CRTI to more diverse members. Additionally, faculty in the program have presented to the Committee on Training to reach training program directors, and they have contacted diverse alumni to recommend CRTI to diverse fellows and junior faculty (King et al., 2016).

PROGRAM TO INCREASE DIVERSITY AMONG INDIVIDUALS ENGAGED IN HEALTH-RELATED RESEARCH

A program with a specific aim of increasing diversity is PRIDE (i.e., Program to Increase Diversity Among Individuals Engaged in Health-Related Research). PRIDE aims to provide intense research and career development mentorship coordinated through a central PRIDE Coordination Core at seven academic sites, each focused on a specific research area. PRIDE at Augusta University in Georgia is focused on "Functional and Translational Genomics of Blood Disorders" and has been funded by NHLBI since 2006. Summer institutes at Augusta University last 2 to 3 weeks and include 3 cohorts of 6–10 mentees. Mentees have monthly contact with mentors with goals focused on grant writing skills. The majority of participants identify as black/African American (80 percent), and the majority of mentees (91.2 percent) conduct SCD research that involves clinical/translation studies. A significant success of the program has been the percentage of extramural grant submissions (75 percent) within 2 years following training completion. Of those participants who submitted grants, 64 percent obtained federal funding (Pace et al., 2017). Furthermore, participants in this mentor and mentee program are exposed to discussions regarding teaching and work–life balance, clinical care, and career plans (Starlard-Davenport et al., 2018).

AMERICAN SOCIETY OF HEMATOLOGY COMMITTEE ON PROMOTING DIVERSITY

Other efforts to increase diversity include the Committee on Promoting Diversity, which is responsible for advising ASH in its efforts to improve minority recruitment into hematology research and practice, attract minority hematologists to become members of the Society, and help develop minority hematologists so they can obtain leadership roles. The committee oversees the selection of applicants for participation and identifies potential mentors. Specific programs include the Medical Student Award Program, the Minority Graduate Student Abstract Achievement Award, the Minority Resident Hematology Award Program, and the ASH-AMFDP, which is a partnership between ASH and the Harold Amos Medical Faculty Development Program of the Robert Wood Johnson Foundation (ASH, 2020).

JOHNS HOPKINS HEMATOLOGY/ MEDICAL ONCOLOGY PROGRAM

There are some existing hematology training models in the United States that have been successful in creating opportunities for individuals who want to pursue a career in benign hematology through structured clinical and research programs that meet the Accreditation Council for Graduate Medical Education (ACGME) requirements. Established in 2005, Johns Hopkins has a Hematology/Medical Oncology program that has a 3-year ACGME accredited single board hematology track that has demonstrated a high retention rate of fellows who remain in clinical and research settings. In 2017, Johns Hopkins formalized its application procedure to allow candidates to apply to the hematology and/or medical oncology tracks. Of the 414 applications, 8 percent of candidates applied to the hematology track only, with half of those candidates expressing a specific interest in benign hematology. Having a hematology track appears to cultivate interest, provide needed role models, and allow fellows to envision a career in the specialty (Naik et al., 2018).

MEDICAL COLLEGE OF WISCONSIN BENIGN HEMATOLOGY CURRICULUM

The benign hematology curriculum at the Medical College of Wisconsin is another example of a training program to increase the number of providers. The development of the curriculum was supported by funding from the ASH Alternative Training Pathway Grant. Specialized features of the program include that the curriculum has a clinical focus on training in benign hematology while still allowing the fellow to be board-eligible for hematology, clinic experiences have an emphasis in non-malignant hematology, and there is a strong foundation for additional (non-ACGME required) research training (Abshire, 2009).

T32 TRAINING GRANT

A multidisciplinary training model for individuals interested in careers in academic hematology research is a T32 Training Grant. The Ruth L. Kirschstein National Research Service Award (T32) supports grants to institutions to develop or enhance research training opportunities. One example is the long-standing Hematology T32 Training Grant at the University of North Carolina at Chapel Hill that trains both M.D. and Ph.D. scientists as adult and pediatric hematology fellows. The 2-year program has tracks in both basic bench and clinical research with scientific and educational interactions between M.D. and Ph.D. trainees in the form of conferences, journal clubs, and symposia. These regular interactions between M.D. and Ph.D. trainees creates an understanding of the goals of biomedical research in hematologic disorders. The foundations of training also include a mentored research project, focused seminars, didactic coursework in clinical research, laboratory methodology, grantsmanship, and navigating academia (UNC School of Medicine, 2020). Improving opportunities and access to T32 grants through additional grant funding would be one step in increasing the workforce in hematology and expanding the knowledge base of providers.

EUROPEAN HEMATOLOGY ASSOCIATION EUROPEAN HEMATOLOGY CURRICULUM

The European Hematology Association also provides a cooperative model for training hematologists that could be adapted in the United

States as their 27 national societies decided to develop a unified curriculum for European hematologists in 2003. The European Hematology Curriculum includes recommendations on minimum levels of competence, knowledge, and skills in hematology. A panel of European experts periodically updates versions to ensure that the curriculum is in line with the new developments in technology, diagnostic methods, and treatment modalities (Ossenkoppele et al., 2012). Of particular importance, they developed an online Curriculum Passport, which is a self-assessment tool that enables continuous survey of competence at individual, national, and European levels. The passport can be used as an educational tool to identify gaps in competence that can then be targeted by attending specific educational events or scientific conferences (Strivens et al., 2013).

SYSTEMS-BASED CLINICAL HEMATOLOGIST

Beyond clinical and research training in hematology, Wallace et al. (2015) have identified opportunities for hematologists to design new models for care delivery. They suggest a role for a "systems-based clinical hematologist," which would be a specialty-trained physician who optimizes individual patient care and the overall health care delivery for patients with blood disorders by creating guidelines for other physicians within the practice to follow. The systems-based hematologist needs to be adaptable and have multiple commitments that could include identifying hematologic issues, developing care pathways, providing input into the appropriate use and interpretation of genomic testing, and counseling of patients with hematologic malignancy.

REFERENCES

Abshire, T. C. 2009. *Curriculum for training in adult benign hematology.* https://www.hematology.org/education/educators/resources-for-training-program-directors/curriculum-for-training-in-adult-benign-hematology (accessed August 26, 2020).

ASH (American Society for Hematology). 2020. *Committee on Promoting Diversity.* https://www.hematology.org/about/governance/standing-committees/diversity (accessed August 26, 2020).

Badawy, S. M., V. Black, E. R. Meier, K. C. Myers, K. Pinkney, C. Hastings, J. M. Hilden, P. Zweidler-McKay, L. C. Stork, T. S. Johnson, and S. R. Vaiselbuh. 2017. Early career mentoring through the American Society of Pediatric Hematology/Oncology: Lessons learned from a pilot program. *Pediatric Blood & Cancer* 64(3):10.1002/pbc.26252.

King, A. A., S. K. Vesely, J. Elwood, J. Basso, K. Carson, and L. Sung. 2016. The American Society of Hematology Clinical Research Training Institute is associated with high retention in academic hematology. *Blood* 128(25):2881–2885.

Naik, R. P., K. Marrone, S. Merrill, R. Donehower, and R. Brodsky. 2018. Single-board hematology fellowship track: A 10-year institutional experience. *Blood* 131(4):462–464.

Ossenkoppele, G., G. Evans-Jones, U. Jaeger, E. Hellström-Lindberg, & Curriculum Update Working Group. 2012. Towards a joint definition of European hematology. *Haematologica* 97(5):636–637.

Pace, B. S., L. H. Makala, R. Sarkar, L., Liu, M. Takezaki, N. Mohandas, G. Dixon, E. M. Werner, D. B. Jeffe, T. K. Rice, N. J. Maihle, and J. González. 2017. Enhancing diversity in the hematology biomedical research workforce: A mentoring program to improve the odds of career success for early stage investigators. *American Journal of Hematology* 92(12):1275–1279.

Starlard-Davenport, A., A. Rich, T. Fasipe, E. I. Lance; K. Adekola, A. Forray, M. Steed, A. Fitzgerald, S. Walker, and B. S. Pace. 2018. Perspective: Sistas in science—Cracking the glass ceiling. *Ethnicity & Disease* 28(4):575–578.

Strivens, J., E. Hellström-Lindberg, O. W. Bjerrum, and C. H. Toh. 2013. A European strategy for targeted education in hematology. *Haematologica* 98(7):1000–1002.

Sung, L., M. Crowther, J. Byrd, S. D. Gitlin, J. Basso, and L. Burns. 2015. Challenges in measuring benefit of Clinical Research Training programs—the ASH Clinical Research Training Institute example. *Journal of Cancer Education* 30(4):754–758.

UNC (University of North Carolina) School of Medicine. 2020. *Overview of the T32 program.* https://www.med.unc.edu/medicine/hemonc/education/training-grants/overview-for-the-t32-program (accessed August 28, 2020).

Wallace, P. J., N. T. Connell, and J. L. Abkowitz. 2015. The role of hematologists in a changing United States health care system. *Blood* 125(16):2467–2470.

Appendix K

Sickle Cell Community-Based Organizations and Patient Groups in the United States

State	Sickle Cell Associations, Nonprofits, and Foundations
National Resources**	• Sickle Cell Disease Association of America
Professional Organization Resources	• American Society of Hematology (ASH), Sickle Cell Adult Provider Network, American Society of Pediatric Hematology/ Oncology, International Association of Sickle Cell Nurses and Professional Associates, Emergency Department Sickle Cell Care Coalition • Foundation for Sickle Cell Disease Research • Sickle Cell Disease Coalition (by ASH) • Sickle Cell Disease Council for CHANGE (supported by Pfizer Rare Disease)
Alabama	• Alabama State Sickle Cell Disease Association • North Alabama Sickle Cell Foundation–Huntsville* • Sickle Cell Disease Association of America–Central Alabama* • Sickle Cell Disease Association of America–Mobile* • Sickle Cell Disease Association–West Alabama, Northport* • Sickle Cell Foundation of The River Region Montgomery* • Southeast Alabama Sickle Cell Association–Tuskegee* • Tri County Sickle Cell Association, Inc.
Arizona	• Sickle Cell Anemia Society of Arizona
Arkansas	• Arkansas Foundation for Sickle Cell Support • Future Builders–Sickle Cell Awareness, Education, and Outreach Initiative

continued

State	Sickle Cell Associations, Nonprofits, and Foundations
California	• Axis Advocacy • Cayenne Wellness Center* • Genetic Disease Resource Center of California State Department of Health Services • Hina Patel Foundation • The K.I.S. Foundation • Pacific Sickle Cell Regional Collaborative • Sickle Cell Anemia Awareness San Francisco • Sickle Cell Community Advisory Council of Northern California • Sickle Cell Community Health Network • Sickle Cell Disease Association of America-San Diego* • Sickle Cell Disease Foundation of California • Sickle Cell Disease Foundation of Orange County • Tracking California's Sickle Cell Data Collection Program • World Sickle Cell Federation
Colorado	• Colorado Department of Public Health and Environment Laboratory Services Division • Colorado Sickle Cell Association-Denver* • Colorado Sickle Cell Foundation • Sickle Cell Adult Provider Network
Connecticut	• Citizens for Quality Sickle Cell Care-New Britain/Hartford* • Sickle Cell Disease Association of America-Southern Connecticut-Bridgeport/New Haven* • Sickle Cell Disease Association of America-Southern Connecticut-Stamford Office* • Southern Regional Sickle Cell Association
Delaware	• Tova Community Health* • William E. Proudford Sickle Cell Fund, Inc.
Florida	• Sickle Cell Association of Hillsborough County* • Sickle Cell Disease Association of America-Broward County-Ft. Lauderdale* • Sickle Cell Disease Association of America-Dade County, Miami* • Sickle Cell Disease Association of America-Escambia and Santa Rosa Counties, Pensacola* • Sickle Cell Disease Association of America-Northeast Florida* • Sickle Cell Disease Association of America-Palm Beach County and Treasure Coast* • Sickle Cell Disease Association of America-St. Petersburg* • Sickle Cell Disease Association of America-Tri-County, Orlando* • Sickle Cell Disease Association of America-Upper Pinellas, Pasco, Hernando Counties* • Sickle Cell Disease Association of America-Volusia County-Daytona Beach* • Sickle Cell Disease Association of America of Levy/Marion Counties-Ocala* • Sickle Cell Disease Association of Florida-Tampa* • Sickle Cell Disease Association of Tri-County–Orlando* • Sickle Cell Foundation of the Big Bend • Sickle Cell Foundation-Tallahassee*
Georgia	• Huisman Sickle Cell Foundation of Augusta, Georgia • Sickle Cell Foundation of Georgia-Atlanta*
Illinois	• Have a Heart for Sickle Cell Anemia Foundation • Sickle Cell Disease Association of America Illinois-Chicago*

State	Sickle Cell Associations, Nonprofits, and Foundations
Indiana	• Martin Center, Inc.–Indianapolis*
Kansas	• Uriel E. Owens Sickle Cell Disease Association of the Midwest
Kentucky	• Christian County Sickle Cell Foundation • The Sickle Cell Association of Kentuckiana
Louisiana	• Baton Rouge Sickle Cell Anemia Foundation • Louisiana Regional Sickle Cell Foundation Alexandria Sickle Cell Anemia Foundation • Northeast Louisiana Sickle Cell Anemia Foundation–Monroe* • Sickle Cell Disease Association of America–Northwest Louisiana* • Southwest Louisiana Sickle Cell Anemia, Inc.–Lake Charles*
Maryland	• Howard University Center for Sickle Cell Disease • Lauren D. Beck Sickle Cell Foundation • Maryland Sickle Cell Disease Association* • Sickle Cell Disease Association of America, Inc.* • William E. Proudford Sickle Cell Fund, Inc.
Massachusetts	• Greater Boston Sickle Cell Disease Association, Inc.* • New England Pediatric Sickle Cell Consortium
Michigan	• Sickle Cell Disease Association of America, Michigan–Detroit*
Minnesota	• Sickle Cell Disease Advocates of Minnesota
Mississippi	• Cure Sickle Cell Foundation • Mississippi Sickle Cell Foundation
Missouri	• Adult Sickle Cell Disease Treatment Program • Bureau of Genetics and Healthy Childhood • Missouri Department of Health and Senior Services • Sickle Cell Association of St. Louis*
Nevada	• Nevada Childhood Cancer Foundation–Las Vegas*
New Jersey	• Sickle Cell Disease Association of New Jersey–Newark*
New Mexico	• Sickle Cell Council of New Mexico–Albuquerque* • University of New Mexico Children's Hospital
New York	• Falling Angels Sickle Cell Foundation* • Queens Sickle Cell Advocacy Network–Queens Village* • Sickle Cell Thalassemia Patients Network*
North Carolina	• Bridges Pointe Sickle Cell Foundation–Durham* • Community Health Interventions and Sickle Cell Agency, Inc.–Fayetteville* • North Carolina Sickle Cell Syndrome Program • Operation Sickle Cell • Piedmont Health Services and Sickle Cell Agency–Greensboro* • Sickle Cell Disease Association of America–Eastern North Carolina Chapter–Jacksonville* • Sickle Cell Partners of the Carolinas–Charlotte NC
Ohio	• American Sickle Cell Anemia Association* • Dayton/Springfield Sickle Cell Affected Families Association • Kincaid's Kindred Spirits • Ohio Sickle Cell and Health Association–Columbus* • Sickle Cell Awareness Group of Greater Cincinnati • Sickle Cell Project of Northwest Ohio

continued

State	Sickle Cell Associations, Nonprofits, and Foundations
Oklahoma	• Oklahoma Sickle Cell Warriors Foundation
Oregon	• Sickle Cell Anemia Foundation of Oregon–Portland*
Pennsylvania	• Children's Sickle Cell Foundation, Inc.–Pittsburgh* • Ryan Clark's Cure League • Sickle Cell Disease Association of America–Philadelphia/ Delaware Valley Chapter* • Sickle Cell Society, Inc.–The Murray-Irvis Genetic Disease Center • The South-Central PA Sickle Cell Council–Harrisburg*
South Carolina	• C.O.B.R.A. Sickle Cell Program • James R. Clark Memorial Sickle Cell Foundation–Columbia* • Louvenia D. Barksdale Sickle Cell Anemia Foundation • Orangeburg Area Sickle Cell Foundation
Tennessee	• The Sickle Cell Foundation of Tennessee–Memphis*
Texas	• The Otis Uduebor Sickle Cell Foundation • Sickle Cell Association of Houston* • Sickle Cell Association of Texas–Marc Thomas Foundation* • Sickle Cell Disease Association of America of Tarrant County–Fort Worth*
Virginia	• Living with Sickle Cell RVA • Sickle Association Inc.–Norfolk* • Sickle Cell Association–Hampton Roads Chapter • Sickle Cell Association of the Peninsula
Washington	• Metropolitan Seattle Sickle Cell Task Force • Northwest Sickle Cell Collaborative
Washington, DC	• Sickle Cell Association of the National Capital Area
Other Advocacy Organizations	• Bold Lips for Sickle Cell • MTS Sickle Cell Foundation • Sickle Cell 101 • The Sickle Cell Community Consortium • Sickle Cell Warriors • Sick Cells
Virtual Only Organization	• Chade SC (Sickle Cell Disease Network) • Excelling with Sickle Cell • Supporters of Families w/ Sickle Cell Disease, Inc.

* A member of the Sickle Cell Disease Association of America.

** National Resources as identified on the Centers for Disease Control and Prevention's website.

NOTES: List compiled on October 7, 2019. The committee was unable to identify sickle cell associations, nonprofits, or foundations for the following states: Alaska, Hawaii, Idaho, Iowa, Maine, Montana, Nebraska, New Hampshire, North Dakota, Rhode Island, South Dakota, Utah, Vermont, West Virginia, Wisconsin, and Wyoming. Organizations listed here are not all-inclusive and represent organizations that were identifiable on public online platforms. Although the committee is aware of additional groups, there is no available comprehensive list or registry of sickle cell disease community-based organizations or advocacy groups.

SOURCES: CDC, 2019; SCDAA, 2019.

REFERENCES

CDC (Centers for Disease Control and Prevention). 2017. *Sickle cell disease (SCD): National resources directory.* http://medbox.iiab.me/modules/en-cdc/www.cdc.gov/ncbddd/ sicklecell/map/map-nationalresourcedirectory.html (accessed August 28, 2020).

SCDAA (Sickle Cell Disease Association of America). *2019. Find member organizations.* https:// www.sicklecelldisease.org/support-and-community/find-member-organizations (accessed August 28, 2020).

Appendix L

Summary Table of Strategic Plan and Blueprint for Sickle Cell Disease Action

The Office of the Assistant Secretary for Health at the U.S. Department of Health and Human Services (HHS) should appoint a team of experts from across HHS agencies to advance the strategic plan.

Specific Actions/Recommendations	Actors	Timeframe for Action
Strategy A: Establish a national system to collect and link data to characterize burden of disease, outcomes, and the needs of those with SCD across the life span.		
Recommendation 3-1 Develop state public health surveillance systems to support a national longitudinal registry of all persons with sickle cell disease (SCD).	The Centers for Disease Control and Prevention (CDC) and state public health departments	1–2 years
Recommendation 3-2 Develop a clinical data registry for SCD in order to identify best practices for care delivery and outcomes.	HHS (specifically, the Health Resources and Services Administration [HRSA], National Institutes of Health [NIH], and Agency for Healthcare Research and Quality [AHRQ])	1–2 years
Recommendation 3-3 Establish a working group to identify existing and disparate sources of data that can be immediately linked and mined.	Office of the Assistant Secretary for Health (OASH)	1–2 years
Strategy B: Establish organized systems of care that ensure both clinical and nonclinical supportive services to all persons living with SCD.		
Recommendation 2-1 Review disability insurance qualifications to ensure that the qualification criteria reflects the burden of the disease borne by SCD patients.	Social Security Administration	1–2 years
Recommendation 2-2 Expand and enhance vocational rehabilitation programs for individuals with SCD who need additional training in order to actively participate in the workforce.	States	2–3 years

Recommendation 5-1	Convene a panel of relevant stakeholders to delineate the elements of a comprehensive system of SCD care, including community supports to improve health outcomes, quality of life, and health inequalities.	HHS (Office of Minority Health and OASH), stakeholders such as National Minority Quality Forum, American Society of Pediatric Hematology/Oncology, American Academy of Pediatrics (AAP), American Society of Hematology (ASH), Sickle Cell Disease Association of America, Inc., Sickle Cell Adult Provider Network, and other key clinical disciplines and stakeholders engaged in SCD care, health systems, and parents and individuals living with SCD	2–3 years
Recommendation 5-2	Develop and pilot reimbursement models for the delivery of coordinated SCD health care and support services.	Centers for Medicare & Medicaid Services (CMS), State Medicaid programs, and private payers	3–4 years
Recommendation 5-3	Develop educational materials to provide guidance for teachers, school nurses, school administrators, and primary care providers to support the medical and academic needs of students with SCD.	U.S. Department of Education, state departments of education, and local school boards	1–2 years

Strategy C: Strengthen the evidence base for interventions and disease management and implement widespread efforts to monitor the quality of SCD care.

| Recommendation 4-1 | Fund and conduct research to close the gaps in the existing evidence base for SCD care to inform the development of clinical practice guidelines and indicators of high-quality care. | Private and public funders and health professional associations | 3–5 years |
| Recommendation 5-4 | Foster the development of quality improvement collaboratives. | National Heart, Lung, and Blood Institute (NHLBI); HRSA; CDC; U.S. Food and Drug Administration (FDA); ASH; Pediatric Emergency Care Applied Research Network; Patient-Centered Outcomes Research Institute | 3–5 years |

continued

Specific Actions/Recommendations		Actors	Timeframe for Action
Recommendation 6-1	Fund researchers and professional associations to develop and track a series of indicators to assess quality of SCD care including patient experience, prevention of disease complications, and health outcomes.	AHRQ, NHLBI, HRSA, CDC, FDA	1–2 years[a] 3–5 years[b]
Recommendation 6-2	Require the reporting of expert consensus-driven SCD quality measures and other metrics of high-quality health care for persons with SCD.	CMS and private payers	3–5 years
Recommendation 6-3	Fund efforts to identify and mitigate potentially modifiable disparities in mortality and health outcomes for vulnerable groups (e.g., young adults in transition, pregnant women, older adults).	HHS	1–2 years
Strategy D: Increase the number of qualified health professionals providing SCD care.			
Recommendation 6-4	Disseminate information about NIH and HRSA loan repayment programs and designate SCD as a Population Health Professional Shortage Area under the National Health Service Corps program and create a Loan Repayment Program for health care professionals working with SCD populations.	NIH, HRSA	1–2 years[c] 3–5 years[d]

Recommendation 6-5	Convene an Academy of SCD Medicine to support SCD providers through education, credentialing, networking, and advocacy.	Health professional associations (ASH, American College of Obstetricians and Gynecologists, American College of Emergency Physicians, American Academy of Family Physicians, AAP, National Medical Association, American College of Physicians, and organizations for other relevant health professionals such as advanced practice providers and nurses)	2–3 years
Recommendation 6-6	Develop early and effective mentoring programs to link early career health professionals with seasoned providers to generate interest in SCD care.	Health professional associations, graduate and professional schools	3–5 years

Strategy E: Improve SCD awareness and strengthen advocacy efforts.

Recommendation 2-3	Improve awareness about the disease and address misconceptions about the disease and those impacted.	HHS, media, health care providers, patient advocacy groups and community-based organizations (CBOs), health professional associations, and state health departments	1–2 years
Recommendation 8-1	Translate and disseminate emerging clinical research information to people living with SCD and their families in order to improve health literacy and empower them to engage in the care and treatment decision-making process.	HHS, health professional associations, health care providers, CBOs, and patient advocates	2–3 years
Recommendation 8-2	Engage the SCD population in designing educational and advocacy programs and policies and in disseminating information on health and community services to individuals living with SCD and their caregivers.	HHS, state health departments, health care providers, and CBOs	1–2 years

continued

Specific Actions/Recommendations		Actors	Timeframe for Action
Strategy F: Address barriers to accessing current and pipeline therapies for SCD.			
Recommendation 7-1	Identify approaches to financing the up-front costs of curative therapies.	CMS and private payers	2–3 years
Recommendation 7-2	Encourage and reimburse the practice of shared decision making and the development of decision aids for novel, high-risk, potentially highly effective therapies for individuals living with SCD.	NIH, FDA, pharmaceutical industry, and research community	1–2 years[e] 3–5 years[f]
Recommendation 7-3	Establish an organized, systematic approach to encourage participation in clinical trials by including affected individuals in the design of trials, working with CBOs to disseminate information and recruit participants, and other targeted activities.	NIH, FDA, pharmaceutical industry, research community, and CBOs	2–3 years
Strategy G: Implement efforts to advance understanding of the full impact of SCT on individuals and society.			
Recommendation 3-4	Standardize the communication and use of newborn screening positive results in genetic counseling and create a mechanism for communicating this information across the life span.	HRSA and states	2–3 years
Recommendation 4-2	Fund research to elucidate the pathophysiology of sickle cell trait (SCT).	NIH	2–3 years
Recommendation 4-3	Disseminate information to promote awareness and education about the potential risks associated with SCT.	OASH, CBOs, media, and other relevant stakeholders	1–2 years

Strategy H: Establish and fund a research agenda to inform effective programs and policies across the life span.

The oversight body appointed by OASH should appoint a research task force to develop the research agenda and identify sources of funding.	OASH, federal and private funders, and researchers	1–2 years to develop research agenda 3–5 years to disseminate funding opportunities for researchers

[a] Define (i.e., identify and develop) list of indicators.

[b] Implement monitoring program to track performance on those indicators.

[c] Disseminate information about existing loan repayment programs (e.g., for health disparities work).

[d] Develop criteria for loan repayment programs for health professionals working specifically with SCD populations.

[e] Identify and synthesize the criteria for the use of recently approved medications.

[f] Develop guidance for shared decision making and tools for implementation.

Appendix M

Summary Table of Sickle Cell Trait Discussion in Report

Chapter	Description of Information
3	Newborn screening and sickle cell trait (SCT) Communicating results from screening State-level approaches to screening Role of genetic counseling Reproductive decision making Screening of subpopulations (National Collegiate Athletic Association athletes; service members)
4	SCT health complications Future research needed for SCT Need for a national approach to SCT Conclusion 4-4 Recommendation 4-4
5	Services for individuals living with SCT Sickle Cell Disease Treatment Demonstration Program
6	Importance of using appropriate screening test Lack of quality indicators or consensus guidelines for genetic counseling Need for national reporting guidelines Committee proposed SCT core measures set
8	Relevant federal agencies involved with SCT activities Confusion between diagnoses of SCT and sickle cell disease Community-based organization services available for individuals living with SCT Public education and awareness about SCT

Appendix N

Glossary

Acidosis: A condition in which there is too much acid in the body fluids. It is the opposite of alkalosis (a condition in which there is too much base in the body fluids).

Acute Hypoxemia: Severe arterial hypoxemia that is refractory to supplemental oxygen. It is caused by intrapulmonary shunting of blood resulting from airspace filling or collapse.

Adenotonsillectomy: The surgical removal of the adenoids and tonsils, a combination of adenoidectomy and tonsillectomy.

Allodynia: Pain sensitization (increased response of neurons) following normally non-painful, often repetitive stimulation. Can lead to triggering of a pain response from stimuli that do not normally provoke pain.

Amniocentesis: A test conducted at 15–20 weeks of pregnancy that tests the amniotic fluid during pregnancy for sickle cell disease and sickle cell trait.

Amygdala: A roughly almond-shaped mass of gray matter inside each cerebral hemisphere, involved with the experiencing of emotions.

Avascular Necrosis: A condition in which poor blood supply to an area of bone leads to bone death. Also known as aseptic necrosis and osteonecrosis.

Benzodiazepines: Any of a class of heterocyclic organic compounds used as tranquilizers and are commonly used in the treatment of anxiety, such as librium and valium.

Central Sensitization: An increase in sensitivity to pain and in the responsiveness of neurons.

Cerebral Ischemia: A condition that occurs when there is not enough blood flow to the brain to meet metabolic demand. This leads to limited oxygen supply, or cerebral hypoxia, and leads to the death of brain tissue, cerebral infarction, or ischemic stroke. It is a subtype of stroke along with subarachnoid hemorrhage and intracerebral hemorrhage.

Cerebral Vasculopathy: This is vasculitis (inflammation of the blood vessel wall) involving the brain and occasionally the spinal cord. It affects all of the vessels: very small blood vessels (capillaries), medium-size blood vessels (arterioles and venules), or large blood vessels (arteries and veins). If blood flow in a vessel with vasculitis is reduced or stopped, the parts of the body that receive blood from that vessel begin to die. It may produce a wide range of neurological symptoms, such as headache, skin rashes, feeling very tired, joint pains, difficulty moving or coordinating part of the body, changes in sensation, and alterations in perception, thought, or behavior, as well as the phenomena of a mass lesion in the brain leading to coma and herniation. Some of its signs and symptoms may resemble multiple sclerosis.

Chorionic Villus Sampling: A testing process that is conducted between 10–13 weeks of pregnancy. A needle is inserted into the cervix or the abdomen to retrieve samples of the chorionic villi. The samples can then be tested for hemoglobin S and sickle cell trait.

Chronic Care Model: An organizational approach to caring for people with chronic disease in a primary care setting. The system is population-based and creates practical, supportive, evidence-based interactions between an informed, activated patient and a prepared, proactive practice team.

Chronic Splenomegaly: An abnormal enlargement of the spleen.

Cirrhosis of the Liver: A late stage of scarring (fibrosis) of the liver caused by many forms of liver diseases and conditions, such as hepatitis and chronic alcoholism.

Comorbidities: The simultaneous presence of two or more chronic diseases or conditions in a patient.

Crizanlizumab: A monoclonal antibody developed by Novartis targeted toward P-selectin. It was announced by the company as an effective drug to prevent vaso-occlusive crisis in patients with sickle cell anemia.

Dyspepsia: Also known as indigestion. A condition characterized by upper abdominal symptoms that may include pain or discomfort, bloating, feeling of fullness with very little intake of food, feeling of unusual fullness following meals, nausea, loss of appetite, heartburn, regurgitation of food or acid, and belching.

Erythrocytes: A red blood cell that (in humans) is typically a biconcave disc without a nucleus. Erythrocytes contain the pigment hemoglobin, which imparts the red color to blood, and transport oxygen and carbon dioxide to and from the tissues.

Functional Asplenia: Occurs when splenic tissue is present but does not work well (e.g., sickle cell disease, polysplenia). Such patients are managed as if asplenic, while in anatomic asplenia, the spleen itself is absent.

HbS: Sickle hemoglobin that results from a genetic mutation in the red blood cells.

HbSC: A moderate clinical severity of sickle cell disease (SCD). People with this form of SCD inherit a sickle cell gene HbS from one parent and a gene for an abnormal hemoglobin called HbC from another parent.

HbSS: Also known as sickle cell anemia, HbSS is a severe or moderately severe genotype of sickle cell disease. This term is also used to refer to sickled hemoglobin.

Hematopoietic Stem Cell Transplantation: The intravenous infusion of hematopoietic stem and progenitor cells designed to establish marrow and immune function in patients with a variety of acquired and inherited malignant and nonmalignant disorders.

Hematuria: The presence of blood in a person's urine. The two types of hematuria are gross hematuria, when a person can see the blood in his or her urine, or microscopic hematuria, when a person cannot see the blood in his or her urine yet it is seen under a microscope.

Hemoglobin: An iron-containing respiratory pigment of vertebrate red blood cells that consists of a globin composed of four subunits, each of which is linked to a heme molecule that functions in oxygen transport to the tissues after conversion to oxygenated form in the gills or lungs, and that assists in carbon dioxide transport back to the gills or lungs after surrender of its oxygen.

Hemolysis: The rupture or destruction of red blood cells.

Hemophilia: A medical condition in which the ability of the blood to clot is severely reduced, causing the sufferer to bleed severely from even a slight injury. The condition is typically caused by a hereditary lack of a coagulation factor, most often factor VIII.

Hyperalgesia: Excessive sensitivity and a raised threshold to painful stimuli.

Hyperviscosity: A group of symptoms triggered by an increase in the viscosity of the blood. Symptoms of high blood viscosity include spontaneous bleeding from mucous membranes, visual disturbances due to retinopathy, and neurologic symptoms ranging from headache and vertigo to seizures and coma.

Ischemia Reperfusion: Reperfusion injury, sometimes called ischemia-reperfusion injury or reoxygenation injury, is the tissue damage caused when blood supply returns to tissue (re- + perfusion) after a period of ischemia or lack of oxygen (anoxia or hypoxia).

Ketorolac: Sold under the brand name Toradol, among others, is a nonsteroidal anti-inflammatory drug used to treat pain. Specifically, it is recommended for moderate to severe pain. Common side effects include sleepiness, dizziness, abdominal pain, swelling, and nausea.

Methylprednisolone: Sold under the brand names Depo-Medrol and Solu-Medrol, among others, is a corticosteroid medication used to suppress the immune system and decrease inflammation.

Mindfulness-Based Stress Reduction: An 8-week evidence-based program that offers secular, intensive mindfulness training to assist people with stress, anxiety, depression, and pain.

Myelosuppression: A condition in which bone marrow activity is decreased, resulting in fewer red blood cells, white blood cells, and platelets. Myelosuppression is a side effect of some cancer treatments. When myelosuppression is severe, it is called myeloablation.

Obstructive Sleep Apnea: A sleep-related breathing disorder that involves a decrease or complete halt in airflow despite an ongoing effort to breathe. It occurs when the muscles relax during sleep, causing soft tissue in the back of the throat to collapse and block the upper airway.

Oophorectomy: A surgical procedure to remove one or both ovaries. When an oophorectomy involves removing both ovaries, it is called bilateral oophorectomy.

Pharmacogenomics: The study of the role of the genome in drug response. Its name reflects the combination of pharmacology and genomics. Pharmacogenomics analyzes how the genetic makeup of an individual affects his or her response to drugs.

Pica: A craving for something that is not normally regarded as nutritive, such as dirt, clay, paper, or chalk. Pica is a classic clue to iron deficiency in children, and it may also occur with zinc deficiency. Pica is also seen as a symptom in several neurobiological disorders, including autism and Tourette's syndrome, and it is sometimes seen during pregnancy.

Pre-eclampsia: A condition in pregnancy characterized by high blood pressure, sometimes with fluid retention and proteinuria.

Priapism: A prolonged, unwanted erection of the penis. It is usually painful and not related to sexual stimulation or arousal.

Prolonged Exposure: A form of behavior therapy and cognitive behavioral therapy designed to treat posttraumatic stress disorder. It is characterized by two main treatment procedures—imaginal and in vivo exposures.

Renal Medullary Carcinoma: A rare type of cancer that affects the kidney. It tends to be aggressive, difficult to treat, and is often metastatic at the time of diagnosis.

Renal Osteodystrophy: A bone disease that occurs when the kidneys fail to maintain proper levels of calcium and phosphorus in the blood. It is common in people with kidney disease and affects most dialysis patients.

Rhabdomyolysis: A serious syndrome due to a direct or an indirect muscle injury. It results from the death of muscle fibers and release of their contents into the bloodstream. This can lead to serious complications such as renal (kidney) failure.

Sickle Cell Disease: A group of genetic blood disorders resulting from point mutations on the beta globin gene that produces in hemoglobin variants that alone or in combination cause early death and profound debilitation.

Sickle Cell Trait: Sickle cell trait is not the disease but occurs when an individual has inherited one sickle cell gene and has one unaffected beta globin gene.

Small Gestational Age for Infants: A term used to describe a baby who is smaller than the usual amount for the number of weeks of pregnancy. Small gestational age babies usually have birthweights below the 10th percentile for babies of the same gestational age.

Somatosensory: Relating to or denoting a sensation (e.g., pressure, pain, or warmth) that can occur anywhere in the body, in contrast to one localized at a sense organ (e.g., sight, balance, or taste).

Spirometry: The most common of the pulmonary function tests. It measures lung function, specifically the amount and/or speed of air that can be inhaled and exhaled. Spirometry is helpful in assessing breathing patterns that identify conditions such as asthma, pulmonary fibrosis, cystic fibrosis, and chronic obstructive pulmonary disease.

Splenic Infarction: A condition in which blood flow supply to the spleen is compromised, leading to partial or complete infarction (tissue death due to oxygen shortage) in the organ. Splenic infarction occurs when the splenic artery or one of its branches are occluded, for example, by a blood clot.

Spontaneous Epidural Hematoma: Manifests from blood accumulating in the epidural space, compressing the spinal cord and leading to acute neurological deficits.

Supraspinal: Means above the spine, and may refer to above the spinal cord and vertebral column or the brain.

Transcranial Doppler: A non-invasive ultrasound method used to examine the blood circulation within the brain.

Venous Thromboembolism: A blood clot that starts in a vein.